OXFORD MEDICAL PUBLICATIONS

Oxford Desk Reference
Endocrinology

Oxford Desk Reference: Acute Medicine
Edited by Richard Leach, Derek Bell, and Kevin Moore

Oxford Desk Reference: Cardiology
Edited by Hung-Fat Tse, Gregory Y. Lip, and Andrew J. Stewart Coats

Oxford Desk Reference: Clinical Genetics, Second Edition
Helen V. Firth and Jane A. Hurst

Oxford Desk Reference: Critical Care
Carl Waldmann, Neil Soni, and Andrew Rhodes

Oxford Desk Reference: Endocrinology
Edited by Helen E. Turner, Richard Eastell, and Ashley Grossman

Oxford Desk Reference: Geriatric Medicine
Edited by Margot Gosney, Adam Harper, and Simon Conroy

Oxford Desk Reference: Major Trauma
Edited by Jason Smith, Ian Greaves, and Keith Porter

Oxford Desk Reference: Nephrology
Jonathan Barratt, Kevin Harris, and Peter Topham

Oxford Desk Reference: Obstetrics and Gynaecology
Edited by Sabaratnam Arulkumaran, Lesley Regan, Aris Papageorghiou, Ash Monga, and David Farquharson

Oxford Desk Reference: Oncology
Edited by Thankamma V. Ajithkumar, Ann Barrett, Helen Hatcher, and Natalie Cook

Oxford Desk Reference: Respiratory Medicine
Edited by Nick Maskell and Ann Millar

Oxford Desk Reference: Rheumatology
Edited by Richard Watts, Gavin Clunie, Frances Hall, and Tarnya Marshall

Oxford Desk Reference: Toxicology
Edited by Nicholas Bateman, Robert Jefferson, Simon Thomas, John Thompson, and Allister Vale

Oxford Desk Reference
Endocrinology

Edited by

Helen E. Turner, MA, MD, FRCP

Consultant in Endocrinology
The Oxford Centre for Diabetes, Endocrinology and Metabolism
Oxford University Hospitals NHS Foundation Trust
Churchill Hospital
UK

Richard Eastell, MD, FRCP FRCPath, FMedSci

Professor of Bone Metabolism
Head of the Academic Unit of Bone Metabolism
Director of the Mellanby Centre for Bone Research
University of Sheffield
UK

Ashley Grossman, BA, BSc, MD, FRCP FMedSci

Emeritus Professor of Endocrinology, University of Oxford
Fellow, Green-Templeton College, UK
Honorary Consultant Physician
Oxford University Hospitals NHS Trust, UK
Consultant NET Endocrinologist
Royal Free London, UK
Professor of Neuroendocrinology,
Barts and the London School of Medicine, UK

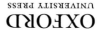
OXFORD
UNIVERSITY PRESS

OXFORD
UNIVERSITY PRESS

Great Clarendon Street, Oxford, OX2 6DP,
United Kingdom

Oxford University Press is a department of the University of Oxford.
It furthers the University's objective of excellence in research, scholarship,
and education by publishing worldwide. Oxford is a registered trade mark of
Oxford University Press in the UK and in certain other countries

Published in the United States of America by Oxford University Press
198 Madison Avenue, New York, NY 10016, United States of America

British Library Cataloguing in Publication Data
Data available

Library of Congress Control Number: 2018933147

ISBN 978-0-19-967283-7

Printed and bound by
CPI Group (UK) Ltd, Croydon, CR0 4YY

Preface

Endocrinology is a broad discipline encompassing many areas such as pituitary, adrenal, thyroid, and gonadal disease, as well as endocrine oncology, neuroendocrine tumours, and disorders of bone, with many diverse forms of presentation. Whilst many endocrinologists see all types of endocrine disease, others may have a more general practice, and yet others may be very specialized; however, all may not infrequently come across areas of specialist endocrinology with which they are not totally familiar. We believe that there has been a need for a readily accessible handbook for clinicians—succinct, practical, and authoritative—which covers all aspects of endocrinology. This would allow for rapid access to contemporary expert opinion and advice in every aspect of endocrinology. It should be of value to all endocrinologists, both in training and in practice, at all levels of knowledge and experience. The handbook has been written by more than 100 national and international authorities, with a view to providing such expert, first-line advice. With the clinic in mind, we have included a readily accessible 'speedy reference' section, diagrams to aid in patient explanation, and information on patient self-help organizations. In addition, we have included specialist sections on areas less frequently covered in major textbooks, such as medico-legal aspects, sports, and 'possible endocrine syndromes', as well as transitional and old-age endocrinology. We hope and trust that this will help deliver expert care to all our patients.

Helen Turner
Richard Eastell
Ashley Grossman
Oxford and Sheffield

Foreword

In this very well-crafted volume, the editors have assembled an expert team of global authors in endocrinology and related specialties to present a concise and functional approach to understanding principles of clinical endocrinology. Authors have nicely distilled important information from current materials, and present the contents in an easily readable functional format. This book offers a welcome and very practical addition to the well-accepted literary armamentarium available in large comprehensive textbooks of endocrinology. The busy clinician is inundated with information overload, and this user-friendly, yet rigorously written, concise guide elucidates important underpinnings of topical endocrine disease pathogenesis, diagnosis, and management, and appropriate use of ancillary diagnostic and therapeutic modalities. Each chapter is short, well written, and referenced. As a desktop or even pocket reference text, it will be a handy and highest quality accompaniment for medical students, specialty physicians-in-training, investigators, and endocrine nurses, as well as endocrinologists, gynaecologists, oncologists, radiologists, pathologists, and surgeons encountering patients with disordered hormone production or action.

The editors and authors have provided the endocrine community with a handy educational tool likely to be frequently used in enhancing the quality of care. This fresh approach to efficiently transmitting relevant medical knowledge is to be applauded.

Shlomo Melmed
Los Angeles, CA

Brief contents

Detailed contents

Contributors

S Faisal Ahmed Samson Gemmell Chair of Child Health, University of Glasgow Royal Hospital for Children, Greater Glasgow and Clyde Health Board, Glasgow, UK

TV Ajithkumar Consultant Clinical Oncologist, Cambridge University Hospitals, Cambridge, UK

Krystallenia Alexandraki Consultant Endocrinologist, Department of Pathophysiology, Laiko University Hospital Medical School, National and Kapodistrian University of Athens, Greece

Josephine Arendt Professor Emeritus, Endocrinology, Faculty of Health and Medical Sciences, University of Surrey, Guildford, UK

Wiebke Arlt William Withering Chair of Medicine, Institute of Metabolism and Systems Research, University of Birmingham, and Consultant Endocrinologist, Centre for Endocrinology, Diabetes and Metabolism, Birmingham Health Partners, Birmingham, UK

Paul Arundel Consultant in Paediatric Metabolic Bone Disease, Academic Unit of Child Health, Sheffield Children's Hospital, Sheffield, UK

Simon Aylwin Consultant Endocrinologist, King's College Hospital London, UK

Ravikumar Balasubramanian Assistant Professor of Medicine, Reproductive Endocrine Unit and Department of Medicine, Massachusetts General Hospital, Harvard Medical School, Boston, MA, USA

Stephen Ball Professor of Medicine and Endocrinology, Department of Endocrinology, Manchester University Hospitals NHS Trust, Manchester, UK

Birke Bausch Internist, Department of Medicine II, Freiburg University Medical Center, Albert–Ludwigs University, Freiburg, Germany

Paolo Beck-Peccoz Professor Emeritus, University of Milan, Italy

John S Bevan Consultant Endocrinologist and Honorary Professor of Endocrinology, Department of Endocrinology, Aberdeen Royal Infirmary, Aberdeen, UK

Kristien Boelaert Reader in Endocrinology, Institute of Metabolism and Systems Research, University of Birmingham, and Consultant Endocrinologist, Centre for Endocrinology, Diabetes and Metabolism, Birmingham Health Partners, Birmingham, UK

Michael Brada Professor of Radiation, Oncology Department of Molecular and Clinical Cancer Medicine, University of Liverpool and Department of Radiation Oncology, Clatterbridge Cancer Centre NHS Foundation Trust, Bebington, Wirral, UK

Karin Bradley Consultant Endocrinologist, University Hospitals Bristol NHS Foundation Trust, Bristol Royal Infirmary, Bristol, UK

Marcello D Bronstein Professor of Endocrinology, Division of Endocrinology and Metabolism, Hospital das Clinicas, University of São Paulo Medical School, São Paulo, SP, Brazil

James V Byrne Professor of Neuroradiology, Nuffield Department of Surgical Sciences, University of Oxford, UK

Matilde Calanchini Oxford Centre for Endocrinology, Diabetes and Metabolism, Churchill Hospital, Oxford University Hospitals NHS Trust, UK

Dominic Cavlan Consultant Endocrinologist, Department of Endocrinology, St Bartholomew's Hospital, Barts Health NHS Trust, London, UK

Harvinder Chahal Consultant Endocrinologist, Department of Endocrinology, Imperial College Healthcare NHS Trust, London, UK

Roland Chapurlat Professor of Rheumatology, Université de Lyon, Hôpital E Herriot, Lyon, France

Evangelia Charmandari Professor of Pediatric and Adolescent Endocrinology Division of Endocrinology, Metabolism and Diabetes, First Department of Pediatrics, National and Kapodistrian University of Athens Medical School, 'Aghia Sophia' Children's Hospital, Athens, Greece

Tim Child Associate Professor in Reproductive Medicine, University of Oxford, Honorary Consultant Gynaecologist, John Radcliffe Hospital, Oxford, and Founding Director, The Fertility Partnership, Oxford, UK

George Chrousos Professor and Chairman of the Department of Paediatrics, Greece First Department of Pediatrics, University of Athens Medical School, 'Aghia Sophia' Children's Hospital, Athens, Greece

Adrian Clark Emeritus Professor of Endocrinology, St George's University of London, and Honorary Professor of Endocrinology, Queen Mary University of London, UK

Roderick Clifton-Bligh Consultant Endocrinologist, Head, Department of Endocrinology, and Co-Head, Cancer Genetics Unit, Kolling Institute, Royal North Shore Hospital, St Leonards, Sydney, Australia

Gerard S Conway Professor of Reproductive Endocrinology, Reproductive Medicine Unit, Institute for Women's Health, University College London, UK

Mark S Cooper Professor of Medicine, ANZAC Research Institute, University of Sydney, Concord Repatriation General Hospital, Sydney, Australia

Kathryn Cox Paediatric Registrar, Royal Hospital for Sick Children, Edinburgh, UK

Simon A Cudlip Consultant Neurosurgeon, Department of Neurosurgery, John Radcliffe Hospital, Oxford University Hospitals NHS Foundation Trust, UK

Wouter W de Herder Professor of Endocrine Oncology, Department of Internal Medicine, Sector of Endocrinology, Erasmus University Medical Center, Rotterdam, The Netherlands

Rebecca Deans Consultant Gynaecologist and Fertility Specialist, University of New South Wales Royal Hospital for Women, Sydney Children's Hospital, Genea Ltd, Sydney, Australia

WM Drake Professor of Clinical Endocrinology, St Bartholomew's Hospital, London, UK

Maralyn Druce Professor of Endocrine Medicine, Centre for Endocrinology, Barts and the London School of Medicine and Dentistry, Queen Mary University of London, UK

Richard Eastell Professor of Bone Metabolism, Director of the Mellanby Centre for Bone Research, University of Sheffield, UK

Charis Eng ACS/Hardis Professor and Chair, Genomic Medicine Institute, Cleveland Clinic, and Professor and Vice Chair, Department of Genetics and Genome Sciences, Case Western Reserve University, Cleveland, OH, USA

Shereen Ezzat FACP Professor of Medicine and Oncology Consultant, Endocrine Site Group, Princess Margaret Cancer Centre, University Health Network, University of Toronto, Canada

Martin Fassnacht Head of Division, Professor for Medicine, Division of Endocrinology, University Hospital Würzburg, Germany

Muhammed Fatum Honorary Senior Clinical Lecturer in Obstetrics, Gynaecology and Reproductive Medicine, Institute of Reproductive Sciences, Nuffield's Department of Women's and Reproductive Health Oxford University, Oxford, UK

Nick Finer Honorary Clinical Professor, National Centre for Cardiovascular Prevention and Outcomes, Institute of Cardiovascular Science, University College London, UK

Ivar Følling Senior Consultant Endocrinologist, Department of Endocrinology, Akershus University Hospital and University of Oslo, Norway

William D Fraser Professor of Medicine, Norwich Medical School, University of East Anglia, Norfolk, UK

Seiji Fukumoto Project Professor, Division of Molecular Endocrinology, Fujii Memorial Institute of Medical Sciences, Institute of Advanced Medical Sciences, Tokushima University, Japan

John W Funder Distinguished Scholar, Hudson Institute and Professor of Medicine, Monash University, Clayton, 3168, Victoria, Australia

Neil Gittoes Consultant Endocrinologist and Honorary Professor, Centre for Endocrinology, Diabetes and Metabolism, Queen Elizabeth Hospital Birmingham, University Hospitals Birmingham NHS Foundation Trust, UK

Helena Gleeson Consultant Endocrinologist, Department of Endocrinology, Queen Elizabeth Hospital Birmingham, University Hospitals Birmingham NHS Foundation Trust, UK

Andrea Glezer Consultant Endocrinologist, Division of Endocrinology and Metabolism, Hospital das Clinicas, University of São Paulo Medical School, São Paulo, SP, Brazil

Karen E Gomez-Hernandez Staff Physician, Division of Endocrinology, and University Health Network Assistant Professor, Department of Medicine, University of Toronto, Canada

Stephen CL Gough Visiting Professor of Diabetes, Oxford Centre for Diabetes, Endocrinology, and Metabolism, Oxford University, and Honorary Consultant Physician, Oxford University Hospital NHS Foundation Trust, UK

Mark Gurnell Clinical SubDean and Honorary Consultant Physician, University of Cambridge School of Clinical Medicine and Wellcome Trust–MRC Institute of Metabolic Science, Addenbrooke's Hospital, Cambridge University Hospitals NHS Foundation Trust, UK

Ken Ho Chair, Centre for Health Research, Princess Alexandra Hospital, and the University of Queensland, Brisbane, Australia

Eva Horvath Department of Laboratory Medicine, Division of Pathology, St. Michael's Hospital, Toronto, Canada

Claire Hughes Consultant Paediatric Endocrinologist, Department of Paediatric Endocrinology, Barts Health NHS Trust, London, UK

Ieuan Hughes Emeritus Professor Paediatrics, Department of Paediatrics, University of Cambridge, UK

Penny Hunt Consultant Endocrinologist, Department of Medicine and Endocrinology, University of Otago, Christchurch Hospital, New Zealand

Steve Hyer Consultant Endocrinologist, Department of Endocrinology, St Helier Hospital, Epsom and St Helier University Hospitals NHS Trust, Carshalton, and Royal Marsden NHS Foundation Trust, and Honorary Senior Lecturer, St George's, London, UK

Warrick Inder Senior Staff Specialist, Princess Alexandra Hospital, and Associate Professor, Faculty of Medicine, University of Queensland, Brisbane, Australia

Bahram Jafar-Mohammadi Consultant Endocrinologist, Oxford Centre for Diabetes, Endocrinology and Metabolism, Churchill Hospital, Oxford University Hospitals NHS Foundation Trust, UK

Sakunthala Jayasinghe Registrar in Clinical Biochemistry, Department of Clinical Biochemistry, The John Radcliffe Hospital, Oxford University Hospitals NHS Trust, UK

T Hugh Jones Consultant Endocrinologist and Honorary Professor of Andrology, Robert Hague Centre for Diabetes and Endocrinology, Barnsley Hospital NHS Trust, and Department of Oncology and Metabolism, University of Sheffield, UK

Gregory Kaltsas Professor of Endocrinology, Medical School, National and Kapodistrian University of Athens, Greece

Niki Karavitaki Senior Clinical Lecturer and Consultant Endocrinologist, Institute of Metabolism and Systems Research, University of Birmingham, and Centre for Endocrinology, Diabetes and Metabolism, Birmingham Health Partners, UK

Fredrik Karpe Professor of Metabolic Medicine and Honorary Consultant Physician, Oxford Centre for Diabetes, Endocrinology and Metabolism, Radcliffe Department of Medicine, University of Oxford, UK

Peter King Reader in Molecular Endocrinology, Centre for Endocrinology, William Harvey Research Institute, Barts and the London School of Medicine and Dentistry, Queen Mary University of London, UK

Katja Kiseljak-Vassiliades Assistant Professor, Division of Endocrinology, Department of Medicine, University of Colorado School of Medicine, Aurora, CO, USA

Anne Klibanski Laurie Carrol Guthart Professor of Medicine, Harvard Medical School, and Chief, Neuroendocrine Unit, Massachusetts General Hospital, Boston, MA, USA

Márta Korbonits Professor of Endocrinology and Metabolism, Centre for Endocrinology, Barts and the London School of Medicine and Dentistry, Queen Mary University of London, UK

Kalman Kovacs Emeritus Professor of Pathology, Department of Laboratory Medicine, Division of Pathology, St. Michael's Hospital, Toronto, Canada

Satoshi Kuwabara Department of Neurology, Graduate School of Medicine, Chiba University, Japan

Bente L Langdahl Professor and Consultant Endocrinologist, Department of Endocrinology and Internal Medicine, Aarhus University Hospital, Denmark

Elizabeth A Lawson Neuroendocrine Unit, Massachusetts General Hospital, and Associate Professor of Medicine, Harvard Medical School, Boston, MA, USA

Diana L Learoyd Endocrinologist and Associate Professor, Sydney Medical School, Northern Campus, Royal North Shore Hospital, Sydney, Australia

William Ledger Vice Dean and Head of Discipline of Obstetrics and Gynaecology, Faculty of Medicine, School of Women's and Children's Health, Sydney, Australia

Andy Levy Professor of Endocrinology and Honorary Consultant Physician, University of Bristol and University Hospitals Bristol NHS Foundation Trust, UK

Miles Levy Consultant Endocrinologist Department of Endocrinology, Leicester Royal Infirmary, University Hospitals of Leicester NHS Trust, UK

Kari Lima Consultant Endocrinologist, Department of Endocrinology, Akershus University Hospital and Clinic of Pediatric and Adolescent Medicine, Women and Children Division, Oslo University Hospital, Norway

Carolyn Lowe Partner, Clinical Negligence Department, Freeths, Oxford, UK

Angelica Malinoc Department of Nephrology and General Medicine Pathology, University Medical Center, Albert-Ludwigs-University, Freiburg, Germany

Victoria L Martucci Predoctoral Research Fellow, Developmental Endocrine Oncology and Genetics Affinity Group, Eunice Kennedy Shriver National Institute of Child Health and Human Development, National Institutes of Health, Bethesda, MD, USA

Alexandre Mathy Neurology Registrar, Nuffield Department of Clinical Neurosciences, John Radcliffe Hospital, Oxford University Hospital NHS Trust, UK

Pat McBride Head of Patient and Family Services, The Pituitary Foundation, Bristol, UK

Chris McCabe Professor of Molecular Endocrinology, Institute of Metabolism and Systems Research, University of Birmingham, UK

Ann McCormack Consultant Endocrinologist, Department of Endocrinology, St Vincent's Hospital, Sydney, Australia

Karim Meeran Professor of Endocrinology, Division of Diabetes, Endocrinology and Metabolism, Imperial College, London, UK

Moises Mercado Director, Experimental Endocrinology Unit, Hospital de Especialidades, Centro Médico Nacional S. XXI, Instituto Mexicano del Seguro Social, Mexico City, Mexico

Radu Mihai Consultant in Endocrine Surgery, Honorary Senior Clinical Lecturer, Churchill Hospital, Oxford University Hospitals NHS Trust Oxford, UK

Anna Louise Mitchell NIHR Academic Clinical Lecturer, Institute of Genetic Medicine, Newcastle University, Newcastle upon Tyne, UK

David Mole NIHR Research Professor and Consultant Nephrologist, Nuffield Department of Medicine, University of Oxford, Oxford, UK

Mark E Molitch Martha Leland Sherwin Professor of Endocrinology, Division of Endocrinology, Metabolism and Molecular Medicine, Department of Medicine, Northwestern University Feinberg School of Medicine, Chicago, IL, USA

Phillip J Monaghan Consultant Clinical Scientist, The Christie Pathology Partnership, The Christie NHS Foundation Trust, Manchester, UK

Emma Mortimer Graphic Illustrator, Oxford, UK

Leif Mosekilde Clinical Professor, Department of Endocrinology and Metabolism, Aarhus University, Denmark

JJ Mukherjee Senior Consultant in Endocrinology and Diabetes, Department of Medicine, Apollo Gleneagles Hospital, Kolkata, India

Lois Mulholland Consultant Clinical Oncologist, Ulster Hospital, Southeastern Trust, Northern Ireland

Atif Munir Consultant Diabetologist and Endocrinologist, Department of Medicine, Fatima Memorial Hospital, Lahore, Pakistan

Robert D Murray Consultant Endocrinologist, Leeds Centre for Diabetes and Endocrinology, St James's University Hospital, Leeds Teaching Hospitals NHS Trust, and Honorary Associate Professor, University of Leeds, UK

Nicola Neary Consultant in Diabetes and Endocrinology, and Acute Medicine, Department of Medicine, St. George's University Hospitals NHS Foundation Trust, London, UK

Hartmut Neumann Emeritus Professor, Section for Preventive Medicine, Department of Nephrology and General Medicine, University Medical Centre, Albert–Ludwigs University of Freiburg, Germany

Kate Newbold Consultant Clinical Oncologist, Institute of Cancer Research and the Royal Marsden NHS Trust, London, UK

John Newell-Price Chair of Endocrinology and Honorary Consultant Physician, Department of Oncology and Metabolism, University of Sheffield, UK

Paul Newey Senior Lecturer in Endocrinology, Division of Molecular and Clinical Medicine, Ninewells Hospital and Medical School, University of Dundee, UK

Joanne Ngeow Head and Senior Consultant, Cancer Genetics Service, National Cancer Centre, Singapore

Lynnette Nieman Senior Investigator, National Institutes of Health, Bethesda, MD, USA

Onyebuchi Okosieme Consultant Endocrinologist, Diabetes Department, Prince Charles Hospital, Cwm Taf University Health Board, Merthyr Tydfil, UK

Karel Pacak Senior Investigator and Chief, Section on Medical Neuroendocrinology; Head, Developmental Endocrine Oncology and Genetics Affinity Group; Professor of Medicine, Eunice Kennedy Shriver National Institute of Child Health and Human Development, National Institutes of Health, Bethesda, MD, USA

Socrates Papapoulos Professor of Medicine, Center for Bone Quality, Leiden University Medical Center, The Netherlands

Chrysoula Papastathi Consultant Endocrinologist, Department of Endocrinology and Diabetes, Pourtalès Hospital, Neuchâtel, Switzerland

Neel Patel Consultant Radiologist, Department of Radiology, Churchill Hospital, Oxford University Hospitals NHS Trust, UK

Simon HS Pearce Professor of Endocrinology and Honorary Consultant Physician, Institute of Genetic Medicine, Newcastle University, Newcastle upon Tyne, UK

Ilias Perogamvros Consultant Endocrinologist and Honorary Research Fellow, Division of Endocrinology and Gastroenterology, School of Medical Sciences Faculty of Biology, Medicine and Health University of Manchester, UK

Marija Pfeifer Professor in Internal Medicine and Endocrinology, Department of Endocrinology, University Medical Centre Ljubljana, Medical Faculty, University of Ljubljana, Slovenia

Veronica Preda Consultant Endocrinologist and Clinical Lecturer, Kolling Institute Royal North Shore Hospital, University of Sydney, St Leonards, Australia

Richard Quinton Consultant and Senior Lecturer in Endocrinology, Newcastle University and Newcastle Hospitals, NHS Trust Royal Victoria Infirmary, Newcastle upon Tyne, UK

Sir Peter Ratcliffe Professor of Medicine and Director of the Target Discovery Institute, University of Oxford, and Director of Clinical Research, The Francis Crick Institute, London, UK

Narendra L Reddy Consultant Endocrinologist and Honorary Senior Lecturer, Leicester Royal Infirmary and University of Leicester, UK

Nicole Reisch Consultant Endocrinologist and Assistant Professor, Department of Endocrinology, Medizinische Klinik IV, Klinikum der Universität München, Munich, Germany

Rodney Reznek Emeritus Professor of Radiology, Barts and the London School of Medicine and Dentistry, London, UK

David Riley Formerly at Newcastle Hospitals NHS Trust

Sophie Roberts Specialist Diabetes Dietitian, Oxford Centre for Diabetes, Endocrinology and Metabolism, Churchill Hospital, Oxford University Hospitals NHS Trust, UK

Bruce Robinson Professor of Endocrinology, Cancer Genetics, Kolling Institute, Department of Endocrinology, Royal North Shore and University of Sydney, Australia

Stephen Robinson Consultant Endocrinologist, St Mary's Hospital, Imperial College Healthcare NHS Trust, London, UK

Andrea Rockall Consultant Radiologist, Imaging Department, Royal Marsden Hospital, London, UK

Angela Rogers Consultant Endocrinologist, Horton General Hospital, Oxford University Hospitals NHS Foundation Trust, UK

Gian Paolo Rossi Chair of Internal Medicine and Head, Clinica dell'Ipertensione Arteriosa, Coordinator International PhD Program in Arterial Hypertension and Vascular Biology, University of Padua Department of Medicine–DIMED, University Hospital of Padua, Italy

Fabio Rotondo Senior Investigator, Research manager, Department of Laboratory Medicine, Division of Pathology, St. Michael's Hospital, Toronto, Canada

Anju Sahdev Reader and Consultant in Imaging, Department of Radiology, St Bartholomew's Hospital Barts Health NHS Trust, London, UK

Brian Shine Consultant Chemical Pathologist, Department of Clinical Biochemistry, John Radcliffe Hospital, Oxford University Hospitals NHS Trust, UK

Matthew Simmonds Senior Lecturer, School of Life Sciences, College of Science, University of Lincoln, UK

Paul Smith Neurosurgeon, Brain and Spine Specialist, Victoria Parade Neurosurgery, East Melbourne, and Consultant Neurosurgeon, St Vincent's Private, Melbourne, Australia

Noel P Somasundaram Consultant Endocrinologist, Diabetes and Endocrine Unit, National Hospital of Sri Lanka, Colombo, Sri Lanka

Constantine A Stratakis Scientific Director, Eunice Kennedy Shriver National Institute of Child Health and Human Development, National Institutes of Health, Bethesda, MD, USA

Rieko Tadokoro-Cuccaro Research Assistant, Department of Paediatrics, University of Cambridge, UK

Garry Tan Consultant Physician, Oxford Centre for Diabetes,Endocrinology and Metabolism (OCDEM), NIHR Biomedical Research Centre, Churchill Hospital, Oxford University Hospitals NHS Foundation Trust, Oxford, UK

Massimo Terzolo Full Professor, Internal Medicine, and Head, Department of Internal Medicine, San Luigi Gonzaga Hospital, University of Turin, Italy

Gaya Thanabalasingham Locum Consultant Diabetes and Endocrinology, London North West University Healthcare NHS Trust, UK

Vivien Thornton-Jones Senior Research Nurse, Oxford Centre for Diabetes, Endocrinology and Metabolism, Churchill Hospital, Oxford University Hospitals NHS Trust, UK

Andy Toogood Consultant Endocrinologist, Department of Endocrinology, Queen Elizabeth Hospital Birmingham, University Hospitals Birmingham NHS Foundation Trust, UK

Christos Toumpanakis Consultant in Gastroenterology and Neuroendocrine Tumours, Neuroendorine Tumour Unit, ENETS Centre of Excellence, Royal Free Hospital London, UK

Peter J Trainer Professor of Endocrinology, Department of Endocrinology, Manchester Academic Health Science Centre, Christie NHS Foundation Trust, UK

Rachel Troke Diabetes and Endocrinology, Department of Endocrinology, Charing Cross Hospital, Imperial College Healthcare NHS Trust, London, UK

Marina Tsoli Endocrinologist, Laiko Hospital, National and Kapodistrian University of Athens, Greece

Helen Turner Consultant in Endocrinology, Oxford Centre for Endocrinology, Diabetes and Metabolism, Churchill Hospital, Oxford University Hospital NHS Trust Oxford, UK

Rosa Vargas-Poussou Département de Génétique, Hôpital Européen Georges Pompidou, Paris, France

Theo J Visser Professor, Department of Internal Medicine, Erasmus University Medical Center, Rotterdam, The Netherlands

Lisa Walker Consultant in Clinical Genetics Oxford Centre for Genomic Medicine Oxford University Hospitals NHS Foundation Trust Oxford UK

Jennifer S Walsh Clinical Senior Lecturer in Bone Metabolism, Mellanby Centre for Bone Research, University of Sheffield, UK

Susan M Webb Endocrinology/Medicine Department, Centro de Investigación Biomédica en Red de Enfermedades Raras, U 747, ISCIII, Research Center for Pituitary Diseases, Hospital Sant Pau, IIB-Sant Pau, and Universitat Autònoma de Barcelona, Spain

Anthony Weetman Emeritus Professor of Medicine, Department of Oncology and Metabolism, University of Sheffield, UK

Philip Weir Consultant Neurosurgeon, Department of Neurosciences, Royal Victoria Hospital, Belfast Trust, UK

Margaret E Wierman Chief of Endocrinology, Denver VAMC Professor in Medicine, Physiology and Biophysics and OBGYN, University of Colorado School of Medicine, Aurora, CO, USA

Paraskevi Xekouki Clinical Lecturer in Endocrinology, Endocrine Department, King's College Hospital, King's College Hospital NHS Foundation Trust, London, UK

Symbols and abbreviations

↑	Increased
↓	Decreased
5-HTP	5-Hydroxytryptophan
99mTc	Technetium-99m
ABP	Athlete Biological Passport
ACE inhibitor	Angiotensin-converting enzyme inhibitor
acetyl CoA	Acetyl coenzyme A
ADHH	Autosomal-dominant hypocalcaemic hypercalciuria
AES–PCOS	Androgen Excess and Polycystic Ovary Syndrome Society
AIDS	Acquired immune deficiency syndrome
ALT	Alanine aminotransferase
APC	Antigen-presenting cell
ApoA1	Apolipoprotein A1
ApoB	Apolipoprotein B
AST	Aspartate aminotransferase
ATP	Adenosine triphosphate
BMI	Body mass index
BMU	Basic multicellular unit
bpm	Beats per minute
BRRS	Bannayan–Riley–Ruvalcaba syndrome
cAMP	Cyclic AMP
CaSR	Calcium-sensing receptor
CATS	Controlled Antenatal Trial Study
CBG	Corticosteroid-binding globulin
CMR	Cardiac magnetic resonance
CMV	Cytomegalovirus
CNS	Central nervous system
CNV	Copy number variant
COPD	Chronic obstructive pulmonary disease
CRH	Corticotrophin-releasing hormone
CRP	C-reactive protein
CSF	Cerebrospinal fluid
CT	Computed tomography
CTX	C-terminal cross-linking telopeptide of type 1 collagen
CVD	Cyclophosphamide, vincristine, and dacarbazine
DHEA	Dihydroepiandrosterone
DHEAS	Dehydroepiandrosterone sulphate
DST	Dexamethasone suppression test
DVLA	Driver and Vehicle Licensing Agency
DXA	Dual-energy X-ray absorptiometry
EBV	Epstein–Barr virus
ECG	Electrocardiogram
EEG	Electroencephalogram
eGFR	Estimated glomerular filtration rate
ELISA	Enzyme-linked immunosorbent assay
EMS	External masculinization score
ENaC	Epithelial sodium channel
ESA	Employment and Support Allowance
ESR	Erythrocyte sedimentation rate
FDA	^{18}F-fluorodopamine
FDA	Food and Drug Administration
FDG	^{18}F-fluorodeoxyglucose
FDH	Familial dysalbuminaemic hyperthyroxinaemia
FDOPA	^{18}F-fluorodopa
FGD	Familial glucocorticoid deficiency
FGF23	Fibroblast growth factor 23
FGFR1	Fibroblast growth factor receptor 1
FGFR3c	Fibroblast growth factor receptor 3c
FGFR4	Fibroblast growth factor receptor 4
FOP	Fibrodysplasia ossificans progressiva
FSG	Fasting serum gastrin
FSH	Follicle-stimulating hormone
FT3	Free triiodothyronine
FT4	Free thyroxine
GFR	Glomerular filtration rate
GHRH	Growth-hormone-releasing hormone
GMP	Guanosine monophosphate
GnRH	Gonadotrophin-releasing hormone
GP	General practitioner
GPCR	G-protein-coupled receptor
GST	Glucagon stimulation test
GTP	Guanosine-5′-triphosphate
GTT	Gestational transient thyrotoxicosis
GWAS	Genome-wide association screening
HAMA	Human anti-mouse antibody
hCG	Human chorionic gonadotrophin
HDL	High-density lipoprotein
HFTC	Hyperphosphataemic familial tumoural calcinosis
hGR	Human glucocorticoid receptor
HIF	Hypoxia-inducible factor
HIV	Human immunodeficiency virus
HLA	Human leukocyte antigen

hMG	Human menopausal gonadotrophin		NSAID	Non-steroidal anti-inflammatory drug
HMG-CoA	Beta-hydroxy beta-methylglutaryl coenzyme A		NTX	N-terminal cross-linking telopeptide of type 1 collagen
HPA	Hypothalamo-pituitary–adrenal		OMIM	Online Mendelian Inheritance in Man
HRQoL	Health-related quality of life		OR	Odds ratio
HRT	Hormone replacement therapy		P1NP	Procollagen type 1 N-terminal propeptide
HSV	Herpes simplex virus		PCOS	Polycystic ovary syndrome
HTLV-1	Human T-cell lymphotrophic virus 1		PCR	Polymerase chain reaction
HU	Hounsfield unit		PDE5	Phosphodiesterase 5
ICSI	Intracytoplasmic sperm injection		PET	Positron emission tomography
IED	Improvised explosive device		PHA1	Pseudohypoaldosteronism type 1
IgA	Immunoglobulin A		PHTS	*PTEN* hamartoma tumour syndrome
IgE	Immunoglobulin E		PMS	Premenstrual syndrome
IGF	Insulin-like growth factor		PNMT	Phenylethanolamine N-methyltransferase
IgG	Immunoglobulin G		PPAR	Peroxisome proliferator-activated receptor
IPEX	Immunodysregulation polyendocrinopathy enteropathy X-linked syndrome		PPNAD	Pigmented nodular adrenocortical disease
ITT	Insulin tolerance test		PSA	Prostate-specific antigen
IVF	In vitro fertilization		ptd-FGFR4	Pituitary-tumour-derived fibroblast growth factor receptor 4
KDIGO	Kidney Disease: Improving Global Outcomes		PTH	Parathyroid hormone
LCH	Langerhans cell histiocytosis		PTH1R	Parathyroid hormone 1 receptor
LD	Linkage disequilibrium		PTH2R	Parathyroid hormone 2 receptor
LDL	Low-density lipoprotein		PTRrP	Parathyroid-hormone-related protein
LH	Luteinizing hormone		RANKL	Receptor activator of nuclear factor kappa-B ligand
LNSC	Late-night salivary cortisol		rhGH	Recombinant human growth hormone
Lp(a)	Lipoprotein(a)		RRA	Radioiodine remnant ablation
MAF	Minor allele frequency		rT3	Reverse triiodothyronine
MCM	Minichromosome maintenance		SF-1	Steroidogenic factor 1
MCR2	Type 2 melanocortin receptor		SHBG	Sex hormone-binding globulin
MGMT	O-6-methylguanine-DNA methyltransferase		SLE	Systemic lupus erythematosus
MHC	Major histocompatibility complex		SMR	Standard mortality rate
MIBG	Metaiodobenzylguanidine		SMV	Superior mesenteric vein
MRAP	Melanocortin-2 receptor accessory protein		SNP	Single nucleotide polymorphism
MRI	Magnetic resonance imaging		SPECT	Single-photon-emission computed tomography
mTESE	Microtesticular sperm extraction		SSRI	Selective serotonin reuptake inhibitor
NADH	Nicotinamide adenine dinucleotide		SVC	Superior vena cava
NADPH	Nicotinamide adenine dinucleotide phosphate		T2	Diiodothyronine
NHS	National Health Service		T3	Triiodothyronine
NICE	National Institute for Health and Care Excellence		T4	Thyroxine
NICHD	National Institute of Child Health and Human Development		TART	Testicular adrenal rest tissue
NIH	National Institutes of Health		TB	Tuberculosis
NK	Natural killer		TBG	Thyroxine-binding globulin
NPT2a	Type 2a sodium–phosphate cotransporter		TCR	T-cell receptor
			TFT	Thyroid function test

TGF	Transforming growth factor
TmP/GFR	Maximal renal tubular reabsorption capacity for phosphate per litre glomerular filtrate
TNF	Tumour necrosis factor
TR-alpha	Thyroid hormone receptor alpha
TR-alpha RTH	Thyroid hormone receptor alpha resistance to thyroid hormone
TR-beta	Thyroid hormone receptor beta
TR-beta RTH	Thyroid hormone receptor beta resistance to thyroid hormone
TRH	Thyrotrophin-releasing hormone

TSH	Thyroid-stimulating hormone
UFC	Urinary free cortisol
UICC	Union for International Cancer Control
UV	Ultraviolet
UVB	Ultraviolet light B
VEGF	Vascular endothelial growth factor
VFA	Vertebral fracture assessment
VLDL	Very low density lipoprotein
WADA	World Anti-Doping Agency
WHI	Women's Health Initiative
WHO	World Health Organization

Chapter 1

Principles of endocrinology

Chapter contents

1.1 Hormones, receptors, and signalling

Introduction

There are two main ways of controlling the almost un-governable complexity of the thirty seven trillion cells that comprise a human being, one rapid, the other gradual. The nervous system acts quickly via electro-chemical signalling, eliciting direct responses. The endo-crine system, by way of utter contrast, is frequently slow, almost deliberately indirect, and acts via blood-borne molecules that instigate effects at remote sites in the body. Despite the apparent differences in speed, the two systems nonetheless coalesce, as evidenced by the complex interaction between the hypothalamus and the pituitary. But the CNS is just one system that hor-mones modulate. In fact, the endocrine system interacts with virtually all bodily systems at some level. Broadly, hormones control reproduction, growth, and devel-opment, the maintenance of the internal environment, and the regulation of energy balance. Aberrant signalling, therefore, can have wide-ranging implications, including causing metabolic, neurological, and developmental dis-orders, as well as profound influences upon cancer, im-mune illnesses, diabetes, and obesity. Understanding the complexities of endocrine signalling thus lies at the heart of future therapeutic advances.

The endocrine glands

Endocrine glands, in contrast to exocrine glands, which generally act directly via ducts, secrete via the blood-stream. The central endocrine glands are the pituitary, the thyroid, the adrenal glands, the ovaries, the testes, the parathyroid, and the pineal gland, but any organ or cell system capable of secreting hormones may be broadly considered to act as an endocrine gland. Generally, endo-crine organs are intensely vascularized. Given that the vasculature links all human organs, it represents an ideal conduit via which signals can be transmitted to the fur-thest universes of the body. But hormones do not need to act remotely. Cells are able to govern their own hor-monal responsiveness via autocrine mechanisms; rather than being secreted into the bloodstream, hormones may act via receptors expressed on or in the secretory cell itself. Cells are also able to influence the activity of their neighbours, via paracrine signalling. Thus, hormones may autoregulate, may influence their surrounding en-vironment within endocrine glands, and may trigger re-sponses at distant, far-flung junctures.

Hormone structures

Hormones come in multiple shapes and sizes, and are ar-ranged into three broad classes. First, many derive from single amino acids, and are known collectively as amines. These include the neurological hormones epineph-rine and dopamine, and the thyroid hormones 3,5,3′-triiodothyronine (T3) and 3,5,3′,5′-tetraiodothyronine (T4, or thyroxine), all of which owe their existence to the amino acid tyrosine. Second, numerous hormones are classified as proteins and peptides. These range spectacularly in size, from thyrotrophin-releasing hor-mone (three amino acids) to follicle-stimulating hor-mone (~200 amino acids). Protein hormones can show intricate three-dimensional folding and post-translational processing, to form the final active hormone. The third discrete classification of hormonal structure describes the steroids. Steroid hormones are direct or indirect descendants of cholesterol, and vary according to often subtle manipulations of their chemical structure, being categorized into progestins, mineralocorticoids, gluco-corticoids, androgens, and oestrogens.

The chemical structure of each class of hormone dic-tates its biological mode of action. For example, hor-mones which are unable to cross the plasma membrane of cells must rely on receptors which span the membrane and instigate intracellular signalling upon specific binding, and are generally unbound in the blood, often resulting in relatively short half-lives. Complex protein hormones need to be processed in the correct manner and at the correct moment for their biological activity to be most acutely felt. Prehormones or preprohormones are often cleaved, glycosylated, and packaged into secretory gran-ules, and hence the timing of their release from the cell is critical and hormone specific.

By contrast, hormones which can pass easily through the lipid-based plasma membrane are able to reach re-ceptors already lying in wait within the cell cytoplasm or nucleus. However, the potential promiscuity of such hor-mones needs to be kept in check via chaperone proteins, which shepherd them around the vasculature. Hormones which can be readily interconverted confer other signalling issues and complexities. In addition to receptor availability, the expression of the enzyme responsible for interconversion must be tightly regulated and tissue spe-cific to ensure the correct steroid hormone is active in the appropriate tissue. Thus, the chemical nature of the signalling molecule to some degree dictates the system which controls its production, release, and transport, and, critically, reacts to its message.

Hormone receptors

Governing all of the complexity of hormonal signalling is a pantheon of cellular receptors. These can be nu-clear, cytoplasmic, or located in the plasma membrane. But the very specific interaction between a hormone and its receptor is the fundamental node at which precision is achieved amongst the apparent noise of endocrine signalling. The expression and localization of a receptor confers spatial and temporal accuracy; the same hor-mone is able to have its desired effect upon the requisite cell at the correct moment because its receptor is avail-able and correctly localized within the cell.

Nuclear hormone receptors

Essentially, hormones are gene regulators. Whether this is direct or indirect, at the level of mRNA or protein, activating or repressing, the ultimate function of a hormone is to reach its target cell and change the expression and/or signalling properties of its inherent genes. The specificity of a nuclear receptor is dictated by its amino acid sequence within the ligand-binding domain. Also critical to the subsequent regu-lation of genes by nuclear receptors is the sequence of the transactivation domain, which facilitates interaction with the transcriptional complexes which ultimately open tightly bound chromosomal DNA up to the possibility of transcrip-tion. Nuclear receptors mediate the transcription of target genes by binding to the response elements of genes, often at sites which are surprisingly distant from the transcrip-tional start site. This facilitates transcriptional complexes comprised of co-regulatory proteins which, via chromatin remodelling and epigenetic modifications, ultimately switch a gene on or off. Nuclear receptor members include those for hydrophobic molecules such as steroid hormones (e.g. oestrogens, glucocorticoids, vitamin D_3), retinoic acids, and thyroid hormones.

Membrane hormone receptors

As peptide and polypeptide hormones are unable to cross the plasma membrane, signalling is contingent upon integral membrane proteins being expressed and correctly localized within target cells. In contrast to nuclear receptors, binding of the hormone thus occurs outside the cell, and results in the activation of the receptor, which in turn transmits a signal generally in the form of pathway activation. A central family of membrane receptors is the G-protein-coupled-receptor (GPCR) family, which illustrates the principle of an external hormone binding and subsequently precipitating internal cellular activity. The system specifically recognizes a hormonal signal, amplifies it, and transmits to the intracellular cAMP-dependent effector proteins. The GPCR thus acts as a conduit to provide the transduction of hormonal signals from the extracellular ligand-binding site to the G proteins located at the cytoplasmic side of the plasma membrane. The binding of a polypeptide hormone such as glucagon, growth hormone, or TSH stimulates the ubiquitously expressed G-alpha protein Gs alpha, resulting in a direct modulation of adenylate cyclase activity, and hence a change in the cAMP cascade. An alternative mode of secondary activation is demonstrated by the receptor tyrosine kinases, another well-characterized class of membrane receptors. Responsive to polypeptides such as insulin, receptor tyrosine kinases also bind their ligands extracellularly, and elicit kinase—as opposed to cAMP—activation, and hence the phosphorylation of downstream cellular targets.

Redundancy and complexity

Irrespective of their chemical composition, hormones circulate at relatively low concentrations, of the order of 10^{-7} to 10^{-12} M. The implication is that hormonal signalling is specific in its mode of action. Hormones must find their respective receptors and elicit a precise order of events, which are governed with exquisite sensitivity and control. Thus, even small changes in the sequence of hormone receptors have been shown in vivo and in experimental models to have drastic consequences for hormonal signalling.

There remains, however, abundant redundancy in the endocrine system. It is possible for one hormone to instigate very different biological processes in different tissues, despite specifically targeting the same receptor. This is particularly exemplified by oestrogen, which has broad roles in cell proliferation, bone turnover, and neurological function. Thus, it is critical to look beyond the receptor, in order to understand that hormonal action relies on and is modulated by other factors, such as transcriptional corepressors and coactivators, or on the interaction with other intracellular signalling cascades such as protein phosphorylation or cAMP activation.

Redundancy and complexity also reside in the observation that several hormones can regulate the same biological process. A primary example exists within the multifaceted control of lipolysis, which can be stimulated by a range of endocrine signalling molecules, including prolactin, glucagon, and catecholamines. Further, endocrine glands are rarely confined to the secretion of a single hormone, and within a gland, different cell types and structures may mediate the production or interconversion of a range of discrete hormones. The adrenal gland, for example, produces cortisol, aldosterone, and androstenedione, all in the cortex, and epinephrine and norepinephrine in the medulla. Similarly, the anterior pituitary produces a diverse range of stimulating hormones (e.g. TSH, follicle-stimulating hormone, and growth hormone), whilst the posterior lobe produces others (e.g. vasopressin and oxytocin). The multiple cell types of the anterior pituitary are generally—but not exclusively—geared up to produce a single hormone (prolactin in lactotrophs; adrenocorticotrophic hormone in corticotrophs), whereas in the thyroid, T3 and T4 are both produced by the same follicular epithelial cells. However, reinforcing the inherent complexity of the endocrine system, there are no hard and fast rules. Cell types may produce a sole hormone or many; glands may confine themselves to a single signalling molecule or a diverse spectrum; hormones may act locally as well as distantly; signalling may occur quickly or slowly; and different hormones may recognize the same receptor (glucocorticoids bind the mineralocorticoid receptor). But, within all of this, current endocrinology is really starting to understand at all levels how hormones signal, how they are regulated, and exactly what goes wrong in endocrine disorders.

Conclusion

Directly or indirectly, hormones influence virtually every major component of cellular function in every organ system, from cell division and differentiation to migration and adhesion, via gene expression and signal transduction. Collectively, these signalling events alter human metabolism, growth, reproduction, homeostasis, and neural function. Hormones are diverse chemical entities, and their individual modes of action reflect the properties of their structures, their modifications, and their cellular processing. They exert their effects at the prereceptor, receptor, and secondary messenger level, in modes of action which may be fleeting or chronic, and constitutive or episodic. Even relatively subtle perturbations in such systems can therefore elicit a broad range of clinical manifestation spanning the entirety of human disorders.

Being now a little over 100 years old, the study of endocrinology is coming of age. Our ability to manipulate, interpret, and characterize the endocrine system is now extraordinary. Insights into the finite mechanisms of hormone signalling continue to illuminate our knowledge of normal physiology and disease. Gaps in our knowledge are closing, and endocrine therapies are being developed to meet the inherent challenges. Never has this been more immediate than in twenty-first-century life, given that the endocrine system is acutely sensitive to our environment and readily disrupted. But our evolving knowledge enables us to understand the endocrine system as never before.

Further reading

Jameson JL. 'Principles of endocrinology', in Jameson JL and De Groot L, eds, *Endocrinology* (7th edition), 2016. Elsevier, pp. 3–15.

1.2 Hormone measurements: Assays

Introduction

The practice of modern endocrinology relies on the accurate measurement of hormones in various biological matrices, including blood, urine, and saliva. Clinicians must therefore have an appreciation of the different formats of laboratory assay employed for hormone measurement and, more importantly, recognize the factors that may confound their accurate measurement in clinical practice. Robust analytical methodology is the cornerstone of biochemical endocrinology, and selection of the most appropriate assay is in part dependent on the chemical properties of the hormone to be analysed. Comprehensive analytical service provision by the laboratory cannot be achieved when based only on a single methodology; therefore, a combination of techniques is essential to accommodate the wide range of endocrine tests available and to attain appropriate turnaround times for test results.

Immunoassay

The basic principles of immunoassay were first elaborated by the independent research of two laboratories on either side of the Atlantic. The work of Rosalyn Yalow and Solomon Berson in New York in the late 1950s culminated in their seminal 1960 paper describing a radioimmunoassay for plasma insulin, work that led to Yalow being awarded the Nobel Prize in Physiology and Medicine in 1977 for the development of radioimmunoassay of peptide hormones. This scientific discovery essentially coincided with the independent work of Roger Ekins, whose pioneering research in London led to the development of a competitive radiolabeled 'saturation assay' for serum thyroxine.

Immunoassay methodology harnesses nature by exploiting the properties of immunoglobulins (i.e. antibodies) to confer the immunoassay with exceptional analytical specificity (measuring only the hormone the assay purports to measure) and sensitivity (the smallest amount of hormone in a sample that can be accurately measured by the assay). These characteristics enable the routine measurement of picomolar (10^{-12}) concentrations of hormones in complex heterogeneous matrices such as blood samples. The range of endogenous and exogenous molecules (i.e. antigens) that immunoglobulins are able to bind with high affinity makes the immunoassay a versatile technique amenable to most hormone measurement applications.

Immunoassay design
Competitive immunoassay

There is an array of different approaches to immunoassay design, yet all are based on the fundamental principle that labelled molecules generate a signal which in turn is modulated by antibody occupancy, whether or not the labelled molecule is bound to antibody. A comprehensive description of immunoassay principles and techniques is beyond the scope of this chapter, and the reader should consult specialist texts for further reading.

Small molecules such as steroid hormones necessitate a 'competitive immunoassay' format whereby only one reagent antibody (immobilized on a solid phase) is used, in limited quantity. The other critical component of this format is the addition of a labelled analyte sometimes called the tracer (e.g. a target analyte labelled with a signal-generating material). The endogenous analyte competes for binding of limited antibody sites with the tracer; therefore, the proportion of antibody-bound tracer (i.e. the immunoassay signal generated) is inversely proportional to the concentration of analyte in the sample (Figure 1.1).

Immunometric assay

For larger hormones, such as peptide hormones, which have a greater surface area and are thus able to accommodate simultaneous binding of two molecules of antibody, the 'immunometric assay' (also referred to as the sandwich assay) is used. In this format, the first antibody (the 'capture' antibody) is immobilized onto a solid support and binds analyte in the sample; a second antibody that is specific for a different epitope site on the analyte and which is also labelled for immunoassay signal generation is present in the reaction to form a sandwich complex, with the antigen bound to both the first and second antibodies. Any unbound labelled antibody is washed away prior to quantification of the generated signal, which in this particular format is directly proportional to the analyte concentration in the sample (Figure 1.2).

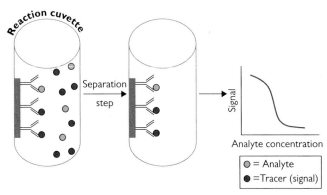

Fig 1.1 Principle of the competitive immunoassay.

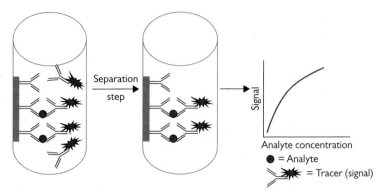

Fig 1.2 Principle of the immunometric assay.

Reporter system
There are many different types of labels to permit signal generation in an immunoassay, including radiolabels, such as iodine-125, which are employed in radioimmuno-assay. However, the conventional isotopic immunoassay has largely been supplanted by the use of non-isotopic labels for general safety, ease of use, and safe disposal. Enzymes are now one of the commonest non-isotopic labels used for signal generation in an immunoassay. The catalytic properties of enzymes also lend enhanced sensitivity to the immunoassay; a single enzyme catalysing the conversion of multiple substrate molecules to generate coloured or fluorescent product (i.e. label) therefore acts to amplify the signal generated by the immuno-assay, resulting in enhanced sensitivity. One format of immunoassay that uses enzymes chemically conjugated to antibodies is known as the enzyme-linked immuno-sorbent assay (ELISA; Figure 1.3).

Free-hormone assays
The development of immunoassays for 'free-hormone' analysis has been spearheaded by the measurement of free thyroxine (FT4) and free triiodothyronine (FT3) in

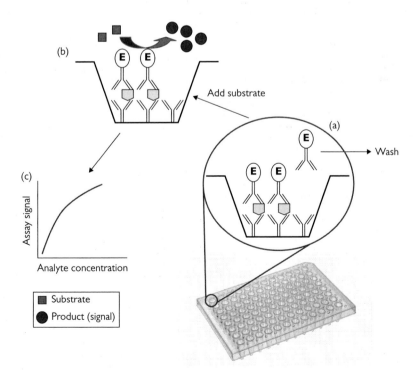

Fig 1.3 Principle of the enzyme-linked immunosorbent assay (ELISA). These assays are often performed using a 96-well plate format.

serum for the diagnosis of thyroid disease; it is the unbound, biologically active hormone component in serum as implied by the free-hormone concept. However, the accurate measurement of free thyroid hormones presents a challenge since the vast majority of thyroid hormone (>99.5%) is protein bound, with the remaining free fraction present at picomolar levels, necessitating highly sensitive assays for detection and quantification of free hormone.

The procedure of equilibrium dialysis is considered the 'gold standard' for free-hormone analysis and constitutes a preliminary separation step by use of a semipermeable membrane to physically separate the free fraction from the protein-bound fraction prior to free-hormone quantification. Until recently, this method has been considered not practicable for routine free-hormone measurement, and its use has been confined to specialist laboratories. However, modern equilibrium dialysis methods are now becoming available that employ high surface-to-volume ratio to reduce the time taken to attain equilibrium and are automation compatible to improve efficiency, thus having potential for future routine application.

The concept of free-hormone assays for T3 and T4, due to the low molecular weight of these target analytes, are based on the competitive immunoassay format which, critically, is designed to conserve the equilibrium between free and protein-bound hormone in serum during the assay process, to ensure that the assay signal generated reflects the 'free' rather than the 'total' hormone concentration. Commercial free-hormone assays for thyroid hormone measurement are based on either a 'one-step analogue' or a 'two-step' immunoassay format. In the one-step assay, a labelled T4 (or T3) analogue is employed which has binding affinity for the reagent antibody but, critically, has minimal affinity for endogenous serum-binding proteins. During the assay reaction, labelled analogue tracer competes for antibody-binding sites with endogenous hormone, and the subsequent assay signal generated is inversely proportional to the serum free-hormone concentration. The two-step format in contrast employs a separation step whereby a small quantity of reagent antibody is first incubated with serum to bind free hormone with minimal perturbation to the serum-free and protein-bound hormone equilibrium. This incubation is followed by a wash step to remove serum from the immobilized antibody, and then subsequent addition of tracer for measurement of free-hormone concentration.

Assays for free-hormone measurement are potentially confounded by factors that affect the serum free-to-bound hormone equilibrium. These factors include the heparin-mediated activation of endothelial lipoprotein lipase; this activation results in the production of free fatty acids that displace albumin-bound thyroid hormone. Additionally, genetic variants of binding proteins such as observed in familial dysalbuminaemic hyperthyroxinaemia (FDH), in which mutations of the albumin gene increase the affinity of albumin for T4 by approximately 60-fold, leading to overestimation of the FT4 concentration (particularly when measured by one-step analogue assays). In suspected cases of FDH, measurement of FT4 by equilibrium dialysis is appropriate for the elimination of FT4 assay interference.

Immunoassay in practice

Immunoassay methods are readily adaptable to automated analysers and subsequently require limited technical input by laboratory staff. In addition, automation enables rapid throughput and turnaround of laboratory test results, making automated immunoassays ideally suited to routine hormone measurement. However, immunoassays have a number of potential analytical pitfalls, including an inherent vulnerability to interference from anti-reagent antibodies and endogenous autoantibodies, susceptibility to cross-reactivity with structurally related compounds, macro-complex interference, and the high-dose hook effect (Table 1.1). These susceptibilities may give rise to false-positive or false-negative results, some examples of which are now briefly discussed. Interference in immunoassays due to anti-reagent antibodies can be categorized by the type of interfering antibody: (1) human anti-mouse antibodies (HAMAs), which are produced by the immune system in response to a direct antigenic stimulus and are sometimes observed in patients who work closely with animals, or in patients who have received therapeutic mouse monoclonal antibodies for imaging or treatment purposes; (2) heterophilic antibodies that, in contrast to HAMAs, are polyclonal and have variable affinities for antibody epitopes, so that immunoassay interference by heterophiles is generally less pronounced than that caused by HAMAs; and (3) rheumatoid factor autoantibodies that bind to the Fc portion of IgG, resulting in interference in the immunoassay and which are often found in the sera of patients with rheumatoid conditions.

Interference in thyroglobulin immunoassay from endogenous thyroglobulin autoantibodies can be particularly problematic, as such autoantibodies are often present in patients with autoimmune thyroid disease and differentiated thyroid carcinoma. Depending on whether the thyroglobulin–autoantibody complex partitions into the free or bound immunoassay fraction, the assay will generate a spuriously high or low result. Such interference has obvious clinical implications, since an undetectable thyroglobulin result after TSH stimulation is a marker of remission of differentiated thyroid carcinoma.

The specificity of reagent antibodies in an immunoassay formulation will determine the assay's vulnerability to structurally related compounds that harbour common cross-reactive epitopes with the analyte of interest. Cross-reacting substances may be (1) an endogenous compound with close structural homology with the target analyte (e.g. human chorionic gonadotrophin (hCG) cross-reactivity in a luteinizing hormone (LH) assay (both hCG and LH having a common alpha subunit)); (2) an endogenous compound that is a precursor in a metabolic pathway (e.g. in patients receiving the 11-beta-hydroxylase inhibitor metyrapone for the medical management of Cushing's syndrome, circulating levels of the cortisol precursor 11-deoxycortisol may accumulate, potentially leading to subsequent unrecognized hypoadrenalism due to spuriously elevated cortisol immunoassay results as a consequence of 11-deoxycortisol cross-reactivity); or (3) an exogenous medication (e.g. cross-reactivity of the growth hormone receptor antagonist pegvisomant in a growth hormone assay; insulin analogues that may cross-react in an insulin assay; and prednisolone cross-reactivity in a cortisol assay).

Macromolecular complexes, as exemplified by macroprolactin, which comprises prolactin bound to an anti-prolactin IgG autoantibody, give rise to hyperprolactinaemia in the absence of pituitary disease and may lead to medical mismanagement of

Table 1.1 Potential analytical interferences in immunoassays

Interference	Mechanism	Example
Cross-reactivity	Structurally-related compounds in the specimen are detected by the IA and generate a false test result.	- Prednisolone cross-reactivity in cortisol assay. - hCG cross-reactivity in LH assay
Anti-reagent antibodies	*Anti-reagent antibodies bind to the capture and/or detection Ab in the IA causing false test result.	- Human anti-mouse antibodies (HAMA) - Heterophilic antibodies - Rheumatoid factor
Autoantibodies	Autoantibody-analyte complex formation causing false test result.	Immunoassays that may be affected by autoantibodies include thyroglobulin, insulin and thyroid hormone assays.
Hereditary binding protein abnormalities	Genetic variants of binding proteins that may cause false test results.	**Albumin variant in FDH has altered binding affinity for T4 causing elevated FT4 result.
Macro-complexes	Immunoglobulin-analyte complex causing a falsely elevated test result.	- Macroprolactin is the most well documented example. Other reported complexes include: - Macro-TSH - Macro-CK (a macroenzyme).
High-dose hook effect	At very high analyte concentration, capture and detection Ab in two-site immunometric assays become saturated, inhibiting sandwich complex formation causing a falsely low test result.	Potential to affect compounds that circulate at very high concentration in the pathophysiological state, including hCG, prolactin and thyroglobulin.

Abbreviations: Ab, antibody; FDH, familial dysalbuminaemic hyperthyroxinaemia; FT4, free thyroxine; hCG, human chorionic gonadotrophin; IA, immunoassay; LH, luteinizing hormone; macro-CK, macro-creatine kinase; macro-TSH, macro-thyroid-stimulating hormone; T4, thyroxine.

*More likely to affect two-site immunometric assay format.

**More likely to affect one-step analogue assays.

patients. Prolactin circulates predominantly as a monomeric 23 kDa form; however, the high molecular weight macroprolactin form may have significant immunoreactivity in conventional prolactin immunoassays yet is minimally bioactive in vivo. It is pertinent to note that macroprolactin may be present in patients with elevated monomeric prolactin, and screening for macroprolactinaemia above an agreed serum prolactin cut-off concentration is widely practised by clinical laboratories. Additionally, prolactin is by no means the only hormone for which macromolecular phenomena have been described; isolated elevations in TSH may, in very rare cases, be caused by macro-TSH that can confound the interpretation of thyroid function test results in the absence of thyroid symptoms.

The high-dose hook effect (sometimes referred to as the pro-zone effect) occurs when analyte is present at very high concentration, leading to the saturation of reagent antibodies in an immunoassay. This is observed in two-site immunometric assays in which the capture and detection antibodies are added to the reaction simultaneously, and the risk is obviously greatest for hormones that have a wide (patho)physiological concentration range, such as hCG, prolactin, and thyroglobulin. Indeed, the effect may be so great that results hook back to within the normal reference range.

Clinical laboratories utilize a variety of testing strategies to investigate possible interference in immunoassays but communication between clinical and laboratory staff is vital when results are incongruent with the clinical picture. Ultimately, minimizing the risk of interference in immunoassays is a shared responsibility. A thorough description of immunoassay interference is beyond the

scope of this chapter and the reader is referred to comprehensive reviews in this area for further reading.

Mass spectrometry

Since the turn of the millennium, liquid chromatography–tandem mass spectrometry has become increasingly prominent in clinical laboratories for the accurate quantification of low-molecular-weight molecules, such as endogenous metabolites, drugs for therapeutic monitoring, and, in the context of endocrinology, steroid hormones. This technique commands exquisite analytical sensitivity and specificity by virtue of its ability to detect and discriminate ions based on mass:charge ratio (m/z), acting as a 'molecular sieve' to filter and quantify the analyte of interest. The dominant detector configuration in current clinical diagnostic applications is the tandem mass spectrometer. Liquid chromatography is used at the front end of the instrument to separate compounds and thus minimize matrix effects and isobaric interferences. The subsequent column eluent undergoes ionization to form charged ions (e.g. m/z of a singly charged ion $[M + H]^+$ = molecular weight +1) before infusion into the ion source of the mass spectrometer. This tandem configuration permits the selection of a precursor ion (parent ion) for stable trajectory through the first quadrupole (MS1), where it is directed into the second quadrupole (the collision cell), where it undergoes fragmentation via collision-induced dissociation. The resulting ion fragments, which are indicative of the structure of the parent molecule enter the third quadrupole (MS2), which is tuned to permit a selected product ion (i.e. the daughter ion) to traverse it for quantification at the detector (see Figure 1.4).

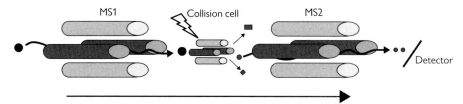

Fig 1.4 Tandem mass spectrometry; the parent ion passes through the first quadrupole (MS1), where it is directed into the second quadrupole (the collision cell), where it undergoes fragmentation via collision-induced dissociation. The resulting ion fragments that are indicative of the structure of the parent molecule enter the third quadrupole (MS2), which is tuned to permit a selected product ion (i.e. the daughter ion) to traverse it for quantification at the detector.

Mass spectrometry in practice

The ability of mass spectrometry to identify and quantify analytes based on their molecular weight offers enhanced analytical specificity. Additionally, recent advances in both mass spectrometry and online sample preparation technology (pre-analytics) has progressed the analytical sensitivity of this methodology to the extent that modern mass spectrometry applications are now comparable to conventional immunoassay methods in this regard. Additionally, mass spectrometry is now entering the arena of peptide quantification, exemplified by the availability of mass spectrometry-based assays for plasma renin activity by measurement of the peptide angiotensin I. Furthermore, protein quantification by mass spectrometry is now possible, with the recent documentation of mass spectrometry assays for insulin-like growth factor 1.

Like immunoassays, mass spectrometry is not impervious to the potential for analytical error. For example, mass spectrometry applications in clinical diagnostic laboratories are generally developed 'in house' and, consequently, mass spectrometry methods for the same target analyte may differ significantly in their application protocols, with potential variables including chromatography strategy, ionization process, mass transitions employed, and the use of different internal standards. As such, differing mass spectrometry method protocols may introduce analytical bias between different laboratories. The potential sources of interference in mass spectrometry are as follows:

- ionization: the presence of compounds in the sample that affect the efficiency of the ionization process prior to starting mass spectrometry; such matrix effects cause ion suppression/enhancement which may differentially impact the target analyte and internal standard, resulting in inaccurate test results
- internal standard: deuterated internal standard may have the same mass as a naturally occurring isotope within the mass distribution of the target analyte; thus, the naturally occurring isotope will increase the amount of internal standard detected, therefore decreasing the relative response for the target analyte and causing the analyte concentration to be underestimated
- mass transition selection: isobaric compounds that share the same *m/z* as the target analyte may lead to incorrect test results; chromatography should be optimized to eliminate this type of interference

Mass spectrometry methods for clinical applications must be rigorously validated prior to implementation into clinical care, and potential sources of bias must be ascertained and systematically addressed. Mass spectrometry is a sequential analytical technique and, consequently, analysis times are generally longer in comparison to automated high-throughput multichannel immunoassay methods. However, for medium-to-high-throughput laboratories, mass spectrometry offers the potential for operational cost savings.

Conclusion

It is important for clinicians to have an understanding of the principles and pitfalls of hormone measurement. This knowledge is a great asset towards the appropriate requesting and interpretation of hormone tests.

There is currently great debate in the biochemical endocrinology community regarding the appropriate use of assays and, indeed, which methodology is best suited to the diagnostic laboratory. The decision as to whether to use immunoassays or mass spectrometry has polarized opinion; advocates of immunoassays have extolled the ease of use and high sample throughput that automated immunoassay platforms offer, whilst mass spectrometrists have praised the superior analytical robustness of mass spectrometry, which lends excellent analytical sensitivity and specificity with minimal susceptibility to assay interference. The truth is that both of these techniques offer advantages for the clinical laboratory, and the individual strengths of each method can be complimentary when applied in the appropriate manner for endocrine investigations.

Further reading

Kay R, Halsall DJ, Annamalai AK, et al. A novel mass spectrometry-based method for determining insulin-like growth factor 1: Assessment in a cohort of subjects with newly diagnosed acromegaly. *Clin Endocrinol* 2013; 78: 424–30.

Kushnir MM, Rockwood AL, Roberts WL, et al. Liquid chromatography tandem mass spectrometry for analysis of steroids in clinical laboratories. *Clin Biochem* 2011; 44: 77–88.

Midgley JEM. Direct and indirect free thyroxine assay methods: Theory and practice. *Clin Chem* 2001; 47: 1353–63.

Monaghan PJ, Owen LJ, Trainer PJ, et al. Comparison of serum cortisol measurement by immunoassay and liquid chromatography-tandem mass spectrometry in patients receiving the 11β-hydroxylase inhibitor metyrapone. *Ann Clin Biochem* 2011; 48: 441–6.

Sturgeon CM and Viljoen A. Analytical error and interference in immunoassay: Minimizing risk. *Ann Clin Biochem* 2011; 48: 418–32.

Wild D, ed. *The Immunoassay Handbook* (2nd edition), 2001. Nature Publishing Group.

1.3 Hormone measurements: Hormone-binding proteins

Introduction

Most hormones circulate in blood extensively bound to proteins. This protein binding results in only a small fraction of the hormone being unbound and available to have biological effects and therefore modulates hormone bioavailability. The amount of protein-bound hormone is variable, but generally hormone assays measure the total (i.e. bound and unbound) hormone concentration in the circulation. Therefore, protein binding is an important determinant, and often caveat, in hormone measurement, as it defines what exactly is measured and how. In this section, known physiological and pathophysiological roles of hormone-binding proteins are briefly described. The significance of protein binding in hormone measurement is then highlighted. Although most hormones have a protein-binding system, the stress of this section is on the binding proteins that are most studied. More specifically, corticosteroid-binding globulin (CBG) is used as the main example, as it typifies the role of most specific hormone-binding proteins.

Carrier proteins and hormone reservoirs

Steroid and thyroid hormones are hydrophobic molecules that require a transfer system in plasma in order to remain soluble, circulate, and reach their target tissues. Hormone-binding proteins can be divided into hormone-specific systems, which usually bind hormones with high affinity and low capacity, and non-hormone-specific binding proteins, which bind with low affinity but high capacity due to their much higher concentrations in serum. The major non-hormone-specific binding protein is albumin, which, along with transthyretin, binds lipophilic hormones. The most extensively studied major hormone-specific binding proteins are CBG, sex hormone-binding globulin (SHBG), and thyroxine-binding globulin (TBG). Although specific binding proteins have been described for other hormones, such as growth hormone and prolactin, here we will use CBG as an example, since the physiological role of CBG is better understood.

CBG is the main plasma transporter for glucocorticoids and binds up to 90% of cortisol. Furthermore, various other endogenous steroids bind to CBG with lower affinity, including testosterone and progesterone. The binding of exogenous glucocorticoids is variable and, although some bind significantly, like prednisolone, others, such as dexamethasone, do not. Critically, CBG acts as a circulating steroid buffer, protecting tissues from steep oscillations in adrenal production of cortisol. The amount of cortisol bound to CBG defines the bioavailable fraction and acts as a readily releasable steroid reservoir.

Modulators of hormone action

CBG is a typical example of a hormone-binding protein that has an active role in modulating hormone action. Detailed structural and functional studies of CBG have revealed a biological role that extends beyond that expected from a simple carrier molecule. As a member of the serine proteinase inhibitor (serpin) family of proteins, CBG undergoes a defined conformational change upon interaction with target proteinases, and this change influences its functionality as a steroid-binding protein. More specifically, when human CBG is cleaved by

neutrophil elastase, this causes a structural rearrangement and substantial loss of cortisol-binding activity, providing a mechanism by which CBG regulates the local delivery of cortisol to target tissues during inflammation. Moreover, CBG behaves as a negative acute phase protein during acute inflammation. Interleukin 6 directly inhibits CBG gene transcription and protein secretion, and exogenous interleukin 6 administration decreases serum CBG concentration by 50%, with levels normalizing after 7 days following a single injection. As a result of reduced hepatic synthesis and increased degradation by elastase, substantial decreases in plasma CBG levels occur in patients with systemic infections, sepsis, severe burns, and myocardial infarction, and this likely ensures that end organs receive a maximal supply of glucocorticoids at multiple levels to control inflammation, gluconeogenesis, and stress.

Significance in hormone measurement

The unbound hormone fraction defines the biological hormone action and, therefore, the feedback regulation of hormone production. As an example, when protein binding is increased, the unbound moiety transiently decreases and this causes increased production of the hormone, due to positive feedback regulation of the hormone axis. This results in a rise in the total circulating hormone concentration, whereas the opposite is observed for reduced protein binding. These changes in CBG and total serum cortisol concentrations are not associated with a phenotypical change, as the unbound bioavailable cortisol remains unaltered. The concentration of binding proteins is regulated by several factors that control production, secretion, and clearance, and this section refers to the most common factors encountered in clinical practice.

CBG has a long half-life of 5–6 days, and factors that modulate secretion but not clearance only affect circulating CBG levels after prolonged exposure. Among the factors that have a clinically relevant effect on CBG and total serum cortisol concentration (Table 1.2), the oestrogen-related increase in CBG is probably the most well documented, contributing to the observed increase of measured total serum cortisol in women treated with oral contraceptives or who are pregnant. Pregnancy-associated CBG glycoforms with increased sialic acid groups have also been identified, possibly resulting in slower clearance. Mitotane, an adrenolytic agent used in the management of adrenal cancer, has oestrogenic properties and causes an increase in total serum cortisol; this increase has to be accounted for in treatment monitoring. In a similar manner, alterations in SHBG concentration affect the total testosterone concentration without changing the corresponding free or bioavailable testosterone concentration. Conditions that alter circulating SHBG concentration are shown in Table 1.3. When protein binding is altered, it is generally accepted that the unbound hormone fraction is not affected and retains normal pharmacokinetics; therefore, this should influence the choice of hormone measurement. This is described in more detail in Section 1.4. Genetic variations in binding-protein concentration and/or binding affinity also impact on total hormone concentration to a clinically important extent.

Table 1.2 Factors affecting circulating corticosteroid-binding globulin concentration

Factors	Effect on CBG	Mechanism
Oestrogens	↑	S
Pregnancy	↑	S,C
Mitotane	↑	S
SERMs	↑	S
IL-6	↓	S,C
Insulin, IGF-I	↓	S
Thyroid hormones	↓/↔	S
Glucocorticoids	↓	S
Cirrhosis	↓	S
Nephrotic syndrome	↓	C

Individual factors that affect corticosteroid-binding globulin secretion (S) and/or clearance (C) are shown, together with their individual effect and mechanism of action.

Abbreviations: CBG, corticosteroid-binding globulin.

Source: Reprinted by permission from Macmillan Publishers Ltd: *Nature Reviews Endocrinology*, Perogamvros I, Ray DW, and Trainer PJ. Regulation of cortisol bioavailability—effects on hormone measurement and action, Volume 8, Issue 12, pp. 717–727, copyright (2012), Rights Managed by Nature Publishing Group.

Routine hormone measurement currently relies on the quantification of total hormone, although realization of the significant effects of protein binding is currently driving

Table 1.3 Factors affecting circulating sex hormone-binding globulin concentration

Decreased SHBG concentration	Increased SHBG concentration
Obesity, diabetes mellitus	Ageing
Nephrotic syndrome	Cirrhosis
Androgens, progestogens, and glucocorticoids	Oestrogens
Hypothyroidism	Hyperthyroidism
Acromegaly	Antiepileptic drugs
Familial SHBG deficiency	Calorie restriction

Abbreviations: SHBG, sex hormone-binding globulin.

a transition to the preferential measurement of unbound hormone. This is further described in Section 1.4.

Further reading

Klieber MA, Underhill C, Hammond GL, et al. Corticosteroid-binding globulin, a structural basis for steroid transport and proteinase-triggered release. *J Biol Chem* 2007; 282: 29594–603.

Mendel CM. The free hormone hypothesis: A physiologically based mathematical model. *Endocr Rev* 1989; 10: 232–74.

Perogamvros I, Ray DW, and Trainer PJ. Regulation of cortisol bioavailability: Effects on hormone measurement and action. *Nat Rev Endocrinol* 2012; 8: 717–27.

Rosner W. The functions of corticosteroid-binding globulin and sex hormone-binding globulin: Recent advances. *Endocr Rev* 1990; 11: 80–91.

1.4 Hormone measurements: Biological matrices for hormone measurement

Introduction

There are various biological matrices in which hormones can be accurately measured by the clinical laboratory. Each of these diagnostic fluids offers advantages dependent upon the clinical setting. Historically, the most common matrices for the measurement of hormones have been blood (plasma/serum) and urine. More recently, hormone measurement in saliva has gained significant attention and is becoming increasingly popular to aid the endocrinologist in certain clinical scenarios. All three aforementioned matrices are now routinely used in current clinical practice for the diagnosis of Cushing's syndrome (see Chapter 3, Section 3.7) and this example will be used to elaborate on the advantages and disadvantages of hormone measurement in each of serum, urine, and saliva.

Serum

The measurement of cortisol in serum is recommended in first-line diagnostic testing for Cushing's syndrome in the form of the dexamethasone suppression test (DST). The measurement of cortisol in serum is simple for the clinical laboratory to perform using automated immunoassay analysers, yet the validity of DST results may be affected by the variable absorption and metabolism of dexamethasone, particularly in patients receiving cytochrome P450 enzyme inducers such as anticonvulsant therapies. Moreover, routine serum cortisol immunoassays measure the total hormone concentration; consequently, false-positive results may be observed for female patients concomitantly taking the oral contraceptive pill, which increases circulating CBG concentration and thus increases total serum cortisol. For this reason, oestrogen-containing medications should be stopped for 6 weeks prior to testing.

In recent years, a transition in the assessment of the hypothalamic–pituitary–adrenal (HPA) axis has been underway, from total serum cortisol to free serum cortisol, in the same way that FT4 as opposed to total T4 is measured by most laboratories. The novel technologies developed, including ultrafiltration and mass spectrometry, have provided methods that can directly measure free serum hormones, are fast, reliable, accurate, and specific, and can be carried out within hours in an acute clinical setting. The practical utility and cost of these assays are, however, important considerations, and salivary biomarkers (see 'Saliva') can provide useful surrogates. The assays need to be validated in large populations and in a range of clinical settings before they can be adopted in clinical practice. The measurement of free serum hormones is especially indicated in selected groups of patients who have alterations in binding proteins.

Urine

Urinary free cortisol (UFC) measurement offers an integrated assessment of cortisol secretion over a 24-hour period and is an accepted first-line investigation for Cushing's syndrome. This test requires a complete 24-hour urine collection and, to ensure accuracy, the patient must be educated to ensure that the collection is performed correctly. Furthermore, as UFC concentrations are variable in patients with Cushing's syndrome, a minimum of two collections should be performed.

Unlike serum cortisol measurement, UFC is unaffected by changes in CBG concentration. However, UFC measurement does have limitations in the fact that the test reflects renal filtration; false-negative results may occur in moderate-to-severe renal impairment. Furthermore, UFC may be within the normal range in patients with mild Cushing's syndrome; for such patients, the measurement of salivary cortisol may be advantageous.

Saliva

In healthy individuals, the circadian rhythm of adrenal cortisol production dictates that circulating cortisol reaches a zenith at 07:00–09:00 h and steadily declines throughout the rest of the day to a nadir at approximately midnight, when the person is unstressed and asleep. A consistent biochemical signature of Cushing's syndrome (see also Chapter 3, Section 3.7) is the loss of normal circadian rhythm, and this physiological phenomenon provides the basis for late-night salivary cortisol (LNSC) measurement. The absence of a late-night cortisol nadir assessed through salivary cortisol measurement is an accepted first-line test for Cushing's syndrome, with patients required to collect two LNSC samples on separate evenings for analysis.

Salivary cortisol measurement offers a variety of advantages for both the patient and clinician. This diagnostic fluid is collected in a simple, non-invasive manner that is convenient for patients. The unbound biologically active form of cortisol in the blood is in equilibrium with cortisol in the saliva, as lipophilic molecules such as steroid hormones enter the saliva from the blood by passive diffusion; measurement of LNSC is therefore unaffected by changes in CBG and provides the endocrinologist with an accurate surrogate marker of circulating free cortisol. Caution must be taken in the interpretation of LNSC results from patients who may have a perturbed diurnal rhythm, such as shift workers, individuals crossing widely different time zones, or patients with variable bed times. In such cases, the LNSC collection time may have to be adjusted. Cigarette smoking has also been demonstrated to cause elevation in LNSC measurement and this should therefore be avoided prior to saliva collection. Likewise, both liquorice and chewing tobacco contain glycyrrhizic acid, which inhibits the enzyme 11 beta-hydroxysteroid dehydrogenase type II isoform which is present in salivary glands and oxidizes cortisol to the inactive metabolite cortisone; therefore, inhibition of this enzyme may lead to false elevation of LNSC values.

Future developments: Hormone measurement in target tissues

Hormones act at a cellular level and affect the tissues that the cells constitute. Therefore, it is clinically important to quantify their concentration in target tissues and cells. As the mechanisms of steroid action are intracellular, tissue steroid concentrations are more physiologically relevant than circulating concentrations. In recent years' microdialysis, a semi-invasive technique has been used for the measurement of unbound endogenous or exogenous analytes in the extracellular fluid. Cell-based bioassays have also been developed to measure gluco-corticoid bioavailability in serum by using transfected cells. These assays are still being validated on research grounds, although it is predicted that they will increasingly influence our understanding of hormone action and, therefore, clinical practice.

Each biological matrix described carries advantages and disadvantages that the endocrinologist must consider when choosing the appropriate biochemical test. It is also important to ensure that the diagnostic laboratory has the appropriate assays that have been thoroughly validated for hormone measurement in the biological matrix of interest.

Further reading

Gröschl M. Current status of salivary hormone analysis. *Clin Chem* 2008; 54: 1759–69.

Nieman LK, Biller BM, Findling JW, et al. The diagnosis of Cushing's syndrome: An Endocrine Society clinical practice guideline. *J Clin Endocrinol Metab* 2008; 93: 1526–40.

Raff H. Update on late-night salivary cortisol for the diagnosis of Cushing's syndrome: Methodological considerations. *Endocrine* 2013; 44: 346–9.

1.5 Autoimmunity and the endocrine system

Introduction

The immune system plays a vital role in protecting the body against attack from bacteria, viruses, and other foreign bodies. Essential to this function is its ability to distinguish between self and non-self. Breakdown in this ability can occur, causing an inappropriate immune response against self-tissues and organs, known as autoimmunity. Endocrine autoimmunity is characterized by autoantibody production against components of the endocrine system (Table 1.4), resulting in a variety of conditions including, for example, type 1 diabetes, Graves' disease, Hashimoto's thyroiditis, Addison's disease, and autoimmune polyendocrine syndrome type 1. Although, the exact organ/s targeted for autoimmune attack vary from disease to disease, co-clustering of different endocrine diseases within individuals and families, and the identification of shared immunological genetic susceptibility loci between diseases, suggest the presence of common pathogenic pathways. This section will focus on how disruption in the following immunological pathways contributes to disease onset:

- Breakdown in ability to distinguish self from non-self
- Disruption in antigen presentation to T cells
- Alterations in T-cell activation/signalling
- Variation in B-cell function
- Environmental impact on the immune system

Breakdown in ability to distinguish self from non-self

Constant monitoring of antigens is performed by T lymphocytes and is essential to ensure that foreign antigens are recognized quickly and an immune response mounted. A T cell's ability to distinguish self from non-self is key to this process and is achieved through central tolerance.

Central tolerance

CD4+ T helper (Th) cells, which activate B cells to produce antibodies, and CD8+ T cells, which produce cytotoxic T cells and natural killer (NK) cells, start off as common progenitor CD4−/CD8− T cells within the bone marrow. Progenitor CD4−/CD8− T cells undergo random rearrangement of their T-cell receptor (TCR) gene, creating precursor CD4+/CD8+ T cells. Random TCR rearrangements provide a mature T-cell repertoire capable of binding a vast array of antigens. Inevitably, however, some non-functional and self/autoreactive precursor T cells are generated. Before entering the peripheral immune system, precursor T cells move to the thymus to undergo positive and negative selection.

Positive selection

Precursor CD4+/CD8+ T cells' TCR functionality is tested by determining binding to human leukocyte antigen (HLA) molecules presenting antigens. Precursor T cells that bind antigen-presenting HLA molecules

Table 1.4 Different autoantigens identified in the endocrine autoimmune diseases

Disease	Autoantigen	Percentage (%) prevalence of autoantibodies directed against autoantigen in disease versus control subjects	
		Disease cases	Control subjects
Type 1 diabetes	Islet cell antibody (antigen unknown)	70	1
	GAD_{65}	70–90	1–2
	GAD_{67}	10–20	1
	Insulin	40–70	1
	IA-2 and IA-2β proteins of protein tyrosine phosphatase	25–60	1
Graves' disease	TSHR	95–100	5
	TPO	90	10–30
	Tg	70	18–30
Hashimoto's Thyroiditis	Tg	95–100	18–30
	TPO	95–100	10–30
Autoimmune hypoparathyroidism	Ca-SR	60	0
Addison's disease	Steroid 21-hydroxylase	70	1
	Steroid 17α-hydroxylase	5	1
	cytP450scc	9	1
APS-1 and APS-2	Organ specific antigens relating to disease component	Variable	

GAD = glutamic acid decarboxylase; TSHR= thyroid-stimulating hormone receptor; TPO = thyroid peroxidase; Tg = thyroglobulin; Ca-SR = calcium-sensing receptor; cytP450scc = cytochrome P450 side chain cleavage enzyme.

Adapted from Wass JAH, Stewart PM, Amiel SA. et al., *Oxford Textbook of Endocrinology and Diabetes*, 2nd edition, Table 1.6.2, pp. 34–44 Copyright © 2011, with permission from Oxford University Press.

receive a survival signal, whereas TCRs that do not bind receive no survival signal and so die.

Negative selection

Precursor T cells that survive positive selection are then retested to determine if they bind HLA molecules presenting an array of self-antigens. Any T cells that recognize self-antigens too strongly, suggesting autoreactivity, undergo TCR editing to alter antigen specificity or undergo apoptosis. Under normal circumstances, only functional, non-autoreactive CD4+/CD8+ precursor T cells mature into CD4+ Th cells or CD8+ T cells and are released into the periphery.

Autoimmunity: A case of bad education?

Many endocrine antigens are expressed outside of the thymus, raising the question as to whether precursor T cells have been educated to recognize them. The protein encoded by *AIRE*, defects in which were originally detected as the genetic cause of autoimmune polyendocrine syndrome type 1, was found to transcribe otherwise tissue-restricted antigens in the thymus, including several thyroid and pancreas antigens. Support for a role of disrupted central tolerance in autoimmune disease came from screening a variable number of tandem repeats upstream of the insulin gene in type 1 diabetes. The region consists of 14–15 base pairs of consensus sequence clustered into Class I (30–60 repeats), Class II (60–120 repeats), and Class III (120–170 repeats) alleles. The presence of Class I alleles predisposes for type 1 diabetes, whereas presence of Class III alleles protects against type 1 diabetes. Functional studies demonstrated that Class III alleles encode 200%–300% higher insulin transcription in the thymus, compared to Class I alleles, suggesting that variation in the thymic transcript levels of endocrine genes could affect how successfully negative selection removes autoreactive T cells.

Disruption in antigen presentation to T cells

The constant processing and display of antigens by HLA molecules on the surface of antigen-presenting cells (APCs) in the periphery is essential for T-cell screening and, if appropriate, the generation of an immune response (see Figure 1.5). Processing of endogenous (internal) and exogenous (external) antigens is achieved through two distinct pathways. Endogenously derived proteins, including viral proteins, are initially ubiquitinated and then degraded by the cytosolic pathway. This leads to the generation of peptides which enter the endoplasmic reticulum, where they become bound by HLA class I molecules. Antigen-bound HLA class I molecules exit the endoplasmic reticulum and move to the APC surface for presentation to CD8+ T cells. If the antigen is recognized as non-self, the CD8+ T cell becomes activated, leading to generation of cytotoxic T cells, which destroy infected cells, and NK cell activation, which produces lymphokines, cytokines, and chemokines essential for immune cell recruitment and cell destruction. Exogenous proteins, such as those

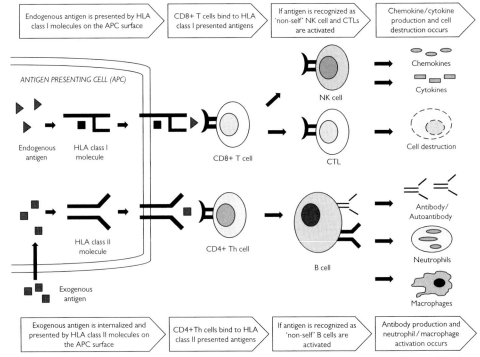

Fig 1.5 The role of T and B cells in monitoring antigens and mounting an immune response against any non-self antigen; HLA, human leukocyte antigen; Th, T helper; NK, natural killer, CTL, cytotoxic T lymphocyte.

from bacteria, have to be internalized into the APC. Once internalized, exogenous proteins navigate between a series of increasingly acidic compartments, known as the endocytic pathway, leading to the generation of antigens. These antigens are bound by HLA class II molecules, which exit the endocytic pathway and are displayed on the APC surface for recognition by CD4+ Th cells. If the antigen is recognized as non-self by the CD4+ Th cell this leads to B-cell activation/antibody production and macrophage activation. The vital role of the HLA region in the immunological defence system is only possible because of the highly variable nature of its encoding genes, which enable the human population to encounter and survive such a wide array of antigenic threats. Some of these variants, however, can predispose to the autoimmune disease process.

Variation in exogenous antigen presentation by HLA class II molecules

Variation within the HLA class II region-encoded HLA-DR molecule (composed of a HLA-DRB1 chain and the almost non-polymorphic HLA-DRA1 chain) and the HLA-DQ molecule (composed of a HLA-DQB1 chain and a HLA-DQA1 chain) has been examined, with the DRB1*03 variant being strongly associated with Graves' disease and type 1 diabetes, and DRB1*04 being strongly associated with type 1 diabetes and Hashimoto's thyroiditis. Due to linkage disequilibrium among DRB1, DQB1, and DQA1 (see Chapter 4), the haplotypes containing DRB1*03 and DRB1*04, known as the DR3 and DR4 haplotypes, respectively, are also strongly associated with autoimmune disease. Regression analysis of DRB1–DQB1–DQA1 haplotypes in Graves' disease revealed the association was due exclusively to DRB1 and DQA1. When comparing the DRB1*03 molecule, which predisposes to Graves' disease, to the DRB1*07 molecule, which protects against Graves' disease, change at amino acid position 74, from a positively charged arginine to a non-charged glutamine, respectively, was observed, in an area which forms part of the HLA antigen-binding domain. Variation at position 74 also differentiated DRB1*0403 and DRB1*0406 molecules, which contain negatively charged glutamic acid at that position and confer a low risk for type 1 diabetes, from high-risk alleles, including DRB1*0401, which contain non-charged polar amino acids at that position. Several hypotheses have been suggested to explain how variation in antigen-binding pockets of HLA class II molecules could lead to auto-immune onset. These include:

- variation in the antigen-binding domain of the HLA molecule may cause preferential selection of a limited set of self-peptides during negative selection, allowing more autoreactive T cells to escape central tolerance
- preferential binding by a given DR/DQ molecule in heterozygous individuals may lead to presentation of specific antigens, depending on whether it is predisposing, neutral, or protective
- although HLA class II molecules present exogenous antigens, cross-presentation of endogenous antigens (normally presented by HLA class I molecules) can occur, and vice versa, potentially altering how exogenous antigens are recognized by the immune system

Variation in endogenous antigen presentation by HLA class I molecules

Association of HLA class I molecules, such as HLA-A, HLA-B, and HLA-C, with many autoimmune endocrine conditions has been detected, with several hypothesis attempting to explain how they could be linked to autoimmunity:

- viral antigens preferentially presented by certain HLA class I molecules may be similar to self-antigens; an immune response mounted against these viral antigens could unintentionally cross-react with similar self-antigens
- viruses presented by HLA class I molecules can trigger strong immune responses that could unintentionally cross-react with self-antigens
- HLA class I molecules interact with killer-cell immunoglobulin-like receptors which help control NK cell activation, and variation in these interactions could cause inappropriate NK cell activation
- variation in HLA class I molecules could cause alterations in central tolerance mechanisms and affect T-cell education and/or the production of T regulatory cells

Variation in T-cell activation/signalling

For T-cell activation to occur, this requires not only binding of the TCR to the antigen presented by HLA molecules on the surface of APCs, but also co-stimulatory signals. These signals come from accessory molecules such as CD28, which promotes signalling, and CTLA-4, which downregulates signalling. CTLA-4 is upregulated during T-cell signalling and has been proposed to block signalling through numerous pathways. These include the following:

- binding of CD28 to co-stimulatory molecules CD80/CD86 can be blocked by CTLA-4
- CTLA-4 can alter lipid raft and microcluster formation, thus aiding downstream TCR signal transduction
- CTLA-4 also produces negative signals to prevent T-cell activation
- CTLA-4 can alter the stability and strength of TCR and APC interactions by decreasing adhesion molecules required for such interactions

Genetic variants within CTLA-4 have been associated with multiple autoimmune disorders, including type 1 diabetes and Graves' disease (see also Chapter 2, Section 2.4) and have been shown to alter the ratio of full-length CTLA-4 to a soluble isoform. As it has been suggested that the soluble isoform may provide greater inhibition of T-cell activation than the full-length isoform, changes in the expression of the soluble isoform could alter T-cell activation thresholds. Other inhibitors of T-cell activation have also been associated with endocrine autoimmunity. Variation within *PTPN22* has been shown to encode a change from arginine to tryptophan at amino acid position 620 (referred to as R620W) of the LYP molecule encoded by *PTPN22*. The presence of the LYP620W variant has been shown to impair LYP interaction with Csk, an important intracellular inhibitor of the T-cell signal transducer Lck, causing greater inhibition of T-cell signalling. The presence of LYP620W could lead to stronger downstream inhibition of T-cell signalling, potentially altering autoreactive T-cell activity during central tolerance and thus affecting negative selection.

Table 1.5 Proposed environmental impacts on autoimmune endocrine disease and how they are believed to impact on the immune system

Environmental factor	How environmental factor is proposed to alter immune system
Viruses and bacteria	Birth rate data from type 1 diabetes and Graves' disease patients show peaks in autumn and winter, when viruses and bacteria are more virulent, compared to birth rates peaks in the summer and spring in the general population; however, more recently, work in several large Caucasian Graves' disease collections failed to show a peak in birth rates in summer and spring, casting doubt over the role of month of birth effects on autoimmune disease onset
Improved hygiene	Humans have developed strong, highly effective immune systems to enable them to survive any foreign threat encountered; due to increases in hygiene, coupled with changes in social behaviour, the body is encountering less foreign insults and, as a result, our highly primed immune systems could turn against us, causing autoimmune onset
Stress and smoking	These have immunosuppressive effects on the immune system by stimulating the hypothalamic–pituitary–adrenal axis, downregulating immune responsiveness and regulation
Exposure to cow's milk early in life	Exposure to cow's milk early in childhood, rather than breast milk, which provides immune support, has been proposed to contribute to type 1 diabetes, as the immune systems could trigger a response against cow insulin that may cross-react with human insulin; however, to date, no clear evidence of a role for cow's milk in increasing rates of type 1 diabetes has been established

Although central tolerance removes the majority of autoreactive T cells before they enter the periphery, inevitably some autoreactive T cells do enter the periphery. T regulatory cells (a form of CD4+ Th cells expressing high CD25 and foxp3 levels) account for 6%–7% of the mature CD4+ Th cell population and suppress the activation and expansion of autoreactive T cells in the periphery. Not only could variation in *CTLA-4* and *PTPN22* affect the function of T regulatory cells but variation in CD25 levels has also been associated with Graves' disease and type 1 diabetes. This leads to alterations in interleukin 2 binding (CD25 forms part of the interleukin 2 receptor), which is involved in the development of T regulatory cells and their ability to cause autoreactive T cells to undergo apoptosis. With evidence emerging for a role for foxp3 variation in autoimmune disease onset, taken together this suggests alterations in policing of peripheral T-cell autoreactivity could contribute to autoimmunity.

Variation in B-cell function

For many years it has been postulated that B cells are merely involved in initiating autoimmunity by producing antibodies, whereas T cells progress disease. Increases in our knowledge of B-cell function has identified additional roles in the immune system, including acting as APCs to CD4+ Th cells in low-antigen environments, controlling inflammation through cytokine production, being directly activated by Toll-like receptor ligands, such as bacterial DNA, independently of T cells and through the possible existence of B regulatory cells. A role for variation in molecules involved in B-cell signalling, such as B-cell activating factor and Fc receptor-like molecules, has been identified in disease, suggesting that the role of B cells in autoimmunity may be more complex than first envisaged.

Environmental impact on the immune system

It has been estimated that environmental factors make up >20% of the contribution to endocrine disease, and several of those identified, including viral and bacterial infection, increased hygiene, stress, smoking, and early intake of cow's milk, have been proposed to alter immune function (Table 1.5).

Manipulating our understanding of immune disruption to create improved therapeutics

Insights into the immune dysfunction behind autoimmune endocrine disease not only provides greater understanding of disease onset and progression but also identify immune pathways upon which therapeutic intervention could be undertaken. Whilst still in its infancy, breakthroughs in immune modulation of autoimmune disease pathways are starting to be reported and will undoubtedly in the future provide improved therapeutic options for these diseases.

Further reading

Bennett ST, Lucassen AM, Gough SC, et al. Susceptibility to human type 1 diabetes at IDDM2 is determined by tandem repeat variation at the insulin gene minisatellite locus. *Nat Genet* 1995; 9: 284–92.

Bottini N, Vang T, Cucca F, et al. Role of PTPN22 in type 1 diabetes and other autoimmune diseases. *Semin Immunol* 2006; 18: 207–13.

Chentoufi AA and Polychronakos C. Insulin expression levels in the thymus modulate insulin-specific autoreactive T-cell tolerance: The mechanism by which the IDDM2 locus may predispose to diabetes. *Diabetes* 2002; 51: 1383–90.

Gough SCL and Simmonds MJ. The HLA region and autoimmune disease: Associations and mechanisms of action. *Curr Genomics* 2007; 8: 453–65.

Gough SCL, Walker LS, and Sansom DM. CTLA4 gene polymorphism and autoimmunity. *Immunol Rev* 2005; 204: 102–15.

Lowe CE, Cooper JD, Brusko T, et al. Large-scale genetic fine mapping and genotype-phenotype associations implicate polymorphism in the IL2RA region in type 1 diabetes. *Nat Genet* 2007; 39: 1074–82.

Simmonds MJ. 'Evaluating the role of B cells in autoimmune disease: More than just initiators of disease?', in Berhardt LV, ed., *Advances in Medicine and Biology*, 2012. Nova Science Publishers, pp. 151–76.

Simmonds MJ and Gough SCL. 'Endocrine autoimmunity', in Wass JAH and Stewart PM, eds, *Oxford Textbook for Endocrinology and Diabetes* (2nd edition), 2011. Oxford Univerisity Press, pp. 34–44.

Simmonds MJ, Howson JM, Heward JM, et al. Regression mapping of association between the human leukocyte antigen region and Graves disease. *Am J Hum Genet* 2005; 76: 157–63.

Ueda H, Howson JM, Esposito L, et al. Association of the T-cell regulatory gene CTLA4 with susceptibility to autoimmune disease. *Nature* 2003; 423: 506–11.

1.6 Genetic endocrine disorders

Introduction

Most common endocrine diseases are caused by a combination of environmental and genetic factors, with genetic factors accounting for ~80% of the predisposition to disease. Due to the difficulties of accessing multiple, in some cases long-term, environmental impacts upon the endocrine system, greater progress has been made in identifying genetic variation at the heart of these disorders. In this section, we will detail the different techniques employed to detect genetic variation over the years, the limitations encountered, and how this has informed the design of current studies. Due to the genetics of type 2 diabetes being extensively reviewed elsewhere, this section will focus on the autoimmune endocrine diseases.

Linkage studies

Linkage studies involved using microsatellite markers, sequences of 2–6 base pairs of DNA repeated in tandem, located throughout the genome, within families with affected (those with the endocrine disease of interest) and unaffected members. The aim was to detect markers that occurred more frequently (co-segregated) in affected individuals and, once identified, employ a 'reverse genetics' approach to narrow down the association signal to a specific gene within the surrounding region.

Applying linkage studies to complex endocrine diseases
Linkage studies were first successfully employed in monogenic (single gene) disorders, identifying among others the role of *AIRE* in autoimmune polyendocrine syndrome type 1 (see Chapter 6, Section 6.13). Most common autoimmune endocrine diseases, including type 1 diabetes and Graves' disease, are complex diseases caused by multiple genetic effects. Linkage studies were also employed to identify the genetic components of complex endocrine diseases, although with limited success. Many signals that were detected failed to reach statistically significance levels, due in part to the small numbers of families screened. Of the positive linkage signals detected, many failed to be replicated between studies and, as for the remainder, due to sparse microsatellite coverage across the genome, it was difficult to narrow down the signal to a specific gene within the surrounding area, which could contain hundreds/thousands of genes. This lack of success of linkage studies in complex disease lead to those leading the field abandoning this approach.

Lessons learnt from linkage studies
The following lessons have been learnt from linkage studies:
- linkage studies were successful for monogenic disease but not complex disease
- for complex diseases, it is difficult to collect large numbers of family pedigrees, affecting the statistical power
- sparse microsatellite coverage throughout the genome made it difficult to narrow down associations to a specific gene

Case control studies

Case control studies involve the analysis of a group of 'cases' with the endocrine disease of interest and a group of matched 'controls'. The frequency of genetic variants (usually common single nucleotide polymorphisms (SNPs) with a minor allele frequency (MAF) >5%) which are thought likely to play a role in endocrine disease due to their known/assumed function are examined. If a specific SNP variant is increased in the cases compared to the controls, this suggests that this SNP variant, or another variant in close proximity, is involved in disease. Similarly if a SNP variant is increased in the controls compared to the cases, that SNP variant, or another in close proximity, is protective against disease onset.

Applying case control studies to complex endocrine disease
Case control studies first undertaken in the early 1970s detected the role of the HLA class II gene region (see Chapter 1, Section 1.5) in numerous autoimmune endocrine conditions. Effect sizes for this relationship, as measured by the odds ratio (OR), ranged from 2.00 to 3.50, making it possible to detect the association of this locus with disease in data sets containing as few as 100–200 cases and controls. Over the next 30 years, additional susceptibility loci were found for endocrine disorders (Table 1.6) via this approach. However, progress was slow, because (i) the ORs for these subsequent gene–disease associations were <1.50, requiring collection of larger data sets in order for these associations to be detected; (ii) many initial demonstrations of associations failed to be replicated in independent data sets; (iii) due to the limited knowledge of the genome, not all common variants within candidate genes were being screened; and (iv) genetic variants are not always inherited independently, as sets of nearby variants can be inherited together (known as linkage disequilibrium (LD)) making it difficult to determine if multiple associations in nearby genes were simply due to LD.

Publication of the first draft of the human genome and the HapMap project within the early 2000s provided a road map of all common variation within the genome and the LD between variants. This enabled the identification of sets of SNPs in LD with each other and the assignment of a single tag SNP which, when typed, could be used to infer the genotype at the other variants, reducing the number of variants required to screen the whole gene (Figure 1.6). Combined with the establishment of fluorescent-based genotyping, enabling faster, more accurate, assessment of gene variation, and the collection of data sets containing >1000 cases and controls, tag SNP case control studies identified numerous additional susceptibility loci for endocrine disease, including some previously 'excluded' by earlier case control studies (Table 1.6). The downside to this technique was that, for every gene detected, tens or hundreds of other genes screened showed no association with disease. With 20,000–25,000 genes within the human genome, selecting candidate genes purely on known/hypothesized gene function, with an inbuilt bias against genes with currently unknown function, was slowing down progress in identifying genetic contributors to endocrine disease.

Lessons learnt from case control studies
The following lessons were learnt from case control studies:
- initial case control studies had some success at detecting susceptibility loci for endocrine disease, with ORs > 1.50; including for example, the HLA region

Table 1.6 Details of the technique used to identify genetic-susceptibility loci for common endocrine disorders such as type 1 diabetes, Graves' disease, Hashimoto's thyroiditis, and Addison's disease

Technique employed to find genetic-susceptibility loci	Type 1 diabetes susceptibility gene/gene region			Graves' disease and Hashimoto's thyroiditis susceptibility gene/gene region		Addison's disease susceptibility gene/gene region
Initial case control studies	HLA region			HLA region		HLA region
	INS			CTLA-4		MICA
	CTLA-4			PTPN22		CTLA-4
	PTPN22					PTPN22
						CYP21
						CYP27B1
						VDR
						FCRL3
Tag SNP case control studies	IL2-RA			TSHR*		CLEC16A
	IFIH1			IL-2RA		NLRP1
						PDL1
Genome-wide association studies and the Immunochip study	1q32.1	IKZF1	CTSH	VAV3†	Tg	
	IL10	7p12.1	DEXI	MMEL1	FOXE1†	
	2p23.3	GLIS3	IL27	FCRL3	ABO	
	AFF3	RBM17/IL2RA	16q23.1	SLAMF6	11q21	
	2q13	PRKCQ	ORMDL3/GSD	TRIB2	PRICKLE1	
	IFIH1	NRP1	17q21.2	LPP	14q32.2	
	STAT4	10q23.31	17q21.31	GDCG4p14	ITGAM	
	CCR5	BAD	PTPN2	BACH2	GPR174-ITM2A	
	4p15.2	CD69	CD226	6q27	C1QTNF6-RAC2	
	4q27	ITGB7	TYK2			
	4q32.3	12q13.2	19q13.32			
	IL7R	CYP27B1	FUT2			
	BACH2	SH2B3	20p13			
	6p22.32	GPR183	UBASH3A			
	TNFIAP3	14q24.1	22q12.2			
	TAGAP	14q32.2	C1QTNF6/RAC2			
	6q27	DLK1	Xq28			
	7p15.2	RASGRP1				

Note: For type 1 diabetes, several genes were detected by initial case control studies and tag SNP case control studies. The onset of genome-wide association studies, however, led to the identification of numerous new gene/gene regions with >50 independent loci now known (see http://www.t1dbase.org for greater details about gene regions associated with type 1 diabetes). For Graves' disease, several genes were detected by initial case control studies and tag SNP case control studies, with additional genes detected by genome-wide association studies and additional follow-on studies such as the Immunochip (Cortes and Brown, 2011; Simmonds, 2013). For Addison's disease, due to the rarity of the condition, only case control studies and tag SNP studies have been undertaken to search for genetic-susceptibility loci (Mitchell and Pearce, 2012).

* Gene only associated with Graves' disease and not Hashimoto's thyroiditis.

† Genes only associated with Hashimoto's thyroiditis and not Graves' disease.

- tag SNP screening of all common variation within a specific gene region proved highly successful at identifying additional susceptibility loci
- as more genes were detected, effect sizes with ORs > 1.50 gave way to those with ORs < 1.30, necessitating the collection of larger data sets
- common autoimmune endocrine diseases are caused by a combination of shared genetic-susceptibility loci and disease-specific loci, such as the insulin gene in type 1 diabetes, and the TSH receptor gene in Graves' disease

Genome-wide association studies

Linkage and case control studies supported the idea that complex endocrine disease was due to a series of common variants, known as the common variant, common disease hypothesis, suggesting that screening all common variation in the genome would identify the majority of the genetic contribution to complex endocrine disease. Several advances within the early 2000s came together to enable genome-wide association screening (GWAS) to become a reality. Assigning tag SNPs across the genome showed that around 500,000

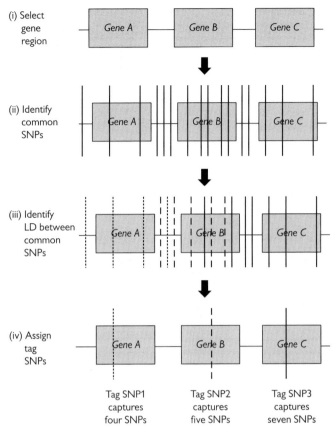

(i) Select gene region

Gene A   Gene B   Gene C

(ii) Identify common SNPs

Gene A   Gene B   Gene C

(iii) Identify LD between common SNPs

Gene A   Gene B   Gene C

(iv) Assign tag SNPs

Gene A   Gene B   Gene C

Tag SNP1 captures four SNPs

Tag SNP2 captures five SNPs

Tag SNP3 captures seven SNPs

Fig 1.6 Use of tag single nucleotide polymorphisms (SNPs) to screen all common variation within a given gene region: (i) select your gene region of interest; (ii) use HapMap to identify all common SNPs within the gene region of interest; (iii) identify the linkage disequilibrium (LD) between all SNPs; (iv) for each set of SNPs in LD, assign a single tag SNP which when typed can be used to infer genotype at all the other LD SNPs, thus reducing the amount of genotyping required to screen this region.

tag SNPs could be used to screen >80% of common variation within the genome (representing 3 million SNPs), including screening non-coding regions and gene 'deserts'. Generation of genotyping chip technology enabled screening of >500,000 SNPs within a timely and cost-effective manner, and the collection of large data sets and replication cohorts (<2000 cases and controls) provided the statistical power to detect genetic associations with ORs <1.30. Application of statistical rigour to avoid false positives (a low P-value association threshold <10^{-7} was applied), and the use of replication to confirm any new susceptibility loci detected, enabled GWAS to become a powerful tool for screening the genome.

Applying GWAS to complex disease
GWAS revolutionized the world of complex genetics by identifying numerous novel genetic associations for most common endocrine diseases (Table 1.6). In type 1 diabetes, pre-GWAS, five genes were known to play a role in disease; but, 3 years' post-GWAS, >40 susceptibility loci were known (with this figure increasing to >50 susceptibility loci currently and counting). Interestingly,

modelling the contribution of the >40 type 1 diabetes susceptibility loci to disease showed they still only accounted for 10% of the genetic contribution to disease, although other studies suggest that this percentage is likely to be higher. This has been mirrored in several other complex endocrine diseases, suggesting that the common variant, common disease hypothesis could not account for all the genetic contribution to complex disease and that other approaches will be required to find the remaining 'missing' genetic heritability.

Lessons learnt from GWAS
The following lessons were learnt from GWAS studies:
• GWAS studies did not find any novel gene associations which had ORs > 1.40 and which had not already been detected by case control studies
• many newly detected susceptibility genes/gene regions were located in poorly characterized or non-coding regions of the genome
• the common variant, common disease hypothesis could not account for all the genetic contribution to common endocrine diseases

Finding the 'missing' heritability

Several hypotheses are currently being investigated to explain where the 'missing' heritability for complex disease could be located; these include:

- low-frequency and rare variants
- copy number variants
- sharing of susceptibility loci
- trans-ethnic mapping
- fine mapping
- gene–gene interaction
- different disease subtypes
- additional influences on genetic susceptibility

Low-frequency and rare variants

Low-frequency (MAF = 1%–5%) and rare (MAF <1%) variants have been suggested to have large effects on complex disease, in a similar manner to that seen in monogenetic disease. The development of next-generation sequencing and establishment of the 1000 Genomes Project, set up to catalogue all genomic variation down to an MAF >1% whilst capturing numerous variants with MAF <1%, has enabled the assessment of low-frequency and rare variants in complex disease to become a reality. Studies in the common type 1 diabetes susceptibility locus *IFIHI* identified several independent rare protective variants, supporting a role for rare variants in complex disease. More recent dense re-sequencing of 20 known autoimmune disease susceptibility loci in 24,892 cases of autoimmune disease (including cases of type 1 diabetes and Graves' disease) did not detect any rare variant effects within these regions, suggesting that rare variants may not account for a significant proportion of the missing heritability.

Copy number variants

Large genomic variations such as inversions, deletions, and duplications exist throughout the genome and can substantially alter the functional copy number of a given gene/gene region within an individual. Screening of 3432 common copy number variants (CNVs) in 2000 cases from eight common complex diseases, including type 1 diabetes, and 3000 shared controls, revealed that the only CNV associated with type 1 diabetes was located within the HLA region and was shown to be in LD with previously detected common variants within the region. Although these initial data cast doubt over the role for CNVs in complex disease, the 3432 CNVs tested only represented 42%–50% of common CNVs within the genome, and no low-frequency or rare CNVs were screened, with work currently ongoing to further assess the role of CNVs in disease.

Sharing of susceptibility loci

Case control studies and GWAS studies highlighted the sharing of genetic susceptibility between related yet different endocrine diseases. As such, bespoke genotyping chips, such as the Immunochip, have been created to screen >180 gene regions previously associated with 12 autoimmune diseases, including type 1 diabetes and Graves' disease, providing hereto unimaginable information about the sharing of susceptibility loci, or lack thereof, between related diseases.

Trans-ethnic mapping

Genetic variation and LD patterns vary between different ethnic groups, and so studying them could provide an opportunity to detect additional susceptibilities in specific ethnic groupings. Whilst initially most genetic analysis of complex endocrine disease was undertaken in Caucasian populations, more recently GWAS data has been coming through from non-Caucasian populations, enabling additional susceptibility loci to be identified.

Fine mapping

Whilst we usually assign a susceptibility locus by the name of the gene in which it was detected, it is not until the whole region has been fine mapped that it is possible to state where the aetiological variant is located or, indeed, whether it resides within the gene in which it was originally identified.

Gene–gene interaction

Gene effects are looked at in isolation but the reality is that many susceptibility loci occur within the same or related pathways. Due to redundancy and compensation within key biological pathways, several small effect gene variants working together within a pathway could have a larger additive impact on disease susceptibility.

Different disease subtypes

For some endocrine diseases, numerous different clinical presentations can be encapsulated under the same name. In type 1 diabetes, for example, it is likely that there are numerous subtypes of disease triggered by different combinations of gene effects and environmental factors. Dissecting out the entire genetic architecture of a disease will help define different subtypes of disease and may ultimately help target specific therapeutic approaches.

Additional influences on genetic susceptibility

A series of other potential modifiers of genetic association include gene–environment interactions, genetic and regulatory element interactions within the genome, trans-generation genetic modifications inherited from previous generations, and parent of origin effects, whereby the genetic association can be modified depending on whether the gene responsible was inherited from the mother or the father. Assessing these types of variation presents its own unique challenges. Recently published information on regions of transcription, the location of transcription factors, chromatin structure, and histone modifications across the human genome are providing the tools to enable us to determine how variation within these regions can impact upon how different genes function and will undoubtedly provide further important insights into disease development.

Final take-home messages

This section concludes with the following take-home messages:

- linkage studies were successful for determining gene associations in monogenic diseases but not in complex diseases
- refinement of the case control approach and GWAS studies has identified numerous genetic-susceptibility loci for most complex endocrine diseases
- the hunt for the remaining 'missing' genetic heritability is now on and will provide further insights into disease pathogenesis

References and further reading

Barrett JC, Clayton DG, Concannon P, et al. Genome-wide association study and meta-analysis find that over 40 loci affect risk of type 1 diabetes. *Nat Genet* 2009; 41: 703–7.

Cooper JD, Simmonds MJ, Walker NM, et al. Seven newly identified loci for autoimmune thyroid disease. *Hum Mol Genet* 2012; 21: 5202–8.

Cortes A and Brown MA. Promise and pitfalls of the Immunochip. *Arthritis Res Ther* 2011; 13: 101.

Craddock N, Hurles ME, Cardin N, et al. Genome-wide association study of CNVs in 16,000 cases of eight common diseases and 3,000 shared controls. Nature 2010; 464: 713–720.

Eichler EE, Flint J, Gibson G, et al. Missing heritability and strategies for finding the underlying causes of complex disease. *Nat Rev Genet* 2010; 11: 446–50.

Gough SCL and Simmonds MJ. The HLA region and autoimmune disease: Associations and mechanisms of action. Curr Genomics 2007; 8: 453–65.

Hunt KA, Mistry V, Bockett NA, et al. Negligible impact of rare autoimmune-locus coding-region variants on missing heritability. *Nature* 2013; 498: 232–5.

Manolio TA, Collins FS, Cox NJ, et al. Finding the missing heritability of complex diseases. *Nature* 2009; 461: 747–53.

Mitchell AL and Pearce SH. Autoimmune Addison disease: Pathophysiology and genetic complexity. *Nat Rev Endocrinol* 2012; 8: 306–16.

Nejentsev S, Walker N, Riches D, et al. Rare variants of IFIH1, a gene implicated in antiviral responses, protect against type 1 diabetes. *Science* 2009; 324: 387–9.

Robertson CC and Rich SS. Genetics of Type 1 diabetes. *Curr Opin Genet Dev* 2018; 50: 7–16.

Simmonds MJ. GWAS in autoimmune thyroid disease: Redefining our understanding of pathogenesis. *Nat Rev Endocrinol* 2013; 9: 277–8.

1.7 Geographic and ethnic variation in endocrine disorders

Introduction

Marked variation can be seen in the prevalence and presentation of common endocrine and metabolic disorders across ethnic and geographic boundaries. Factors that influence variations in endocrine disorders include:

- genetic factors
- physical characteristics:
  - hip morphometry
  - skin pigmentation
- environmental factors:
  - iodine content
  - exposure to sunlight
  - pollution (e.g. chemical and radiation)
- the availability of screening tests for early detection

Thyroid disorders

Iodine deficiency and endemic goitre

Mountainous regions

Most mountainous areas in the world have been or still are endemic goitre regions. Iodine deficiency and endemic goitre may be seen in the Andes, Himalayas, Alps, Greece, Middle Eastern countries, the highlands of China, and Papua New Guinea. In mountainous regions, the soil has been leached of iodine over aeons by glacial formation and melting.

Non-mountainous regions

There are non-mountainous endemic regions, such as the central African region, central Europe, and parts of Brazil.

In these plains, iodine has been leached over time by recurrent flooding.

In most of the endemic regions, iodization programmes have been implemented and goitre is seen predominantly in the adult population (and not in children). However, pockets remain where the entire population is at risk.

Other goitrogenic factors

Although iodine deficiency is the main cause of endemic goitre, other factors may also be involved. These include:

- genetic predisposition in inbred communities
- dietary goitrogens (e.g. cyanogenic glucosides, thioglucosides, thiocyanate, and goitrin)
- autoimmune mechanisms

Iodine deficiency and endemic cretinism

In the most severely iodine-deficient environments (iodine intake <25 µg per day), endemic cretinism can occur (see Figure 1.7). It is seen in North India, Indonesia, China, Papua New Guinea, Zaire, and South America (Ecuador, Peru, Bolivia). Clinical features of endemic cretinism include:

- neurologic syndrome:
  - mental deficiency
  - deaf mutism
  - spastic diplegia
- stunting of growth
- hypothyroidism
- goitre (may or may not occur)

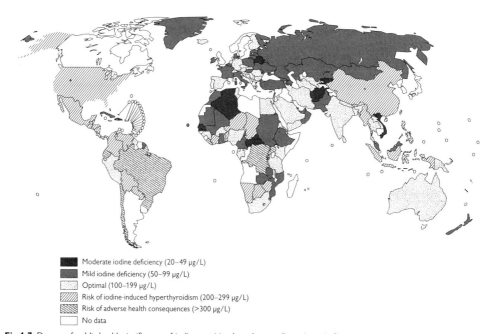

Moderate iodine deficiency (20–49 µg/L)
Mild iodine deficiency (50–99 µg/L)
Optimal (100–199 µg/L)
Risk of iodine-induced hyperthyroidism (200–299 µg/L)
Risk of adverse health consequences (>300 µg/L)
No data

Fig 1.7 Degree of public health significance of iodine nutrition based on median urinary iodine.
Reproduced with permission from De Benoist B, McLean E et al., Iodine deficiency in 2007: Global progress since 2003, *Food and Nutrition Bulletin*, Volume 29, Issue 3, pp. 195–201, Copyright © 2008, © SAGE Publications.

Impact of iodization programmes on health

Iodization has many benefits, and these benefits outweigh the risks. However, iodization of an iodine-deficient population has been shown to result in changes in the pattern of thyroid diseases (Slowinska-Klencka et al., 2002; Teng et al., 2006). These include an increase in the incidence of:

- iodine-induced hyperthyroidism
- chronic autoimmune thyroiditis
- an increase in the ratio of papillary to follicular thyroid carcinoma

Thyroid cancer

The annual incidence of thyroid cancer varies considerably and is highest in Iceland and Hawaii.

Disorders of bone metabolism

Hyperparathyroidism

In developed countries

In developed countries, primary hyperparathyroidism has become a common endocrine disorder. A four- to fivefold increase in the incidence of primary hyperparathyroidism has been observed since the introduction of the auto-analyser. Primary hyperparathyroidism is usually diagnosed in its preclinical stage.

In developing countries

In developing countries, primary hyperparathyroidism is usually diagnosed with florid manifestations, as routine testing is not available.

Paget's disease of bone

The striking feature of the epidemiology of Paget's disease is its great variability across countries and even within one country:

- the prevalence is relatively high in the populations of England, USA, Australia, New Zealand, Canada, South Africa, and France
- it is rare in Asia and Scandinavia
- even within the UK, a Lancashire focus is seen

Hip fracture rates

The incidence of hip fracture varies among populations, with a north–south gradient:

- the rates are higher in the north and highest in Scandinavia
- rates are markedly lower in the black and Asian races
- in Western populations, hip fracture incidence increased until around 1980; thereafter, the rates have reached a plateau or are decreasing (Cooper et al., 2011)
- in Asia, age-specific rates are increasing

Vitamin D deficiency

Vitamin D deficiency has emerged as a worldwide health problem. Severe vitamin D deficiency (defined as <25 nmol/L (<10 ng/mL)) appears to be most common in the Middle East and South Asia despite plenty of sunshine and favourable latitude. Skin pigmentation, sun avoidance behaviour, clothing patterns, and environmental pollution in the cities are some of the key factors that cause vitamin D deficiency. Despite an abundance of sunshine, the Middle East and Africa have the highest rates of rickets worldwide (Mithal et al., 2009).

Pituitary disease

In developing countries, pituitary and parasellar tumours tend to be diagnosed later than in the developed countries. The tumours tend to be larger at diagnosis.

Multiple endocrine neoplasia

Multiple endocrine neoplasia is mainly described in Caucasians and is very rare in Asians. It is not clear as to whether this is a true ethnic difference or is secondary to decreased case identification.

Diabetes and insulin resistance

The prevalence of both type 1 and type 2 diabetes varies dramatically across the globe. In addition, recently published data suggest that there may in fact be 5 subgroups of diabetes, but currently it is not clear as to how these vary geographically.

Type 1 diabetes

Worldwide patterns of incidence for type 1 diabetes

The worldwide patterns of incidence for type 1 diabetes are as follows (also see Figure 1.8):

- incidence rates are very high in the Scandinavian countries, such as Finland
- rates are very low in the Oriental populations, such as China and Japan
- Estonia has an incidence rate 25% that of Finland, despite their geographic proximity
- even within countries, variation in incidence across geographical areas can be observed

The vulnerability for developing type 1 diabetes occurs from an interaction between

- genetic factors (e.g. HLA on Chromosome 6) and
- environmental factors (e.g. viral infections or environmental and dietary toxins).

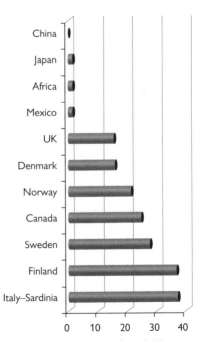

Fig 1.8 Age-standardized incidence of type 1 diabetes in children <14 years of age (per 100,000 per year).
Data from Karvonen M, Kajander MV et al. Incidence of Childhood Type 1 Diabetes Worldwide. *Diabetes Care*, 2000; Volume 23, pp. 1516–1526.

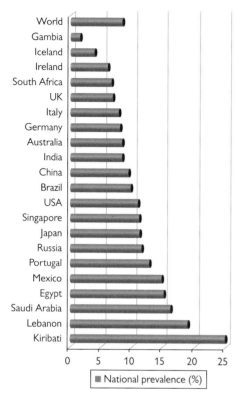

Fig 1.9 Prevalence (%) of type 2 diabetes in adults (20–79 years).
Data from *IDF Diabetes Atlas*, 5th edn. Brussels, Belgium: International Diabetes Federation, 2011. http://www.idf.org/diabetesatlas.

Type 2 diabetes
A dramatic rise in the prevalence of type 2 diabetes has been observed in the developing countries across the globe. The causes include:
- a rapid change in lifestyle, including:
  - an increase in calorie intake
  - a decrease in physical activity

- genetic predisposition: Asians develop more marked insulin resistance and have higher central adiposity, compared to the Caucasians of the same BMI

The prevalence of type 2 diabetes is as follows (also see Figure 1.9):
- many Pacific islands and Middle Eastern and Central American countries have prevalences in excess of 15%
- China, most parts of Asia, the USA, and South America have a prevalence of 9%–12%
- in Europe and Canada, the prevalence is 5%–8%
- in Africa, the prevalence is lower than 5%
- even in low-prevalence countries, the numbers are much higher in urban populations

Polycystic ovary disease
Polycystic ovary disease is much more common and more severe in the South Asians and Caribbean Hispanics than in Caucasians.

References and further reading

Ahlqvist E, Storm P, Käräjämäki A, et al. Novel subgroups of adult-onset diabetes and their association with outcomes: a data-driven cluster analysis of six variables. *Lancet Diabet* 2018; in press.

De Benoist B, McLean E, Andersson M, et al. Iodine deficiency in 2007: Global progress since 2003. *Food Nutri Bull* 2008; 29: 195–201.

Cooper C, Cole ZA, Holroyd CR, et al. Secular trends in hip and other osteoporotic fractures. *Osteoporos Int* 2011; 22: 1277–88.

International Diabetes Federation. IDF Diabetes Atlas (5th edition), 2015. Available at http://www.idf.org/diabetesatlas (accessed 3 Oct 2017).

Karvonen M, Kajander MV, Moltchanova E, et al. Incidence of childhood type 1 diabetes worldwide. *Diabetes Care* 2000; 23: 1516–26.

Mithal A, Wahl DA, Bonjour JP, et al. Global vitamin D status and determinants of hypovitaminosis D. *Osteoporos Int* 2009; 20: 1807–20.

Slowinska-Klencka D, Klencki M, Sporny, S, et al. Fine needle aspiration biopsy of the thyroid in an area of endemic goiter. *Eur J Endo* 2002; 146: 19–26.

Teng W, Shan Z, Teng, X, et al. Effect of iodine intake on thyroid disease in China. *N Engl J Med* 2006; 354: 2783–93.

Chapter 2

Thyroid hormone metabolism

Chapter contents

2.1 Physiology

Introduction

In healthy humans with a normal iodine intake, the thyroid follicular cells produce predominantly the prohormone T4, which is converted in peripheral tissues to the bioactive hormone T3 or the inactive metabolite 3,3′,5′-triiodothyronine (reverse T3 (rT3)). The bioavailability of thyroid hormone in target tissues depends to a large extent on the supply of plasma T4 and T3, the activity of transporters mediating the cellular uptake, and/ or the efflux of these hormones, as well as the activity of deiodinases which catalyse their activation or inactivation. Thyroid function is regulated most importantly by TSH, which is also called thyrotrophin. In turn, TSH secretion from the anterior pituitary is stimulated by the hypothalamic factor thyrotrophin-releasing hormone (TRH). TSH secretion is downregulated by the negative feedback action of thyroid hormone on the hypothalamus and the pituitary. The contribution of locally produced T3 versus plasma T3 is much greater for some tissues such as the brain and the pituitary than for other tissues. In this chapter, we briefly discuss (a) the neuroendocrine regulation of thyroid function, (b) the biosynthesis of thyroid hormone, (c) the activation and inactivation of thyroid hormone in peripheral tissues, and (d) the mechanism by which T3 exerts it biological activity. For further information on this topic, please see the *Oxford Textbook of Endocrinology* [1].

Regulation of thyroid function
TRH

A schematic overview of the hypothalamus–pituitary–thyroid axis is presented in Figure 2.1. TRH is a tripeptide with the structure pGlu-His-ProNH$_2$. Hypophysiotrophic TRH is produced in neurons located in the paraventricular nucleus of the hypothalamus. The biosynthesis

of TRH involves the production of a precursor protein (proTRH) containing six copies of the TRH progenitor sequence Gln-His-Pro-Gly. Following processing and transport to the median eminence, TRH is released into the portal vessels of the pituitary stalk. In the anterior lobe of the pituitary, TRH stimulates the production and secretion of TSH (and prolactin). TRH is rapidly degraded in blood and different tissues, in particular by a specific TRH-degrading ectoenzyme, TRH-DE, which catalyses the cleavage of the pGlu-His bond. TRH-DE activity is increased in hyperthyroidism and decreased in hypothyroidism and contributes to the negative feedback control of TSH secretion by thyroid hormone.

TRH effects are initiated by binding to a GPCR expressed on the thyrotroph (and the lactotroph). The human TRH receptor is a protein consisting of 398 amino acids, and binding of TRH induces activation of phospholipase C. which stimulates the generation of multiple intermediate factors, leading to the increased synthesis and secretion of TSH (and prolactin).

TSH

TSH is a glycoprotein produced by the thyrotrophic cells of the anterior pituitary. Like the other pituitary hormones LH and FSH, it is composed of two subunits. The alpha subunit is identical and the beta subunit is homologous among the three hormones. Although hormone specificity is conveyed by the beta subunit, dimerization with the alpha subunit is required for biological activity. Human TSH consists of 205 amino acids and three complex carbohydrate groups; the structures of the latter are important for the biological activity of TSH and depend on the stimulation of the thyrotroph by TRH.

The TSH receptor is a specific GPCR expressed on thyroid follicular cell, which in humans consists of 764 amino acids and an exceptionally long extracellular N-terminal domain. Binding of TSH to its receptor results in the activation of adenylate cyclase and thus stimulates production of the second messenger cAMP and, consequently, an increase in thyroid activity. In particular, the expression of key genes for thyroid hormone production is increased through mechanisms which also involve the thyroid-specific transcription factors TTF1/NKX2.1, TTF2/FOXE1, and PAX8. Stimulation of the TSH receptor with high TSH concentrations also results in the activation of the phospholipase C pathway, which is also involved in the regulation of thyroid function and growth.

Biosynthesis of thyroid hormone

The functional unit of the thyroid gland is the follicle, which is composed of a single layer of epithelial cells surrounding a colloidal lumen where thyroid hormone synthesis and storage take place. The biosynthesis of thyroid hormone comprises the following steps, which are depicted schematically in Figure 2.2:

- uptake of iodide at the basolateral membrane through the Na/I symporter, which is a glycoprotein containing 13 transmembrane domains and transports iodide and sodium ions in a stoichiometry of 1:2
- export of iodide at the apical membrane through (among others) pendrin, a transporter mutated in patients with Pendred syndrome, which is characterized by deafness, due to a cochlear defect, and

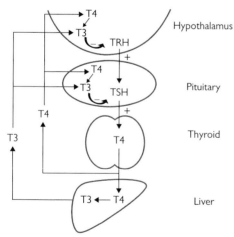

Fig 2.1 Schematic overview of the regulation of the production and metabolism of thyroid hormone in the hypothalamus-pituitary-thyroid-periphery axis, showing the liver as a major triiodothyronine-producing tissue; T3, triiodothyronine; T4, thyroxine; TRH, thyroid-releasing hormone; TSH, thyroid-stimulating hormone.

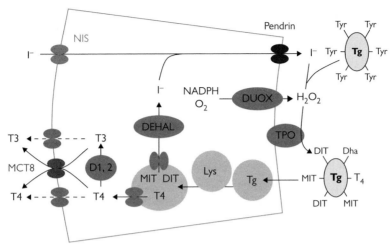

Fig 2.2 Schematic presentation of a thyroid follicular cell and important steps in the synthesis of thyroid hormone; D1, type 1 deiodinase; D2, type 2 deiodinase; DEHAL, iodotyrosine dehalogenase; DIT, diiodotyrosine; DUOX2, dual oxidase; H_2O_2, hydrogen peroxide; I^-, iodide ion; Lys, lysine; MIT, monoiodotyrosine; NADPH, nicotinamide adenine dinucleotide phosphate; NIS, sodium-iodide symporter; O_2, oxygen; T3, triiodothyronine; T4, thyroxine; Tg, thyroglobulin; TPO, thyroid peroxidase; Tyr, tyrosine.

hypothyroidism, due to a thyroid hormone synthesis defect; pendrin is capable of transporting bicarbonate, chloride, and iodide.

- clustering of thyroglobulin, the dual oxidase DUOX2, and thyroid peroxidase in a 'thyroxisome' at the luminal surface of the apical membrane:
  - thyroglobulin is an exceptionally large glycoprotein consisting of two identical subunits with a molecular weight each of ~330 kDa
  - DUOX2 is a complex glycoprotein embedded in the apical membrane and contains multiple functional domains; functional expression of DUOX2 requires the presence of the maturation factor DUOXA2
  - thyroid peroxidase is a glycoprotein featuring a single transmembrane domain; the larger part of thyroid peroxidase is exposed on the luminal surface of the apical membrane and contains a haem-binding domain, which is the active centre of the enzyme
- generation of H_2O_2 by DUOX2, involving the oxidation of NADPH from the cytoplasm and the delivery of the product H_2O_2 to the luminal surface of the apical membrane
- H_2O_2-dependent iodination of tyrosine residues in thyroglobulin by thyroid peroxidase; this involves the two-electron oxidation of I^- to I^+ which is incorporated into susceptible Tyr residues, with the formation initially of monoiodotyrosine and subsequently of diiodotyrosine
- H_2O_2-dependent coupling of iodotyrosine to iodothyronine residues in thyroglobulin by thyroid peroxidase, probably involving the single-electron oxidation of both donor and acceptor iodotyrosine residues, generating radicals that rapidly combine to produce iodothyronine residues:

- coupling two diiodotyrosines results in the formation of T4 (the major product)
- coupling a monoiodotyrosine with a diiodotyrosine yields T3 (the minor product)
- at this stage, T4 and T3 are still integral parts of thyroglobulin
- endocytosis and proteolysis of thyroglobulin:
  - after modification by thyroid peroxidase, thyroglobulin is resorbed from the lumen by receptor-mediated endocytosis
  - subsequently, the endosomes fuse with lysosomes, generating so-called phagolysosomes, in which thyroglobulin is hydrolysed by lysosomal proteases, resulting in the liberation of T4, a small amount of T3, as well as excess monoiodotyrosine and diiodotyrosine
- release of iodotyrosines and iodothyronines (predominantly T4) from vesicles through unidentified transporter(s)
- deiodination of monoiodotyrosine and diiodotyrosine by iodotyrosine dehalogenase, which is located in the endoplasmic reticulum and uses NADH as a cofactor; the iodide released is reutilized for the iodination of thyroglobulin
- partial deiodination of T4 to T3 by type 1 and type 2 iodothyronine deiodinases expressed in the thyroid
- secretion of T4 (and T3) in particular through the thyroid hormone transporter MCT8; the involvement of MCT8 in thyroid hormone secretion has been demonstrated recently in studies of Mct8 knockout mice [2, 3].

On average, T4 and T3 are secreted in a ratio of about 15:1, that is, about 100 μg (130 nmol) T4 and 6 μg (9 nmol) T3 per day. The latter represents ≈20% of daily total T3 production. Hence, most T3 is produced by the deiodination of T4 in peripheral tissues.

Table 2.1 Characteristics of T4-binding proteins in human plasma

Protein	Concentration in plasma		Dissociation constant (K_d)	T4 distribution
	(mg/L)	(µmol/L)	(mol/L)	(%)
TBG	≈15	≈0.3	≈10^{-10}	75
TTR	≈250	≈5	10^{-8}	10
Albumin	≈40,000	≈600	10^{-6}–10^{-5}	15

Abbreviations: TBG, T4-binding globulin; TTR, transthyretin.

Transport of thyroid hormone

Plasma transport

In plasma, thyroid hormone is bound to three proteins: TBG, transthyretin, and albumin, which are all produced by the liver (Table 2.1). Human TBG is a 54 kDa glycoprotein with a single iodothyronine-binding site, encoded by a gene located on the X chromosome. Transthyretin is composed of four identical subunits, consisting each of 127 amino acids. It has a cigar-shaped structure with two identical binding channels, with ligand entry sites at opposite ends of the transthyretin molecule. Transthyretin also binds retinol-binding protein and thus also plays an important role in vitamin A transport. Albumin has multiple low-affinity binding sites for thyroid hormone.

The affinity of the binding proteins for T4 decreases in the order TBG > transthyretin > albumin, and their plasma concentration decreases in the opposite order: albumin > transthyretin > TBG. As a result, ~75% of plasma T4 is bound to TBG, ~15% to albumin, and ~10% to transthyretin. The total binding capacity is so high that only ~0.02% of plasma T4 is free. The affinity of T3 for the different proteins is roughly tenfold lower, so that ~0.2% of plasma T3 is free. Thus, whilst the mean normal plasma total T4 (~100 nmol/L; ~8 µg/dL) and T3 (~2 nmol/L; ~130 ng/dL) levels differ ~50-fold, the difference in mean normal FT4 (~20 pmol/L; ~1.5 ng/dL) and FT3 (~5 pmol/L; ~0.3 ng/dL) concentrations is only ~4-fold.

Perturbation of plasma iodothyronine binding provokes an adaptation of the hypothalamus–pituitary–thyroid axis until normal FT4 and FT3 concentrations are again obtained. Therefore, measurement of plasma FT4 rather than total T4 levels is, together with analysis of plasma TSH, the cornerstone of the diagnosis of thyroid disorders.

Tissue transport

Thyroid hormone metabolism and action are intracellular processes which require cellular uptake of iodothyronines across the plasma membrane (Figure 2.3). It has now been established that tissue thyroid hormone uptake does not take place by diffusion but is mediated by specific plasma membrane transporters. A number of thyroid hormone transporters have been identified at the molecular level. These include NTCP, different members of the OATP family, the L-type amino acid transporters, and members of the MCT family. Probably the most important of these for thyroid hormone homeostasis are OATP1C1, MCT8, and MCT10. OATP1C1 shows a high preference for T4 as the ligand, and almost exclusive expression in the brain, especially in the choroid plexus and

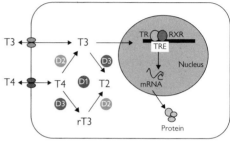

Fig 2.3 Importance of transporters and deiodinases in the regulation of intracellular triiodothyronine levels in a thyroid hormone target cell; D1, type 1 iodothyronine; D2, type 2 iodothyronine; D3 type 3 iodothyronine; rT3, reverse T3; RXR, retinoid X receptor; T2, diiodothyronine; T3, triiodothyronine; T4, thyroxine; TR, T3 receptor; TRE, T3 response element.

in astrocytes, where it makes T4 available for conversion to T3.

MCT8 and MCT10 are the most effective thyroid hormone transporters known to date. Of these, MCT10 also transports aromatic amino acids, but so far only iodothyronines have been identified as substrates for MCT8. MCT8 and MCT10 are homologous, nonglycosylated proteins containing 12 transmembrane domains, which are encoded by genes located on the X chromosome and Chromosome 6. MCT8 and MCT10 show wide but distinct tissue distributions. Among others, MCT8 is importantly expressed in brain, where it is localized in the choroid plexus, the capillaries, and neurons in different brain areas. MCT8 is essential for thyroid hormone transport in the CNS and is thus crucial for thyroid hormone action during brain development. Hemizygous mutations in MCT8 in males result in the Allan–Herndon–Dudley syndrome, which is characterized by severe psychomotor retardation in combination with low T4 and high T3 levels. These thyroid hormone alterations are explained at least in part by impaired thyroidal T4 secretion and increased T4 to T3 conversion in the thyroid, liver, and kidney [2–4].

Metabolism of thyroid hormone

A small amount of T3 is secreted by the thyroid but most circulating T3 is produced by enzymatic outer ring deiodination of T4 in peripheral tissues. Alternatively, inner ring deiodination of T4 produces the inactive metabolite rT3, thyroidal secretion of which is negligible. T3 and rT3 are also further metabolized largely by deiodination. T3 undergoes inner ring deiodination to

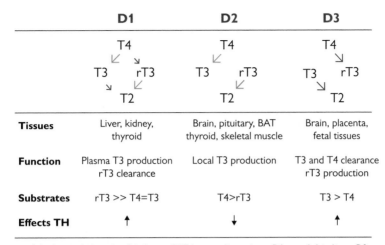

	D1	**D2**	**D3**
Tissues	Liver, kidney, thyroid	Brain, pituitary, BAT thyroid, skeletal muscle	Brain, placenta, fetal tissues
Function	Plasma T3 production rT3 clearance	Local T3 production	T3 and T4 clearance rT3 production
Substrates	rT3 >> T4=T3	T4>rT3	T3 > T4
Effects TH	↑	↓	↑

Fig 2.4 Properties of the three iodothyronine deiodinases; BAT, brown adipose tissue; D1, type 1 deiodinase; D2, type 2 deiodinase; D3 type 3 deiodinase; rT3, reverse T3; T2, diiodothyronine; T3, triiodothyronine; T4, thyroxine; TH, thyroid hormone.

the inactive compound 3,3′-diiodothyronine, which is also produced by outer ring deiodination of rT3. Thus, the bioactivity of thyroid hormone is importantly determined by enzyme activities catalysing the outer ring deiodination (activation) or inner ring deiodination (inactivation) of iodothyronines.

Three iodothyronine deiodinases, deiodinases 1–3, are involved in the reductive deiodination of thyroid hormone (Figure 2.4). They are homologous proteins consisting of 249–278 amino acids, with a single transmembrane domain located at the N terminus. The deiodinases are inserted in cellular membranes, with their active centre exposed on the cytoplasmic surface, providing the reductive environment required for deiodination. The most remarkable feature of all three deiodinases is the presence of a selenocysteine residue in the active centre of these enzymes.

D1 is a membrane-bound enzyme expressed predominantly in the liver, the kidneys, and the thyroid. It catalyses the outer ring deiodination and/or the inner ring deiodination of a variety of iodothyronine derivatives, although it is most effective in the outer ring deiodination of rT3. Hepatic D1 is probably a major site for the production of plasma T3 and clearance of plasma rT3. D1 activity in the liver and the kidneys is increased in hyperthyroidism and decreased in hypothyroidism, representing the regulation of D1 activity by T3 at the transcriptional level.

D2 is expressed primarily in the brain, the anterior pituitary, brown adipose tissue, thyroid, and, to some extent, in skeletal muscle. In the brain, D2 has been localized predominantly in astrocytes. D2 has only outer ring deiodination activity, with a preference for T4 over rT3 as the substrate. The amount of T3 in the brain, the pituitary, and brown adipose tissue is derived to a large extent from the local conversion of T4 by D2. The enzyme, which is located in the anterior pituitary and the hypothalamus, is essential for the negative feedback of T4 on TSH and TRH secretion. In general, D2 activity is increased in hypothyroidism and decreased in hyperthyroidism. This is explained in part by substrate (T4, rT3)-induced inactivation of D2 by the ubiquitin–proteasome system. D2 polymorphisms are common, and some have suggested that genotyping may explain differences in patient responsiveness.

D3 activity has been detected in different human tissues such as the brain, the skin, the liver, and the intestine, where activities are much higher in the fetal stage than in the adult stage. D3 is also abundantly expressed in the placenta and the pregnant uterus. D3 has only inner ring deiodination activity, catalysing the inactivation of T4 and T3. D3 in tissues such as the brain is thought to play a role in the regulation of intracellular T3 levels, whilst its presence in the placenta, the pregnant uterus, and fetal tissues may serve to protect developing organs against undue exposure to active thyroid hormone. Also in adults, D3 is an important site for clearance of plasma T3 and production of plasma rT3. In the brain, but not in the placenta, D3 expression is increased in hyperthyroidism and decreased in hypothyroidism.

Patients have not been identified with disorders caused by mutations in deiodinases. However, a multisystem disorder has been described which is caused by mutations in SBP2, a protein required for the synthesis of selenoproteins, and thus also for deiodinases. Among others, these patients show impaired T4 to T3 conversion and disturbed feedback regulation of TSH by T4 [5, 6].

Other, minor pathways of thyroid hormone metabolism include side-chain modification to iodothyronamine and iodothyroacetic acid derivatives, and conjugation of the phenolic hydroxyl group with glucuronic acid or sulphate. These metabolic pathways are described in more detail elsewhere [1].

Thyroid hormone action

Thyroid hormone is essential for the development of different tissues, in particular the brain, and for the regulation of energy expenditure and thermogenesis throughout life. Most actions of thyroid hormone are initiated by binding of T3 to nuclear receptors, which belong to the superfamily of ligand-dependent transcription factors. T3 receptors are encoded by two genes: *THRA*, which is located on chromosome 17, and *THRB*, which is located on chromosome 3; these give rise to different receptor isoforms, in particular TRα1, TRα2, TRβ1, and TRβ2. Through alternative splicing, TRα2 has lost part of the ligand-binding domain and is unable to bind T3. The receptor isoforms show distinct tissue distributions. TRα1 is the predominant receptor expressed in brain, heart, and bone, whereas TRβ1 is the major receptor in other tissues, including the liver, skeletal muscle, the kidneys, and fat. TRβ2 is expressed especially in the anterior pituitary and the hypothalamus, where it is involved in the feedback inhibition of TSH and TRH secretion by thyroid hormone.

Regulation of the expression of T3-responsive genes involves the binding of these receptors, usually as a heterodimer with the retinoid X receptor, to so-called T3 response elements in the promoter region of these genes. T3 response elements usually consist of two half-sites with the 'consensus' sequence AGGTCA arranged as repeats or palindromes. Binding of T3 to its receptor results in a change in the interaction with cofactors, leading to the altered expression of thyroid hormone-responsive genes. A large number of patients have been reported with thyroid hormone resistance due to mutations in *THRB*; this is associated, among other effects, with impaired negative feedback regulation of TSH secretion, and hence with a combination of elevated thyroid hormone and non-suppressed TSH levels. Only recently, the first patients have been described with thyroid hormone resistance due to mutations in *THRA*. They show marked growth retardation, delayed bone development, mildly abnormal motor and mental development, and constipation [7, 8]. These different clinical phenotypes reflect the different tissue expression pattern of the T3 receptors.

References and further reading

1. Visser TJ. 'Biosynthesis, transport, metabolism, and actions of thyroid hormone' in Wass JAH, ed., *Oxford Textbook of Endocrinology and Metabolism*, 2010. Oxford University Press, pp. 309–23.
2. Trajkovic-Arsic M, Müller J, Darras VM, et al. Impact of monocarboxylate transporter-8 deficiency on the hypothalamus-pituitary-thyroid axis in mice. *Endocrinology* 2010; 151: 5053–62.
3. Di Cosmo C, Liao XH, Dumitrescu AM, et al. Mice deficient in MCT8 reveal a mechanism regulating thyroid hormone secretion. *J Clin Invest* 2010; 120: 3377–88.
4. Trajkovic-Arsic M, Visser TJ, Darras VM, et al. Consequences of monocarboxylate transporter 8 deficiency for renal transport and metabolism of thyroid hormones in mice. *Endocrinology* 2010; 151: 802–9.
5. Dumitrescu AM, Liao XH, Abdullah MS, et al. Mutations in SECISBP2 result in abnormal thyroid hormone metabolism. *Nat Genet* 2005; 37: 1247–52.
6. Schoenmakers E, Agostini M, Mitchell C, et al. Mutations in the selenocysteine insertion sequence-binding protein 2 gene lead to a multisystem selenoprotein deficiency disorder in humans. *J Clin Invest* 2010; 120: 4220–35.
7. Bochukova E, Schoenmakers N, Agostini M, et al. A mutation in the thyroid hormone receptor alpha gene. *N Engl J Med* 2012; 366: 243–9.
8. Van Mullem A, van Heerebeek R, Chrysis D, et al. Clinical phenotype and mutant TRα1. *N Engl J Med* 2012; 366: 1451–3.

2.2 Thyroid investigations

Biochemical investigations

Thyroid function testing

The hormones of the hypothalamic–pituitary–thyroid axis that are commonly measured for diagnostic purposes include serum TSH, FT4, and FT3. Assays of total serum thyroid hormone concentration have been largely superseded because their interpretation is significantly confounded by circulating levels of thyroid hormone-binding proteins.

The first step in the investigation of suspected thyroid disease is to establish the level of serum TSH. Measurement of serum TSH alone has high utility as a screening tool because the finding of a normal TSH effectively excludes a primary thyroid problem. On the whole, an elevated serum TSH (>5.0 mU/L) indicates hypothyroidism, while TSH suppression (<0.1 mU/L) is consistent with hyperthyroidism. However, in a number of clinical conditions, particularly in the case of pituitary disease, measurement of TSH alone can be misleading (Box 2.1).

Biochemically, the hallmark of primary hypothyroidism is an elevated serum TSH. In symptomatic, overt hypothyroidism, FT4 is frequently below the lower limit of the laboratory reference range. However, FT3 may be normal, even in quite profound hypothyroidism. A state of subclinical hypothyroidism is defined by an elevation in serum TSH (generally between 5.0–10.0 mU/L) associated with normal FT4 and FT3 levels. With this pattern of tests, a repeat TSH measurement can be normal in as many as 50% of cases. Furthermore, people with subclinical hypothyroidism are frequently asymptomatic, or have only very mild or equivocal symptoms attributable to hypothyroidism. Nevertheless, there are other rarer causes of an elevated serum TSH. One rare but important cause is a TSH-secreting adenoma of the pituitary (TSH-oma) which causes secondary hyperthyroidism where the TSH is elevated or at the upper end of the laboratory reference range, with elevated FT4 and FT3 levels. In addition, an elevated TSH, or a TSH level that is inappropriately normal in the context of elevated FT4 and FT3 levels, is found in thyroid hormone resistance.

During prolonged primary hyperthyroidism, there is functional atrophy of the pituitary thyrotroph cells, leading to an enduring suppression of serum TSH. However, while a suppressed serum TSH (<0.1 mU/L) is the hallmark of hyperthyroidism, a low or suppressed TSH may also be observed in a number of other circumstances. Thus, in overt primary hyperthyroidism, the TSH is suppressed, with an elevation of serum FT3 and FT4. A less severe state of hyperthyroidism, known as T3 thyrotoxicosis, is also defined by a suppressed TSH with elevation of serum FT3 but normal FT4. Subclinical hyperthyroidism is present when the serum TSH is below the reference range (<0.4 mU/L), but there is normal serum FT4 and FT3. Patients with subclinical hyperthyroidism are rarely symptomatic, and this pattern of tests may also be found as a consequence of several different drugs (e.g. opiates, steroids, overtreatment with levothyroxine) as well as in non-thyroidal illness. A similar pattern, with suppressed TSH, high FT4, but often normal FT3 is also observed in *thyrotoxicosis factitia* (levothyroxine abuse). During treatment of hyperthyroidism with anti-thyroid drugs, or in the immediate aftermath of radioiodine therapy, serum TSH can remain suppressed for several months following normalization of the serum thyroid hormone levels, while pituitary thyrotroph function recovers. Low TSH levels may also be seen in pituitary disease (secondary hypothyroidism), where the low TSH is typically accompanied by low FT4 levels. Non-thyroidal illness (sick-euthyroid syndrome) frequently causes low TSH levels, classically associated with low serum FT3 and, if severe or prolonged, a low serum FT4. In the recovery phase, there may be a transient rise in serum TSH.

A suppressed serum TSH is found in about 10% of healthy pregnancies, during the first trimester. This is due to increased circulating levels of hCG, which shares a common alpha subunit with TSH and therefore can weakly stimulate the TSH receptor. Pregnancy-specific reference ranges for TSH should therefore be adopted (<2.5 mU/L in the first trimester; 0.1–3.0 mU/L thereafter).

Using the common screening approach of measuring TSH alone, the finding of an abnormal TSH always needs to be followed up by measuring circulating thyroid hormone levels. In the case of high TSH, the FT4 should be measured; FT3 is unhelpful in the diagnosis of primary hypothyroidism. In the case of a low TSH, the serum FT3 is the next most sensitive test for thyrotoxicosis. In all circumstances, the clinical picture should be considered when interpreting thyroid function tests (TFTs) as an assay artefact can result in spurious results. A one-off test result which is not in keeping with the clinical picture should be repeated. A summary of common TFT patterns is shown in Box 2.1

Box 2.1 Common patterns of thyroid function tests

Primary hypothyroidism: TSH ↑ FT4 ↓ FT3 ↓/ ↔ clinically hypothyroid
Primary hyperthyroidism: TSH ↓ FT3 ↑ FT4 ↑ clinically hyperthyroid
Secondary hypothyroidism, e.g. pituitary disease: TSH ↓/ ↔ FT4 ↓ FT3 ↓/ ↔ clinically hypothyroid
Secondary hyperthyroidism, e.g. TSH-oma: TSH ↑/ ↔ FT4 ↑ FT3 ↑ clinically hyperthyroid
T3 thyrotoxicosis: TSH ↓ FT4 ↔ FT3 ↑ clinically hyperthyroid
Subclinical hypothyroidism: TSH ↑ FT4 ↔ FT3 ↔ euthyroid/mild hypothyroid symptoms
Subclinical hyperthyroidism: TSH ↓ FT4 ↔ FT3 ↔ euthyroid/mild hyperthyroid symptoms
Thyroid hormone resistance: TSH ↑/↔ FT4 ↑ FT3 ↑ clinically variable

Laboratory reference ranges

It is important to remember that 'laboratory reference ranges' represent the 95% prediction interval of measurements from healthy individuals within a population. Therefore, there is a 2.5% chance that a sample will have a value which is less than the lower reference limit, and a 2.5% chance that a sample will have a value greater than the upper reference limit, simply by chance. 'Healthy person' reference ranges actually do vary with factors such as age, gender, and ethnicity. It is particularly important to interpret TFTs with caution in the very young, the very elderly, and pregnant women.

When healthy elderly individuals are studied, a proportion will have TFT results that fall outside of the quoted reference range. This suggests that there are physiological changes which occur within the hypothalamic–pituitary–thyroid axis with increasing age. Treating these healthy elderly individuals on the basis of reference ranges constructed from the data of young adults is counterintuitive and may indeed be counterproductive. For example, in several studies, it has been shown that the upper limit of the reference range for TSH in healthy older people is about 7.0 mU/L. Interestingly, a TSH above the normal 'younger person's' reference range has been associated with a survival benefit in older people. At present, age-specific references ranges for the elderly are not applied and therefore TFTs from this group should be interpreted with caution, and the clinical status of each patient carefully considered. In neonates, infants, and children, age-specific reference ranges are often quoted by laboratories, facilitating interpretation.

Technical problems with assays

See also Chapter 1, Section 1.2. Rarely, spontaneously occurring natural antibodies (termed heterophilic antibodies) can interfere with commonly used immunoassay reagents, which rely on the binding of a diagnostic antibody to the substrate of interest. This phenomenon most frequently affects assays for FT4 and FT3, resulting in either spuriously high or spuriously low results. This leads to a puzzling picture for the clinician to interpret. Thus, it is imperative that TFT results should always be viewed in light of the clinical picture, and the onus is on clinicians to be aware of the possibility of assay artefact and to be suspicious of TFT results that are not consistent with the clinical scenario. In this case, discussion with the laboratory can be extremely helpful to determine if a problem has arisen which can be resolved. Other human error problems include specimen mislabelling, or misassigning results. In all cases, puzzling TFTs should be repeated for verification. In some cases, if the result remains counterintuitive, it is necessary to use an independent assay to verify the result, or remeasure using a method incorporating equilibrium dialysis.

Thyroid autoantibodies

Autoimmune thyroid disease is the commonest cause of thyroid dysfunction. Circulating autoantibodies to thyroid peroxidase and the TSH receptor are the immunological hallmarks of autoimmune hypothyroidism and Graves' disease, respectively (see also Chapter 1, Section 1.3). Between 5% and 15% of euthyroid women, and approximately 2% of euthyroid men, have positive thyroid autoantibodies, increasing in an age-related fashion. Longitudinal studies have demonstrated that euthyroid individuals positive for thyroid-peroxidase autoantibodies are at increased risk of developing overt thyroid disease in the future.

Thyroid peroxidase autoantibodies

Almost all patients with autoimmune hypothyroidism, and approximately 90% of those with Graves' disease, have autoantibodies against the thyroid peroxidase enzyme, which is a membrane-bound haem-containing protein responsible for the iodination of tyrosine residues on thyroglobulin. Thyroid peroxidase antibodies are generally of IgG subclass 1, 2, or 4 and are directed against two regions of the thyroid peroxidase molecule: the myeloperoxidase-like and the complement control protein-like domains. In vitro, thyroid peroxidase antibodies can fix complement and target thyrocytes for cell-mediated cytotoxicity. Indeed, thyroid peroxidase autoantibodies have been detected in thyroid follicles of individuals with autoimmune hypothyroidism, suggesting that these antibodies might have a direct pathogenic role in the condition. However, they do not appear to inhibit thyroid peroxidase enzyme activity directly. Similarly, studies of the Rag 1-deficient mouse (which has no mature B cells and is therefore unable to produce autoantibodies), which develops spontaneous hypothyroidism with histological changes of thyroiditis, suggests that thyroid peroxidase antibodies are not necessary per se for disease development. In addition, thyroid peroxidase antibodies are commonly detected in 'healthy' individuals with no apparent signs of thyroid disease.

TSH receptor autoantibodies

More than 95% of patients with Graves' disease have detectable circulating TSH receptor autoantibodies. TSH receptor autoantibodies are classically IgG1 subclass and they typically circulate in concentrations 1000-fold lower than that of thyroid peroxidase antibodies. They target an epitope in the N-terminal region of the leucine-rich repeat motif in the extracellular domain of the TSH receptor. Autoantibody binding to the TSH receptor triggers the cAMP and phospholipase-C pathways: a cascade of intracellular events that finally leads to thyrocyte hyperplasia and increased thyroid hormone synthesis. TSH receptor autoantibodies, in addition to being stimulating, can also be 'blocking' in nature, preventing receptor activation, which can result in hypothyroidism. A mixture of blocking and stimulating antibodies may be present in a single person, and this can result in fluctuating thyroid status. TSH receptor antibodies are highly sensitive for Graves' disease but they are not commonly measured directly. Instead, the TSH-binding inhibitory immunoglobulin is commonly measured as an indirect measure of TSH-stimulating antibodies.

Other autoantibodies

Antibodies directed against thyroglobulin, a large glycoprotein which is the scaffold molecule that is iodinated to form the precursors of thyroid hormones, are also observed in autoimmune thyroid disease. They are found in up to half of individuals with Graves' disease and in approximately 60% of individuals with autoimmune hypothyroidism. However, they are rarely seen without thyroid peroxidase antibodies and therefore they are not measured in routine practice. Nevertheless, in differentiated thyroid cancer patients, endogenous anti-thyroglobulin antibodies can interfere with measurement of serum thyroglobulin, which is used as a tumour marker post thyroidectomy. In a small numbers of patients

(20%–40% of those with autoimmune hypothyroidism), antibodies to the sodium iodide symporter and the apical iodide transporter, pendrin, have also been reported but these are not measured routinely.

Genetic investigations

Several thyroid disorders have strong genetic contributions to their pathogenesis (see also Chapter 1, Section 1.6). Moreover, levels of serum thyroid hormones and TSH within the healthy reference range are also determined to a significant extent by genetic variants. Those clinical disorders that are directly genetic can be divided into conditions that are monogenic, those which arise as a result of chromosomal abnormalities, and those which are thought to be complex traits, resulting from the interaction of multiple genetic variants with environmental factors.

Monogenic thyroid disorders

Monogenic conditions are typically inherited in a strict Mendelian fashion. Monogenic disorders of the thyroid most commonly manifest shortly after birth or in early childhood as congenital hypothyroidism and this is the rationale for national screening programmes, which consist, in the UK, of a single capillary blood TSH measurement between the fifth and eighth days of life.

Congenital hypothyroidism can be divided into disorders of dyshormonogenesis, and disorders of thyroid ontogeny and migration. These conditions are frequently autosomal recessive and may be associated with other extra-thyroidal abnormalities such as cleft lip and palate, sensorineural deafness, and musculoskeletal abnormalities. Monogenic thyroid disorders may be subclassified according to the level at which the defect arises within the hypothalamic–pituitary–thyroid axis, as shown in Table 2.2.

Thyroid hormone resistance

See also Chapter 16, Section 16.1. Until recently, thyroid hormone resistance was thought to be solely due to mutations arising in the gene that encodes the beta subunit of the nuclear thyroid hormone receptor TRB. These mutations result in an autosomal dominant disorder characterized by elevated FT4 and FT3 levels in the context of a normal or elevated serum TSH; this is termed 'thyroid hormone resistance'. Clinically, these patients are euthyroid but may have a goitre, a mild reduction in IQ, tachycardia, and delayed skeletal maturation. In these individuals, hypothyroidism due to an unresponsive TRB is partially overcome by higher levels of circulating thyroid hormones. In approximately one-fifth of individuals, the mutation arises de novo. Making the diagnosis in these cases does not alter the management, as these individuals do not generally require any treatment. However, correct diagnosis prevents unnecessary treatment for misdiagnosed hyperthyroidism, and allows genetic counselling to take place.

Recently, mutations in the gene encoding the thyroid hormone receptor alpha isoform have also been described. The affected individuals who have been described to date have a more severe phenotype than individuals with beta subunit mutations, with features of congenital hypothyroidism including skeletal dysplasia, developmental delay, and slow transit constipation. In these individuals, treatment with thyroid hormone replacement therapy seems, at least in part, to ameliorate the phenotype.

Euthyroid excess of serum total thyroid hormones: Familial dysalbuminaemic hyperthyroxinaemia

DNA sequence analysis may also be helpful in confirming the presence of mutations in the thyroid transport protein genes (thyroid binding globulin, transthyretin, and albumin). The most common of these conditions is familial dysalbuminaemic hyperthyroxinaemia. These conditions are characterized by increased total T4 and T3 levels, but with normal free hormone levels, with a normal TSH. These conditions now rarely result in diagnostic difficulty, as free thyroid hormone assays are now routine. A family history is often given, in which an autosomal dominant pattern of inheritance is observed, and no treatment is required.

Thyroid conditions associated with chromosomal abnormalities

A number of syndromes resulting from chromosomal abnormalities are associated with thyroid diseases. Trisomy 21 (Down's syndrome) is frequently associated with thyroid disease: autoimmune hypothyroidism affects approximately one-fifth of adults with Down's syndrome, while congenital hypothyroidism occurs in 2% of infants with trisomy 21. The prevalence of Graves' disease in this population is similar to that in the general population.

Turner's syndrome (also known as 45XO) is also strongly associated with autoimmune thyroid disease (see also Chapter 7, Section 7.7). Similar to Down's syndrome, approximately 15% of girls with Turner's syndrome have autoimmune hypothyroidism, many with high thyroid autoantibody titres.

DiGeorge syndrome, which results from deletion of a portion of the long arm of Chromosome 22 (22q11), is associated with Graves' disease in one-fifth of cases.

Complex genetic disorders of the thyroid

The common autoimmune thyroid diseases, autoimmune hypothyroidism (Hashimoto's thyroiditis) and Graves' disease, do not have an underlying monogenic aetiology. Instead, they are thought to have a complex genetic aetiology, where multiple genomic variants interact with non-genetic factors, such as environmental or hormonal influences (e.g. smoking, pregnancy).

Graves' disease

Graves' disease is an autoimmune thyroid condition with a complex genetic aetiology. A large Danish twin study estimated that about 80% of the propensity to develop Graves' disease is attributable to genetic factors. In addition, Graves' disease clusters within families, supporting its genetic basis. Up to 25% of people with Graves' disease have a first-degree relative with autoimmune thyroid disease.

A number of genetic loci have been shown to contribute to the susceptibility to Graves' disease. The genes that have been implicated encode proteins within biological pathways that regulate immune system activity or thyroid biology. The strongest and most widely replicated association in Graves' disease has been with the major histocompatibility (MHC) region on Chromosome 6p21. The MHC region is associated with multiple autoimmune conditions. The HLA genes found within the MHC region play a vital role in pathogen and self-peptide recognition, and therefore have a clear role in immunity and in establishing and maintaining immune tolerance. In European populations, the primary association between MHC and Graves' disease is with the Class II MHC allele,

Table 2.2 Monogenic thyroid disorders

Disorder	Phenotype	Gene	Inheritance
Hypothalamic-pituitary defect			
Insensitivity to TRH	Hypothyroidism with no response to TRH stimulation	TRH-R	AR
Combined pituitary hormone deficiency	Hypothyroidism	POU1F1, PROP1	AR, AD
			AR
	With rigid cervical spine	LHX3	AR
	With septo-optic dysplasia	HESX1	AR, AD
	With testicular enlargement & variable hypoprolactinaemia	IGSF1	XR
Isolated TSH deficiency	Hypothyroidism	TSH-B	AR
Thyroid gland development defect			
Thyroid agenesis	Hypothyroidism, midline facial defects, choanal atresia	FOXE1 (TTF2)	AR
	Hypothyroidism, cleft palate, choanal atresia		
Thyroid dysgenesis	Hypothyroidism, ectopic or hypoplastic thyroid	PAX8	AD
	Pulmonary hypoplasia and choreoathetosis	NKX2-1 (TTF1)	PD
Thyroid hormonogenesis defect			
Thyroglobulin defect	Variable hypothyroidism, goitre	thyroglobulin	AR
	Simple goitre	thyroglobulin	AD
Hydrogen peroxide generation defect	Permanent or transient hypothyroidism	DUOX2	AR/ PD
	Mild hypothyroidism	DUOXA2	AR
Iodide transport defect	Hypothyroidism, goitre	SCL5A5 (NIS)	AR
Thyroidal iodide recycling	Goitre and hypothyroidism after the neonatal period	IYD (DEHAL1)	AR (rarely AD)
Total organification defect	Hypothyroidism, goitre	thyroid peroxidase	AR
Partial organification defect	Transient neonatal hypothyroidism, goitre, sensorineural deafness (Pendred's syndrome)	SCL26A4 (PDS)	AR
TSH-receptor signalling defect			
Complete TSH resistance	Hypothyroidism, thyroid hypoplasia	TSH-R	AR
Partial TSH resistance	Euthyroid hyperthyrotropinaemia	TSH-R	AR
	Pseudohypoparathyroidism type 1a (parathyroid hormone resistance, osteodystrophy)	GNAS2	AD/paternal imprinting
Hereditary toxic thyroid hyperplasia	Congenital hyperthyroidism and goitre	TSH-R activation	AD
Familial gestational hyperthyroidism	Hyperthyroidism in pregnancy	TSH-R	AD
Thyroid Hormone transport			
Euthyroid hypothyroxinaemia	Thyroid hormone binding globulin deficiency	TBG	XR
Euthyroid, excess serum total thyroid hormone levels	Familial dysalbuminaemic hyperthyroxinaemia	Albumin	AD
	Familial dysalbuminaemic hypertriiodothyroninaemia	Albumin	AD
	Excess of thyroid hormone binding globulin	TBG duplication	XR
	Increased transthyretin affinity	TTR	AD
Transmembrane defect	Low T4, high T3, hypotonia, nystagmus, developmental delay	MCT8	XR
End organ resistance			
Thyroid hormone resistance	High T4 and T3, inappropriately normal or raised TSH, goitre	TR-β	AD
	Normal-high FT3, normal-low FT4, normal TSH. Growth restriction, developmental delay, constipation.	TR-α	AD

Abbreviations: AD, autosomal dominant; AR, autosomal recessive; PD, partial dominant or haploinsufficient (a heterozygote, with one mutant and one normal allele, displays a phenotype because the wild-type allele alone does not produce sufficient product to result in a normal phenotype; TTR, transthyretin; XR, X-linked recessive.

Adapted from Braverman L.E. and Utiger R.D., *Werner & Ingbar's The Thyroid*, 9th edition, pp. 408–409. Copyright (2004) with permission from Wolters Kluwer.

HLA-DR3. The *DR3* allele is detected twice as frequently in Graves' disease subjects as it is in healthy controls (i.e. 50% of Graves' disease subjects vs 25% of controls) and this allele is thought to more readily allow self-peptides into the binding pocket to be presented to lymphocytes, inducing an autoimmune response. However, approximately 50% of individuals with Graves' disease do not have the *HLA-DR3* allele, implying that there are other factors at play in this condition.

In addition to MHC, a number of other loci have been associated with Graves' disease; however, two have been robustly and widely replicated and are worthy of further mention. Polymorphisms within *CTLA-4* (Chromosome 2q33) have been associated with Graves' disease. *CTLA-4* encodes a co-stimulatory molecule expressed on activated T lymphocytes. This molecule plays an important role in downregulating T-cell responses and modulating T-cell activation. A SNP downstream from the 3′ untranslated region (*CT60*) was found to influence Graves' disease susceptibility (OR 1.5) and was thought to be a causative factor; however, the functional effects of this variant remain poorly defined. The *CTLA-4* autoimmune 'susceptible' haplotype is also found in approximately 50% of individuals from healthy European populations; therefore, it is clear that other factors must also be at play. *CTLA-4* polymorphisms are not specific to Graves' disease: they have also been found to contribute to susceptibility to type 1 diabetes, autoimmune Addison's disease, and rheumatoid arthritis.

Another widely and robustly replicated association with Graves' disease is *PTPN22* on Chromosome 1p13. This gene encodes LYP, which, like CTLA-4, is involved in the regulation of T-cell activation. In Graves' disease, a coding variant (*R620W*) was found more frequently in Caucasians with Graves' disease than in controls (13% vs 7%, respectively, OR 1.8). This variant has been demonstrated to result in an enzyme that is short-lived, compared to the wild-type, resulting in the inhibition of T-cell receptor signalling. This variant has also been found to contribute to susceptibility to rheumatoid arthritis and autoimmune Addison's disease.

Autoimmune hypothyroidism

Autoimmune hypothyroidism, like Graves' disease, is a complex genetic condition. Evidence for heritability in this condition comes from familial clustering. A number of studies have suggested that autoimmune hypothyroidism has a greater genetic contribution than Graves' disease does. Should a healthy individual have a sibling with Graves' disease, it is estimated that their relative risk is around 10, which is similar to that for type 1 diabetes. In autoimmune hypothyroidism, the relative risk is estimated to be between 10 and 45. Autoimmune hypothyroidism and Graves' disease are thought to share some genetic susceptibility factors; this may explain why is it common to see a mixture of Graves' disease and autoimmune hypothyroidism in families prone to autoimmune thyroid disease. In common with Graves' disease, both the MHC class II alleles (*DR3*, *DR4*, and *DR5* alleles) and *CTLA-4* variants have been associated with autoimmune hypothyroidism susceptibility. Other loci implicated in autoimmune hypothyroidism susceptibility include the tumour necrosis factor alpha gene *TNFA*, *PTPN22*, *CYP27B1*, TCR genes, and several immunoglobulin genes and cytokine regulatory genes. Further studies on larger patient cohorts are needed to clarify the underlying genetic aetiology of this common condition.

Genetic contributions towards TSH and FT4 values within the reference range

Several studies have suggested that common genomic variants, or polymorphisms, contribute to serum TSH and free thyroid hormone concentrations within the normal range. A host of loci have so far been associated with TSH and FT4 levels, each contributing modestly to variation within the normal range. Interestingly, significant differences between males and females have been reported at some loci, with researchers speculating that this may provide clues as to why the prevalence of thyroid pathology differs between the sexes. Contrary to expectations, alleles that contribute to higher TSH levels do not necessarily have reciprocal effects on FT4 concentration, suggesting that the TSH and FT4 set points are independently regulated. The reported loci, as a whole, currently explain less than a quarter of the trait variance. Thus, it is clear that our current understanding of the regulation of the hypothalamic–pituitary–thyroid axis is incomplete and requires further study.

Further reading

Bochukova E, Schoenmakers N, Agostini M, et al. A mutation in the thyroid hormone receptor alpha gene. *New Eng J Med* 2012; 366: n243–9.

Franklyn JA and Boelaert K. Thyrotoxicosis. *Lancet* 2012; 379: 1155–66.

McLachlan SM and Rapoport B. Thyroid peroxidase as an autoantigen. *Thyroid* 2007; 17: 939–48.

Porcu E, Medici M, Pistis G, et al. A meta-analysis of thyroid-related traits reveals novel loci and gender-specific differences in the regulation of thyroid function. *PLoS Genet* 2013; 9: e1003266.

Refetoff S and Dumitrescu AM. Syndromes of reduced sensitivity to thyroid hormone: Genetic defects in hormone receptors, cell transporters and deiodination. *Best Pract Res Clin Endocrinol Metab* 2007; 21: 277–305.

Pearce SH. 'Graves' disease', in Weetman, AP, ed., *Autoimmune Diseases in Endocrinology*, 2008. Humana Press, pp. 117–35.

Ueda H, Howson JM, Esposito L, et al. Association of the T-cell regulatory gene CTLA4 with susceptibility to autoimmune disease. *Nature* 2003; 423: 506–11.

Vaidya B and Pearce SH. Management of hypothyroidism in adults. *BMJ* 2008; 337: a801.

Velaga MR, Wilson V, Jennings CE, et al. The codon 620 tryptophan allele of the lymphoid tyrosine phosphatase (LYP) gene is a major determinant of Graves' disease. *J Clin Endocrinol Metab* 2004; 89: 5862–5.

2.3 Imaging and localization of the thyroid

Introduction

The anatomy and function of the thyroid gland can be assessed by a variety of imaging modalities including ultrasound, CT, MRI, and radionuclide imaging. Of these, ultrasound and radionuclide imaging are the mainstays for evaluation of thyroid disease.

Modalities

Ultrasound

The superficial location of the thyroid, among other endocrine glands, facilitates the use of high-resolution ultrasound in the assessment of it and associated structures within the neck, such as lymph nodes. The additional use of spectral Doppler imaging allows evaluation of the vasculature in thyroid diseases. Ultrasound can also provide information on the consistency of tissue via elastography techniques, although this is not widely available and generally is not used in routine clinical practice.

Ultrasound is the most sensitive modality for identifying and characterizing nodules within the thyroid and combined with fine-needle aspiration cytology is the initial investigation for thyroid nodules.

Radionuclide imaging

Radionuclide imaging is the standard modality for functional assessment of thyroid disease. The most common radioisotopes used are ^{123}I and technetium-99m (^{99m}Tc)-pertechnetate. Their principle of action lies in acting as a surrogate of thyroid handling of dietary iodine, therefore reflecting thyroid function. Pertechnetate is trapped in a similar manner to iodine through the sodium iodide symporter; however, it is not organified by the thyroid. It has the advantage over radioiodine of being cheap and easily available and therefore is more preferably used. ^{131}I can also be used for imaging; however, it is primarily used for the treatment of thyroid cancer and hyperthyroidism, as it gives a high thyroid and total body radiation dose from its beta emission.

Radionuclide imaging also involves PET using ^{18}[F]-fluorodeoxyglucose (FDG). This is used in thyroid imaging predominantly for detecting recurrent thyroid cancer, particularly in the context of negative radioiodine scans (Figure 2.5a, b).

CT and MRI

CT and MRI also have a role to play in thyroid imaging; they are, however, less sensitive than ultrasound at detecting thyroid nodules. They are better at determining the extension of retrosternal thyroid masses and assessing distant spread of thyroid carcinoma.

Indications

Congenital abnormalities

Identifying the site of thyroid tissue is best performed with radionuclide imaging which can detect ectopic thyroid tissue in its location from between the tongue base to the anterior mediastinum. Radionuclide imaging also is used in conjunction with ultrasound to investigate congenital hypothyroidism, to help identify the presence and site of the thyroid. A defect in organification can be demonstrated by early uptake of ^{123}I (or ^{99m}Tc); however, delayed scanning (at 24 hours) shows little or no activity in the thyroid due to washout of trapped ^{123}I. Thyroglossal duct cysts may also be detected by radionuclide imaging; however, they are often cystic and better identified with ultrasound, CT, or MRI.

Goitre

See also Section 2.8. A euthyroid goitre can be familial, due to iodine deficiency, or due to compensatory hypertrophy. Imaging can be used to define the size of the goitre, with MRI and CT best at assessing mediastinal extension. Radionuclide imaging offers poor spatial resolution, but is specific in characterizing mediastinal masses as thyroid tissue. If used, ^{123}I is preferred to ^{99m}Tc due to a better signal-to-noise ratio.

Nodules and malignancy

See also Section 2.8. The main role for ultrasound in thyroid imaging is the evaluation of thyroid nodules for malignancy. Nodules within the thyroid are usually distinct from the thyroid parenchyma, and are manifestations of a variety of disease processes. Many are incidentally discovered, and are so common that it is not feasible to get a tissue sample of each one.

Features of thyroid nodules that can be elucidated from ultrasound include echogenicity, shape, margins, whether it is solid/cystic, comet-tails, vascularity, and calcification. No individual feature can completely characterize a nodule with full sensitivity and specificity, but rather it is a combination of features which determines the likelihood of malignancy and requirement for fine-needle aspiration cytology. Nodules that do not require tissue sampling are as follows:

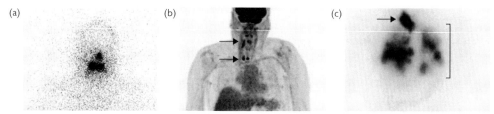

(a)   (b)   (c)

Fig 2.5 Radionuclide imaging of thyroid cancer. (a) A patient with thyroid cancer and normal physiological uptake of ^{131}I within the head and neck; however, ^{18}F-fluorodeoxyglucose (FDG) PET (b) demonstrates residual nodal disease (arrows). This highlights the fact that some poorly differentiated thyroid cancers do not take up iodine but are metabolically active and take up FDG. (c) An ^{131}I scan in a different patient, demonstrating uptake in residual thyroid cancer within the right neck (arrow) and multiple, bilateral lung metastases (square bracket).

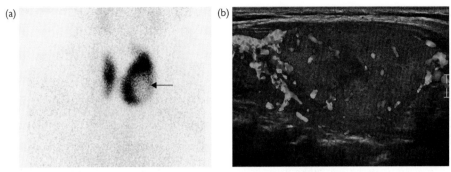

Fig 2.6 (a) A pertechnetate scan of a patient with hyperthyroidism, demonstrating globally increased uptake within the thyroid, as is associated with Graves' disease. In the left lobe, there is a photopaenic defect (arrow) suggesting a cold nodule. The presence of a nodule is confirmed on an ultrasound scan (b), which also shows hypervascularity on Doppler in surrounding thyroid tissue, as is characteristic of Graves' disease.

small cystic, colloid nodules with comet-tail artefacts

nodules with an internal honeycombed or spongiform cystic appearance

large predominantly cystic nodules

diffuse, numerous small nodules with intervening hypoechoic bands (known as giraffe skin appearance), which are associated with Hashimoto's thyroiditis

Radionuclide imaging can help assess thyroid nodules when cytology results are indeterminate, as hyperfunctioning thyroid nodules are almost always benign (>99%). In contrast, a non-functioning or 'cold' nodule has around a 20% chance of being malignant, which rises to around 40% when other risk factors such as prior neck radiation exist. Rarely, nodules are hot on ^{99m}Tc-pertechnetate imaging but cold on 24-hour ^{123}I imaging and are termed discordant. This represents trapping but failure of organification within the nodule and, in some cases, is associated with malignancy.

Radionuclide imaging is also used post thyroidectomy, when ^{131}I is used to treat residual thyroid malignancy and to ablate remaining thyroid tissue. Whole body scans can be used to assess the extent of disease and then to follow up for recurrence (Figure 2.5c).

Thyroid function

Imaging to assess thyroid function is predominantly performed in the setting of hyperthyroidism when TSH is suppressed. In this scenario, radionuclide imaging uses thyroid uptake of tracer to determine if the thyroid gland is functioning autonomously, and to help differentiate between Graves' disease, hyperfunctioning nodules, subacute thyroiditis, or factitious hyperthyroidism. When interpreting the results of a thyroid scan, correlation with clinical and drug history, and biochemical and ultrasound findings, are important.

Graves' disease

See also Section 2.5. On radionuclide imaging, the thyroid often appears enlarged and has homogeneously increased uptake throughout the gland. The presence of Graves' disease does not exclude the presence of thyroid nodules, which have relatively decreased uptake (Figure 2.6a). When Graves' disease is found with a hyperfunctioning nodule, this is known as Marine–Lenhart syndrome.

Ultrasound in Graves' will demonstrate marked hypervascularity on Doppler; this appearance is described as a 'thyroid inferno' (Figure 2.6b). Such an appearance may also occasionally be seen in Hashimoto's thyroiditis. MRI may show increased T1 in the thyroid; the reason for this is unknown.

Hyperfunctioning nodules

See also Section 2.5. Radionuclide imaging of hyperfunctioning or toxic nodules (Figure 2.7) will demonstrate increased uptake with partial or complete suppression of normal thyroid tissue. Ultrasound cannot

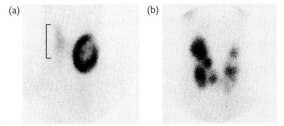

Fig 2.7 Pertechnetate scans demonstrating hyperfunctioning (toxic) nodules. (a) A solitary toxic nodule (Plummer's syndrome) with almost complete suppression of uptake in the remainder of the thyroid gland (square bracket). (b) Multiple hyperfunctioning nodules in an enlarged thyroid gland, in keeping with a toxic multinodular goitre.

(a)   (b)

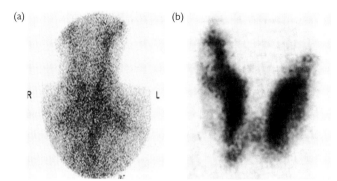

R   L

Fig 2.8 Pertechnetate scan thyroid scans of thyroiditis. (a) Subacute thyroiditis with no uptake within the thyroid. Only background soft tissue uptake in the neck is seen. (b) Patchy thyroid uptake in Hashimoto's thyroiditis.

differentiate nodules that are hyperfunctioning from those that are not.

Thyroiditis

Subacute thyroiditis

See also Section 2.6. Subacute most commonly refers to de Quervain's thyroiditis. which usually presents as a painful swollen gland and is diagnosed clinically without the need for imaging. In less clear-cut cases, radionuclide imaging can help confirm the diagnosis by demonstrating little or no uptake of radiotracer (Figure 2.8a). This is due to an intact pituitary feedback mechanism rather than damage to the thyroid gland. Ultrasound has little role to play in diagnosis, but can help distinguish subacute thyroiditis from Graves' disease by the absence of increased vascularity.

Hashimoto's thyroiditis

Hashimoto's thyroiditis is the most common chronic inflammatory disease of the thyroid. Acutely, Hashimoto's can demonstrate either small hypoechoic, avascular, poorly defined nodules or a micronodular appearance on a background of an avascular gland. The small nodules represent a lymphocytic infiltrate and sometimes can be mistaken for a mass lesion. In chronic states, the thyroid can be enlarged and hypervascular, similar to the appearances of Graves' disease. The gland can also contain multiple hypoechoic regions delineated by fibrous septa which are echogenic. End-stage Hashimoto's demonstrates a small, atrophic, heterogeneous, and avascular thyroid gland.

On radionuclide imaging, Hashimoto's may have increased uptake acutely followed by coarse patchy uptake in chronic disease (Figure 2.8b).

Acute thyroiditis

Acute thyroiditis is usually bacterial, and imaging has little role to play in evaluation.

Amiodarone-induced thyroiditis

Amiodarone is an iodine-rich drug which may induce two distinct types of thyroiditis. Type I is iodine induced and occurs in patients with latent or pre-existing thyroid disorders. Type II occurs in the normal thyroid and leads to a destructive thyroiditis. Ultrasound demonstrating Doppler flow, increased gland size, and nodularity is more in keeping with type I, whereas an ultrasound showing no vascularity is more in keeping with type II. On radionuclide imaging, type I classically has increased or normal uptake whereas type II has little or no uptake. In practice, this is confounded by the fact that high systemic iodine levels may compete with uptake of radiotracer in the thyroid and lead to decreased uptake in type I.

2.4 Approach to the assessment of disorders of thyroid hormone homeostasis

Thyroid hormone homeostasis

Thyroid hormone homeostasis depends not only upon normal functioning of the multiloop hypothalamic–pituitary–thyroid feedback system but also on normal functioning of the thyroid gland itself, including controlled synthesis, secretion, transport, and metabolism of thyroid hormones. The net effect is to maintain the peripheral thyroid hormone concentrations within the relatively narrow normal limits necessary to maintain optimal health. A large number of conditions can influence one or more aspects of thyroid hormone homeostasis; many, but not all, result in ill health.

The hypothalamic–pituitary–thyroid axis

The activity of the thyroid gland is regulated primarily by TSH, which is synthesized and released by the anterior pituitary thyrotroph cells. TSH synthesis and release is regulated by TRH, which is synthesized in the supraoptic and paraventricular nucleus of the hypothalamus and stored in the median eminence. The hormones produced by the thyroid gland, namely T4 and T3, in turn, interact with the hypothalamus and pituitary in a classic multiloop negative feedback system, affecting the release of TSH and TRH, thereby maintaining normal peripheral thyroid hormone concentrations. Under normal conditions, the feedback effect is primarily exerted by circulating T4, which is taken up by the thyrotroph cells and deiodinated intracellularly to T3.

Synthesis, secretion, transport, and metabolism of thyroid hormones

See also Chapter 2.1. Thyroid hormone synthesis starts with the active transport of iodide into the thyroid follicle cells. This is followed by the oxidation of iodide, which then gets organified by iodination of the tyrosyl residues within thyroglobulin. Iodination of tyrosyl residues results in the formation of mono- and diiodotyrosines in the presence of thyroid peroxidase and hydrogen peroxide; coupling of iodotyrosines results in the formation of T4 and T3, which are then released in to the blood following proteolytic cleavage from thyroglobulin within the thyroid follicle cell. T4 in the peripheral circulation arises primarily from direct secretion from the thyroid gland, whereas T3 in the peripheral circulation is mostly generated by the peripheral conversion of T4 to T3 by monodeiodination.

A unique feature of thyroid hormone homeostasis is the ability of the gland to store large amounts of hormones, such that peripheral thyroid hormone concentrations do not get depleted for a few days despite cessation of synthesis. This explains the delay in the onset of action of anti-thyroid medications that affect synthesis of thyroid hormones, and underlies the need for not only the administration of agents that inhibit release of hormones (such as iodine) should rapid control of peripheral hormone concentrations be desired (thyroid storm, preparation for urgent surgery in hyperthyroid patients), but also for the administration of beta blockers for the first few weeks after the initiation of anti-thyroid medications to control symptoms.

Thyroid hormones that circulate in the blood are bound to several proteins synthesized in the liver; these include TBG, transthyretin (pre-albumin) and albumin. A very small proportion of T4 and T3 circulate in the free form. Altered concentrations of binding proteins affect the concentration of T4 and T3 in the peripheral circulation, but not the concentration of the free hormones.

Conditions that affect thyroid hormone homeostasis

The following conditions affect thyroid hormone homeostasis:

A. *Regulatory dysfunction (hypothalamic-pituitary-thyroid axis dysfunction):*
- abnormalities in hypothalamic TRH secretion
- abnormalities in pituitary TSH secretion (hypopituitarism, TSH-oma)

B. *Thyroid gland dysfunction:*
- hypothyroidism due to thyroid gland hypofunction
- thyrotoxicosis due to thyroid gland or ectopic thyroid tissue hyperfunction, or thyroiditis

C. *Factors affecting the transport and metabolism of thyroid hormones:*
- euthyroid hyperthyroxinaemia (increased T4 values but normal thyroid function):
  - increased TBG
  - resistance to thyroid hormones (see also Section 16.1)
  - non-thyroidal illness
  - drugs
- euthyroid hypothyroxinaemia (decreased T4 values but normal thyroid function):
  - decreased TBG
  - drugs

D. *Miscellaneous conditions (affecting homeostasis at one or more levels):*
- age
- gender
- pregnancy
- environmental temperature
- nutritional status
- deficiency or excess availability of iodine
- glucocorticoids
- pharmacological agents
- non-thyroidal illness

Approach to assessment of disorders of thyroid hormone homeostasis

Correct interpretation of an abnormal set of TFTs is mostly straightforward, as discussed in the subsequent chapters on hypo- and hyperthyroidism. However, a number of conditions other than dysfunction of the thyroid gland or a defect in the hypothalamic–pituitary–thyroid axis might result in abnormal TFTs. The following can cause abnormal TFT results in subjects without thyroid disease:

1. *Laboratory artefacts:*
- due to antibodies to TSH or thyroid hormones, or to the use of pharmacological agents such as heparin (results in artefactual elevation of FT4; see also Chapter 1, Section 1.5)

2. *Chronic malnutrition/undernutrition:*
   - results primarily in a decrease in serum T3, normal or mildly decreased serum T4, but mostly normal or marginally low serum TSH
3. *Non-thyroidal illness (sick euthyroid syndrome):*
   - results from a disruption in thyroid hormone homeostasis due to acute illness (such as acute febrile illness, uncontrolled diabetes, acute myocardial infarction), major surgical intervention, trauma, or moderate or severe chronic illness
   - the fundamental defect is a decrease in T4 to T3 conversion, resulting in low T3 values
   - T4 values might be increased or normal initially but, with more protracted illness, they fall too
   - serum TSH is mostly normal or low in non-thyroidal illness, except in the late recovery phase, when it can rise temporarily for a few weeks
   - the most confusing scenario is seen in patients in the intensive care unit, when T3, T4, and TSH values are all low, mimicking secondary hypothyroidism; further investigations including assessment of serum cortisol might be necessary
4. *Acute psychiatric illness:*
   - results in an elevation in T4 and FT4 values in some patients, together with normal or increased T3
   - the values return to normal after a few weeks without any intervention
5. *HIV infection:*
   - results in elevated TBG, leading to elevated T4, together with normal or borderline low T3 value
6. *Drugs:*
   - can affect thyroid homeostasis in numerous ways and result in:
     - hypothyroidism: lithium, iodide, amiodarone, methimazole, propylthiouracil
     - hyperthyroidism: iodide, amiodarone
     - hypothyroidism in patients treated with thyroxine, either by affecting the absorption of T4 (iron, aluminium hydroxide, sucralfate, cholestyramine) or by enhancing T4 metabolism by stimulating hepatic microsomal enzyme activity (phenobarbitone, rifampicin, carbamazepine, phenytoin)
     - euthyroid hyperthyroxinaemia resulting from elevated TBG (oestrogens, methadone, mitotane, fluorouracil) or inhibition of peripheral conversion of T4 to T3 (iopanoic acid, sodium ipodate, glucocorticoids, amiodarone, propranolol)
     - euthyroid hypothyroxinaemia resulting from decreased TBG (glucocorticoids, androgens, nicotinic acid, anabolic steroids) or inhibition of binding of T4 to TBG (high-dose furosemide and salicylates)
7. *Atypical clinical situations:*
   - thyrotoxicosis factitia (usually unprescribed intake of exogenous thyroid hormone): elevated FT4 and suppressed TSH, depressed thyroid uptake on scintigraphy, low thyroglobulin
   - struma ovarii (ovarian teratoma containing hyperfunctioning thyroid tissue): biochemical picture of thyrotoxicosis, depressed thyroid uptake on scintigraphy
   - trophoblast tumours (hCG structural homology with TSH results in mild hyperthyroidism
   - hyperemesis gravidarum (see Chapter 10, Section 10.1)

Further reading

Gardner DF, Kaplan MM, Stanley CA, et al. Effect of triiodothyronine replacement on the metabolic and pituitary responses to starvation. *N Engl J Med* 1979; 30: 579–84.

Larsen PR. Feedback regulation of thyrotropin secretion by thyroid hormones. Thyroid–pituitary interaction. *N Engl J Med* 1982; 306: 23–32.

Refetoff S. Syndromes of thyroid hormone resistance. *Am J Physiol* 1982; 243: E88–98.

Tan MJ, Tan F, Hawkins R, et al. A hyperthyroid patient with measurable thyroid stimulating hormone concentration: A trap for the unwary. *Ann Acad Med Singapore* 2006; 35: 500–3.

Surks MI and Sievert R. Drugs and thyroid function. *N Engl J Med* 1995; 333: 1688–94.

Wartofsky L and Burman KD. Alterations in thyroid function in patients with systemic illness: The 'euthyroid sick syndrome'. *Endocr Rev* 1982; 3: 164–217.

2.5 Hyperthyroidism

Definition

Hyperthyroidism is a disorder of excess synthesis and secretion of thyroid hormones resulting in typical clinical manifestations of thyrotoxicosis. Two main thyroid hormones are released by the thyroid gland: T4 and T3. T4 is a prohormone which is produced in higher concentrations than T3, the biologically active hormone. Thyrotoxicosis can occur without hyperthyroidism, usually when stored thyroid hormones are released in the circulation as part of inflammatory disease (thyroiditis).

In primary hyperthyroidism there is increased thyroid hormone secretion by the thyroid gland, whereas increased secretion of TSH from the pituitary or TRH from the hypothalamus results in secondary hyperthyroidism.

Hyperthyroidism is common, with a population prevalence of 2% in women and 0.2% in men in the UK. The incidence of hyperthyroidism increases with age and is higher is white populations and in areas of iodine deficiency.

Aetiology

The most common cause of *overt hyperthyroidism* is Graves' disease, an autoimmune condition in which autoantibodies bind to TSH receptors on follicular thyroid cells, resulting in the excess production of T3 and T4. In iodine-sufficient areas, Graves' disease accounts for about 80% of cases of hyperthyroidism. The next most common cause is toxic nodular hyperthyroidism, in which one (solitary toxic adenoma) or more (toxic multinodular goitre) thyroid nodules cause autonomous overproduction of thyroid hormones. This accounts for 50% of cases of hyperthyroidism in iodine-deficient areas. Thyroiditis, or inflammation of the thyroid gland, is responsible for about 10% of thyrotoxicosis and represents a condition of thyroid cell destruction resulting in release of excess thyroid hormones in the circulation. The common and less common causes of hyperthyroidism and thyrotoxicosis are displayed in Table 2.3.

Subclinical hyperthyroidism (see Chapter 20, Section 20.1) is a biochemical diagnosis in which serum TSH concentrations are below normal with normal circulating thyroid hormone concentrations. Based on the degree of serum TSH suppression, this is often further classified as undetectable serum TSH and low but detectable concentrations. Subclinical hyperthyroidism may be endogenous or exogenous (due to excessive doses of levothyroxine replacement).

Graves' hyperthyroidism

Pathophysiology

- Graves' disease is one of the most prevalent autoimmune diseases and often coexists with other autoimmune conditions such as rheumatoid arthritis. A low threshold for screening for associated autoimmune conditions is advisable.
- Long-acting stimulating antibodies to the TSH receptor are the pathognomonic hallmark of Graves' disease.
- Almost 50% of patients with Graves' thyrotoxicosis have a family history of thyroid dysfunction.
- Graves' disease is caused by an interplay between genetic and environmental factors (see Section 2.2 and Chapter 1, Sections 1.5, and 1.6); 80% of the susceptibility can be attributed to genetic factors.

Environmental factors include smoking, infections, stress, and pregnancy.

Clinical features

- Excess thyroid hormone concentrations affect nearly every physiological system.
- Symptoms and signs relating to the cardiovascular system are often present. Many patients complain of palpitation, and sinus tachycardia is usually present. Development of atrial fibrillation is one of the most feared consequences of hyperthyroidism and is an independent predictor of mortality.
- Weight loss despite increased appetite, together with fatigue, heat intolerance, nervousness, irritability, muscle weakness, and increased frequency of bowel movement are common symptoms of thyrotoxicosis.
- Shortness of breath and reduced exercise capacity are caused by a combination of cardiovascular abnormalities and respiratory muscle weakness.
- Clinical signs include the presence of a smooth goitre, fine tremor, sinus tachycardia, warm moist skin, and hyperreflexia.
- Roughly 50% of patients with Graves' disease have ophthalmopathy which is characterized by eye lid retraction and lag, proptosis, conjunctival injection and periorbital oedema. In severe cases this may result in ophthalmoplegia. It is estimated that around 5% of patients with Graves' disease develop severe ophthalmopathy.
- Other extra-thyroidal manifestations of Graves' disease include pretibial myxoedema and thyroid acropachy.
- Thyrotoxic periodic paralysis is a serious complication of hyperthyroidism, characterized by muscle paralysis and hypokalaemia. This condition is more common in Asian populations.
- Overall, the frequency and severity of symptoms are related to the degree of circulating thyroid hormone abnormality. Older people have fewer symptoms and signs with the exception of weight loss, shortness of breath, and atrial fibrillation.

Investigations

- Table 2.4 illustrates the main diagnostic criteria for Graves' disease.
- Measurement of serum TSH is the most sensitive screening test to exclude thyrotoxicosis. In overt hyperthyroidism, serum TSH is usually undetectable because of negative feedback of high levels of circulating thyroid hormones on the anterior pituitary.
- The serum FT4 concentration is usually raised in overt hyperthyroidism except in more rare cases of T3 toxicosis.
- The patient's history and clinical features often confirm the diagnosis, especially if extra-thyroidal manifestations are present.
- A diagnosis of Graves' disease can be confirmed by measurement of TSH receptor antibodies, and anti-thyroperoxidase antibodies are present in 75% of patients with Graves' disease.
- Isotope imaging (with technetium or radioactive iodine) may help distinguish Graves' disease from other causes of thyrotoxicosis.

Table 2.3 Aetiology of hyperthyroidism and thyrotoxicosis

Type of thyrotoxicosis	Pathogenic mechanism
Common causes	
Thyrotoxicosis associated with hyperthyroidism	
Graves' disease	TSH-receptor stimulating antibody
Toxic multinodular goitre	Activating mutations in TSH receptors or G proteins
Solitary toxic adenoma	Focus of functional autonomy
	Benign tumour
Thyrotoxicosis not associated with hyperthyroidism	Release of stored hormones
Silent (painless) thyroiditis (including postpartum)	Autoimmune destruction of thyroid cells
Subacute thyroiditis	Probable viral infection
Exogenous thyroid hormone	Excess ingestion of thyroid hormone (iatrogenic or factitious)
Uncommon causes	
Thyrotoxicosis associated with hyperthyroidism	
TSH-secreting pituitary adenoma	Hyperplasia of TSH-producing pituitary cells
Pituitary resistance to thyroid hormone	Mutated thyroid hormone beta receptor with greater expression in the pituitary compared with peripheral tissues
Neonatal Graves' disease	Thyroid-stimulating immunoglobulins
Choriocarcinoma	hCG secretion
Hyperemesis gravidarum	
Congenital hyperthyroidism	Activating mutations in the TSH receptor
Struma ovarii	Toxic adenoma in dermoid tumour of ovary
Metastatic follicular thyroid carcinoma	Foci of functional autonomy
Iodine, iodine-containing drugs (amiodarone), and radiographic contrast agents	Jod–Basedow, excess iodine resulting in unregulated thyroid hormone production
Thyrotoxicosis not associated with hyperthyroidism	Destruction of thyroid follicles
Drug-induced thyroiditis (amiodarone, interferon alpha, lithium)	Direct toxic drug effects
Acute infectious thyroiditis	Thyroidal infection (bacterial, fungal, etc.)
Radiation thyroiditis	Cell destruction caused by radioactive iodine
Infarction of thyroid adenoma	Release of stored hormones
'Hamburger' thyrotoxicosis	Ingestion of contaminated food

Table 2.4 Differential diagnosis of thyrotoxicosis

Diagnostic tool	Graves' disease	Toxic nodular hyperthyroidism	Thyroiditis
Patient's history	Symptoms of thyrotoxicosis	Symptoms of thyrotoxicosis	Symptoms of thyrotoxicosis
	Extra-thyroidal symptoms		Recent viral infection
			Painful neck swelling
			Recent delivery of child
Clinical examination	Signs of thyrotoxicosis	Signs of thyrotoxicosis	Signs of thyrotoxicosis
	Extra-thyroidal manifestations (particularly signs of ophthalmopathy)	Single nodule or multinodular goitre	Painful diffuse goitre
	Diffuse goitre		
Thyroid function and other laboratory tests	TSH undetectable	TSH undetectable	TSH undetectable
	FT4 and FT3 raised	FT4 and FT3 raised	FT4 and FT3 raised
		(only FT3 raised in T3 toxicosis)	Raised inflammatory markers (ESR, CRP)
Immunological tests	TSH-receptor antibodies raised		TPO antibodies may be raised
	TPO antibodies raised		
Radio-isotope scan	Diffuse uptake of tracer	Focal pattern of tracer uptake with reduced uptake in remainder of thyroid gland	Minimal uptake of tracer

Abbreviations: FT3, free triiodothyronine; FT4, free thyroxine; TPO, thyroid peroxidase.

Treatment

If thyrotoxicosis is suspected or confirmed, treatment with beta-adrenoceptor blockers is effective in controlling symptoms of tremor, palpitation, and anxiety.

Once a diagnosis of Graves' disease has been confirmed, it is necessary to choose between three treatment options: anti-thyroid drugs, radioiodine administration, or surgery. There is significant geographical variation between preferred therapeutic choices with radioiodine administration being the preferred option in the US, and anti-thyroid drugs the most commonly used modality in Europe. Guidelines recommend a discussion of the treatment options, considering advantages and disadvantages, between patient and physician. Table 2.5 summarizes the indications, advantages, and disadvantages of the therapeutic strategies for hyperthyroidism.

Anti-thyroid drugs

- Thionamides are the drugs of choice for the treatment of hyperthyroidism. Carbimazole is most frequently used in the UK: its active metabolite methimazole is the drug of choice in the US. Propylthiouracil is the other anti-thyroid drug, which is used much less commonly.
- These drugs act by inhibiting the action of thyroid peroxidase and hence the synthesis of thyroid hormones.
- Carbimazole is administered once daily and compliance is therefore better than with propylthiouracil, which has to be administered twice or thrice daily.
- A recommended starting dose of carbimazole is 10–20 mg daily, an equivalent dose of propylthiouracil being 100–200 mg daily in two to three divided doses. Higher doses may be needed if thyrotoxicosis is severe.

- If a dose titration regime is used, the dose of anti-thyroid drugs is reduced as serum FT4 concentrations normalize. Initially, regular 4–6-weekly thyroid functioning testing is required to avoid overtreatment and once maintenance doses are used, this can be done less frequently (every 2–3 months).
- Some centres prefer a block-replace regime in which high doses of anti-thyroid drugs are used to block thyroid function in combination with levothyroxine replacement. This approach does not improve remission rates and is associated with more side effects.
- If anti-thyroid drugs are used to induce remission of Graves' disease—evidenced by normal thyroid function 1 year after discontinuation of drugs—then a prolonged 12–18 month course is advised.
- Overall, long-term remission rates of Graves' hyperthyroidism after a prolonged course of anti-thyroid drugs are 30%–50%. Factors predicting poor response include severe biochemical disease, male gender, younger age, smoking, presence of a large goitre, and high concentrations of TSH-receptor antibodies.
- Minor and often transient side effects occur in around 3% of patients on anti-thyroid drugs. These include rashes, arthralgia, fever, and gastrointestinal upset.
- The most feared severe side effect of both carbimazole and propylthiouracil is agranulocytosis, which occurs in 0.2%–0.5% of subjects taking these drugs. Treatment with anti-thyroid drugs should not be restarted when a patient develops agranulocytosis, and alternative treatment options should be considered. Patients should be warned about this risk and a record made in the notes.
- Propylthiouracil is associated with antineutrophil cytoplasmic antibody-positive vasculitis and with acute

Table 2.5 Treatment modalities in hyperthyroidism

Treatment modality	Indications	Advantages	Disadvantages
Anti-thyroid drugs	Newly diagnosed Graves' disease	Non-invasive	Low cure rates
		Outpatient therapy	Adverse effects (1%–5%)
	Before radioiodine or surgery (short term)	Low cost	Frequent follow-up and compliance required
	Children	Low risk of permanent hypothyroidism	
	Pregnancy	Possible immune-modulatory effects	
Radioactive iodine (^{131}I)	Relapsed Graves' disease	Effective cure	Slow cure
	Toxic nodular hyperthyroidism	Outpatient therapy	Induction of permanent hypothyroidism
	Newly diagnosed Graves' disease	Reduction in goitre size	Potential worsening of ophthalmopathy
			Defer pregnancy for 6 months
			Adherence to radiation protection guidance required
Surgery	Large goitres	Rapid control of hyperthyroidism	Invasive
	Current pregnancy	Relief of compressive symptoms	Expensive
	Significant ophthalmopathy	100% cure	Permanent hypothyroidism
	Severe adverse effects of anti-thyroid drugs		In-patient treatment
			Risk of complications
			Scar

liver failure, which is estimated to occur in 1 per 10,000 adults taking this drug. Experts recommend that propylthiouracil should only be used as first-line treatment during the first trimester of pregnancy, in thyroid storm, or if there are significant side effects from carbimazole and alternative therapeutic options are not suitable options.

Radioiodine treatment

- This is the treatment of choice in relapsed Graves' disease and is increasingly used as first-line therapy. It is a safe and effective treatment option with cure rates of up to 85% after a single dose.
- The aim of treatment is to restore a euthyroid state with or without hypothyroidism. The majority of patients will be rendered hypothyroid following a standard dose of 400–600 MBq.
- Contraindications include pregnancy or lactation; desire for pregnancy within 6 months of treatment; suspicion or diagnosis of coexisting thyroid cancer; and inability to comply with radiation protection regulations.
- Most centres use a single fixed dose, and the use of calculated doses has not proven to be cost-effective.
- Most UK centres pretreat patient with anti-thyroid drugs to provide symptomatic relief and to avoid exacerbations (thyroid storm). Anti-thyroid drugs are usually discontinued for 2–14 days prior to the administration of radioactive iodine, and may be recommenced after treatment.
- Patients will be advised on precautions regarding contact with children /pregnant women and public travel in the immediate period after treatment with radioactive iodine.
- Graves' ophthalmopathy is a relative contraindication and many centres administer radioactive iodine in those with inactive thyroid eye disease under steroid prophylaxis. Liaison with a specialist ophthalmologist is advisable when considering this treatment in subjects with eye involvement.
- Monitoring of thyroid function is required 4–6-weekly after radioiodine administration initially in view of the risk of hypothyroidism. Once euthyroidism is achieved, annual thyroid function testing is advised.
- Fears about the development of cancer after radioiodine have not been realized, although Graves' disease itself may be associated with a slight increase in the risk of thyroid cancer.

Surgery

- Surgery is used infrequently to treat hyperthyroidism. Total thyroidectomy is advised, and complication rates are low in the hands of experienced surgeons.
- Relative indications include large goitres (especially if thyroid cancer is suspected), pregnancy, and pronounced ophthalmopathy.
- Complications include bleeding, scar, infection, permanent hypoparathyroidism, and recurrent laryngeal nerve damage.
- Pretreatment with anti-thyroid drugs is required to render the patient euthyroid prior to surgery.

Graves' orbitopathy

Extra-thyroidal manifestations of Graves' disease include Graves' orbitopathy, dermopathy (or pretibial myxoedema), and acropachy. The latter two are rare, but clinically detectable ophthalmopathy is present in about 25% of patients with Graves' disease at presentation and is usually mild. Moderate to severe orbitopathy develops in 5% of patients and rarely may progress to sight-threatening forms.

Epidemiology and clinical features

- Most of the clinical signs and symptoms of Graves' orbitopathy are due to proliferation of orbital fibroblasts, expansion of fat tissue, enlargement of extraocular muscles due to infiltration of inflammatory cells, and increased glycosaminoglycan resulting in an increased volume of the orbital content.
- Graves' orbitopathy is an autoimmune disorder and linked to the thyroid by shared antigens between thyroidal and orbital tissues. It is triggered by antibodies to the TSH receptor and the IGF-1 receptor.
- Identified risk factors include cigarette smoking, thyroid dysfunction (both hyper- and hypothyroidism), radioiodine therapy, higher levels of TSH receptor antibodies, and oxidative stress.
- The incidence of Graves' orbitopathy is 42.2 per million per year, with the peak incidence in individuals aged 40–60 years. It is five times more common in women than in men.
- Common clinical features include diplopia or symptoms related to exophthalmos and corneal exposure, including photophobia, tearing, grittiness, and pain. Soft tissues changes such as eyelid oedema and hyperaemia, conjunctival hyperaemia, chemosis, and caruncle oedema may be present in moderate to severe ophthalmopathy.
- Decreased colour sensitivity, decreased visual acuity, and visual field defects are worrying clinical features.
- Quality of life is often significantly affected, even in patients with mild Graves' orbitopathy.

Assessment of Graves' orbitopathy

- Both the activity and severity of Graves' orbitopathy should be assessed using standardized criteria, and Graves' orbitopathy should be classified as active or inactive and as mild, moderate to severe, or sight threatening.
- There are several classification systems, including the Graves' orbitopathy clinical activity score, NOSPECS, and the European Group on Graves' orbitopathy classification.
- Box 2.2 displays the most commonly accepted criteria for the classification of Graves' orbitopathy activity and severity.

General management principles in Graves' orbitopathy

- A patient-focused treatment approach should be adopted, encompassing the effects of the disease and its treatment on quality of life and psychological well-being.
- Graves' orbitopathy should be managed by a multidisciplinary team of endocrinologists, ophthalmologists, radiologists, orbital surgeons, and radiotherapists.
- Except for the mildest cases, which improve with normalization of thyroid function and local lubricants, patients should be referred to combined thyroid–eye clinics or specialized centres.
- Euthyroidism should be promptly restored and maintained in all patients with Graves' orbitopathy.
- All patients with Graves' disease should be encouraged to refrain from smoking whether Graves' orbitopathy is present or not.

Box 2.2 Standardized criteria to assess Graves' orbitopathy activity and severity

---

Assessment of Graves' orbitopathy severity (European Group on Graves' orbitopathy)

1. MILD: one or more of (i) minor lid retraction (<2 mm), (ii) mild soft-tissue involvement, (iii) exophthalmos <3 mm above normal for race and gender. No or intermittent diplopia and corneal exposure responsive to lubricants.
2. MODERATE TO SEVERE: two or more of (i) lid retraction ≥2 mm, (ii) moderate or severe soft-tissue involvement, (iii) exophthalmos ≥3 mm above normal for race and gender. Inconstant or constant diplopia.
3. SIGHT-THREATENING: patients with dysthyroid optic neuropathy or corneal breakdown.

Assessment of Graves' orbitopathy activity (clinical activity score)

Score 1 point for each of the following:

1. Spontaneous retrobulbar pain
2. Pain on upward or downward gaze
3. Redness of eyelids
4. Redness of conjunctiva
5. Swelling of caruncle or plica
6. Swelling of eyelids
7. Swelling of conjunctiva (chemosis)

INACTIVE Graves' orbitopathy = clinical activity score < 3
ACTIVE Graves' orbitopathy = clinical activity score ≥ 3

Adapted from Bartalena L, Baldeschi L, Dickinson A et al., Consensus statement of the European Group on Graves' orbitopathy (EUGOGO) on management of GO, *European Journal of Endocrinology*, 2008, Volume 158, Issue 3, pp. 273–285. Copyright © 2008, European Society of Endocrinology, published by BioScientifica Ltd. Data from Mourits MP, Koornneef L, Wiersinga WM et al., Clinical criteria for the assessment of disease activity in Graves' ophthalmopathy: a novel approach, *British Journal of Ophthalmology*, 1989, Volume 73, Issue 8, pp. 639–644.

- Oral prednisolone prophylaxis, starting with daily dose of 0.3–0.5 mg prednisone/kg body weight should be given in radioiodine-treated patients at high risk of progression or de novo development of Graves' orbitopathy. Lower-dose prednisone can be used in lower-risk patients treated with radioiodine.
- Patients with inactive Graves' orbitopathy can safely receive radioiodine without steroid cover, as long as hypothyroidism is avoided and if other risk factors for Graves' orbitopathy progression, particularly smoking, are absent.
- Radioiodine should be avoided in patients with moderate to severe and active Graves' orbitopathy.

Specific management principles for Graves' orbitopathy, according to severity

- All patients with Graves' orbitopathy should be treated extensively with non-preserved artificial tears with osmoprotective properties at all times and, if corneal exposure is present, more protective gels or ointments should be offered.
- Six-month selenium supplementation should be given to patients with mild Graves' orbitopathy of relatively short duration.
- High-dose intravenous glucocorticoids are the first-line treatment in patients with moderate to severe and active Graves' orbitopathy, and this treatment should be given in specialist centres.
- A standard regime consists of methylprednisolone 0.5 g once weekly for 6 weeks, followed by 0.25 g once weekly for 6 weeks (4.5 g cumulative dose).

Some centres use steroid-sparing agents (e.g. methotrexate or ciclosporin) after initial methyl prednisolone.

- Elective rehabilitative surgery should be offered to patients with Graves' orbitopathy when the disease is associated with a significant impact on visual function or quality of life after the disease has been inactive for at least 6 months.
- If more than one surgical procedure is required, orbital decompression should precede squint surgery and be followed by lid surgery.
- Severe corneal exposure needs to be treated medically or by surgery as soon as possible in order to avoid progression to corneal breakdown.
- Dysthyroid optic neuropathy should be treated immediately with very high doses of intravenous glucocorticoids (500–1000 mg methylprednisolone for 3 consecutive days or on alternate days during the first week), and urgent orbital decompression should be performed if response is absent or poor within 2 weeks.

Targeted therapies in Graves' orbitopathy

- Rituximab, which depletes CD20-positive B cells, is currently being investigated as a potential treatment for Graves' orbitopathy. Results from small uncontrolled studies appear are promising, although outcomes from larger-scale randomized trials are awaited.
- Anti-cytokine therapies, such as treatments against tumour necrosis factor alpha and interleukin 6 have shown potential promise but are not used routinely.
- Small studies have shown exciting results using blocking monoclonal antibodies and small molecule antagonists against TSH and IGF-1 receptors, and larger multicentre trials are being conducted.

Prognosis

The treatment modalities for Graves' hyperthyroidism, which accounts for the vast majority of cases of hyperthyroidism in the UK, are aimed at stopping excess thyroid hormone production and ablating the thyroid gland. A prolonged course of antithyroid drugs induces a lasting remission in 30%–50% of subjects. The other treatment modalities results in permanent hypothyroidism, requiring replacement treatment with levothyroxine in most. Future efforts are likely to concentrate on novel and safe ways to modulate the underlying immune processes.

A long-term increase in all cause and vascular mortality after treatment of hyperthyroidism has been described. Induction of hypothyroidism after radioiodine treatment reduces the risk, possibly since hypothyroidism is the best marker of reversal of adverse tissue effects.

Toxic nodular hyperthyroidism

- Toxic nodular hyperthyroidism is more prevalent in older subjects. In addition to clinical features of hyperthyroidism, a palpable multinodular goitre or solitary thyroid may be present. Occasionally an autonomous thyroid nodule secretes only excess T3, resulting in T3 toxicosis (Table 2.4).
- The principles of treatment for hyperthyroidism due to toxic nodular adenoma and toxic nodular goitre are the same as those for Graves' hyperthyroidism. The underlying disease process does not remit and antithyroid drugs should therefore only be used in preparation of radioiodine administration of surgery.
- Low-dose long-term treatment with anti-thyroid drugs may be indicated in subjects with a short life expectancy and who are unfit for surgery or radioiodine therapy.
- Total thyroidectomy is the treatment of choice in those with large goitres, especially if compressive features are present. More limited surgery is indicated in those with a toxic adenoma.
- Cure rates following radioiodine administration are similar to those in Graves' disease, although rates of hypothyroidism are lower because radioisotope uptake is confined to autonomous nodules.

Thyroiditis

- Thyroiditis is an inflammation of the thyroid gland and results in thyrotoxicosis as a consequence of thyroid cell destruction (See Table 2.4 for diagnostic features).
- Subacute (de Quervain's) thyroiditis is associated with thyroid tenderness, fever, and malaise as well as features of thyrotoxicosis. Uptake of radioisotope is typically low on scans. Treatment is symptomatic with beta-adrenoceptor blockers and non-steroidal anti-inflammatory agents. Following a hyperthyroid state, there may be transient hypothyroidism but euthyroidism is usually restored after 4–6 weeks.
- Silent or painless thyroiditis is associated with lymphocytic infiltration of the thyroid, and levels of thyroid antibodies may be raised. Treatment with anti-thyroid drugs is contraindicated. Following a thyrotoxic state, there usually is a hypothyroid state which may resolve, although many subjects will develop permanent hypothyroidism.

Thyrotoxicosis during pregnancy and the post-partum period

Thyrotoxicosis in pregnancy

See also Chapter 9, Section 9.1.

- Graves' hyperthyroidism complicates 1 in 500 pregnancies. Normal pregnancy is associated with changes in thyroid function test results and, ideally, trimester-specific reference ranges should be used when evaluating thyroid function in pregnancy.
- A differential diagnosis with gestational thyrotoxicosis should be made in patient presenting with hyperthyroidism in pregnancy. This often complicates pregnancies associated with hyperemesis gravidarum and is driven by high levels of hCG stimulating the TSH receptor on thyroid cells. Clinical features such as the presence of a goitre or signs of Graves' ophthalmopathy point towards a diagnosis of Graves' disease rather than transient gestational thyrotoxicosis.
- Propylthiouracil is the anti-thyroid drug of choice in the first trimester of pregnancy, since it is associated with less teratogenic effects. If anti-thyroid drugs are required during the second trimester, a swap to carbimazole is advisable because of the potential liver failure associated with propylthiouracil.
- Radioactive iodine treatment is contraindicated, and surgery is rarely indicated. If thyroidectomy is required, this should be performed in the second trimester.
- Maternal TSH receptor antibodies may cross the placenta and result in fetal thyrotoxicosis. Guidelines recommend measurement of these antibodies at 20–24 weeks gestation in pregnant women with previous or existing Graves' thyrotoxicosis.

Thyrotoxicosis in the post-partum period

See also Chapter 9, Section 9.1.

- Whilst Graves' hyperthyroidism typically improves during pregnancy, relapse of this condition is common in the postpartum period.
- A differential diagnosis with postpartum thyroiditis needs to be established. This affects up to 10% of pregnancies and results in permanent hypothyroidism in up to 50%. It is likely to recur in subsequent pregnancies (up to 80%). Measurement of TSH receptor antibodies and radioisotope uptake scans may aid in establishing the differential diagnosis.
- Administration of carbimazole is safe during breastfeeding. Since anti-thyroid drugs will be excreted in breast milk, it is advisable to take these in divided doses and to monitor the baby's thyroid function when total doses of 20 mg (or 200 mg propylthiouracil) are taken.

Amiodarone-associated thyrotoxicosis

See also Section 2.6.

- Amiodarone is an iodine-containing drug, use of which frequently induces TFT abnormalities. A slight increase in FT4, transient increase in TSH, and decrease in FT3 are common and do not reflect thyroid dysfunction.
- Amiodarone-associated thyrotoxicosis is present in 6%–10% of subjects taking this drug and is associated with worsening of cardiovascular complications. Serum TSH should be suppressed, and FT4 as well as FT3 should be raised, to establish the diagnosis.
- Type 1 amiodarone-associated thyrotoxicosis is induced by the iodine load and occurs in people

predisposed to thyroid autoimmunity or if pre-existing thyroid nodules are present. This is best treated with high doses of carbimazole (a minimum of 40 mg daily).

- Type 2 amiodarone-associated thyrotoxicosis is a destructive thyroiditis as a consequence of toxic effects of amiodarone on the thyroid. This is best treated with prednisolone (40 mg daily), often in combination with anti-thyroid drugs.
- The distinction between both types may be difficult and many patients have features of both. Colour flow Doppler ultrasonography may detect increased vascularity in type 1 but in type 2.
- Discontinuation of amiodarone may be contraindicated and requires liaison between endocrinologist and cardiologist. Control of thyrotoxicosis may be achieved whilst amiodarone is continued.
- Radioiodine treatment is unfeasible because iodine uptake is low in both types due to the iodine load of the drug. Amiodarone needs to be discontinued for 6–12 months before considering radioiodine therapy in view of the long half-life of the drug.
- Thyroidectomy may be used in cases resistant to anti-thyroid drugs, but is often relatively contraindicated in view of significant coexisting cardiac morbidity.

Subclinical hyperthyroidism
See also Chapter 20, Section 20.1.

- Subclinical hyperthyroidism is a condition of slight thyroid hormone excess which may be associated with important adverse effects. It is characterized by a low serum TSH concentration with normal circulating thyroid hormone concentrations.
- These biochemical changes are commonly found in elderly patients in whom the prevalence is around 2%. It is more common in women and in areas of iodine deficiency.
- It is important to establish that the abnormalities are persistent and not due to non-thyroidal illness or to the taking of drugs such as glucocorticoids, especially if TSH is low but detectable.
- Over-replacement with thyroid hormones results in exogenous subclinical hyperthyroidism and should be managed by reducing the dose of replacement therapy until serum TSH normalizes.
- Graves' disease is the most common cause of subclinical hyperthyroidism in young patients and toxic nodular goitre or autonomous nodules become more prevalent with increasing age. Transient or persistent subclinical hyperthyroidism may occur following treatment of overt hyperthyroidism with anti-thyroid drugs or with radioactive iodine. If the underlying cause is not clear based on clinical features, an isotope scan may reveal a hot nodule.
- There is increasing evidence for an association with adverse clinical outcomes including atrial fibrillation, coronary heart disease, and increased mortality in subjects with underlying heart disease. Some, but not all, meta-analyses have demonstrated increased risks of all-cause mortality.
- Subclinical hyperthyroidism has also been associated with reduced bone mineral density and increased fracture risks especially in post-menopausal women. There

are conflicting results linking low serum TSH concentrations to reduced cognitive function and dementia.
- The need for treatment of subclinical hyperthyroidism remains controversial, especially since there are no randomized clinical trials demonstrating beneficial clinical outcomes following treatment. Expert panels recommend treating those with persistently undetectable serum TSH, those aged over 65 years, and those with cardiac risk, heart disease, or osteoporosis.
- If treatment is considered, administration of radioiodine is the therapeutic option of choice, especially in those with toxic nodular goitre. Long-term low-dose treatment with carbimazole is an option, especially if radioiodine treatment is not feasible. Large-scale randomized trials are needed to inform treatment decisions for patients with subclinical hyperthyroidism.

Further reading
Bartalena L, Baldeschi L, Dickinson A, et al. Consensus statement of the European Group on Graves' Orbitopathy (EUGOGO) on management of GO. *Eur J Endocrinol* 2008; 158: 273–85.

Bartalena L, Baldeschi L, Kostas B, et al.The 2016 European Thyroid Association/European Group on Graves' Orbitopathy guidelines for the management of Graves' orbitopathy. *Eur Thyroid J* 2016; 5: 9–26.

Boelaert K, Maisonneuve P, Torlinska B, et al. Comparison of mortality in hyperthyroidism during periods of treatment with thionamides and after radioiodine. *J Clin Endocrinol Metab* 2013; 98: 1869–82.

Boelaert K, Torlinska B, Holder RL, et al. Older subjects with hyperthyroidism present with a paucity of symptoms and signs: A large cross-sectional study. *J Clin Endocrinol Metab* 2010; 95: 2715–26.

Boelaert K. Thyroid dysfunction in the elderly. *Nat Rev Endocrinol* 2013; 9: 194–204.

Bogazzi F, Bartalena L, and Martino E. Approach to the patient with amiodarone-induced thyrotoxicosis. *J Clin Endocrinol Metab* 2010; 95: 2529–35.

Cooper DS and Biondi B. Subclinical thyroid disease. *Lancet* 2012; 379: 1142–54.

Franklyn JA and Boelaert K. Thyrotoxicosis. *Lancet* 2012; 379: 1155–66.

Perros P, Dayan CM, Dickinson AJ, et al. Management of patients with Graves' orbitopthy: Initial assessment, managemenmt outside specialised centres and referral pathways. *Clin Med* 2015; 15: 173–8.

Perros P and Wiersinga WM. The Amsterdam declaration on Graves' orbitopathy. *Thyroid* 2010; 20; 245–6.

Ross DS, Burch HB, Cooper DS, et al. 2016 American Thyroid Association guidelines for diagnosis and management of hyperthyroidism and other causes of thyrotoxicosis. *Thyroid* 2016; 26: 1343–1420.

Salvi M, Vannucchi G, Curro N, et al. Efficacy of B-cell targeted therapy with rituximab in patients with active modearte to severe Graves' orbitopathy: A randomized controlled study. *J Clin Endocrinol Metab* 2015; 100; 422–31.

Stagnaro-Green A, Abalovich M, Alexander E, et al. Guidelines of the American Thyroid Association for the diagnosis and management of thyroid disease during pregnancy and postpartum. *Thyroid* 2011; 21: 1081–125.

Tunbridge WM, Evered DC, Hall R, et al. The spectrum of thyroid disease in a community: The Whickham survey. *Clin Endocrinol (Oxf)* 1977; 7: 481–93.

2.6 Thyroiditis

Definition

Thyroiditis is defined as inflammation of the thyroid gland, and may result in temporary or permanent thyroid dysfunction.

General clinical features of thyroiditis

Many patients have few specific symptoms and are diagnosed following abnormal TFT results. Others present with clinical symptoms of hyper- or, more usually, hypothyroidism, and some have a history of neck pain.

Thyroiditis-induced hyperthyroidism

Inflammatory destruction of the thyroid may lead to release of thyroid hormones and transitory hyperthyroidism. Distinguishing this from hyperthyroidism due to increased thyroid hormone synthesis may be challenging (Table 2.6). Graves' ophthalmopathy is specific and so can be a useful diagnostic observation. Most patients with hyperthyroidism due to thyroiditis do not require treatment; a minority may benefit from beta-adrenoceptor blockade to control the adrenergic symptoms. Thionamides, which inhibit thyroid hormone synthesis for use in autoimmune hyperthyroidism, are not effective in thyroiditis, but when given in cases of diagnostic uncertainly usually do not have adverse effect.

Thyroiditis-induced hypothyroidism

Patients with thyroiditis commonly develop hypothyroidism, which is treated with T4 replacement. The goal of this therapy is to normalize the TSH levels. The hypothyroidism may be temporary, especially with post-partum or subacute thyroiditis. Therefore, consideration should be given to withdrawing T4 and re-assessing thyroid status.

Causes of thyroiditis

The causes of thyroiditis are diverse (Box 2.3) and each pathological entity will be discussed individually.

Autoimmune-mediated thyroiditis

Hashimoto's thyroiditis

Hashimoto's thyroiditis is the most common autoimmune disorder and is, in iodine-replete populations, the most common cause of hypothyroidism. It was first described in 1912 as a painless enlargement of the thyroid with lymphocytic infiltration and germinal centre formation, occurring mainly in elderly women. The autoimmune response is thought to be triggered by the activation of thyroid-antigen-specific helper T-cells. Once activated, these helper T-cells induce B-cells to make anti-thyroid antibodies. The anti- thyroid antibodies most frequently measured are anti-thyroid peroxidase antibodies and anti-thyroglobulin antibodies; these antibodies are complement fixing, and their presence tends to correlate with thyroidal damage and lymphatic infiltration.

The landmark epidemiological Wickham study, a cross-sectional study of 2779 subjects living in rural and urban communities, was performed in North East England in the 1970s. The prevalence of spontaneous hypothyroidism was 1%–2%, was ten times more common in women than men, and was even more prevalent in older women (Vanderpump et al., 2002): 60% of subjects with a TSH > 6 were positive for anti-thyroid antibodies. Subsequent studies in Europe, Japan, and the US confirmed these findings, indicating that they have wide applicability to iodine-replete populations.

A significant proportion of the population has circulating anti-thyroid antibodies (anti-thyroid peroxidase and/or anti-thyroglobulin) but is biochemically euthyroid (see also Chapter 1, Section 1.5). Interestingly, positivity for anti-thyroid antibodies correlates with the presence of focal thyroiditis on thyroid biopsy and at post-mortem. In a 20-year follow-up of the Wickham study, with data from 1277 known survivors, the mean incidence of spontaneous hypothyroidism was 3.5/1000 per year in women, and 0.6/1000 per year for men. An elevated TSH at baseline was associated with an OR of developing hypothyroidism that was 8 for women and 44 for men. Positivity for anti-thyroid antibodies was associated with an OR of 8 for women and 25 for men; when accompanied by elevated TSH, it is associated with an OR of 38 for women and 178 for men. Thus, positivity for anti-thyroid antibodies, and elevated TSH, predict a risk of future hypothyroidism, both individually and even more strongly together.

Clinically, in Hashimoto's thyroiditis there may be a firm, bumpy, symmetrical, painless goitre or, in about 10% patients, the thyroid is atrophic. Whilst some patients may develop transient hyperthyroidism, or 'Hashitoxicosis', the majority are hypothyroid. Anti-thyroid peroxidase antibodies should be measured and are positive in 90% of patients. Anti-thyroglobulin antibodies are present in fewer patients (20%–50%) and may be less useful clinically. Although thyroid lymphoma is rare, the relative risk is increased in Hashimoto's by over 60-fold. Patients with Hashimoto's thyroiditis may also develop papillary and follicular thyroid cancers, although there is no clear evidence of an increased risk compared with the general population. As in all patients, thyroid nodules should undergo consideration for fine-needle aspiration with cytological examination.

Table 2.6 Distinguishing destructive thyroiditis-induced thyrotoxicosis from hyperthyroidism due to Graves' disease or toxic nodular goitre

	Graves'	Toxic nodular goitre	Thyroiditis
T3/T4 ratio	Increased	Increased	Reduced
TSH receptor antibody	Usually elevated	Negative	Negative
Thyroid uptake scan	Homogeneous increased uptake	Discrete area(s) of increased uptake	Suppressed uptake
Clinical course (without therapy)	Persistent hyperthyroidism	Persistent hyperthyroidism	Progression to euthyroidism and possibly hypothyroidism

---

Box 2.3 Causes of thyroiditis

- Autoimmune:
  - Hashimoto's thyroiditis
  - post-partum thyroiditis
- Subacute thyroiditis
- Drug induced
- Radiation induced
- Acute infectious thyroiditis
- Riedel's chronic sclerosing thyroiditis

Box 2.4 Clinical features of subacute thyroiditis

- Prodrome of generalized myalgias, pharyngitis, low-grade fever, and fatigue
- Weight loss; appetite is inhibited with the viral illness whilst metabolism is increased related to thyroid function
- Severe neck pain and/or swelling
- Markedly elevated ESR and elevated CRP
- Usually negative thyroid antibodies
- Thyrotoxicosis in about 50% patients
- May develop hypothyroidism lasting 4–6 months

For the vast majority of patients with Hashimoto's thyroiditis, the treatment is lifelong T4 replacement for hypothyroidism.

Post-partum thyroiditis
See also Section 10.1. Post-partum thyroiditis may be defined as the occurrence of de novo thyroid disease, excluding Graves' disease, in the first year post partum. There is a large variation in the prevalence of post-partum thyroiditis, ranging from 1.1% to 16.7%. Post-partum thyroiditis is thought to be autoimmune mediated because the majority patients with post-partum thyroiditis are positive for anti-thyroid antibodies, and the immunological rebound following pregnancy may be the precipitant. Cytology from fine-needle aspiration shows lymphocytic thyroiditis, as seen in Hashimoto's. In patients with Hashimoto's thyroiditis and post-partum thyroiditis, there is an increased incidence of HLA subtypes DR3, DR4, and DR5. Patients with autoimmune diseases such as type 1 diabetes mellitus and systemic lupus erythematosus (SLE) have a greater risk of developing post-partum thyroiditis. TFT screening for post-partum thyroiditis should be considered at 3 months post partum in patients with type 1 diabetes or other autoimmune disease, a history of anti-thyroid peroxidase antibodies, or a history of miscarriage, or who develop post-partum depression.

The classical clinical course is of hyperthyroidism 2–10 months post partum for 2–3 months, which may need symptomatic beta-adrenoceptor blockade. Hypothyroidism (2–12 months post partum) follows or may be the only feature, which is treated with T4, and then there may be spontaneous resolution to euthyroidism. Not all patients go through all three phases.

Following post-partum thyroiditis, there is a 20%–40% incidence of permanent hypothyroidism. Women who are not considering pregnancy at the time should be given a trial of T4 therapy withdrawal with monitoring of thyroid function. Thereafter, annual TFT screening should be performed.

Subacute thyroiditis
Subacute thyroiditis is the most common cause of thyroid pain. It is a self-limiting process that usually follows an upper respiratory tract infection. A viral cause has therefore been suggested and HTLV-1, enterovirus, rubella, mumps virus, HSV, EBV, and parvovirus have been identified in patients with subacute thyroiditis. However, there is no clear evidence of a causative effect. The features can be local thyroidal inflammatory symptoms, those of a generalized viral illness, or those of a thyroid function disorder (see Box 2.4).

The treatment for the hyperthyroid phase is symptomatic and includes NSAIDs for neck pain, and glucocorticoids for severe neck pain (e.g. prednisolone 40 mg tapering over 4–6 weeks). Beta-adrenoceptor blockers are used to treat adrenergic symptoms. The hypothyroid phase tends to be transitory; hence, T4 therapy is not usually required but can be given to symptomatic patients. The majority of patients recover completely. Subacute thyroiditis has a low incidence of permanent hypothyroidism of about 5% and an even lower rate of recurrence of 2%.

Drug-induced thyroiditis
Patients on the medications shown in Box 2.5 should have TFTs and anti-thyroid peroxidase antibodies measured at baseline and thereafter every 6–12 months. Whilst amiodarone may need to be discontinued in consultation with the cardiologist, the other medications are usually continued and the thyroid dysfunction treated.

Amiodarone
Amiodarone inhibits the peripheral conversion of T4 to T3, routinely causing a slight rise in TSH. Significant thyroid dysfunction occurs in 15%–20% patients on amiodarone, and there is a relatively higher proportion of hypothyroidism in iodine-deficient areas. In a study of 303 consecutive Dutch patients treated with amiodarone, 6% developed hypothyroidism, which was predicted by elevated baseline TSH but not gender, and 8% developed thyrotoxicosis, which was predicted only by younger age (<62 years). There are two, potentially overlapping, aetiologies of amiodarone-induced hypothyroidism: type 1, which is attributable to amiodarone's high iodine content and occurs in an 'abnormal thyroid', such as a nodular goitre; and type 2, which is a destructive inflammatory

---

Box 2.5 Drugs that may induce thyroiditis

Drugs that may induce thyroiditis include:
- amiodarone
- lithium
- interferon alfa
- interleukin 2
- biological therapies (alemtuzumab, ipilimumab, nivolumab, pembrolizumab)
- tyrosine kinase inhibitors

Table 2.7 Type 1 and Type 2 amiodarone-induced thyroiditis

	Type 1	Type 2
Aetiology	Iodine load on 'abnormal thyroid'	Destructive inflammatory thyroiditis
Thyroid uptake scan	May be low in iodine-replete populations	Very low
Ultrasound	Increased vascularity	Decreased vascularity
Treatment	Stop amiodarone if feasible	High-dose glucocorticoids, e.g. prednisolone 30–50 mg daily
	Thionamides	

thyroiditis that may occur in a normal thyroid (Table 2.7). Thyrotoxicosis poses a significant risk to patients with underlying cardiac disease, and therefore euthyroidism should be restored as quickly as possible. However, the large fat stores of amiodarone mean that, even if the drug can be discontinued, continued release of amiodarone can stimulate thyroiditis for many months, hampering treatment.

Numerous investigations have been suggested to allow the differential diagnosis of the type of amiodarone-induced hypothyroidism and guide management, although none has been definitive. Theoretically, the treatment of type 1 amiodarone-induced hypothyroidism is with thionamides, whereas type 2 is treated with corticosteroids. A management protocol based on a therapeutic trial rather than insensitive investigations, as described by Vanderpump, has proved very useful. At diagnosis, amiodarone is discontinued if possible: 40 mg carbimazole and 40 mg prednisolone a day are used for 2 weeks. If the serum T3 is unchanged. diagnose type 1 amiodarone-induced hypothyroidism and stop the prednisolone. Surgery or radioactive iodine could be considered at a later stage. If the serum T3 is decreased by >50%, diagnose type 2 amiodarone-induced hypothyroidism and stop the carbimazole.

Lithium
Lithium is concentrated by the thyroid and inhibits thyroid hormone release. In a study of 718 patients on lithium, 10% were found to be hypothyroid; thus, patients on lithium require baseline and monitoring of TFTs every 12 months. Whether lithium alters thyroid autoimmunity is controversial. Analysis is complicated by the fact that lithium is often be given to middle-aged women who have a relatively high rate of baseline thyroid autoimmunity.

Interferon alfa
Interferon alfa is a central component of therapy for patients with chronic hepatitis C, in addition to its use in multiple sclerosis. Symptomatic hypothyroidism was observed in 3% of interferon-treated patients, and 20% patients were found to have abnormal TSH. In up to 15% patients without thyroid autoimmunity, anti-thyroid peroxidase antibodies will develop during interferon antibody therapy, and this may lead to a destructive thyroiditis or, less commonly, Graves' disease. Thyroid function usually resolves at the end of cytotoxic therapy, but patients are at risk of autoimmune thyroiditis in the future.

Tyrosine kinase inhibitors
Tyrosine kinase inhibitors, such as sunitinib, have been associated with thyroid dysfunction, which may be due to antibody-negative destructive thyroiditis.

Radiation-induced thyroiditis
Radiation-induced thyroiditis is a relatively uncommon event, compared to atrophy of the thyroid following radiotherapy.

Acute infectious thyroiditis
Acute infectious thyroiditis is usually caused by bacteria, but can be due to viral or fungal infection. The thyroid is usually resistant to infection because of its encapsulation, high iodine content, rich blood supply, and extensive lymphatic drainage. Therefore, infectious thyroiditis is rare but may occur in patients with pre-existing thyroid disease or congenital thyroid abnormalities and in the immunocompromised, particularly in those with HIV and *Pneumocystis jiroveci* infection.

Acute infectious thyroiditis is potentially life-threatening and needs to be diagnosed and treated quickly. Patients with acute bacterial infection tend to be acutely unwell (see Box 2.6). The key diagnostic step is Gram staining and culture of fine-needle aspiration material. First-line therapies include surgical drainage of any abscess and systemic antibiotics, as guided by fine-needle aspiration culture. In contrast, infectious thyroiditis due to fungi, parasites, or opportunistic infections tends to be much more insidious.

Riedel's thyroiditis
Riedel's thyroiditis may be defined as progressive fibrosis of the thyroid gland, which may extend to surrounding tissues as part of a systemic fibrotic process. In thyroidectomy specimens, Riedel's thyroiditis is only found in 0.05 %, indicating how rarely this occurs. Clinically, patients present with a rock-hard, painless, and immobile goitre. They may have symptoms of oesophageal or tracheal compression or hypoparathyroidism due to infiltration of surrounding tissues. Most patients are euthyroid at diagnosis but become hypothyroid as the fibrosis progresses. Diagnosis is made by open biopsy and the first-line treatment is surgical thyroidectomy, although therapy with glucocorticoids has reported to be effective in the early stages of the disease in isolated cases.

Box 2.6 Clinical features of acute bacterial thyroiditis

- Fever
- Anterior neck pain
- Erythema
- Dysphagia
- Dysphonia
- Elevated ESR, CRP
- Usually normal thyroid function tests

References and further reading

Ahmed S, Van Gelder IC, Wiesfeld AC, et al. Determinants and outcome of amiodarone-associated thyroid dysfunction. *Clin Endocrinol (Oxf)* 2011; 75: 388–94.

Bogazzi F, Bartalena L, and Martino E. Amiodarone-induced thyrotoxicosis. *J Clin Endocrinol Metab* 2010; 95: 2529–35.

De Lange WE, Freling NJ, Molenaar WM, et al. Invasive fibrous thyroiditis (Riedel's struma): A manifestation of multifocal fibrosclerosis? A case report with review of the literature. *Q J Med* 1989; 72: 709–17.

Desai J, Yassa L, Marqusee E, et al. Hypothyroidism after sunitinib treatment for patients with gastrointestinal stromal tumors. *Ann Intern Med* 2006; 145: 660–4.

Desailloud R and Hober D. Viruses and thyroiditis: An update. *Virol J* 2009; 6: 5.

Han TS, Williams GR, and Vanderpump MP. Benzofuran derivatives and the thyroid. *Clin Endocrinol (Oxf)* 2009; 70: 2–13.

Holm L-E, Blomgren H, and Lowhagen T. Cancer risks in patients with chronic lymphocytic thyroiditis. *N Engl J Med* 1985; 312: 601–4.

Iitaka M, Momotani N, Ishii J, et al. Incidence of subacute thyroiditis recurrences after a prolonged latency: 24-year survey. *J Clin Endocrinol Metab* 1996; 81: 466–9.

Kitchener MI and Chapman IM. Subacute thyroiditis: A review of 105 cases. *Clin Nucl Med* 1989; 14: 439–42.

Johnston AM and Eagles JM. Lithium-associated clinical hypothyroidism. Prevalence and risk factors. *Br J Psychiatry* 1999; 175: 336–9.

Pearce EN, Farwell AP, and Braverman LE. Mechanisms of thyroiditis *N Engl J Med* 2003; 348: 2646–55.

Stagnaro-Green A. Clinical review 152: Postpartum thyroiditis. *J Clin Endocrinol Metab* 2002; 87: 4042–7.

Vanderpump MP and Tunbridge WM. Epidemiology and prevention of clinical and subclinical hypothyroidism. *Thyroid* 2002; 12: 839–47.

2.7 Hypothyroidism

Introduction

In primary hypothyroidism, the thyroid gland produces insufficient amounts of thyroid hormones, whilst in secondary hypothyroidism there is inadequate secretion of either TSH from the pituitary or TRH from the hypothalamus. The presentation varies from asymptomatic to, rarely, multisystem organ failure ('myxoedema coma').

Epidemiology

The prevalence of hypothyroidism is approximately 1%–2% in the adult population; there is increasing occurrence with older age (mean age at diagnosis 60 years), and women are affected ten times more than men (Vanderpump et al.,1995; Vanderpump, 2011). The biggest worldwide cause of hypothyroidism is iodine deficiency, which is present in one-third of the world's population (see Chapter 1, Section 1.7). In the developed world, chronic autoimmune (Hashimoto's) thyroiditis is the commonest cause of hypothyroidism, followed by iatrogenic causes and other causes (see Table 2.8).

There is no consensus as to the necessity of population screening for hypothyroidism. However, patients who are planning pregnancy and are at high risk of hypothyroidism should be screened; these include those with:

- maternal age >30 years
- positivity for anti-thyroid peroxidase antibodies
- a family history of thyroid dysfunction
- a history of head and neck irradiation
- type 1 diabetes
- other known autoimmune disease
- a history of unexplained miscarriage
- a history of preterm delivery
- a history of childhood malignancy
- a history of residing in an area of known iodine insufficiency
- a history of infertility

Pathophysiology

The thyroid gland produces T4 and T3, which circulate bound to the carrier proteins TBG, transthyretin, and albumin. The 'free' thyroid hormone levels (i.e. unbound fraction) have become preferred analytes. T3 binds to nuclear thyroid hormone receptors (alpha and beta isoforms) to mediate most biologic actions. T4 is converted to T3 by peripheral deiodination.

Thyroid hormone production is controlled by a negative feedback loop, where the hypothalamic–pituitary–adrenal axis hormones TRH and TSH stimulate the release of T4 and T3, which in turn feedback negatively onto the axis. Dietary iodine >50 µg daily is an essential component of thyroid hormone synthesis (WHO guidelines for pregnancy recommend a dietary and supplemental intake of >250 µg/day). Increased serum TSH (with normal T4) can indicate early hypothyroidism, although providing negative feedback at the pituitary is normal. With progression to overt hypothyroidism, first serum FT4 and then FT3 concentrations become subnormal.

Chronic autoimmune (Hashimoto's) thyroiditis

See also Section 2.6. In chronic autoimmune (Hashimoto's) thyroiditis, the thyroid is destroyed by cytotoxic T cells and cytokines. Antibodies against thyroid peroxidase and thyroglobulin are usually present. Some patients with thyroid antibodies remain euthyroid, and their risk of developing hypothyroidism is 4% per year. However 10%–15% of patients may be antibody negative. A goitre may be present early in the natural history of Hashimoto's disease, progressing to thyroid atrophy over many years. . Histologic studies have shown diffuse lymphocytic and plasma cell infiltration of the thyroid. The compensated or subclinical phase is characterized by an elevated serum TSH with serum FT4 and T3 in the normal range.

The risks of papillary thyroid cancer and malignant thyroid lymphoma are slightly increased in Hashimoto's disease, although lymphomas are very rare.

Silent thyroiditis, including post-partum thyroiditis

This is a variant of autoimmune thyroiditis where anti-thyroid antibodies are often present. Transient hypothyroidism is common, lasting 2–8 weeks, (sometimes preceded by a thyrotoxic phase), before spontaneous recovery. The risk of permanent hypothyroidism is up to 30% at 5 years. The incidence of post-partum thyroiditis is approximately 5% per year and is up to 30% if anti-thyroid antibodies are detected during pregnancy.

Subacute thyroiditis

See also Section 2.5. Hypothyroidism may occur during the recovery phase of subacute thyroiditis but spontaneous recovery is usual and permanent hypothyroidism is rare.

Drug-induced hypothyroidism: Amiodarone, iodine, lithium, interferon alfa, tyrosine kinase inhibitors, and immunomodulators

- Amiodarone contains a large iodine load and can cause many aberrations of thyroid function. For example, in patients taking amiodarone, an initial increase in FT4 with a reduced FT3 may be seen, due to inhibition of peripheral deiodination of T4. Thyroid dysfunction (hypo- or hyper-) may develop in 14%–18% of amiodarone-treated subjects (Martino et al., 2001). Hypothyroidism more commonly occurs in iodine-replete patients. Treatment is withdrawal of the drug if possible, with or without T4.
- Iodine from the diet or other sources, including Lugol's iodine and radiocontrast, can cause the Wolff–Chaikoff effect, a transient 'stunning' of thyroid hormone synthesis and release.
- Lithium inhibits thyroid iodine transport and the release of T4 and T3. This may resolve on drug cessation but permanent hypothyroidism occurs in about 20% of long-term lithium-treated subjects and is more likely in those who are positive for anti-thyroid antibodies.
- Hypothyroidism is seen in around 5% of patients on interferon alfa therapy, and this can persist even after treatment cessation.
- Tyrosine kinase inhibitors such as sunitinib can induce hypothyroidism via a reduction of glandular vascularity and the induction of type 3 deiodinase activity (Kappers et al, 2011). Increased T4 requirements are seen in thyroidectomized patients taking tyrosine kinase inhibitors.
- Immunomodulators such as PD-1 and CTLA-4 inhibitors can also induce hypothyroidism.

Table 2.8 Primary and secondary causes of hypothyroidism

Cause of hypothyroidism		TSH	T4	Other
Primary				
Congenital	Thyroid dysgenesis- defective embryonic formation of gland; complete or partial with lingual/sublingual location.	↑	Normal or ↓	
	Usually sporadic			
	Rarely heritable (autosomal recessive): mutations in *FOXE1, NKX2–1,* or *PAX8*			
	Thyroid dyshormonogenesis; thyroid gland present, but reduced function (typically heritable, autosomal recessive):	↑	Normal or ↓	
	• thyroglobulin defects			
	• TPO defects			
	• sodium–iodine symporter defects			
	• DUOX defects			
	• TSH receptor defects			
	• Pendred syndrome (familial organification syndrome associated with congenital deafness, due to mutation in *PDS*)			
Acquired	Chronic autoimmune (Hashimoto's) thyroiditis	↑	Normal or ↓	anti-TPO and anti-Tg antibodies
	Silent thyroiditis (including post partum)	↑	Normal or ↓	
	Subacute thyroiditis	↑	Normal or ↓	
	Drug induced (e.g. amiodarone, interferon, iodides, thionamides, tyrosine kinase inhibitors (e.g. sunitinib), or biological therapies (e.g. CTLA-4 inhibitor)	↑	Normal or ↓	
	Post-surgical/radiotherapy	↑	Normal or ↓	
Secondary				
Pituitary	Isolated TSH deficiency	Low-normal or ↓	Low-normal or ↓	Other pit profile hormones normal
	Panhypopituitarism	Low-normal or ↓	Low-normal or ↓	↓ Pit profile hormones
Hypothalamic	Congenital	Low-normal or ↓	Low-normal or ↓	
	Infection	Low-normal or ↓	Low-normal or ↓	
	Neoplasia including craniopharyngioma	Low-normal or ↓	Low-normal or ↓	
	Infiltration e.g. sarcoid, lymphocytic, or granulomatous hypophysitis	Low-normal or ↓	Low-normal or ↓	
	Haemorrhagic necrosis (Sheehan's syndrome)	Low-normal or ↓	Low-normal or ↓	

Abbreviations: Tg, thyroglobulin; TPO, thyroid peroxidase.

Congenital hypothyroidism

Congenital hypothyroidism occurs with a frequency of 1 in 3000–4000, a frequency which is geographically constant. The major cause worldwide continues to be iodine deficiency causing endemic cretinism (Delange, 2001).

Other causes of congenital hypothyroidism can be explained by the failure of one or more components of the developing hypothalamic–pituitary–thyroid axis: in 80%–90% of cases, thyroid agenesis, hypoplasia, or ectopy occur and, in 10%, a disorder of thyroid hormone synthesis causes hypothyroidism with goitre (dyshormonogenesis); very uncommonly, secondary or

tertiary hypothyroidism results from pituitary or hypothalamic dysfunction, respectively.

The introduction of neonatal screening programmes in many countries has resulted in a dramatic decline in morbidity due to congenital hypothyroidism. In particular, the dramatic improvement of its neurological sequelae is now possible by prompt and adequate replacement of thyroid hormone, regardless of the cause of its deficiency.

Sick euthyroid syndrome (non-thyroidal illness)

Sick euthyroid syndrome is seen in the context of starvation or severe illness such as severe sepsis, cardiac failure, renal failure, and end-stage malignancy. Tissue thyroid hormone concentrations are very low, and there is low total and FT3, often with low/low-normal T4, and low or low-normal serum TSH, but T4 replacement is generally not indicated as there is no clear evidence that treatment is beneficial or safe (Grozinsky-Glasberg et al. 2006).

Clinical symptoms of hypothyroidism

Clinical symptoms of hypothyroidism include fatigue, weight gain, cold intolerance, constipation, impaired concentration, dry skin, oedema, mood change, myalgias, and menorrhagia. These can be subtle in Hashimoto's disease or more sudden and severe in those who undergo thyroidectomy without thyroid hormone replacement.

Clinical signs of hypothyroidism

Clinical signs of hypothyroidism include weight change, myxoedematous facies, thinning of the hair and eyebrows, bradycardia, diastolic hypertension, reduced deep tendon reflexes with prolongation of the relaxation phase, macroglossia, ataxia, cold peripheries, thickened ridged nails, disinterest/depression, dysphonia, and sleep apnoea.

Biochemical abnormalities in hypothyroidism

Hyponatraemia may be seen in hypothyroidism, due to reduced renal tubular loss or, less commonly, due to coexisting cortisol deficiency. Elevation of LDL, triglycerides, and cholesterol is seen and creatinine kinase is elevated in severe hypothyroidism. Serum prolactin is elevated in primary hypothyroidism, probably due to increased TRH which stimulates pituitary lactotrophs. Anaemia and macrocytosis are described and coexisting vitamin B_{12} deficiency should be considered.

Investigations in hypothyroidism

Investigations in hypothyroidism should include:
- TSH
- FT4
- FT3
- anti-thyroid peroxidase antibodies
- anti-thyroglobulin antibodies
- anti-TSH receptor antibodies (more commonly associated with Graves' thyroid disease)

Imaging in hypothyroidism

Ultrasound is not needed for a diagnosis of autoimmune thyroid disease, but may be useful for assessing thyroid size, echotexture, and the presence of thyroid nodules.

Management of hypothyroidism

Medical management of hypothyroidism

Thyroid hormone replacement with T4 is usually for life. Adult patients typically require 1.6–1.8 μg/kg day^{-1} but smaller doses may suffice in mild cases and in the elderly, and larger doses may be needed in thyroidectomized patients. The goal of therapy is to return TSH into the normal range; serum FT4 should also be within reference range. It takes at least 4 weeks for TSH levels to reach a steady state. In secondary hypothyroidism, measurement of serum TSH is *not* clinically meaningful, and T4 replacement should be titrated to keep serum FT4 in the upper half of the normal range. Patients over 50 years and younger patients with cardiac disease are started on a low dose of 25 μg per day, with clinical and biochemical re-evaluation in 6–8 weeks.

A number of medications interfere with the gastrointestinal absorption of T4, and should be separated from T4 ingestion by at least 1–2 hours. These include calcium carbonate, ferrous sulfate, aluminium hydroxide, and colestyramine.

T4 dose adjustments may be required for patients on long-term proton-pump inhibitors, anticonvulsants, and rifampicin. In addition, patients who have undergone bariatric surgery, have undergone bowel resection with short-bowel syndrome, or have coeliac disease often require increased doses of T4 to maintain the euthyroid state.

Patients with a normal TSH who are positive for anti-thyroid antibodies will need monitoring of TSH every 6–12 months, but antibody titres will not need to be re-measured.

Congenital hypothyroidism detected by neonatal screening should be treated as soon as possible.

Concerning T3 administration, randomized controlled trials do not favour a benefit for levothyroxine combined with liothyronine versus levothyroxine alone, but T3 may be appropriate for initiating therapy in patients with severe (myxoedematous) hypothyroidism and may be used intravenously. Differential expression of thyroid hormone receptor subtypes in brain versus other tissues has led to attempted T3 therapy in patients who feel tired on T4 alone (despite a normal TSH); although this approach is not well supported by evidence, it can be effective in occasional patients.

Treatment of subclinical hypothyroidism is controversial but studies favour treatment if the patient is under 65, has heart failure, or is pregnant or considering conception. Treatment in patients with serum TSH levels of 5–10 mU/L may lead to a reduction in cardiovascular mortality, but this is controversial (Rodondi et al. 2010).

Special scenarios

Pregnancy

Pregnancy induces an increased need for T4 (see also Chapter 10, Section 10.1). Women with hypothyroidism typically require an increase of about 30%–40% in their pre-pregnancy T4 dose in order to maintain serum TSH in the appropriate range. Pregnancy-specific normal ranges apply for serum TSH (Garber et al, 2012); note that a transient reduction in serum TSH levels typically occurs toward the end of the first trimester, secondary to high circulating levels of hCG, which cross-reacts with the TSH receptor. Measurements of TSH in pregnancy are still more accurate than measurements of T4. Target levels are summarized in Table 2.9. The increase in the

Table 2.9 Trimester-specific ranges and targets

Trimester	TSH normal ranges (mIU/L)
First	0.1–2.5
Second	0.2– 3.0
Third	0.3– 3.0

Data from Stagnaro-Green A, Abalovich M, Alexander E, et al. Guidelines of the American Thyroid Association for the diagnosis and management of thyroid disease during pregnancy and postpartum. *Thyroid* 2011; 21: 1081–1125 and De Groot L, Abalovich M, Alexander EK, et al. Management of thyroid dysfunction during pregnancy and postpartum: an Endocrine Society clinical practice guideline. *J Clin Endocrinol Metab* 2012; 97: 2543–2565.

T4 requirement is thought to be due to increased levels of TBG, use by the foetus, and metabolism of T4 by the fetoplacental unit. Return to pre-pregnancy requirements occurs 6–8 weeks post partum.

Myxoedema crisis

Extreme hypothyroidism is uncommon but has a mortality rate of 60%. It may occur with long-standing, undiagnosed hypothyroidism or discontinuation of T4 replacement therapy, or when there is failure to institute T4 replacement after thyroid ablation or surgery. It may be precipitated by intercurrent illness and by drugs that depress the respiratory drive. If a myxoedema crisis occurs, T4 should be administered intravenously or via a nasogastric tube in a loading dose of 4 µg/kg of lean body weight (i.e. about 300–600 µg). A daily maintenance dose should be continued thereafter at 50–100 µg/day; intensive care admission is usually required. Parenteral hydrocortisone is often administered but the evidence base for this is weak.

Persistently elevated TSH despite T4 replacement

Persistently elevated TSH despite T4 replacement most commonly occurs due to lack of compliance; if TSH still elevated when the T4 dose is 1.6 µg/kg per day, consider malabsorption or drug interference. In that case, consider administering a T4 absorption test or supervised weekly dosing, possibly in solution. Also consider interference with TSH assay.

Use of alternative biological preparations

The use of alternative biological preparations in treating hypothyroidism is not recommended, as they are often unphysiological and poorly standardised (e.g. Armour Thyroid can contain a threefold excess of T3 (British Thyroid Association Executive Committee, 2007).

Patient support groups/useful websites

Two patient support groups/useful websites are as follows:

- http://thyroidguidelines.net/hypothyroidism
- http://www.endotext.org/

References and further reading

British Thyroid Association Executive Committee. Armour Thyroid (USP) and Combined Thyroxine/Tri-Oidothyronin as Thyroid Hormone Replacement, 2007. Available at http://british-thyroid-association.org/sandbox/bta2016/bta_statement_on_the_use_of_armour_thyroid_and_combined_t4_and_t3.pdf (accessed 19 Dec 2017).

Delange F. Iodine deficiency as a cause of brain damage. *Postgrad Med J* 2001; 77: 217–20.

Garber JR, Cobin RH, Gharib H, et al. Clinical practice guidelines for hypothyroidism in adults: Cosponsored by the American Association of Clinical Endocrinologists and the American Thyroid Association. *Thyroid* 2012; 22: 1200–35.

Grozinsky-Glasberg S, Fraser A, Nahshoni E, et al. Thyroxine-triiodothyronine combination therapy versus thyroxine monotherapy for clinical hypothyroidism: Meta-analysis of randomized controlled trials. *J Clin Endocrinol Metab* 2006; 91: 2592–9.

Hyland KA, Arnold AM, Lee JS, et al. Persistent subclinical hypothyroidism and cardiovascular risk in the elderly: The cardiovascular health study. *J Clin Endocrinol Metab* 2013; 98: 533–40.

Kappers MH, van Esch JH, Smedts FM, et al. Sunitinib-induced hypothyroidism is due to induction of type 3 deiodinase activity and thyroidal capillary regression. *J Clin Endocrinol Metab* 2011; 96: 3087–94.

Klein I. Subclinical hypothyroidism: Just a high serum thyrotropin (TSH) concentration or something else? *J Clin Endocrinol Metab* 2013; 98: 508–10.

Martino E, Bartalena L, Bogazzi F, et al. The effects of amiodarone on the thyroid. *Endocr Rev* 2001; 22: 240–54.

Okosieme O, Gilbert J, Abraham P, et al. Management of primary hypothyroidism: Statement by the British Thyroid Association Executive Committee. *Clin Endocrinol* 2016; 84: 799–808.

Razvi S, Weaver JU, Butler TJ, et al, Levothyroxine treatment of subclinical hypothyroidism, fatal and nonfatal cardiovascular events, and mortality. *Arch Intern Med* 2012; 172: 811–7.

Rodondi N, Den Elzen WP, Bauer DC, et al. Subclinical hypothyroidism and the risk of coronary heart disease and mortality. *JAMA* 2010; 304: 1365–74.

Tunbridge WM and Vanderpump MP. Population screening for autoimmune thyroid disease. *Endocrinol Metab Clin North Am* 2000; 29: 239–53.

Vanderpump MP. The epidemiology of thyroid disease. *Br Med Bull* 2011; 99: 39–51.

Vanderpump MP, Tunbridge WM, French J, et al., The incidence of thyroid disorders in the community: A twenty-year follow-up of the Whickham Survey. *Clin Endocrinol (Oxf)* 1995; 43: 55–68.

Völzke H, Schmidt CO, John U, et al. Reference levels for serum thyroid function tests of diagnostic and prognostic significance. *Horm Metab Res* 2010; 42: 809–14.

2.8 Thyroid nodules and cancer

Non-toxic goitres

Epidemiology of non-toxic goitres
Thyroid enlargement (goitre) is common; in the original UK Whickham community survey, euthyroid goitre was present in 23% females and 5% of males, becoming less frequent (10% and 2%, respectively) when subjects were reassessed 20 years later. The decreasing frequency of goitre with age contrasts with the increasing frequency of nodules in older patients.

Pathophysiology of non-toxic goitres
Diffuse non-toxic goitre generally arises from prolonged TSH stimulation in response to:
- iodine deficiency
- exposure to goitrogens (drugs such as amiodarone and lithium, and environmental goitrogens such as thiocyanate contained in cassava and cabbage)
- inborn errors of thyroid hormone synthesis
- autoimmune thyroiditis (Hashimoto's disease) in association with hypothyroidism

A diffuse goitre associated with lack of iodine or reduced iodine uptake will often become nodular over time as the thyroid attempts to adapt to iodine deficiency. Nodular goitres are discussed in 'Single thyroid nodules'.

Clinical features of non-toxic goitres
Clinical features of non-toxic goitres include:
- an asymptomatic goitre discovered incidentally, typically at the time of imaging of the neck for unrelated reason (e.g. carotid ultrasound study)
- obstructive symptoms:
  - compression of vital structures in the neck occurs with retrosternal extension of goitres
  - symptoms include dysphagia, dyspnoea, stridor, choking sensation, and hoarseness
- Pemberton's sign:
  - venous engorgement (neck and head veins, flushed) when both arms are raised
  - suggests obstruction to the great veins in the neck

Investigations for non-toxic goitres
The following investigations should be performed for non-toxic goitres:
- assess thyroid function: FT4, FT3, TSH
- assess autoantibody status: anti-thyroid antibodies, especially thyroid peroxidase antibodies
- ultrasound scan: look for nodules (see 'Single thyroid nodules')
- if retrosternal extension is suspected, a flow-volume loop lung-function test and CT scan of neck and thoracic inlet are recommended; neck MRI may also be considered

Treatment of non-toxic goitres
Treatment of non-toxic goitres is as follows:
- medical: routine levothyroxine suppressive treatment is not recommended; monitor TSH in euthyroid autoimmune patients and treat with levothyroxine when TSH >10 mIU/L
- surgery (thyroidectomy): generally offered if there are compressive symptoms or if significant radiological

tracheal narrowing (as opposed to deviation), oesophageal compression, or superior vena cava syndrome is present

Single thyroid nodules

Epidemiology of single thyroid nodules
Palpable thyroid nodules are present in 3%–7% of the population and are more frequent in females. The true prevalence of thyroid nodules is much higher (about 70%) if studied by ultrasound scan.

Pathophysiology of single thyroid nodules Type of single thyroid nodules
There are three types of single thyroid nodules:
- cystic (e.g. simple cyst, cystic adenoma, colloid cyst); may have a solid component
- spongiform: almost always benign
- solid (e.g. hyperplastic nodule, follicular adenoma, follicular neoplasm, papillary neoplasm, Hurthle cell thyroid cancer, anaplastic thyroid cancer, medullary thyroid cancer)

Functional type of single thyroid nodules
There are three functional types of single thyroid nodules:
- hyperthyroid (toxic): may arise from gain of function mutations in the TSH receptor; may be autonomous; usually; benign
- hypothyroid; may be associated with Hashimoto's thyroiditis
- euthyroid (most common)

Clinical features of single thyroid nodules
Nodules may be palpable or discovered incidentally on scan. Risk factors for malignancy are:
- male gender
- age <14 or >70
- history of head or neck irradiation
- the nodule having a firm or hard consistency
- associated lymphadenopathy
- associated dysphonia, dysphagia, or stridor
- rapid growth
- family history (multiple endocrine neoplasia, medullary thyroid cancer, differentiated thyroid cancer)
- TSH > 6 mIU/L

Treatment of single thyroid nodules
Treatment depends on an accurate diagnosis in order to distinguish benign from malignant lesions. Newer modalities such as PET imaging, elastography, and genetic markers are currently being evaluated.

See the algorithms shown in Figures 2.9 and 2.10.

Thyroid cancer

Epidemiology of thyroid cancer
Thyroid cancer represents about 1% of all malignancies. The incidence in the UK is reported as 5.1/100,000 (females) and 1.9/100,000 (males) and appears to be rising. Most of the increase is in small sub-centimetre nodules.

Pathophysiology of thyroid cancer
Thyroid cancer is characterized by the cell type of origin. There are five types of thyroid cancer:

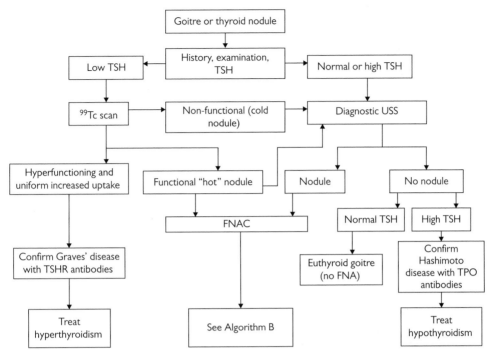

Fig 2.9 Algorithm for diagnosis and treatment of an enlarged thyroid (goitre) or thyroid nodule(s); FNA, fine-needle aspiration; FNAC, fine-needle aspiration cytology; ⁹⁹Tc, technetium-99; TPO, thyroid peroxidase; TSH, thyroid-stimulating hormone; TSHR, thyroid-stimulating hormone receptor; USS, ultrasound scan.
Data from American Thyroid Association Guidelines Task Force, Medullary thyroid cancer: management guidelines of the American Thyroid Association, *Thyroid*, 2009, Volume 19, pp. 565–612.

- differentiated thyroid cancer arising from the thyroid follicular cell:
  - papillary thyroid cancer (85%)
  - follicular thyroid cancer (10%)
  - Hurthle cell (oncocytic follicular, oxyphil) tumours(5%)
- anaplastic thyroid cancer (probably arising from thyroid follicular cells)
- medullary thyroid cancer (arising from parafollicular calcitonin-producing C-cells)
- primary thyroid lymphoma (non-Hodgkin B-cell tumour; usually background of Hashimoto's thyroiditis)
- thyroid sarcoma (arising from stromal tissue)

Ionizing radiation, particularly in childhood (under 5 years) or infancy, is strongly associated with an increased risk of differentiated thyroid cancer. *RET* rearrangements resulting in chimeric genes have been identified in papillary thyroid cancers following the Chernobyl incident.

Medullary thyroid cancer is classified as:
- sporadic (75%) (somatic *RET* mutation)
- familial (25%) (germline *RET* mutation)
- as part of multiple endocrine neoplasia syndrome:
  - multiple endocrine neoplasia type 2A (medullary thyroid cancer + phaeochromocytoma + hyperparathyroidism); rarely, cutaneous lichen amyloidosis or Hirschsprung disease
  - multiple endocrine neoplasia type 2B (medullary thyroid cancer + marfanoid habitus + phaeochromocytoma + multiple mucosal neuromas)

RET germline mutations in medullary thyroid cancer are correlated with clinical features and prognosis (see also Chapter 14, Section 14.8); for example:
- codon 918 and 634 mutations are associated with unilateral or bilateral phaeochromocytoma
- codon 634 mutations are associated with hyperparathyroidism and an aggressive course
- codon 918 mutations are associated with multiple endocrine neoplasia type 2B and the most aggressive course

The plasma calcitonin doubling time also provides prognostic information; a doubling time <1 year is associated with an adverse prognosis. The calcitonin and carcinoembryonic antigen doubling time may act similarly.

Clinical features of thyroid cancer
The clinical features of thyroid cancer are as follows:
- the thyroid nodule is painless and palpable, with especially rapid growth
- the nodule may be hard and fixed to soft tissues
- there may be associated lymph node enlargement
- there may be associated hoarseness or stridor
- especially found in patients >45 or <30
- there may be a history of irradiation in childhood

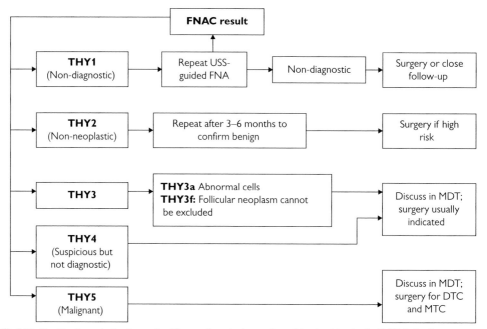

Fig 2.10 Algorithm for evaluating the results of fine-needle aspiration cytology of the thyroid, using the THY1–5 classification system; DTC, differentiated thyroid cancer; FNA, fine-needle aspiration; FNAC, fine-needle aspiration cytology; MDT, multidisciplinary team; MTC, medullary thyroid cancer; USS, ultrasound scan.
Data from British Thyroid Association & Royal College of Physicians, Guidelines for the management of thyroid cancer, *Clinical Endocrinology*, 2014, Volume 81, Supplement 1.

- the nodule may be detected during family screening (particularly medullary thyroid cancer)
- there may be associated features of multiple endocrine neoplasia type 2

Investigations for thyroid cancer
Blood/urine tests
- Assess thyroid function (FT4, FT3, TSH).
- Assess plasma calcitonin (if medullary thyroid cancer suspected).
- Exclude phaeochromocytoma (urine metanephrines) and parathyroid disease (calcium, PTH) for patients with suspected multiple endocrine neoplasia type 2 syndromes.

Note: Serum thyroglobulin is not recommended before surgery.

Cytology
- Perform fine-needle aspiration cytology (see algorithm).

Imaging
- Perform an ultrasound scan; adverse features include increased intralesional Doppler flow, hypoechoicity, microcalcifications, irregular margins, lack of halo around the nodule. There may be associated lymphadenopathy. The use of the U1–U5 grading system is recommended for assessing the risk of malignancy. BTA guidelines (2014) recommend the U classification to standardize ultrasound reports on nodules as benign, suspicious or malignant and help rationalize the use of FNA.

- Perform staging by non-contrast CT (iodine-containing contrast will reduce radioiodine uptake) or MRI in patients with proven thyroid cancer

Other tests
- Perform a flow-volume loop study if upper airway obstruction is suspected.
- Perform vocal cord assessment prior to surgery.

Treatment of thyroid cancer
The management of thyroid cancer should be determined by a multidisciplinary team. Patients should be staged using the TNM classification (seventh edition) and assigned to the appropriate risk group. The risk groups and their associated treatments are as follows:
- very-low-risk differentiated thyroid cancer (T1 (<1 cm) N0 M0): lobectomy and T4 treatment; no need for radioiodine
- low-risk differentiated thyroid cancer (T1–3 N0/1 M0): total thyroidectomy + ablative radioiodine (HiLo study (Mallick et al., 2012); 1.1 MBq is equally effective as 3.7 MBq); T4 dose to maintain TSH between 0.1 and 0.5 mIU/L
- high-risk differentiated thyroid cancer (T4 N1, M1): total thyroidectomy + ablative radioiodine; T4 dose to maintain TSH at undetectable levels
- Hurthle cell tumour: total thyroidectomy; if papillary elements are present in the biopsy, then radioiodine (about 10% take up iodine)

- medullary thyroid cancer: total thyroidectomy + central compartment node dissection; tyrosine kinase inhibitors (TKIs) (e.g. vandetanib, cabozantinib) if there is tumour progression or metastatic medullary thyroid cancer (monitor corrected QT intervals, blood pressure). The levothyroxine dose may need increasing when taking TKIs, and there is a risk of hand–foot syndrome
- radioiodine-refractory progressive differentiated thyroid cancer: TKIs (e.g. sorafenib, lenvatinib) have recently been licensed for this indication and other TKIs are in development
- anaplastic thyroid cancer: external beam radiotherapy improves local control; surgery and radioiodine not usually indicated; trials using TKIs are in progress
- thyroid lymphoma: chemotherapy (not thyroidectomy)
- thyroid sarcoma: total thyroidectomy

References and further reading

American Thyroid Association Guidelines Task Force. Medullary thyroid cancer: Management guidelines of the American Thyroid Association. *Thyroid* 2009; 19: 565–612.

American Thyroid Association Management Guidelines for adult patients with thyroid nodules and differentiated thyroid cancer. *Thyroid* 2016; 26: 1–133.

British Thyroid Association. Guidelines for the management of thyroid cancer. Third edition. *Clin Endocrinol* 2014 81: 1–122.

Gharib H, Papini E, Valcavi R, et al. AACE/AME Task Force on Thyroid Nodules. American Association of Clinical Endocrinologists and Associazione Medici Endocrinologi medical guidelines for clinical practice for the diagnosis and management of thyroid nodules. *Endocr Pract* 2006; 12: 63–102.

Mallick U, Harmer C, Yap B, et al. Ablation with low dose radioiodine and thyrotropin-alpha in thyroid cancer. *N Engl J Med* 2012; 366: 1674–85.

Nikoforov YE and Nikiforova MN. Molecular genetics and diagnosis of thyroid cancer. *Nat Rev Endcorinol* 2011; 7: 569–80.

Perros P, Boelaert K, Colley S, et al. Guidelines for the management of thyroid cancer. *Clin Endocrinol* 2014; 81: 1–122.

Smallridge RC. Approach to the patient with anaplastic thyroid carcinoma. *J Clin Endocrinol Metab* 2012; 97: 2566–72.

Vanderpump MP, Tunbridge WM, French JM, et al. The incidence of thyroid disorders in the community: A twenty-year follow-up of the Whickham Survey. *Clin Endocrinol* 1995; 43: 55–68.

Chapter 3

Pituitary gland

Chapter contents

3.1 Anatomy and physiology

Introduction

The pituitary gland, or hypophysis, is a bean-shaped, bilaterally symmetrical reddish-brown organ, located in the sella turcica at the base of the brain under the hypothalamus. In adults, it weighs on average 0.6 g, ranging between 0.4–0.8 g, and measures approximately 13 mm transversely, 9 mm anterioposteriorly, and 6 mm vertically. It is covered by the sellar diaphragm, which is part of the dura mater, a dense layer of connective tissue which lines the sella turcica. The sellar diaphragm has a small central opening that is approximately 5 mm and is penetrated by the pituitary stalk, which connects the hypothalamus with the pituitary.

The pituitary can be divided into two parts: the adenohypophysis or anterior pituitary and the neurohypophysis or posterior pituitary (see Figure 3.1). The adenohypophysis is larger, making up 80% of the gland, and consists of three parts: the pars distalis, the pars intermedia, and the pars tuberalis. The pars distalis is composed of acini, which are groups of pituitary hormone-producing cells surrounded by reticulin fibres. The neurohypophysis makes up the remaining 20% of the entire gland, is sharply separated from the adenohypophysis, and also consists of three parts: the median eminence of the infundibulum, the hypophysial stalk, and the posterior or neural lobe.

The blood supply of the anterior pituitary comes mainly from the portal vessels, which originate in the infundibulum, and, via the pituitary stalk, terminates in the adenohypophysial capillaries and supplies the adenohypophysis with blood. There is an additional direct arterial supply from the hypophysial artery via the capsular arteries as well. The neurohypophysis receives blood directly from the internal carotid artery via the hypophysial arteries.

Except for a few nerve fibres which penetrate the anterior lobe along the vessels, the adenohypophysis has no direct nerve supply. The posterior lobe is extensively innervated via nerves originating in the hypothalamus.

Hormone synthesis

There are six types of cells in the adenohypophysis: growth hormone-producing somatotrophs, prolactin-producing lactotrophs, adrenocorticotrophic hormone-producing corticotrophs, TSH-producing thyrotrophs, FSH- and LH-producing gonadotrophs, and folliculo-stellate cells. Thyrotrophs and gonadotrophs, the cells producing glycoprotein hormones, consist of two components: alpha and beta subunits. The beta subunits are biologically active; the alpha subunits are assumed to have no biologic activities. Folliculo-stellate cells are spindle-shaped, elongated cells with several functions. They have a sustentacular role, produce several cytokines, and can transform to hormone-producing cells and then retransform back to folliculo-stellate cells. They most likely represent adult stem cells or progenitor cells.

The posterior pituitary extends down into the pituitary stalk and sella turcica and is composed of unmyelinated nerve fibres, an interlacing network of axons, axon terminals, glial cells called pituicytes, and Herring bodies which are swollen axon terminals filled with neurosecretory material. They release two hormones: vasopressin, also known as antidiuretic hormone, and oxytocin. These two hormones are synthesized in the magnocellular portion of the hypothalamic supraoptic nucleus and the magnocellular portion of the paraventricular nucleus and transported with their carrier protein, which is called neurophysin, to the posterior lobe by nerve fibres via the pituitary stalk. Pituicytes, which are located in the posterior lobe, not only store but may also synthesize the two neurohypophysial hormones.

Immunohistochemical and electron microscopic investigation is of fundamental importance for recognizing the cell types and their endocrine activity (see Figure 3.2) The application of molecular/genetic methods opens new avenues for research and may lead to a better understanding of structure–function relations.

Earlier, the one-cell-one-hormone theory was the widely accepted paradigm. According to this interpretation, one adenohypophysial cell can synthesize and release only one hormone. Later studies led to considerable change. There is conclusive evidence that one adenohypophysial cell is capable of producing more than

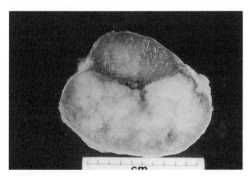

Fig 3.1 Horizontal cross-section of a normal human pituitary, showing the anterior and posterior lobes.

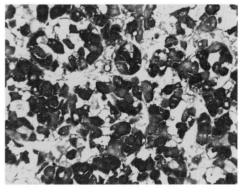

Fig 3.2 Immunohistochemistry demonstrating growth-hormone-immunopositive adenohypophysial cells (magnification, 250×).

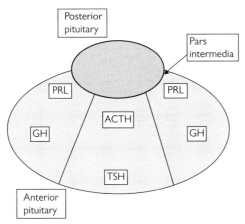

Fig 3.3 Regional distribution of anterior pituitary cells. Somatotrophs are mainly located in the lateral wings, corticotrophs in the central portion of the mucoid wedge, and thyrotrophs in the anteromedial portion of the mucoid wedge. Lactotrophs are mainly located close to the posterior lobe, and gonadotrophs are randomly all around the pars distalis of the adenohypophysis; ACTH, adrenocorticotrophic-hormone-secreting cells; GH, growth-hormone-secreting cells; PRL, prolactin-secreting cells; TSH, thyroid-stimulating-hormone-secreting cells.

one hormone (plurihormonality). The concept of pituitary plasticity was also introduced. According to this interpretation, depending on the need, adenohypophysial cells can transform to another cell type and then retransform back again to the original cell type. These are very intriguing findings which has changed our thinking on pituitary endocrine activity.

The various pituitary cell types are unevenly distributed, as illustrated in Figure 3.3. In the centre of the acini are the pituitary follicles containing folliculo-stellate cells. Depending on their functional status, they may be immunopositive for S-100 protein or glial fibrillary acidic protein (GFAP).

Several recent studies have focused on the regulation of the pituitary gland (see Table 3.1).

The function of the various pituitary hormones is only briefly presented in this short review.

Growth hormone stimulates body growth and plays an important role in metabolism. Prolactin enhances breast development and milk production in females. Its absence leads to impotence and loss of libido in males. Adrenocorticotrophic hormone stimulates the secretion of adrenocortical hormones, mainly cortisol, and gives rise to adrenocortical hyperplasia. TSH stimulates the secretion of thyroid hormones and causes enlargement of the thyroid gland. FSH stimulates oestrogen secretion in females and sperm production in males. LH causes ovulation and corpus luteum formation and stimulates oestrogen and progesterone secretion in females, and

Table 3.1 Hypothalamo-pituitary system

Cell type	Tissue-specific transcription factor	Fetal appearance (weeks)	Hormone	Stimulators	Inhibitors	Target gland or tissue	Trophic effect	Normal range
Somatotroph	PROP1	8	GH	GHRH	Somatostatin	Liver	IGF-1 production	<0.5 µg/L
	PIT1			Ghrelin		Various tissues	Induces growth	
							Insulin inhibitor	
Lactotroph	PROP1	12	PRL	Oestrogen	Dopamine	Breast	Milk production	M<15 µg/L
	PIT1			TRH		Uterus		F<20 µg/L
				VIP				
Corticotroph	TBX19	6	ACTH	CRH	Glucocorticoids	Adrenal	Corticosteroid production	ACTH: 4–22 pg/L
				Vasopressin				
				gp-130 Cytokines				
Thyrotroph	PROP1	12	TSH	TRH	T3	Thyroid	T3, T4 secretion	0.1–5.0 mU/L
	PIT1				T4			
	TEF				Dopamine			
					Somatostatin			
					Glucocorticoids			
Gonadotroph	SF-1	12	FSH/LH	GnRH	Inhibin	Testis	Follicle growth	M: 5–20 IU/L
	DAX1			Activins	Sex steroids	Ovaries	Sex steroid production	F: 5–20 IU/L
							Germ cell maturation	

Abbreviations: ACTH, adrenocorticotrophic hormone; CRH, corticotrophin-releasing hormone; GH, growth hormone; GHRH, growth hormone-releasing hormone; GnRH, gonadotrophin-releasing hormone; GLH, luteinizing hormone; gp-130, glycoprotein 130; PRL, prolactin; SF-1, steroidogenic factor 1; T3, triiodothyronine; T4, thyroxine; TEF, thyrotroph embryonic factor; TRH, thyrotrophin-releasing hormone; VIP, vasoactive intestinal peptide.

stimulates testicular Leydig cells and testosterone secretion in males. (The hormone is called interstitial cell stimulating hormone in males.)

The two posterior pituitary hormones, vasopressin and oxytocin, are produced mainly in the supraoptic and magnocellular portion of the paraventricular nuclei of the hypothalamus, transported along the nerve fibres to the posterior lobe, where they are stored and then released into the circulation if needed.

Vasopressin regulates water metabolism. It acts on the renal tubules and reabsorbs water. In its absence, polyuria and polydipsia develop; the associated disease is called *diabetes insipidus*. Oxytocin causes contraction of the uterine smooth muscle cells, plays an important role in delivery, and promotes milk ejection from the mammary gland.

Future developments

Recent evidence indicates that pituitary hormones and the hypothalamic stimulating and inhibiting hormones play a more widespread role. For example, prolactin receptors are present in endothelial cells and it appears that prolactin can affect angiogenesis.

The regulation of pituitary hormone synthesis and release is much more complex than it was earlier believed. Various hormones can interact; there are several receptors which can affect hormone secretion and endocrine activity. Obviously, much more work is needed to understand the function and regulation of pituitary hormones. New molecular/genetic studies will lead to significant changes in the interpretation of hormone synthesis and release, regulation, hormone action, and endocrine homeostasis.

Further reading

Horvath E and Kovacs K. 'The adenohypophysis', in Kovacs K and Asa S, eds, Functional Endocrine Pathology (2nd edition), 1998. Blackwell Science, pp. 247–81.

Horvath E, Scheithauer BW, Kovacs K, et al. 'Hypothalamus and pituitary', in Graham DI and Lantos PL, eds, *Greenfield's Neuropathology* (7th edition), 2002. Arnold Publishers, pp. 983–1062.

Kovacs K and Horvath E. *Tumors of the Pituitary Gland*, 1986. Atlas of Tumor Pathology, Series 2, Fascicle 21. Armed Forces Institute of Pathology.

Thibodeau GA and Patton KT. 'Endocrine system', in *Anatomy and Physiology* (4th edition), 1999. Mosby, pp. 480–523.

3.2 Genetic testing for pituitary adenomas

Introduction

Pituitary adenomas can be caused by genetic abnormalities. The diseases and genes which are currently known to be involved with inherited or congenital pituitary tumorigenesis are listed in Box 3.1, and an approach to genetic testing in pituitary patients can be seen in Figure 3.4.

General considerations in genetic testing

Genetic testing of selected affected patients should be offered after a careful discussion of the advantages, disadvantages, and possible pitfalls of performing the test; this discussion should take place with the treating endocrinologist or with a clinical geneticist. Genetic counselling of pre-symptomatic family members, ideally conducted by a clinical geneticist or genetic counsellor, should include, in addition to sharing information on the disease and the clinical consequences of the testing, advice on the possible financial implications of the genetic test, such as on insurance policies.

Box 3.1 Diseases and genes known to be associated with inherited or congenital pituitary tumorigenesis

The following diseases and genes are known to be associated with inherited or congenital pituitary tumorigenesis:

- multiple endocrine neoplasia type 1 and type 4:
  MEN1 (encodes menin)
  CDKN2B (encodes p15)
  CDKN2C (encodes p18)
  CDKN1A (encodes p21)
- multiple endocrine neoplasia type 4:
  CDKN1B (encodes p27)
- familial isolated pituitary adenoma:
  AIP (encodes aryl hydrocarbon receptor-interacting protein)
  GPR101 (encodes G-protein coupled receptor 101; germline or somatic microduplication)
- Carney complex:
  PRKAR1A (encodes the regulatory subunit of protein kinase A)
  PRKACA (encodes the catalytic subunit of protein kinase A)
- McCune–Albright syndrome (mosaic condition):
  GNAS1 (encodes Gs alpha)
- DICER1-related syndrome (causing infant pituitary blastoma):
  DICER1 gene
- SDHx-related syndrome (associated with pituitary adenoma and phaeochromocytoma/ paraganglioma):
  SDHA, SDHB, SDHD, SDHC, and *SDHA2F* (encode subunits of the succinate dehydrogenase enzyme)

DNA analysis may involve—depending on the particular disease or gene—sequencing of the exon and of the exon–intron junctions of the gene, using a technique to detect large deletions, such as multiplex ligation-dependent probe amplification; array comparative genomic hybridization, to detect copy number variation; and, more recently, whole exome or whole genome sequencing.

The decision whether a rare or novel sequence variant is a harmless change (polymorphism) or a disease-causing mutation can be complex, and advice from specialist geneticist and laboratories may be needed; in addition, further studies, including RNA and tumour-sample testing, as well as family segregation studies, could be helpful.

Cascade screening of family members of a proband is suggested. Carrier family members may benefit from clinical screening, as early diagnosis may lead to better treatment outcomes, whilst family members free of the family-specific mutation will benefit, as no further tests are needed.

It is important to keep in mind that phenocopies have been described in many genetic disorders, including *MEN1*- and *AIP*-mutation-positive familial isolated pituitary adenoma. The term 'phenocopy' refers to a condition where disease manifestations in keeping with a particular gene mutation are present but are due to a different aetiology, such as a true sporadic disease or another gene mutation. A typical example could be an elderly female who has recent-onset hyperparathyroidism but does not carry the *MEN1* mutation although having relatives who carry a known disease-causing *MEN1* gene mutation.

Genetic testing in multiple endocrine neoplasia type 1 and type 4

See also Chapter 14, Section 14.7. *MEN1* is located on 11q13 and encodes the 610-amino-acid menin protein (Chandrasekharappa et al. 1997; Lemmens et al., 1997; see also Chapter 13, Section 13.7). Patients are heterozygous for the disease-causing mutation, and disease penetrance is over 95% by the age of 50 (Thakker et al., 2012). *MEN1* behaves as a tumour suppressor gene; three-quarters of the mutations lead to a truncated protein, and the majority of *MEN1*-related tumour tissues show loss of heterozygosity at the *MEN1* locus. Menin has extensive interactions with other proteins involved in cell proliferation, cell cycle regulation, and transcriptional regulation, but it is currently unclear how the lack of this protein leads to tumorigenesis in the pituitary or other endocrine organs. There have been over 1300 mutations identified, with a few hotspot mutations being responsible for 20% of the cases, but with no genotype–phenotype correlation. Pituitary adenomas (prolactinoma > somatotrophinoma > corticotrophinoma > non-functioning adenoma) manifest in about 30%–40% of cases (Turner et al., 2010), and pituitary adenoma can be the first manifestation of the disease in 15% of the cases. Prospective screening, however, identified a high proportion of small clinically non-functioning pituitary adenomas (de Laat et al., 2015). Clinically manifesting *MEN1*-related pituitary adenomas are larger and are more difficult to treat than sporadic pituitary adenomas. Somatic mutations of *MEN1* have been commonly described in sporadic neuroendocrine and parathyroid tumours but very rarely in sporadic pituitary adenomas.

MEN1 testing can help to establish the clinical diagnosis in the index patient and can lead to search and early identification of other manifestations. In addition, it can identify other family members with the mutation, and, at the same time, can rule out other family members who therefore do not need any further medical attention in this respect. Indications for MEN1 genetic testing are listed in Table 3.2. Phenocopies are regularly encountered and need to be carefully considered.

Mutations in CDKN1B, which encodes the cyclin-dependent kinase inhibitor p27, are found in 1.5% of patients with multiple endocrine neoplasia type 4, which has a phenotype similar to that seen in multiple endocrine neoplasia type 1 but in the absence of detectable MEN1 mutations. Mutations in other genes encoding cyclin-dependent kinase inhibitors (e.g. CDKN2B (which encodes p15), CDKN2C (which encodes p18), and CDKN1A (which encodes p21)) can be rarely found, accounting, together with CDKN1B mutations, for about 2% of patients who are negative for MEN1 mutations (Pellegata et al., 2006; Agarwal et al., 2009).

Genetic testing in familial isolated pituitary adenoma

Familial isolated pituitary adenoma is a genetically heterogeneous disease with autosomal dominant inheritance pattern. Patients with this disease can be divided into three subgroups, based on their genotypes according to our current knowledge:

- AIP-mutation-associated familial isolated pituitary adenoma
- X-linked acrogigantism
- familial isolated pituitary adenoma with unknown genetic cause

The phenotypes of these three groups are considerably different from each other.

AIP-mutation-associated familial isolated pituitary adenoma
In 17%–20% of families with familial isolated pituitary adenoma, a heterozygous germ-line mutation of AIP can be detected (Vierimaa et al., 2006; Daly et al., 2010; Hernández-Ramírez et al., 2015). Families with AIP mutations typically have at least one member with a growth hormone-secreting tumour, and disease onset is significantly younger (mean age 20–24 years) in these patients, compared to patients with AIP-mutation-negative familial isolated pituitary adenoma or sporadic pituitary adenoma. The disease most often manifests in adolescence, but childhood and young adult cases are also common. Patients usually have large aggressive adenomas. Somatotroph adenomas often show sparsely granulated pattern and poor response to somatostatin analogue treatment. The most common pituitary adenomas are somatotroph tumours, mammosomatotroph tumours, and prolactin-secreting tumours, followed by non-functioning tumours and, rarely, corticotroph or thyrotroph adenomas. The disease can also manifest in patients without an apparent family history, and their phenotype is not different from the familial cases (simplex cases). About 20% of childhood-onset, apparently sporadic, hormone-secreting adenomas are caused by AIP mutations.

AIP is located at 11q13, and codes for a 330-amino-acid protein. AIP is tumour suppressor gene, and loss of heterozygosity has been identified in many AIP mutation-related pituitary adenoma tissues. Whilst a number of proteins have been identified that interact with AIP, the exact tumorigenic mechanism is not known. Over 60 different mutations have been described, the majority leading to truncated protein, with a few genetic hotspots, the most common being a stop mutation affecting amino acid 304 (p.R304*). This particular mutation has been identified in a large number of young-onset acromegaly patients, including one born in the eighteenth century, supporting the data that this is due to a founder effect from about 100 generations ago (Chahal et al., 2011). No somatic mutations have been identified in somatotroph adenomas to date.

AIP testing indications are shown in Table 3.2. Awareness of AIP mutations in affected patients might help to predict the course of disease (Hernández-Ramírez et al., 2015) and could assist decisions on treatment options. As the only clinical manifestation of familial isolated pituitary adenoma is a pituitary adenoma, the presence of pituitary incidentalomas (a common finding in up to 20% of the general population) could make clinical screening more difficult.

X-linked acrogigantism
A subset of patients with very young-onset gigantism harbour duplication of the orphan G protein-coupled receptor GPR101, usually as part of a microduplication at Xq26.3 (Trivellin et al., 2014; Iacovazzo et al., 2016), with this mutation leading to X-linked acrogigantism. This recently described disease has a high, possibly full penetrance. Most cases develop the first signs by the age of 1 and are diagnosed before the age of 5. The majority of the patients are females and harbour a de novo microduplication, although familial cases (Trivellin et al., 2014; Beckers et al., 2015) and, in males, mosaic cases have also been described (Daly et al., 2016; Iacovazzo et al., 2016; Rodd et al., 2016). Patients have growth hormone-secreting pituitary hyperplasia or adenoma, usually with prolactin hypersecretion and characterized by extreme growth velocity and final height unless treated.

Familial isolated pituitary adenoma with unknown genetic cause
In the third and far the largest group of families with familial isolated pituitary adenoma, no disease-causing mutation can be identified to date (Hernández-Ramírez et al., 2015). These patients have an age of onset considerably older than patients with the other two types of familial isolated pituitary adenoma, apparently not dissimilar to sporadic patients. Penetrance is low—less than in AIP-mutation-positive cases. The clinical phenotype is also more variable. About half the families are homogenous (i.e. all family members have the same type of pituitary adenoma), where growth hormone- or prolactin-secreting adenomas predominate, with fewer families with non-functioning adenomas or exceptional adrenocorticotrophic hormone-secreting adenomas. Heterogeneous families can have different types of adenomas, although TSH-omas are exceptionally rare.

Genetic testing in Carney complex

Carney complex is characterized by spotty skin pigmentation; cutaneous, mucosal, and atrial myxomas; and various endocrine overactivities, as well as other tumours (see also Chapter 14, Section 14.4, and the detailed review in Horvath and Stratakis, 2008). Diagnosis is made

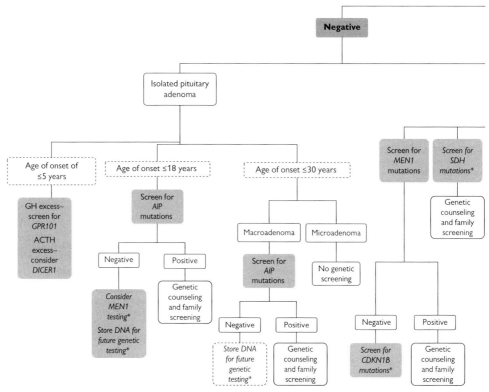

Fig 3.4 Approach for genetic testing in patients with pituitary adenomas.
* Weak evidence for these suggestions.
Reproduced with permission from Hernández-Ramírez LC and Korbonits M, Familial pituitary adenomas. In: *Pituitary Disorders: Diagnosis and Management*, edited by Lawson EA, Ezzat S, Asa AL et al. Copyright © John Wiley and Sons Ltd, 2012.

on clinical grounds. About 60% of all the cases, and 80% of cases involving adrenal Cushing syndrome, are caused by a heterozygous germ-line mutation in *PRKAR1A*, coding for the regulatory subunit of protein kinase A (Kirschner et al., 2000). Disease penetrance is over 95% by the age of 50. *PRKAR1A* is located at 17q22–4, consists of 384 amino-acid residues, and is a typical tumour-suppressor gene, with loss of heterozygosity detected in many human tumour samples. Until now, over 110 mutations have been described, with the majority coding for a truncated protein; in addition, nonsense-mediated decay of the mutant mRNA has been observed. Some genotype–phenotype correlations have been described. Protein kinase A is part of the cAMP pathway, which is activated by growth hormone-releasing hormone in somatotrophs and is known to be altered in somatotroph adenomas associated with mutations in *GNAS1* (the so-called gsp oncogene, which encodes G alpha), thus indicating the mechanism by which such mutations lead to pituitary tumorigenesis. Sequence variants in *PDE11A* may have modifying effects on disease manifestations. More

recently, a few cases have been described with increased copy number of *PRKACA* (Lodish et al., 2015). In some of the *PRKAR1A*-mutation-negative families, linkage studies point to the 2p16 locus.

The pituitary gland is frequently affected in Carney complex, manifesting either as somatotroph and lactotroph hyperplasia with abnormal IGF-I and pro-lactin levels and growth hormone level dynamics, whilst true adenomas occur only in a small proportion of the cases.

Indications for genetic testing are listed in Table 3.2. It is suggested that family members be tested before the age of 6 months. Carrier family members benefit from early clinical screening, whilst family members free of the family-specific mutation do not need further follow up.

Genetic testing in McCune–Albright syndrome

McCune–Albright syndrome is not a familial disease but is caused by an embryonic genetic alteration which results in a mosaic condition (see also Chapter 14, Section 14.1).

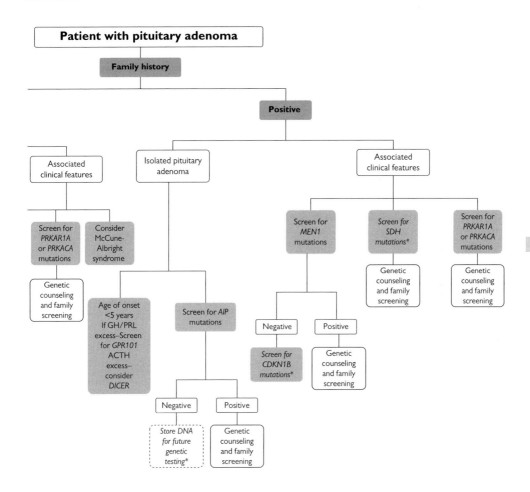

It is not transmitted to the offspring of affected subjects. The manifestations can be variable, depending on what stage of development the mutation occurred in and therefore how many organs and sites are affected. The diagnosis of McCune–Albright syndrome is established on clinical grounds, with patients having at least two features of the triad of polyostotic fibrous dysplasia: café-au-lait skin pigmentation and autonomous endocrine hyperfunction, including precocious puberty, thyrotoxicosis, pituitary gigantism, and Cushing's syndrome. Pituitary disease in McCune–Albright syndrome occurs in 21% of the cases, and around half of these cases manifest as growth hormone- and prolactin-producing cell hyperplasia, whilst the other half has adenomas. The average age of onset is 24 years, and acromegaly is almost always associated with skull base fibrous dysplasia. These patients are difficult to treat, as the surgical approach is difficult, total hypophysectomy is needed, and response to radiotherapy and somatostatin analogues is poor; however, growth-hormone-antagonist treatment is promising (Akintoye et al, 2006; Salenave et al., 2014).

The disease is caused by an activating mutation in Gs alpha, the stimulatory G protein alpha subunit encoded by GNAS1, which is located on 20q13. Gs alpha is a ubiquitously expressed 1037-amino-acid protein. In 15%–40% of sporadic somatotroph adenomas, somatic mutations also affect GNAS1. Gs alpha activates adenylyl cyclase and leads to the generation of excess cAMP. Mutations in McCune–Albright syndrome affect arginine 201 (but usually not residue 227; somatic mutations in sporadic somatotrophs can affect both residues 221 and 227). McCune–Albright syndrome is a clinical diagnosis, and genetic testing is not routinely performed. The disease-causing genetic abnormality can be identified from peripheral leucocytes in about 40% of cases, and in 90% of the cases if the affected tissues are tested. Growth hormone-adenoma tissue testing for somatic GNAS1 mutation or the identification of mutations in McCune–Albright is not performed routinely.

Genetic testing in DICER1 syndrome

Heterozygous germ-line mutations in DICER1 are associated with increased risk for pleuropulmonary blastoma, cystic nephroma, nasal chondromesenchymal hamartoma, ovarian Sertoli–Leydig cell tumours, ciliary body medulloepithelioma, pineoblastoma, pituitary blastoma,

Table 3.2 Indications for genetic testing for pituitary adenomas

Gene	Indication for gene testing	Reference
MEN1	Patient with two or more MEN1-related manifestations	Thakker RV, Newey PJ, Walls GV, et al. Clinical practice guidelines for multiple endocrine neoplasia type 1 (MEN1). *J Clin Endocrinol Metab* 2012; 97: 2990–3011.
	Patient with one MEN1-related manifestation and a first-degree family member with MEN1	
	Patient with suspicious MEN1 (with parathyroid adenomas occurring before the age of 30; or multigland parathyroid disease, gastrinoma, or multiple pancreatic NET at any age)	
	Patient with atypical MEN1: one classical and one non-classical manifestation (adrenal cortical tumour, carcinoid, facial angiofibroma, collagenoma, thyroid tumours, lipomatous tumour, and meningioma)	
	First-degree relative of a carrier of an *MEN1* mutation	
AIP	Patient with familial isolated pituitary adenoma	Korbonits M, Storr H, and Kumar AV. Familial pituitary adenomas: Who should be tested for AIP mutations? *Clin Endocrinol (Oxf)* 2012; 77: 351–6.
	Patient with childhood-onset pituitary adenoma (primarily GH- and/or prolactin-secreting) and no MEN1 and Carney complex-related family history	
	Young-onset (<30 years of age) macroadenoma patient (primarily GH- and/or prolactin-secreting) and no MEN1 and Carney complex-related family history	
	First-degree relative of a carrier of an *AIP* mutation	
Xq26.3 microduplication	Patient with extreme growth starting before the age of 5	Trivellin G, Daly AF, Faucz FR, et al. Gigantism and acromegaly due to Xq26 microduplications and GPR101 mutation. *N Engl J Med* 2014; 371: 2363–74.
	Patient may have a pituitary adenoma, hyperplasia, or an apparently normal-sized pituitary gland on MRI	
PRKAR1A	Patient with Carney complex	Horvath A and Stratakis CA. Clinical and molecular genetics of acromegaly: MEN1, Carney complex, McCune-Albright syndrome, familial acromegaly and genetic defects in sporadic tumors. *Rev Endocr Metab Disord* 2008; 9: 1–11.
	Patient with a Carney complex-related manifestation and a first-degree family member with Carney complex	
	First-degree relative of a carrier of a *PRKAR1A* mutation	
PRKACA copy number variation	In patients with Carney complex and negative *PRKAR1A* sequencing and MLPA tests	Forlino A, Vetro A, Garavelli L, et al. PRKACB and Carney complex. *N Engl J Med* 2014; 370: 1065–67.
DICER1	Infant with large pituitary adenoma which is usually ACTH secreting, and possibly other features of *DICER1* syndrome, such as pleuropulmonary blastoma or kidney cysts	de Kock L, Sabbaghian N, Plourde F, et al. Pituitary blastoma: A pathognomonic feature of germ-line DICER1 mutations. *Acta Neuropathol* 2014; 128: 111–22.
SDHx	Patient with pituitary adenoma and phaeochromocytoma or paraganglioma	O'Toole SM, Denes J, Robledo M, et al. 15 years of paraganglioma: The association of pituitary adenomas and phaeochromocytomas or paragangliomas. *Endocr Relat Cancer* 2015; 22: 105–22.

Abbreviations: ACTH, adrenocorticotrophic hormone; GH, growth hormone; MEN1, multiple endocrine neoplasia type 1; MLPA, multiplex ligation-dependent probe amplification; NET, neuroendocrine tumour.

Data from: Thakker RV, Newey PJ, Walls GV, Bilezikian J, Dralle H, Ebeling PR, Melmed S, Sakurai A, Tonelli F, Brandi ML, Clinical practice guidelines for multiple endocrine neoplasia type 1 (MEN1). *J Clin Endocrinol Metab*. 2012;97:2990–3011; Korbonits M, Storr H, Kumar AV, Familial pituitary adenomas - Who should be tested for AIP mutations? *Clin Endocrinol*, 2012;77:351–356; and Horvath A, Stratakis CA, Clinical and molecular genetics of acromegaly: MEN1, Carney complex, McCune-Albright syndrome and genetic defects in sporadic tumors. *Rev Endocr Metab Disord*. 2008;9:1–11.

nodular thyroid hyperplasia, thyroid carcinoma, and botryoid embryonal rhabdomyosarcoma of the uterine cervix. These tumours could present in isolation or as a syndromic disease. Pituitary blastoma, originally described in 2008 as a separate entity (Scheithauer et al., 2008), is an extremely rare, low-penetrance (<1%), potentially lethal, early childhood (7–24 months old) adrenocorticotrophic hormone-secreting tumour of the pituitary gland. The tissue has an embryonic appearance, and previous cases had 40% lethality (de Kock et al., 2014).

Genetic testing in *SDHx*-mutation-related pituitary adenoma

The coexistence of pituitary adenoma and paraganglioma or phaeochromocytoma is rare, but it has recently been described in a number of patients with *SDH* mutations, most commonly *SDHD* and *SDHB*. The common pathogenesis is supported by data indicating loss of heterozygosity at the *SDHx* loci in the pituitary tissue in the studied cases. The pituitary adenoma is usually a hormone-secreting (prolactin and growth hormone) macroadenoma with relatively aggressive behaviour; a metastatic pituitary carcinoma has also been described (Tufton et al., 2017). An interesting histological feature of vacuolized cells has been observed in these cases. It is important to remember that pituitary adenoma and phaeochromocytoma (but not paraganglioma) can, rarely, be a feature of multiple endocrine neoplasia type 1 (Xekouki et al., 2012; Dénes et al., 2015).

References and further reading

Agarwal SK, Mateo CM, and Marx SJ. Rare germline mutations in cyclin-dependent kinase inhibitor genes in multiple endocrine neoplasia type 1 and related states. *J Clin Endocrinol Metab* 2009; 94: 1826–34.

Akintoye SO, Kelly MH, Brillante B, et al. Pegvisomant for the treatment of gsp-mediated growth hormone excess in patients with McCune-Albright syndrome. *J Clin Endocrinol Metab* 2006; 91: 2960–6.

Beckers A, Lodish MB, Trivellin G, et al. X-linked acrogigantism syndrome: Clinical profile and therapeutic responses. *Endocr Relat Cancer* 2015; 22: 353–67.

Chahal HS, Stals K, Unterlander M, et al. AIP mutation in pituitary adenomas in the 18th century and today. *N Engl J Med* 2011; 364: 43–50.

Chandrasekharappa SC, Guru SC, Manickam P, et al. Positional cloning of the gene for multiple endocrine neoplasia-type 1. *Science* 1997; 276: 404–7.

Daly AF, Tichomirowa MA, Petrossians P, et al. Clinical characteristics and therapeutic responses in patients with germ-line AIP mutations and pituitary adenomas: an international collaborative study. *J Clin Endocrinol Metab* 2010; 95: E373–83.

Daly AF, Yuan B, Fina F, et al. Somatic mosaicism underlies X-linked acrogigantism syndrome in sporadic male subjects. *Endocr Relat Cancer* 2016; 23: 221–33.

de Kock L, Sabbaghian N, Plourde F, et al. Pituitary blastoma: A pathognomonic feature of germ-line DICER1 mutations. *Acta Neuropathol* 2014; 128: 111–22.

de Laat JM, Dekkers OM, Pieterman CR, et al. Long-term natural course of pituitary tumors in patients with MEN1: Results from the DutchMEN1 study group (DMSG). *J Clin Endocrinol Metab* 2015; 100: 3288–96.

Dénes J, Swords F, Rattenberry E, et al. Heterogeneous genetic background of the association of pheochromocytoma/paraganglioma and pituitary adenoma: results from a large patient cohort. *J Clin Endocrinol Metab* 2015; 100: E531–41.

Forlino A, Vetro A, Garavelli L, et al. PRKACB and Carney complex. *N Engl J Med* 2014; 370: 1065–67.

Hernández-Ramírez LC, Gabrovska P, Dénes J, et al. Landscape of familial isolated and young-onset pituitary adenomas: Prospective diagnosis in AIP mutation carriers. *J Clin Endocrinol Metab* 2015; 100: E1242–54.

Horvath A and Stratakis CA. Clinical and molecular genetics of acromegaly: MEN1, Carney complex, McCune-Albright syndrome, familial acromegaly and genetic defects in sporadic tumors. *Rev Endocr Metab Disord* 2008; 9: 1–11.

Iacovazzo D, Caswell R, Bunce B, et al. Germline or somatic GPR101 duplication leads to X-linked acrogigantism: A clinico-pathological and genetic study. *Acta Neuropathol Commun* 2016; 4: 56.

Kirschner LS, Carney JA, Pack SD, et al. Mutations of the gene encoding the protein kinase A type I-alpha regulatory subunit in patients with the Carney complex. *Nat Genet* 2000; 26: 89–92.

Korbonits M, Storr H, and Kumar AV. Familial pituitary adenomas: Who should be tested for AIP mutations? *Clin Endocrinol (Oxf)* 2012; 77: 351–6.

Lemmens I, Van de Ven WJ, Kas K, et al. Identification of the multiple endocrine neoplasia type 1 (MEN1) gene. The European Consortium on MEN1. *Hum Mol Genet* 1997; 6: 1177–83.

Lodish MB, Yuan B, Levy I, et al. Germline PRKACA amplification causes variable phenotypes that may depend on the extent of the genomic defect: molecular mechanisms and clinical presentations. *Eur J Endocrinol* 2015; 172: 803–11.

O'Toole SM, Denes J, Robledo M, et al. 15 years of paraganglioma: The association of pituitary adenomas and phaeochromocytomas or paragangliomas. *Endocr Relat Cancer* 2015; 22:T105–22.

Pellegata NS, Quintanilla-Martinez L, Siggelkow H, et al. Germline mutations in p27Kip1 cause a multiple endocrine neoplasia syndrome in rats and humans. *Proc Natl Acad Sci USA* 2006; 103: 15558–63.

Rodd C, Millette M, Iacovazzo D, et al. Somatic GPR101 duplication causing X-linked acrogigantism (XLAG): Diagnosis and management. *J Clin Endocrinol Metab* 2016; 101: 1927–30.

Salenave S, Boyce AM, Collins MT, et al. Acromegaly and McCune-Albright syndrome. *J Clin Endocrinol Metab* 2014; 99: 1955–69.

Scheithauer BW, Kovacs K, Horvath E, et al. Pituitary blastoma. *Acta Neuropathol* 2008; 116: 657–66.

Thakker RV, Newey PJ, Walls GV, et al. Clinical practice guidelines for multiple endocrine neoplasia type 1 (MEN1). *J Clin Endocrinol Metab* 2012; 97: 2990–3011.

Trivellin G, Daly AF, Faucz FR, et al. Gigantism and acromegaly due to Xq26 microduplications and GPR101 mutation. *N Engl J Med* 2014; 371: 2363–74.

Tufton N, Roncaroli F, Hadjidemetriou I, et al. Pituitary carcinoma in a patient with an *SDHB* mutation. *Endocr Pathol* 2017;

Turner JJ, Christie PT, Pearce SH, et al. Diagnostic challenges due to phenocopies: Lessons from multiple endocrine neoplasia type 1 (MEN1). *Hum Mutat* 2010; 31: E1089–101.

Vierimaa O, Georgitsi M, Lehtonen R, et al. Pituitary adenoma predisposition caused by germline mutations in the AIP gene. *Science* 2006; 312: 1228–30.

Xekouki P, Pacak K, Almeida M, et al. Succinate dehydrogenase (SDH) D subunit (SDHD) inactivation in a growth-hormone-producing pituitary tumor: A new association for SDH? *J Clin Endocrinol Metab* 2012; 97: E357–66.

3.3 Pituitary imaging and localization

Introduction

The small size and location of the pituitary within the sella turcica poses several difficulties for imaging. Traditional high-resolution skull radiographs are unable to demonstrate soft tissue and so, in the past, radiological diagnosis of pituitary tumours relied on showing secondary features such as enlargement of the sella, pathological calcification, or bone destruction. Planar scanning with CT and MRI can demonstrate the gland directly but both techniques have to be optimized to cope with the particular anatomical constraints of the sella region. For CT, which like radiographs, measures density, bone and calcification are easily imaged but the steep density gradients between bone (of the skull base), air in the para-nasal sinuses and soft tissue of the pituitary gland make the computer image reconstructions required to show the gland difficult. For MRI, which relies on obtaining specific resonance signal from different types of tissue, the sella and its contents are more easily imaged. However, multiple measurements are required to obtain adequate signal, and movements (i.e. of patient or carotid arterial pulsation) can easily degrade data and, consequently, image quality.

Imaging the pituitary gland is therefore best performed using dedicated MRI techniques and higher-strength magnets (1.0 tesla or greater), whilst CT is best for showing bone and calcification.

Imaging modalities

MRI is the method of first choice because it avoids use of ionizing radiation, is directly multiplanar, and gives some data on tissue structure. Enhancement with intravenous (external) contrast agents (e.g. gadolinium) depends on tissue blood supply and blood–brain barrier integrity. The normal gland, therefore, enhances, so the value of giving gadolinium to exaggerate differences between the tumour and the gland is limited, but it may help to distinguish other types of pathologies in the pituitary region.

CT is the method of second choice, because it uses ionizing radiation and because it is less sensitive to differences in soft-tissue structure. Modern scanners acquire a volume of data, which are reconstructed as images in orthogonal planes. This latter process reduces their accuracy and resolution. CT is better than MRI for demonstrating bone structure and pathological calcification. Its sensitivity in the detection of microadenoma is only about 20%.

Radionuclide imaging is best performed using PET. This scanning technique demonstrates tissue uptake of administered positron-emitting isotopes and is generally combined with CT to improve localization of the areas emitting the administered radiopharmaceutical. Although challenged by the small scale of pituitary anatomy, the technique has enormous theoretical potential which has yet to be realized in clinical practice. Somatastatin-receptor scintigraphy may be used to distinguish between current or residual tumour and post-operative scar tissue, and thalium-201 uptake has been described in pituitary abscesses.

Other imaging techniques may have a role in special circumstances. Angiography using digital subtraction angiography is used to localize the carotid arteries, to demonstrate vascular disease (e.g. aneurysms), or for inferior petrosal sinus sampling in Cushing's disease. Skull radiographs no longer have a role but fluoroscopy may assist in surgical localization or to monitor the flow of contrast media administered intrathecally for the localization of CSF leakage caused by pituitary tumours or trans-sphenoidal surgery.

Indications and contraindications

Pituitary imaging should be performed in patients with endocrine disturbances suggesting pituitary dysfunction (i.e. hyperprolactinaemia, hypogonadism, and Cushing's disease). Non-endocrine symptoms and signs suggesting pituitary disease are headache, visual symptoms such as blurring and diplopia, and visual field defects indicating compression of the optic chiasm (e.g. bitemporal hemianopia). Additional abnormal symptoms that warrant MRI are palsies of other cranial nerves (third, fourth, and sixth), and other neurological symptoms suggestive of mass lesions in the sella region. Follow-up imaging of patients with a known pituitary mass is the commonest reason for scanning.

Contraindications to MRI are the presence of metallic body implants, which are liable to movement (e.g. vascular clips), and electronic implants such as cardiac pacemakers. Patients may not tolerate MRI if they are claustrophobic or if they are very obese and cannot fit within standard sized scanners. Pregnancy is a relative contraindication. Despite the lack of a known biological hazard, scanning in the first trimester is not recommended.

MRI techniques

The resolution of MRI depends on the ratio of signal to noise. This is improved by increasing the magnet strength, obtaining more data (longer scan times), and using dedicated transmitters and receivers. In practice, MRI scanning protocols are a compromise, performed using 1.5–3.0-tesla magnets, sensible scan times (3–8 minutes per scan), and electronic sequences optimized to reduce movement artefacts (from cavernous sinus pulsation and swallowing; see Figure 3.5). Post-operative imaging is best delayed for 3–6 months to allow surrounding tissues to heal. Trans-sphenoidal surgeons may use a tissue homograft which includes fat to close defects in the anterior sella, and this tissue needs to be distinguished from residual or recurrent tumour. Over 1–2 years, MRI signal from implanted fat (typically bright on the T1-weighted scan) fades.

See Table 3.3 for a typical scan protocol, and Table 3.4 for additional sequences.

Dynamic scanning

This technique is used to identify and/or localize microadenomas by differences in the speed of uptake of gadolinium between the normal pituitary and a small tumour. Images in the coronal plane are made immediately after gadolinium injection so that increasing signal change in the tissues can be observed. In most instances, the uptake in the gland precedes that in tumour by 20–30 seconds. See Table 3.5.

Surveillance scanning

Intervals between follow up scans are usually determined by locally agreed protocols. In general, post-operative

(a) 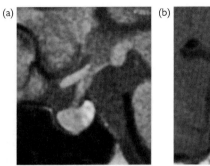 (b)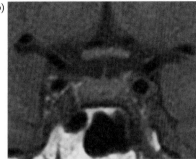

Fig 3.5 A normal pituitary on MRI. (a) Sagittal T1-weighted MRI of a normal pituitary. (b) Coronal T1-weighted MRI of a normal pituitary.
Reproduced from Wass AH, Stewart PM, Amiel SA et al., *Oxford Textbook of Endocrinology and Diabetes*, Second Edition, Fig. 2.3.5.1, Copyright © 2011, with permission from Oxford University Press.

Table 3.3 A typical MRI scan protocol

#1 spin echo	T1 weighted	Coronal plane	Small FOV	5 minutes
#2 spin echo	T1 weighted	Sagittal plane	Small FOV	5 minutes
#3 spin echo	T2 weighted	Axial plane	Large FOV	3 minutes

Abbreviations: FOV, field of view.

Table 3.4 Additional sequences

#4 spin echo	T1 weighted post gadolinium	Coronal plane	Small FOV	5 minutes
#5 spin echo	T1 weighted post gadolinium	Sagittal plane	Small FOV	5 minutes
#6 spin echo	T2 weighted	Coronal plane	Medium FOV	3 minutes

Abbreviations: FOV, field of view.

Table 3.5 Dynamic scanning

| #7 spin echo | T1 weighted | Coronal plane | Small FOV | 2 minutes |

Abbreviations: FOV, field of view.

MRI is delayed for 3–6 months after trans-sphenoidal tumour resection to allow healing and performed to obtain a baseline study. Subsequent imaging should then be performed with the same MRI protocols. Its value for small hypersecting tumours is limited, since biochemical monitoring of treatment is more sensitive, and regular assessments of vision can detect chiasm compression. Follow-up of non-functioning adenoma is generally performed annually for 5 years and then omitted or extended to every other year. The numbers of scans and length of follow-up for patients treated by combined resection and radiotherapy can be less.

Imaging findings in common pathologies

Incidentaloma
Small pituitary masses are common incidental findings on brain MRI with pituitary masses >3 mm reported in about 10% of patients without endocrine symptoms. These so-called incidentalomas are rarely progressive or clinically relevant.

Pituitary adenoma
An arbitrary 1 cm maximum dimension threshold separates microadenoma from macroademona as descriptive terms for tumours of the anterior pituitary.

Macroadenoma
The MRI signal depends on the tumour structure and generally cannot be used to distinguish hormone secreting from non-secreting tumours. Adenomas return signal that is, generally, homogeneous and of similar intensity to that of the anterior lobe. They enhance after gadolinium administration, as does normal gland tissue (see Figure 3.6). However, if they contain cysts, these return lower (darker) signal (on T1-weighted scans), and any dystrophic calcification returns very little signal and so cannot easily be distinguished. Tumour calcification returns hypointensity (dark) on both T1- and T2-weighted scans. Thus, areas of calcification have to be large to be identified on MRI. After tumour necrosis or bleeding within solid tumour tissue or cysts, the signal is heterogeneous. It is usually distinguishable by the

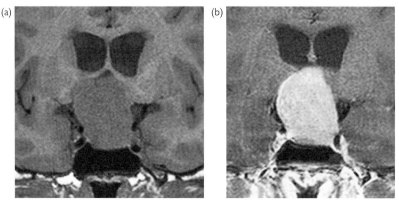

Fig 3.6 Pituitary macroadenoma. (a) Coronal T1-weighted MRI showing a large tumour expanding the pituitary fossa and filling the chiasmatic cistern. (b) The tumour enhances after gadolinium administration.

presence of high-signal areas caused by the breakdown products of haemoglobin or tumour secretions. Thus, areas returning hyperintense or bright signal are seen on T1-weighted sequences after haemorrhage (i.e. apoplexy). This may persist for several months and should not be confused with signal from fat (which is also bright on T1-weighted scans) introduced as a packing material after transphenoidal surgery. MRI can identify invasion of surrounding structures by tumour. Thus, reports should include details of any superior extension and its relationship to the anterior optic pathway (optic chiasm, tracts, or nerves) as well as lateral extension into the cavernous sinuses or invasion of bone and sinuses of the sphenoid. It may be difficult to distinguish invasion of the cavernous sinuses from a tumour bulging laterally and displacing the medial walls of the sinuses. Invasion is diagnosed only if the normal contour of the lateral sinus walls is lost.

Microadenomas

Microadenomas are only evident if they return signal, which contrasts with that of the normal gland. This is usually lower (i.e. darker) but occasionally it may be higher (i.e. brighter) than the normal gland (see Figure 3.7). Gadolinium enhancement and dynamic scanning is useful to demonstrate small adenomas.

Other common pituitary tumours

Craniopharyngioma

On MRI the signal reflects the variable types of tissue that constitute this tumour (Figure 3.8). The adamantinomatous type (predominantly found in children) is likely to contain larger cysts and calcification than the papillary type (predominantly found in adults). Typically centred superior to the gland, these tumours extend into the chiasmatic cistern with both intrasellar and suprasellar involvement. The cysts may contain fluid that is bright on T1-weighted scans due to blood products, cholesterol, or protein. This feature is also seen in *Rathke's cleft cysts*, whose appearance is similar to the cystic components of craniopharyngioma but without solid tumour tissue.

Meningioma

Meningiomas arising from the dura adjacent to the sella may simulate pituitary tumours because they return homogenous signal, like the gland, and often extend into the sella and suprasellar compartments (see Figure 3.9). They may contain calcification and usually show intense enhancement after gadolinium administration. A 'tail' of tumour enhancement extending into the adjacent dura is characteristic and virtually diagnostic.

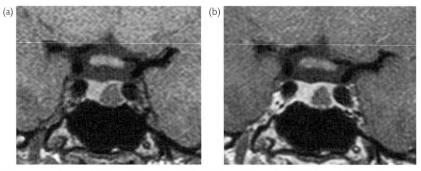

Fig 3.7 Pituitary microadenoma. (a) Coronal T1-weighted MRI. (b) Coronal T1-weighted MRI after gadolinium enhancement.

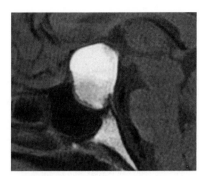

Fig 3.8 Craniopharyngioma (adamantinomatous type).

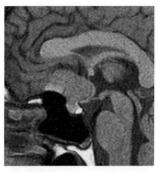

Fig 3.9 T1-weighted MRI showing a meningioma arising from the planum sphenoidale, elevating the frontal lobe, and extending posteriorly to displace the optic chiasm and lamina terminalis. Its signal is slightly darker than that of the anterior pituitary, which is seen under the mass in the sella.

Conclusion

- MRI is the method of first choice, and CT is used principally when MRI is contraindicated or patients cannot tolerate scanning.
- Gadolinium enhancement has a limited role.
- Localizing the extent of tumours relative to the pituitary fossa helps diagnosis and is crucial for treatment planning.

Further reading

Bonneville JF, Bonneville F, and Cattin F. Magnetic resonance imaging of pituitary adenomas. *Eur Radiol* 2005; 15: 543–8.

Byrne JV. 'Imaging of the pituitary', in Wass JHA and Stewart PM, eds, *Oxford Textbook of Endocrinology*, 2011. Oxford University Press, pp. 136–44.

Famini P, Maya MM, and Melmed S. Pituitary magnetic resonance imaging for sellar and parasellar masses: Ten-year experience in 2598 patients. *J Clin Endocrinol Metab* 2011; 96: 1630–41.

Scott WA. *Magnetic Resonance Imaging of the Brain and Spine* (5th edition), 2016. *Lippincott-Raven*, Wolters Kluwer.

3.4 Approach to the assessment of disorders of pituitary hormone homeostasis

Hypopituitarism

Hypopituitarism refers to a state of deficiency of one or more pituitary hormones. There are six recognized anterior hormones (growth hormone, LH, FSH, adrenocorticotrophic hormone, TSH, and prolactin), and two posterior pituitary hormones (vasopressin and oxytocin). All pituitary hormones are under regulatory control from both hypothalamic hormones and negative feedback from the corresponding peripheral hormone or effect. The resultant anterior pituitary hormone secretory patterns are complex with superimposed diurnal and ultradian rhythms. Early diagnosis of hypopituitarism is essential due to its association with increased morbidity, impaired well-being, and excess mortality.

The presentation of hypopituitarism is frequently insidious and comprised of non-specific symptoms such as lethargy, lightheadedness, and alterations in body composition. As a result, delay in diagnosis of hypopituitarism is frequent. More specific symptoms may also occur (amenorrhoea) which may direct investigations towards abnormalities of the hypothalamo-pituitary axes earlier. The pattern by which hormone deficiencies evolve is dependent upon the insult to the hypothalamo-pituitary axis. In the majority of cases (pituitary tumours, parasellar tumours, hypothalamo-pituitary irradiation), pituitary hormone deficits develop in the following order:

- growth hormone
- gonadotrophins
- adrenocorticotrophic hormone
- TSH

This order is less predictable where damage to the hypothalamo-pituitary axes is due, for example, to transcription factor mutations, traumatic brain injury, hypophysitis, or Sheehan's syndrome.

Establishing a diagnosis of hypopituitarism is dependent upon a combination of the following:

- clinical suspicion
- biochemical assessment
- imaging of the pituitary

Full biochemical assessment of hypopituitarism usually requires a combination of baseline and stimulation tests. Basal pituitary hormone assessment incorporates measurement of both the pituitary hormone and the target hormone, most reliably performed at 07.00–09.00 h to aid interpretation. Where these tests do not provide adequate information, a stimulation test may be necessary. Consensus varies as to the most appropriate stimulation test(s) to perform. Intuitively, the use of hypothalamic releasing hormones (corticotrophin-releasing hormone (CRH), gonadotrophin-releasing hormone (GnRH), TRH, and growth-hormone-releasing hormone (GHRH)) to test pituitary-axis integrity would appear sensible; however, these tests have failed to live up to expectations and now have little diagnostic utility in the adult. Stimulation tests have therefore centred around measurement of the peripheral hormone. Although a number of diagnostic thresholds have been established for tests of pituitary function, there is significant dependency on the assay used, and diagnostic thresholds therefore need to be confirmed locally.

The results of biochemical assessment of the hypothalamo-pituitary axes must always be taken within the clinical context. For example, a patient found on routine blood tests to have a slightly low FT4 with a normal TSH may be suggestive of secondary hypothyroidism. This needs to be placed in the context that, in the absence of additional pituitary-hormone deficits, isolated TSH deficiency is rare. This biochemical finding is therefore more likely to represent the patient being one of the 2.5% of normal individuals with an FT4 value below the normative range, heterophile antibody interference, or a concomitant drug effect (i.e. carbamazepine).

The growth-hormone axis

Physiological growth-hormone secretion is pulsatile, with levels below the limit of detection of clinically available growth-hormone assays for the majority of the day. The majority of pulsatile growth-hormone secretion occurs during the first few hours of sleep, associated with slow-wave sleep. Serum IGF-I is a growth-hormone-dependent protein through which growth hormone exerts many of its actions and thus can be used as a surrogate marker for integrated growth hormone secretion. A number of additional factors influence IGF-I secretion, with serum levels being lower in renal dysfunction, hepatic dysfunction, protein malnutrition, and hypothyroidism. Additionally, IGF-I levels fall with aging, reflecting a fall in 24-hour integrated growth-hormone secretion. Levels of the predominant IGF-I binding protein, IGFBP-3, are growth-hormone dependent. IGFBP-3 forms a ternary complex with acid-labile subunit and IGF-I to prolong the half-life of IGF-I, thereby stabilizing IGF-I levels in serum.

Given the dependency of serum IGF-I and serum IGFBP-3 on 24-hour integrated growth-hormone secretion, the utility of both of these proteins has been proposed in the diagnosis of growth-hormone deficiency. The attraction is that the diagnosis could potentially been made on a single blood test, without the need for more complex and labour-intensive growth-hormone stimulation tests or growth-hormone profiling. There is, however, significant overlap between the normative range and that of individuals with severe growth-hormone deficiency (Figure 3.10). The degree of overlap is greater for IGFBP-3 than IGF-I, implicating IGF-I as the more useful of these two proteins. Growth hormone secretion and, consequently, IGF-I levels decrease with ageing, with ambient IGF-I levels becoming relatively less dependent on growth hormone with age. The result is that the IGF-I range for normal individuals and growth-hormone-deficient hypopituitary subjects show increasing overlap with ageing, such that a normal IGF-I level does not exclude a diagnosis of growth-hormone deficiency. Subnormal IGF-I levels are consistent with a diagnosis of growth-hormone deficiency in the absence of confounding factors, and may be sufficient to establish the diagnosis where there is evidence of multiple pituitary hormone deficits.

Formal assessment of the integrity of the growth-hormone axis is dependent on direct quantification of the ability of the hypothalamo-pituitary axis to secrete

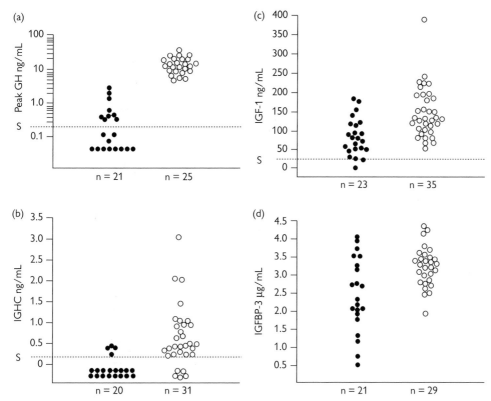

Fig 3.10 Results of tests of growth hormone (GH) deficiency in normal (white dots) and hypopituitary (black dots) subjects. (a) Peak GH response to an insulin tolerance test (ITT). (b) Mean 24-hour GH (24-hour integrated GH concentration (IGHC)); (c) IGF-I concentration; (d) IGFBP-3 concentration. Note the logarithmic scale for ITT; S, assay sensitivity for GH (0.2 ng/mL) and IGF-I (25 ng/mL); n, number of subjects tested.
Reprinted from *The Lancet*, Volume 343, Hoffman DM., O'Sullivan AJ., Ho KKY, et al., Diagnosis of growth-hormone deficiency in adults, pp. 1064–1068, Copyright (1994), with permission from Elsevier.

growth hormone. This requires the use of a growth-hormone stimulation test. A large number of agents have been identified to promote growth-hormone secretion. Those most utilized in clinical practice include the following:

- insulin tolerance test (ITT)
- GHRH–arginine test
- glucagon stimulation test

ITT
Insulin-induced hypoglycaemia is a powerful stimulant to cortisol and growth hormone release. After basal levels are measured, soluble insulin (0.1–0.15 IU/kg) is administered, and blood collected every 15 minutes for 1 hour and every 30 minutes for the following hour for cortisol, growth hormone, and glucose. The patient is observed closely for signs of hypoglycaemia along with regular capillary blood-glucose monitoring. Once hypoglycaemia has been induced, the patient is given oral glucose and a meal to resolve the hypoglycaemia. The test is contraindicated in patients with known ischaemic heart disease, epilepsy, or an abnormal ECG. Many endocrinologists also have an age

threshold of 65 years. The morbidity of this test in experienced hands within an endocrine investigation unit is reassuringly low.

GHRH-arginine test
Following a basal measurement of growth hormone, arginine 0.5 mg/kg (max 30 mg) is infused over 30 minutes, followed by GHRH 1 µg/kg over 2 minutes. Transient flushing is not infrequent following injection of GHRH. Growth hormone levels are measured every 30 minutes for 3 hours.

Glucagon stimulation test
After basal measurements, injection of 1mg glucagon intramuscularly is followed by measurement of both cortisol and growth hormone every 30 minutes for 3–5 hours. It is less potent and a less reliable stimulant than the ITT, and false positive results are not infrequent. Up to 30% of patients experience nausea, with vomiting and abdominal pain occurring less frequently.

Diagnostic thresholds for growth-hormone deficiency are dependent on the stimulation test employed. The ITT shows good separation between growth-hormone-replete individuals, and those patients with severe growth-hormone deficiency (Figure 3.10), with a peak growth-hormone response of <3 μg/L arbitrarily defining severe growth hormone deficiency in the adult. Reproducibility of the ITT is good. Equivalent diagnostic thresholds when using alternate stimulation tests have been established. Notably, peak responses to all growth-hormone stimulation tests are abrogated with increases in abdominal adiposity and BMI. Care must therefore be taken in interpreting the results of stimulation tests performed in overweight and obese individuals. A graduated diagnostic threshold has been suggested for use of the GHRH–arginine test in patients whom are overweight or obese (Corneli et al., 2005). The GHRH–arginine test is a more exuberant stimulant of growth hormone secretion compared with the ITT. A diagnosis of growth hormone deficiency is considered in patients of normal BMI (<25 kg/m^2) with a peak growth-hormone response <11.5 μg/L, whereas the diagnostic threshold where growth hormone deficiency should be considered in patients whom are overweight (BMI 25–30 mg/kg^2) or obese (BMI >30 kg/m^2) is 8.0 and 4.2 μg/L respectively. Additional growth hormone stimulation tests, including clonidine, L-DOPA and arginine, are only weak stimulants of growth hormone, are poorly reproducible, and should therefore not be used to characterize growth hormone status in adults.

In practical terms, the likelihood of growth-hormone deficiency increases with the degree of hypopituitarism. The probability of growth-hormone deficiency where there are 0, 1, or 2/3 additional anterior pituitary hormone deficits is 24%, 55%, and 91% respectively. Thus, in patients with two or three additional anterior pituitary hormone deficits, either a low-IGF-I or subthreshold peak growth-hormone response on stimulation would be considered supportive of a diagnosis of growth-hormone deficiency. In the setting of isolated or one additional anterior pituitary hormone deficit, two supportive tests are ideally required—either a low-IGF-I and a subthreshold peak growth-hormone response to stimulation, or a subthreshold peak growth-hormone response to two separate growth-hormone stimulation tests. Notably, adult-onset isolated growth-hormone deficiency in the absence of an insult to the hypothalamo-pituitary axis has not been substantiated, and care should be taken when considering this as a diagnosis given the false-positive diagnostic frequency of up to 10% with the growth-hormone stimulation tests commonly used in clinical practice.

The reproductive axis

Gonadotrophin deficiency in men displays a continuum from severe deficiency with low gonadotrophins and a clearly subnormal testosterone level, to that of mild androgen deficiency defined by gonadotrophin and testosterone levels both within the lower reaches of the normative range (partial gonadotrophin deficiency). When measuring testosterone, SHBG should also be measured to aid interpretation of 'free' testosterone levels.

Diagnostic difficulties occur only for men with partial gonadotrophin deficiency. Where serum levels are consistent with partial gonadotrophin deficiency and there are additional anterior pituitary hormone deficits, there is evidence for an insult to the hypothalamo-pituitary axis, and the individual is symptomatic, androgen replacement should be considered. As with the diagnosis of growth-hormone deficiency, obesity and abdominal adiposity are confounders to the interpretation of tests of the reproductive axis, as both gonadotrophins and testosterone levels are frequently reduced, particularly if there is concurrent diabetes mellitus (late-onset hypogonadism).

In females, even slight attenuation of gonadotrophin secretion leads to absence of ovulation; anovulatory cycles; and subsequent amenorrhoea. As with men, the diagnosis is clear when both the gonadotrophins and estradiol are suppressed, but is less clear when gonadotrophin and estradiol levels lie in the normative range. The presence of additional anterior pituitary hormone deficits may aid diagnosis. A regular menstrual cycle does not necessarily correlate with ovulation, and measurement of Day 19–25 progesterone levels may be necessary to confirm this.

The glucocorticoid axis

The primary importance of testing the integrity of the hypothalamo-pituitary–adrenal axis lies in ensuring patients with a known insult to the pituitary have sufficient ability to secrete cortisol in times of stress. Testing is also performed where patients exhibit symptoms of adrenal insufficiency. Notably, cortisol requirements for stresses are different from those required to maintain day-to-day health. As such, some patients who fail to produce an adequate response to stimulation may not have enough ambient cortisol in times of stress, although they may not require regular glucocorticoid replacement. Experience in the management and interpretation of the diagnostic tests of these individuals is essential to avoid patients inappropriately commencing lifelong glucocorticoid replacement or, alternately, the patient being left untreated.

Cortisol measurements are almost exclusively undertaken using radioimmunoassays. Hydrocortisone is appropriately quantitated and prednisolone shows a variable degree of cross-reactivity, whereas dexamethasone is not measured using cortisol radioimmunoassays. To assess endogenous cortisol, hydrocortisone and prednisolone should be discontinued for at least 12 and 24 hours, respectively. Around 90% of cortisol is bound to cortisol-binding globulin (CBG), and measurements with radioimmuno assays reflect 'total cortisol'. Levels of cortisol are therefore highly dependent on variables that modulate CBG levels. Levels of CBG increase in response to oestrogen, making it difficult to interpret cortisol levels during pregnancy and in patients receiving oestrogens. Oestrogen-containing preparations should be withdrawn at least 4–6 weeks before assessment of cortisol status. Conversely, falsely low cortisol levels are observed in protein-losing states (malnutrition, nephrotic syndrome, protein-losing enteropathies). Growth hormone can also reduce CBG, resulting in misleadingly low levels in acromegaly.

Measurement of a single early morning cortisol level at 07.00–09.00 h, when cortisol levels are at their highest, can be of value diagnostically. Adequacy of this axis can be inferred from a random cortisol level of more than 400 nmol/L (14.5 μg/dL). A cortisol level of less than 100 nmol/L (3.6 μg/dL) at this time is consistent with cortisol insufficiency, and the patient should be commenced on glucocorticoid replacement immediately. Ideally, confirmation using a stimulation test should be performed electively. The majority of 09.00 h cortisol values, both for healthy individuals and those with hypopituitarism, lie between 100–400 nmol/L (3.6–14.5 μg/dL) and require further evaluation with a stimulation test.

The most frequently used stimulation tests clinically are as follows:

- ITT
- Short Synacthen® test
- glucagon stimulation test

Short Synacthen® test

In hypopituitarism, loss of the trophic action of adreno-corticotrophic hormone leads to atropy of the zona fasciulata over a period of several weeks, and subsequent blunting of the cortisol response to exogenous adrenocorticotrophic hormone. The standard test involves injection of a pharmacological dose of synthetic adrenocorticotrophic hormone (Syn-acth-en, 250 μg) to directly stimulate cortisol production. Blood is taken at baseline and at 30 minutes for assessment of cortisol levels. False-negative results can occur if the test is performed early in the onset of hypopituitarism (e.g. post-apoplexy), such that atrophy of the adrenal gland has not yet occurred. A low-dose Synacthen® test has also been championed, using 1 μg of Synacthen® to reflect a more physiological stimulus. Although the low-dose test has been purported to have some benefits over the standard test, relating to false reassurance of a normal cortisol axis in patients with hypopituitarism, dilution of Synacthen® from a 250 μg vial can lead to errors and lack of reproducibility.

Thresholds for adequacy of cortisol secretory reserve are dependent on the stimulation test performed and assay in use locally. For the ITT a peak cortisol of >500 nmol/L (18.12 μg/dL; depending on assay) is considered consistent with normal cortisol reserve. This threshold reflects levels observed in patients undergoing major abdominal surgery. The ITT is generally accepted as the 'gold standard' for assessment of the hypothalamo-pituitary–adrenal axis, although, as with all tests of cortisol reserve, it requires interpretation within the clinical context.

The thyroid axis

The diagnosis of secondary hypothyroidism is based entirely on measurement of TSH and free-thyroid hormones levels. In profound hypopituitarism, both TSH and the free-thyroid hormone levels are low and the diagnosis is clear. In more equivocal disease, both the TSH and free-thyroid-hormone levels lie in the lower reaches of the normative range. Where this occurs, there is almost always evidence for additional anterior-pituitary-hormone deficits to aid diagnosis. Less commonly in secondary hypothyroidism, a picture of high-normal or mildly elevated TSH levels can occur with low free-thyroid-hormone levels. This results from an increase in immunoactive, but biologically inactive, forms of TSH. Functional abnormalities of TSH secretion are common in hypothalamo-pituitary disease, but are not pathognomic of evolving secondary hypothyroidism. These anomalies include loss of the normal nocturnal TSH surge and delay, or attenuation, of the TSH response to TRH. The use of the TRH test in diagnosis of secondary hypothyroidism has no utility.

Prolactin

Deficiency of prolactin is infrequent, most commonly being observed in transcription factor deficiencies including PROP1 and POU1F1, or post-pituitary surgery. Confirmation of prolactin deficiency can be ascertained using the TRH test. Other than failure of lactation, there are no data to suggest long-term adverse health outcomes of prolactin deficiency.

Anterior pituitary hormone replacement

With the exception of growth hormone, pituitary hormone replacement is undertaken with the peripheral target hormone (sex steroids, cortisol, T4), in preference to the pituitary trophic hormone. Replacement therapy with the pituitary trophic hormones would, in practice, impart a layer of difficulty, as these hormones are proteins and glycoproteins that would require parenteral administration and have only a short half-life. The peripheral hormones, steroids and thyroxines, are more stable with a longer half-life and allow oral administration. Particular care should be taken during pregnancy (see also Chapter 10, Section 10.3).

Sex-steroid replacement

In the setting of gonadotrophin deficiency, consideration has to be given to both sex-hormone replacement and fertility potential. Both of these aspects need to be considered in context for an individual.

For males, androgen replacement should be considered where fertility is not requisite in the forthcoming 12 months. In the majority of cases, androgen replacement will be required for life. Androgens are important in males for sexual health, maintenance of bone and muscle mass, and well-being. Side effects are infrequent with physiological replacement, although they can include mood swings, aggression, increased libido, and polycythaemia. As replacement therapy aims to bring androgen levels back into the normal range, androgenic actions on the prostate should not increase the risk of prostatic hypertrophy or cancer above that of the background male population.

There are a number of modes of delivery of androgens, including oral, transdermal, buccal, and parenteral formulations. Replacement is undertaken and monitored as for primary hypogonadism aiming to place testosterone levels within the normative range. Gonadotrophin levels are of no value in guiding appropriateness of replacement. Where induction of fertility is desired, gonadotrophin therapy is necessary. Therapy is commenced using recombinant LH or highly purified hCG self-administered subcutaneously thrice per week. Once testosterone levels have been optimized and maintained for at least 3 months, a semen analysis can be performed. Where there is little or no improvement in the semen analysis, recombinant FSH or highly purified human menopausal gonadotrophin (hMG) is added to the regimen. It can take up to 2 years to optimize the semen analysis. A normal semen analysis is not requisite for fertility with spontaneous conception often occurring before normal semen concentrations are reached. The use of assisted fertility techniques improve outcomes further.

In females, consideration needs to be given to establishing fertility requirements before sex-hormone replacement is commenced. Where fertility is being considered relatively soon, referral to an assisted fertility unit should be considered. Oestrogen replacement is important in premenopausal women to maintain bone mass and well-being, as well as prevent symptoms of oestrogen deficiency. Sex-steroid replacement should be undertaken with a combination of oestrogen and progesterone in women with an intact uterus, and oestrogens alone where the patient has had a previous hysterectomy.

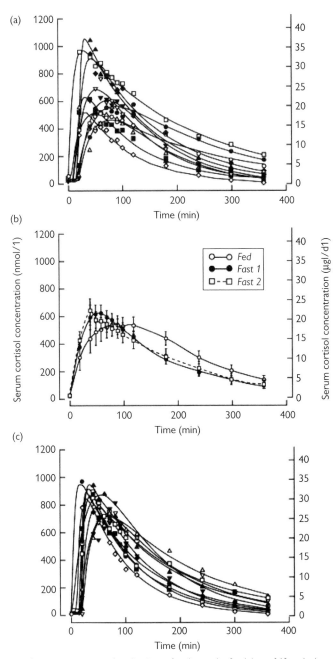

Fig 3.11 (a) Serum cortisol concentrations in ten fasted patients after they took a fixed dose of 10 mg hydrocortisone; (b) mean serum cortisol concentrations following a fixed dose of 10 mg hydrocortisone, in fasting and fed states; and (c) serum cortisol concentration in ten fasted patients after they took a weight-adjusted (0.12 mg/kg) dose of hydrocortisone.
Reproduced with permission from Mah PM, Jenkins RC., Rostami-Hodjegan A. et al., Weight-related dosing, timing and monitoring hydrocortisone replacement therapy in patients with adrenal insufficiency, *Clinical Endocrinology*, Volume 61, Issue 3, pp. 367–375, Copyright (2004) John Wiley and Sons Ltd.

The optimal regimen for sex-steroid replacement has not yet been established. In practice, oestrogen replacement regimens are individualized, taking into account patient preferences. Choices for oestrogen replacement are as follows:

- the combined oral contraceptive pill or hormone replacement therapy
- transdermal or oral oestorgen replacement
- cyclical or continuous oestorgen replacement

Potential side effects of oestrogen replacement include fluid retention, headaches, thromboembolic disease, breast tenderness, and mood swings. Monitoring is clinical for efficacy and side effects. Gonadotrophin and oestrogen levels are suppressed in women taking the oral contraceptive, and are variable in women taking hormone replacement therapy, with the gonadotrophins frequently remaining elevated. Recent guidelines provide helpful information regarding the assessment and treatment of hypothalamic amenorrhoea.

Cortisol

In adrenocorticotrophic-hormone deficiency, replacement of the target hormone, cortisol, is performed using one of several glucocorticoids. The most commonly used glucocorticoids used are hydrocortisone, prednisolone, dexamethasone, and cortisone acetate (outside the UK). Replacement glucocorticoids vary in potency and half-life. Only dexamethasone has no mineralocorticoid activity. Most endocrinologists use hydrocortisone as replacement therapy, as it is molecularly identical to cortisol and is therefore measurable on the cortisol assay. The short half-life of hydrocortisone necessitates taking tablets two or three times per day. The latter provides a closer approximation to daytime physiological cortisol levels, particularly where the dose is adjusted for weight (Figure 3.11); however, this does not replace the physiological cortisol secretion observed in the early hours of the morning. The absence of glucocorticoid on waking is the likely explanation for the lethargy and lack of initiative experienced by adrenal insufficient individuals on waking. A once-daily dual core formulation of hydrocortisone has become available which more closely mimics the daytime physiological profile of cortisol, but not the early morning cortisol release. Early data shows some improvement in metabolic indicies compared with standard hydrocortisone.

Studies of cortisol production rates using stable nucleotides show daily secretion of 5–7 mg/m^2, equating to a daily dosage of 10–15 mg. Patients with hypopituitarism frequently have at least some residual cortisol secretion, and therefore may not require full replacement dosage.

Patient education as to the importance of increasing glucocorticoids with intercurrent illness, physical stress, and surgical procedures is central to management of these individuals. Patients should be provided with hydrocortisone for parenteral administration in times of protracted vomiting, and taught in the use of this. Provision of written information regarding the importance of changing steroid doses in illness and stress is essential, and all patients should be encouraged to have a medical alert bracelet or pendant.

Thyroid hormone replacement

Thyroid hormone replacement is performed exclusively using levothyroxine monotherapy. TSH levels are of no utility in optimizing thyroid hormone replacement, and thus monitoring of levels are dependent exclusively on measurement of FT4 levels. In general, the aim is to place FT4 levels in the upper half of the normal range to ensure adequate replacement.

Prolactin

There is no indication, or provision, for prolactin replacement.

Growth hormone replacement

Growth hormone replacement was not considered as important to the adult until the publication of two seminal studies of adult growth hormone replacement in 1989 (Salomon et al., 1989, Jorgensen et al., 1989). It has since become clear that severe growth-hormone deficiency in adults results in a number of adverse sequelea, including

- excess total and truncal fat mass
- increased total and LDL-cholesterol
- reduced lean body mass
- reduced exercise tolerance
- a procoagulant environment;
- impaired well-being and quality of life

Fracture rates are also increased in these individuals, although data on bone mass are conflicting. Bone mass is decreased in those individuals who developed growth-hormone deficiency during childhood. Initial studies of adult growth-hormone replacement were performed using weight-based dosing regimens which were later replaced by incremental increases in growth hormone dose aiming to optimize the IGF-I level within the upper half of the normative range. In most individuals the growth hormone dose is commenced at 0.2–0.3 mg/day and titrated on the basis of IGF-I levels checked at 2–4 weekly intervals until the maintenance dose is achieved.

Adult growth-hormone replacement leads to increased lean body mass and bone mass, reduced truncal and total body fat mass, reductions in total and LDL cholesterol, plasminogen activator inhibitor-1, fibrinogen, and CRP. Improvements in exercise tolerance and strength are small, and occur over a protracted period of at least 12 months. Quality of life improves, but specifically in those patients with significant impairment at baseline. Notably, at least 50% of patients with severe growth-hormone deficiency do not exhibit significantly impaired quality of life. Effects on fracture rates and mortality have not been established in the setting of clinical trials. Potential side effects include joint pains and fluid retention, which are reversible with dose reduction.

References and further reading

Abdu TA, Elhadd TA, Neary R, et al. Comparison of the low dose short synacthen test (1 microg), the conventional dose short synacthen test (250 microg), and the insulin tolerance test for assessment of the hypothalamo-pituitary-adrenal axis in patients with pituitary disease. *J Clin Endocrinol Metab* 1999; 84: 838–43.

Bates AS, Van't Hoff W, Jones PJ, et al. The effect of hypopituitarism on life expectancy. *J Clin Endocrinol Metab* 1996; 81: 1169–72.

Corneli G, Di Somma C, Baldelli R, et al. The cut-off limits of the GH response to GH-releasing hormone-arginine test related to body mass index. *Eur J Endocrinol* 2005; 153: 257–64.

Esteban NV, Loughlin T, Yergey AL, et al. Daily cortisol production rate in man determined by stable isotope dilution/mass spectrometry. *J Clin Endocrinol Metab* 1991; 72: 39–45.

Gordon CM, Ackerman KE, Berga SL, et al. Functional hypothal-amic amenorrhea: an endocrine society clinical practice guide-line. *J Clin Endocrinol Metab* 2017; 102: 1413–39.

Hoffman DM, O'Sullivan AJ, Baxter RC, et al. Diagnosis of growth-hormone deficiency in adults. *Lancet* 1994; 343: 1064–8.

Johannsson G, Nilsson AG, Bergthorsdottir R, et al. Improved cortisol exposure-time profile and outcome in patients with ad-renal insufficiency: A prospective randomized trial of a novel hydrocortisone dual-release formulation. *J Clin Endocrinol Metab* 2012; 97: 473–81.

Jorgensen JO, Pedersen SA, Thuesen L, et al. Beneficial effects of growth hormone treatment in GH-deficient adults. *Lancet* 1989; 1: 1221–5.

Lee KO, Persani L, Tan M, et al. Thyrotropin with decreased bio-logical activity, a delayed consequence of cranial irradiation for nasopharyngeal carcinoma. *J Endocrinol Invest* 1995; 18: 800–5.

Mah PM, Jenkins RC, Rostami-Hodjegan A, et al. Weight-related dosing, timing and monitoring hydrocortisone replacement therapy in patients with adrenal insufficiency. *Clin Endocrinol (Oxf)* 2004; 61: 367–75.

Plumpton FS and Besser GM. The adrenocortical response to surgery and insulin-induced hypoglycaemia in corticosteroid-treated and normal subjects. *Br J Surg* 1969; 56: 216–9.

Purnell JQ, Brandon DD, Isabelle LM, et al. Association of 24-hour cortisol production rates, cortisol-binding globulin, and plasma-free cortisol levels with body composition, leptin levels, and aging in adult men and women. *J Clin Endocrinol Metab* 2004; 89: 281–7.

Rosen T and Bengtsson BA. Premature mortality due to cardio-vascular disease in hypopituitarism. *Lancet* 1990; 336: 285–8.

Salomon F, Cuneo RC, Hesp R, et al. The effects of treatment with recombinant human growth hormone on body compos-ition and metabolism in adults with growth hormone deficiency. *N Engl J Med* 1989; 321: 1797–803.

Toogood AA, Beardwell CG, and Shalet SM. The severity of growth hormone deficiency in adults with pituitary disease is related to the degree of hypopituitarism. *Clin Endocrinol (Oxf)* 1994; 41: 511–6.

3.5 Prolactinomas

Epidemiology

Prolactinomas are responsible for 51% of pituitary adenomas, and their prevalence is estimated as 500 cases/million inhabitants. They more commonly affect women between the third and fourth decades, in a proportion ten times higher than men up to 50 years of age. Pituitary carcinomas are extremely rare and suspected if the tumour is aggressive and unresponsive to dopamine agonists cases.

Pathophysiology

Prolactin secretion is under the tuberohypophysial dopaminergic neurons inhibitory tonus. Dopamine acts via dopaminergic type 2 receptor, leading to reduction of intracellular calcium and cAMP concentrations paralleled with the impairment of prolactin gene transcription, reducing therefore prolactin secretion. Moreover, the dopaminergic system is also responsible for lactotrophs antiproliferative actions. On the other hand, prolactin secretion is also stimulated by diverse dopaminergic neurons inhibitors such as opioids, neuropeptide Y, and so on, or by factors that directly stimulate prolactin secretion including vasoactive intestinal polypeptide. Nursing stimulus, via intercostal innervation, and stress also have a stimulatory role. Oestrogens directly stimulate prolactin secretion by lactotrophs and also reduce dopamine action.

Hyperprolactinaemia leads to hypogonadotrophic hypogonadism mainly due to inhibition of GnRH pulse secretion, but also to a directly inhibitory effect on steroidogenic activity at the gonads.

Clinical features

Hypogonadism hypogonadotrophic in hyperprolactinaemic patients is characterized by irregular menses and amenorrhea in women, sexual dysfunction, infertility, and loss of bone mineral density in both genders. Galactorrhoea is frequently seen among women; however, it is not a specific sign. Hyperprolactinaemia is an important cause of infertility in clinical practice. In women, it is characterized by a short luteal phase, anovulatory cycles, oligomenorrhoea, and amenorrhea. In men, abnormal spermatogenesis can be found. Hyperprolactinaemic patients may present with reduced bone mineral density which can lead to vertebral fractures in both genders.

An impaired quality of life is reported among patients with hyperprolactinaemia. In women with microadenomas, anxiety and depression are frequently found and related to prolactin levels.

Regarding patients with macroadenomas, tumour mass effect including headache, visual impairment, and hydrocephalus can occur, especially in giant tumours. Hypopituitarism can also occur as a result of pituitary stalk compression or pituitary destruction.

Investigation

Usually, in prolactinomas, prolactin level is proportional to the tumour mass: around 50–300 ng/mL (1000–6000 mIU/L) in microadenomas, and 200–5000 ng/mL (>4000 mIU/L) in macroadenomas (normal values ranging from 2–23 ng/mL to 4–460 mIU/L). The 'hook effect' may be seen in patients with grossly elevated serum prolactin levels, where the assay utilizes one antibody to capture the antigen and one to detect it, thus spuriously lowering the measured prolactin. Stimulation (TRH and metoclopramide) or suppression (L-DOPA) tests are of no utility. In pituitary tumours, except prolactinomas, and in other tumours of the sellar region, pituitary stalk disconnection can occur and interrupt dopamine inhibitory tone, resulting in hyperprolactinaemia. Nevertheless, prolactin levels rarely exceed 100 ng/mL (2000 mIU/L). Prolactin levels in drug-induced hyperprolactinaemia rarely exceed 250 ng/mL (5000 mIU/L). Differential diagnosis is crucial for directing the correct treatment, since in most prolactinomas clinical treatment is the first choice.

Another cause of clinical–laboratorial dissociation is macroprolactinaemia. Prolactin isoforms can be classified according to their molecular weight in monomeric prolactin, dimeric prolactin, and macroprolactin (big-big PRL). Usually, the most prevalent isoform is monomeric, whilst macroprolactin corresponds to less than 5% of the total prolactin. Nevertheless, in 10%–25% of hyperprolactinaemic individuals, the main circulating isoform is macroprolactin, leading to so-called macroprolactinaemia. Macroprolactin has a low biological activity, so macroprolactinaemia is a benign condition. However, macroprolactinaemia may coexist with high serum monomeric prolactin levels, leading to symptomatic hyperprolactinaemia.

Pituitary function evaluation is necessary in patients with macroadenomas, including IGF-1 and growth hormone measurements to evaluate the possibility of a cosecretory tumour. Gonadotrophin levels can be normal or suppressed, reflecting hypogonadotrophic hypogonadism. In patients with prolactinomas, screening for multiple endocrine neoplasia type 1 is also recommended (see also Chapter 14, Section 14.7).

When facing a patient with hyperprolactinaemia, after excluding pregnancy, breast-feeding, pharmacological causes, primary hypothyroidism, renal failure, and liver failure, a sellar MRI is indicated. Sellar imaging can depict a microadenoma (<1 cm) or a macroadenoma (>1 cm). As hypogonadism may cause a reduction in bone mineral density, bone densitometry should be considered and repeated, if necessary.

Although the issue of dopaminergic-agonists-related valvopathy in prolactinomas is still a matter of debate, some recommend performing a transthoracic echocardiogram before and periodically during dopaminergic-agonist treatment, although evidence for dopaminergic-agonist-induced valvulopathy in these patients is minimal or non-existent.

Treatment

The aims of prolactinoma treatment are restoration of eugonadism and fertility, ablation of galactorrhoea, and tumoural mass control in order to reduce mass effect. Treatment modalities include medical treatment and radiotherapy.

Medical treatment

Dopaminergic agonists are the gold-standard treatment for prolactinomas for both hormonal and tumour mass control. Cabergoline, a specific D2-receptor agonist, is the first choice, due to its higher efficacy and better tolerability. Bromocriptine use brings normal prolactin levels in 80% of microadenomas and in 70% of macroadenomas, whilst with cabergoline, this goal is obtained in more than 85% of the cases, and tumour mass reduction is seen in more than 80% of the cases. The most common side effects are nausea, vomiting, and postural hypotension. Cabergoline, in much higher doses than used in hyperprolactinaemia, was related to valvulopathy in patients with Parkinson's disease, as they present a higher prevalence of other risk factors for heart valve disease. Cabergoline is also an agonist for the serotonin receptor 5HT2B, and so can promote fibroblast proliferation and valvular insufficiency, especially in the tricuspid and pulmonary valves. In patients using cabergoline for the treatment of hyperprolactinaemia, valvulopathy due to medication is still controversial. In a recent review, there was no risk of valvular regurgitation associated with cabergoline in the majority of the studies. In only one study, there was a moderate risk dose dependently of tricuspid regurgitation.

Chronic use of dopaminergic agonists can be associated with remission of hyperprolactinaemia. In a recent meta-analysis, Dekkers et al. (2010) showed that a mean of 21% of patients with hyperprolactinaemia, when treated with dopaminergic agonists, remained normoprolactinaemic after drug withdrawal. Therefore, dopaminergic agonists can be withdrawn in patients who are normorprolactinaemic with tumour reduction, especially after 2 years of treatment.

Occasionally, patients, around 10% of those on cabergoline and 25% of those on bromocriptine, may be totally intolerant or resistant (failure to normalize and/or to reduce tumour size by >50%) to dopaminergic-agonist therapy. Treatment options comprise switching to a different dopaminergic agonist, gradual dose escalation, surgery, or radiotherapy. Surgical treatment, usually by the transsphenoidal approach, is indicated for patients without normalization of prolactin levels with high doses of dopaminergic agonists; patients with macroadenomas with chiasmal compression and visual impairment without rapid improvement on clinical treatment; and patients with symptomatic apoplexy and cerebrospinal fluid leakage. In patients with microprolactinomas but who are intolerant of dopaminergic agonists, careful oestrogen replacement therapy can be safe, provided imaging is performed regularly.

Neurosurgical expertise, prolactin levels (<200 ng/mL), and tumour dimensions and invasiveness are the most important factors for successful surgical treatment. Reviewing more than 50 series, Gillam et al. (2006) reported remission in 74.7% of microadenomas and in 34% of macroadenomas, with a recurrence rate of 18% in microadenomas and 23% in macroadenomas.

Debulking is a strategy shown to be useful for other pituitary adenomas, such as somatotrophinomas. In two recent studies, the authors showed that debulking surgery led to higher rate of prolactin control and reduction in cabergoline dose.

Radiotherapy

Prolactinomas are among the most radioresistant of pituitary tumours. However, radiotherapy is indicated to control tumour growth in cases resistant to dopaminergic agonists and not controlled by surgery. Normal serum prolactin levels are reached in 31.4% of the cases, with no difference between techniques and combining therapies. Continuation of dopaminergic agonists should be reconsidered over time, especially after 2 years, and the dose reduced where possible or occasionally withdrawn.

Aggressive prolactinomas are characterized by the presence of expansion/invasion of neighbouring structures, rapid tumour growth, and/or the presence of a tumour with more than 4 cm in its largest diameter. They are more prevalent in males. The initial strategy for treating patients partially resistant to dopaminergic agonists is a stepwise increase in the dose of medication. It has been shown that is it possible to obtain normalization of prolactin levels in 96.2% of patients with a dose of up to 12 mg per week of cabergoline. Nevertheless, the maximum dose of cabergoline on prescribing information is 2 mg weekly. Another strategy which is useful for particularly aggressive prolactinomas is the use of temozolomide, an oral alkylating agent that crosses the blood–brain barrier. In a recent review of the literature, there was a good response in 15 out of 20 prolactinomas.

Other strategies still without clinical trial support are the use of chimeric molecules, the use of a multireceptor ligand somatostatin analogue such as pasireotide, the addition of oestrogen receptor modulators to dopaminergic agonists for partially resistant cases, the development of antagonists of prolactin receptor, and specific targeted agents such as mTOR and tyrosine kinase inhibitors.

During pregnancy, the main concern is tumour growth, due to high levels of oestrogens, leading to visual disturbance and headache (see also Chapter 10, Section 10.3). In microadenomas, the likelihood of tumour growth with these symptoms is less than 5%, and therefore, upon confirmation of pregnancy, dopaminergic agonists should be withdrawn and reintroduced if there is significant tumour growth. However, for patients with macroadenomas the risk of clinically significant tumour growth is 15%–35%. Thus, in patients with large macroadenomas, conception should be delayed until the tumour has shrunk well away from the optic chiasm following treatment with dopaminergic agonists. If tumour reduction does not occur, surgical treatment may be indicated. The maintenance or not of dopaminergic agonists throughout pregnancy should be at expert discretion. In cases where the suspension of dopaminergic agonists resulted in tumour growth, the initial procedure is the reintroduction of the drug. In case of failure, surgical treatment is indicated, preferably during the second trimester. Although bromocriptine is still the preferred drug for pregnancy induction, cumulative data point to equivalent safety with cabergoline, although patients should be warned this is an unlicensed indication in most countries.

Further reading

Bronstein MD, Paraiba DB, and Jallad RS. Management of pituitary tumors in pregnancy. *Nat Rev Endocrinol* 2011; 7: 301–10.

Dekkers OM, Lagro J, Burman P, et al. Recurrence of hyperprolactinemia after withdrawal of dopamine agonists: Systematic review and meta-analysis. *J Clin Endocrinol Metab* 2010; 95: 43–51.

Drake WM, Stiles CE, Howlett TA et al. A cross-sectional study of the prevalence of cardiac valvular abnormalities in hyperprolactinemic patients treated with ergot-derived dopamine agonists. *J Clin Endocrinol Metab* 2014 99: 90–6.

Gillam MP, Molitch ME, Lombardi G, et al. Advances in the treatment of prolactinomas. *Endocr Rev* 2006; 27: 485–534.

Glezer A, Soares CR, Vieira JG, et al. Human macroprolactin displays low biological activity via its homologous receptor in a new sensitive bioassay. *J Clin Endocrinol Metab* 2006; 91: 1048–55.

Melmed S, Casanueva FF, Hoffman AR, et al. Diagnosis and treatment of hyperprolactinemia: An Endocrine Society clinical practice guideline. *J Clin Endocrinol Metab* 2011; 96: 273–88.

Valassi E, Klibanski A, and Biller BM. Potential cardiac valve effects of dopamine agonists in hyperprolactinemia. *J Clin Endocrinol Metab* 2010; 95: 1025–33.

Webster J, Piscitelli G, Polli A, et al. A comparison of cabergoline and bromocriptine in the treatment of hyperprolactinemic amenorrhea. *N Engl J Med* 1994; 331: 904–9.

3.6 Acromegaly

Definitions and epidemiology
Acromegaly results from an excessive secretion of growth hormone (GH) by a pituitary adenoma (very rarely from excess ectopic secretion of Growth hormone releasing hormone). When the growth hormone-secreting adenoma develops before the closure of bone epiphysis, the condition is known as gigantism. Acromegaly has an incidence of 3–4 new cases per year and a prevalence of 20–40 cases per million.

Etiopathogenesis and pathology
In over 90% of the cases, acromegaly is caused by a benign sporadic GH-secreting pituitary adenoma or somatotrophinoma; in 70% of the patients, these are larger than 1 cm (macroadenomas) whereas the remaining third harbours lesions smaller than 1 cm (microadenomas). In 20%–30% of the cases, the adenoma arises from the mammosomatotrope, a less differentiated cell that co-secretes prolactin. GH-secreting carcinomas are exceedingly infrequent.

The molecular pathogenesis of acromegaly includes inactivation of tumour suppressor genes, activation of oncogenes, and perhaps the trophic effect of hypothalamic releasing hormones. Activating somatic point mutations of *GNAS1* can be found in 15%–40% of somatotrophinomas, depending on the ethnic background of the patient. When acromegaly occurs as part of multiple endocrine neoplasia type 1, the molecular alteration consists of inactivating mutations of menin, a tumour suppressor gene located in the short arm of Chromosome 11. More recently, isolated familial acromegaly and the familial pituitary tumour syndrome have been linked to inactivating mutations of *AIP*, a tumour suppressor gene encoding the aryl-hydrocarbon related protein and also located on Chromosome 11.

On rare occasions, acromegaly may result from GHRH-secreting neuroendocrine tumours usually located in the lungs, thymus, or endocrine pancreas; even less frequent are cases of real ectopic growth hormone secretion, usually by pituitary remnants in the sphenoid sinus or by a lymphoma.

Clinical features
Acromegaly is a multisystemic disorder, which develops insidiously over many years (usually 7–10 years before the diagnosis is made). Symptoms and signs can be divided into those resulting from the compressive effects of the tumour and those that are a consequence of the GH and IGF-1 (Insulin-like growth factor-1) excess (see Table 3.6).

Among the compressive symptoms, headache and visual field defects (bitemporal hemi- or quadrantopia) are the most common. Headache results from both an increase in intracranial pressure and the effects of GH itself. Occasionally, large tumours invading laterally into the cavernous sinuses may give rise to cranial nerve syndromes, usually third and sixth and, less commonly, fourth and seventh. The somatic effects of GH and IGF-1 can be seen in every organ system.

Acral enlargement is usually manifested as an increase in ring and shoe size, as well as prominence of the nose-bridge, supraciliary arches, frontal bones, and mandible. This creates the coarse, acromegaloid fascies.

Patients frequently show prognathism as well as dental separation. Arthralgias can be incapacitating and most commonly involve knees, wrists, elbows, and distal interphangeal joints. Paresthesiae of hands and feet and a proximal painful myopathy are frequently reported. Nerve entrapment syndromes such as carpal tunnel syndrome occur in nearly half of the patients. The skin is thick and oily due to seborrhoea and hyperhidrosis. Skin tags and acanthosis nigricans are common.

Arterial hypertension is found in 30% of patients; its pathogenesis includes both hyporeninemic hyperaldosteronism and an increased sympathetic tone. The echocardiogram shows left ventricular and septal hypertrophy with varying diastolic dysfunction. Symptomatic cardiac disease develops in 15% of patients and is usually due to coronary artery disease, heart failure, and arrhythmias. Most patients are loud 'snorers'. A significant proportion have sleep apnoea syndrome, which has both a central and a peripheral/obstructive component.

Chronic GH hypersecretion results in insulin resistance. Glucose intolerance has been reported in 30%–50% of patients and 25%–30% have frank diabetes. Hypertriglyceridaemia is not uncommon. Acromegaly is associated with hypercalciuria and hyperphosphataemia, but osteoporosis does not constitute a major problem except in patients with hypogonadism. GH and IGF-1 are potential mitogens. Adenomatous colonic polyps with malignant potential are more frequent than in the general population and thus colonoscopic surveillance is recommended at diagnosis and at regular intervals, depending on the findings. Well-differentiated thyroid carcinoma has emerged as the most common malignant neoplasm in patients with acromegaly.

Associated endocrine abnormalities are as follows. A euthyroid goitre is frequently found but seldom requires treatment. Hypopituitarism occurs variably, depending on the size and extension of the tumour and whether the patient has undergone surgery or radiation therapy. Hypogonadotrophic hypogonadism is the most common pituitary deficiency in untreated acromegaly, occurring in

Table 3.6 Diagnostic key points

Clinical	Paraclinical
Headaches, visual field defects	Hormonal:
	Elevated age-adjusted IGF-1
Acral enlargement	Glucose-suppressed GH >0.4 ng/mL (ultrasensitive immunoassays), >1 ng/mL (old RIA)
Thick oily skin, hyperhydrosis	
Arthralgias, osteoarthritis	
Paresthesiae, carpal tunnel syndrome	Pituitary reserve: LH; FSH; PRL; testosterone or estradiol; cortisol; TSH; FT4
Glucose intolerance, diabetes	
Snoring, sleep apnoea	Imaging (MRI):
Hypertension, arrhythmias	• microadenomas 25%
Risk of colon polyps and cancer	• macroadenomas 70%
	• invasive tumours 5%

Abbreviations: FT4, free thyroxine; GH, growth hormone; LH, luteinizing hormone; PRL, prolactin; RIA, radioimmunoassays.

20% of the patients. Decreased libido is a common presenting complaint in both males and females; females frequently have menstrual and ovulatory disturbances whereas males complain of impotence and frequently have oligospermia. Although an elevated prolactin is common, it does not always reflect co-secretion, but rather an interruption of the descending dopaminergic tone by the tumour compressing the pituitary stalk. Central hypocortisolism and hypothyroidism are less common but do occur. Acromegaly/gigantism can also develop in patients with McCune–Albright syndrome, multiple endocrine neoplasia type 1, or Carney complex (see Chapter 14).

Investigations

Biochemical diagnosis

Random GH values lower than 0.4 ng/mL exclude the diagnosis (Table 3.6). Most patients with acromegaly fail to suppress their GH levels to less than 1 ng/mL upon ingesting a glucose load. Situations associated with a decreased suppression of growth hormone by glucose include puberty, pregnancy, use of oral contraceptives, poorly controlled diabetes, malnutrition, and renal and hepatic insufficiency.

IGF-1 levels reflect the integrated GH concentrations over 24 hours and correlate well with clinical activity. IGF-1 concentrations decrease with age, reflecting the parallel decline of the somatotrophic axis, and thus need to be adjusted accordingly. Conditions that lower IGF-1 levels include malnutrition, poorly controlled diabetes, and hepatic and renal failure. IGF-1 circulates in plasma bound to different binding proteins that need to be removed before proceeding with the immunoassay.

Genetic investigations

In young patients (<30 years of age) and with gigantism, it is worth considering genetic screening for mutations of *AIP* and possibly other other genes (see Chapter 3, Section 3.2).

Imaging

Pituitary MRI with gadolinium enhancement is the imaging method of choice. The usual protocol consisting of T1-weighted sagittal and coronal sequences allows visualization of lesions as small as 2 or 3 mm in diameter.

Management

The decision as to what treatment modality should be used has to take into account not only medical issues such as the presence of cardiopulmonary co-morbidities that may increase anaesthetic risk, along with the size and extension of the tumour, but also the local characteristics of the centre where the patient is being managed.

Surgery

Trans-sphenoidal removal of the pituitary adenoma remains the treatment of choice (see Table 3.7). In experienced hands, trans-sphenoidal removal achieves biochemical cure (i.e. normalization of IGF-1 and a glucose-suppressed GH <1 ng/mL) in 80%–90% of microadenomas and intrasellar macroadenomas, whereas 40%–50% of larger macroadenomas and less than 10% of invasive tumours are effectively cured by surgery. Preoperative treatment with somatostatin analogues may improve surgical outcome.

Pharmacological therapy

Long-acting, depot formulations of somatostatin analogues, such as octreotide LAR (10–40 mg every 4–8 weeks) and lanreotide autogel (90–120 mg every 4–8 weeks) are the most frequently used medications. These somatostatin analogues have very high affinity for somatostatin receptors 2 and, to a lesser extent, 5, which are precisely the most commonly expressed receptors in GH-secreting adenomas. Adequate biochemical and clinical control is achieved in 25%–50% of patients and, in over 70% of patients, a significant shrinkage of the adenoma can be demonstrated. Treatment success is related to the abundance of these receptors in the tumour. Lower pretreatment GH levels have also been associated with a better response to somatostatin analogues. Side effects of somatostatin analogues, including nausea, abdominal pain, alopecia and biliary sludge in 20% of the patients, seldom require discontinuation of the drug. Pasireotide is a new long-acting somatostatin analogue that targets not only somatostatin receptors 2 and 5 but also somatostatin receptors 1 and 3. Pasireotide appears to be somewhat more effective than octreotide in lowering IGF-1 levels, and might be the treatment of choice in octreotide-resistant patients, but the diabetogenic effects of pasireotide may be treatment limiting. In general, these agents are used as second-line therapy after surgery, but in some circumstances could be considered as primary treatment. More recently, an oral formulation of octreotide has been investigated in Phase III trials, with positive results

Table 3.7 Therapeutic key points

Treatment modalities	Follow-up strategies
Transsphenoidal surgery for microadenomas and intrasellar macroadenomas; to relieve compressive effects and to debulk tumour (if pituitary surgeon available)	Surgical remission: • GH post glucose <0.4 ng/mL *and* normal age-adjusted IGF-1
SA (octreotide, lanreotide): • secondary treatment after failed surgery • primary treatment for inaccessible lesions, contraindications for surgery, or patient's preference	Pharmacological control on SA: • Random GH <1 ng/mL *and* normal age-adjusted IGF-1
Cabergoline may be added in resistant patients	Control of GHR antagonists: • normal age-adjusted IGF-1, GH levels are high
Pegvisomant in non-responders, with tumours >3 mm away from chiasma	Radiotherapy response monitoring: • delayed 2–5 years, check for other anterior pituitary hormone deficiencies at least yearly
Radiotherapy for patients with persistently active disease and visible tumour remnant	

Abbreviations: GH, growth hormone; SA, somatostatin analogues.

Pegvisomant, a mutated form of GH, prevents functional activity of the growth hormone receptor and results in normalization of IGF-1 in 70%–90% of patients, whilst increasing GH levels. Pegvisomant should not be used as primary treatment for acromegaly due to its elevated cost, but rather is indicated in patients who are intolerant of or resistant to somatostatin-analogue therapy. Dopamine agonists such as cabergoline are effective in a proportion of patients, around 30%–50%, particularly when used in combination with somatostatin analogues.

Radiation therapy

Both conventional external-beam radiotherapy and radiosurgery are indicated in patients with persistent disease, with a demonstrable tumour remnant on MRI, and who are either intolerant or resistant to pharmacological treatment. Biochemical success occurs variably from less than 20% to over 60%. An average of 5 years is required to document a biochemical response. Hypopituitarism develops in over 50% of patients within 10 years. Serious adverse effects such as brain necrosis and optic nerve damage seldom occur with modern techniques. Some concern has been recently raised regarding an elevated prevalence of cerebrovascular events and mortality in patients who had undergone radiation therapy.

Mortality and prognosis

Life expectancy in patients with acromegaly is decreased by about 10–15 years in the absence of effective therapy. When managed at highly specialized centres focusing not only on achieving GH and IGF-1 targets but also on managing co-morbidities, the mortality can be successfully reduced to that seen in the general population. The most frequent causes of death have shifted from cardio- and cerebrovascular events to neoplasms, as described in more recently reported series. Hormonal control has a definite impact on survival. Lowering serum GH to less than 1 ng/mL results in a significant reduction in the mortality rate. Other factors associated with an increased mortality include advanced age and the presence of hypertension and diabetes. Where there is discordance between the GH and IGF1 levels, patients need to be considered on a case-by-case basis.

Further reading

Caron P, Bevan JS, Petersenn S, et al. Tumor shrinkage with lanreotide autogel 120 mg as primary therapy in acromegaly. *J Clin Endocrinol Metab* 2014; 99: 1282–90.

Chahal HS, Stals K, Unterländer M, et al. AIP mutation in pituitary adenomas in the 18th century and today. *N Engl J Med* 2011; 364: 43–50.

Colao A, Ferone D, Marzullo P, et al. Systemic complications of acromegaly: Epidemiology, pathogenesis and management *Endocr Rev* 2004; 25: 102–52.

Dekkers AM, Biermasz NR, Pereira AM, et al. Mortality in acromegaly: A meta-analyisis. *J Clin Endocrinol Metab* 2008; 93: 61–7.

Espinosa E, Ramirez C, and Mercado M. The multimodal treatment of acromegaly: Current status and future perspectives. *Endocr Metab Immun Drug Targets* 2014; 14: 169–81.

Espinosa-de-los-Monteros AL, Sosa E, Cheng S, et al. Biochemical evaluation of disease activity after pituitary surgery in acromegaly: A critical analysis of patients who spontaneously change disease status *Clin Endocrinol* 2006; 64: 245–9.

Espinosa-de-los-Monteros, González B, Vargas G, et al. Clinical and biochemical characteristics of acromegalic patients with different abnormalities in glucose metabolism. *Pituitary* 2011; 14: 231–5.

Espinosa de los Monteros AL, Gonzalez B, Vargas G, et al. Octreotide-LAR treatment 'in real life':long term outcome at a tertiary care center. *Pituitary* 2015; 18: 290–6.

Giustina A, Chanson P, Bronstein MD, et al. A consensus on criteria for cure of acromegaly. *J Clin Endocrinol Metab* 2010; 95: 3141–8.

Giustina A, Chanson P, Kleinberg D, et al. Expert consensus document: A consensus on the medical treatment of acromegaly. *Nat Rev Endocrinol* 2014; 10: 243–8.

Kopchick JJ, Parkinson C, Stevens EC, et al. Growth hormone receptor antagonists: Discovery, development, and use in patients with acromegaly. *Endocr Rev* 2002; 23: 623–46.

Melmed S. Acromegaly pathogenesis and treatment. *J Clin Invest* 2009; 119: 3189–202.

Mercado M, Borges F, Bouterfa H, et al. A prospective, multicentre study to investigate the efficacy, safety and tolerability of octreotide LAR® (long-acting repeatable octreotide) in the primary therapy of patients with acromegaly. *Clin Endocrinol* 2007; 66: 859–68.

Mercado M, Gonzalez B, Vargas G, et al. Succesful mortality reduction and control of comorbidities in patients with acromegaly followed at a highly specialized multidisciplinary clinic. *J Clin Endocrinol Metab* 2014; 99: 4438–46.

3.7 Cushing's disease

Definition
Cushing's syndrome results from prolonged, and inappropriate, exposure to excessive circulating free glucocorticoid (cortisol in Cushing's disease).

Pathophysiology
- A corticotroph adenoma of the pituitary gland causes excess secretion of adrenocorticotrophic hormone.
- Excess adrenocorticotrophic hormone drives excess cortisol secretion from the adrenal gland, and the resulting hypercortisolaemia causes the clinical features.

Epidemiology
- The incidence of Cushing's disease is approximately 1/250,000.
- It is three times more common in women.

Clinical features
Patients often have a history of symptoms lasting 1–2 years before confirmation of the diagnosis. Signs that most reliably distinguish Cushing's syndrome are thin skin, easy bruising, and proximal myopathy. It is essential to exclude exogenous glucocorticoids as the cause of a 'Cushingoid appearance'.

Investigations
Who to investigate?
Testing for Cushing's syndrome should be considered in:
- patients with unusual features for age (e.g. osteoporosis and livid striae in young men)
- patients with multiple and progressive features clinical features suggestive of Cushing's syndrome
- children with decreasing height percentile and increasing weight

How to test
Diagnosis of Cushing's disease is a two-step process. It is *essential* that the diagnosis of Cushing's syndrome is confirmed before attempting to determine if Cushing's disease is the cause. Some patients with Cushing's disease exhibit cyclical secretion of cortisol, which may fluctuate and remit spontaneously, sometimes over many years. This can cause considerable diagnostic difficulty, and reinvestigation at intervals, and on several occasions, may be required. Oral oestrogens increase cortisol-binding globulin and therefore lead to falsely elevated serum cortisol levels, and should be stopped for 6 weeks before investigation.

Step 1: Diagnosis of Cushing's syndrome
Three principal tests are commonly used to establish the diagnosis:
- low-dose DST: dexamethasone 0.5 mg orally is administered strictly 6-hourly, and plasma cortisol measured basally and at 48 hours (normal serum cortisol <50 nmol/L (1.8 μg/dL); or overnight dexamethsone test with dexamethasone 1 mg at 2300 h and serum cortisol at 0900 h the next day, with the same cut-off as above.
- late-night salivary or midnight plasma cortisol: normal undetectable or below normative threshold
- 24-hour UFC

At least two concordantly abnormal different tests are needed to establish diagnosis. Midnight serum cortisol is best used to exclude mild cases; it is not indicated in florid Cushing's syndrome, and should not be attempted as an investigation on a busy general ward.

Step 2: Determining the cause of Cushing's syndrome
Basal biochemical tests: Plasma adrenocorticotrophic hormone
After confirmation of Cushing's syndrome, plasma adrenocorticotrophic hormone is measured; to avoid obtaining falsely low results, samples must be cold-centrifuged immediately after sampling, and immediately frozen (−40 °C) before storage for later assay. Levels of adrenocorticotrophic hormone persistently greater than 15 pg/mL can confidently be ascribed to adrenocorticotrophic-hormone-dependent   Cushing's syndrome.

Plasma potassium
Ectopic adrenocorticotrophic hormone secretion is usually associated with higher circulating levels of cortisol than in Cushing's disease. These high levels overwhelm the 11-beta-hydroxysteroid dehydrogenase type 2 enzyme, allowing cortisol to act as a mineralocorticoid in the kidney. Hypokalaemia is consequently more common in ectopic adrenocorticotrophic hormone secretion, but is also present in 10% of patients with Cushing's disease

Further investigation: Where should it be performed?
It is strongly recommended that further investigation be performed in major referral centres:
- adrenocorticotrophic hormone-secreting non-pituitary neuroendocrine tumours (ectopic adrenocorticotrophic hormone) may mimic many of the clinical features of Cushing's disease.
- biochemical evaluation rather than imaging should be relied on to differentiate pituitary from non-pituitary sources of adrenocorticotrophic hormone (although a pituitary macroadenoma found on imaging in the context of adrenocorticotrophic hormone-dependent Cushing's syndrome is highly suggestive of Cushing's disease)

High-dose DST
Dexamethasone 2 mg orally is administered strictly 6-hourly, and plasma cortisol measured basally and at 48 hours. In about 80% of patients with Cushing's disease, cortisol is reduced to less than 50% of the basal level. This is, however, lower than the pretest likelihood of Cushing's disease in women (90%), and thus this test is no longer recommended where there is access to bilateral inferior petrosal sinus sampling.

CRH test
CRH (100 μg or 1 μg/kg in children, intravenously)) stimulates release of adrenocorticotrophic hormone from the corticotrophs of the anterior pituitary. Patients with Cushing's disease typically exhibit an excessive increase in plasma cortisol (>20% above basal) and adrenocorticotrophic hormone, whereas those with ectopic adrenocorticotrophic hormone secretion usually do not.

Desmopressin test
There is lack of availability worldwide of CRH. Desmopressin (10 μg intravenous) is used as an alternative since corticotroph adenoma express the V1b receptor that is also activated by this ligand. It is an

inferior test, and the use of CRH is recommended where available.

Bilateral inferior petrosal sinus sampling

Bilateral inferior petrosal sinus sampling is a highly specialized, invasive investigation, but is the most reliable test for differentiating pituitary and non-pituitary sources of adrenocorticotrophic hormone. Cannulas are placed in each inferior petrosal sinus for simultaneous sampling of adrenocorticotrophic hormone from this central area and a peripheral sample at the same time. If the source of CRH is of a pituitary origin, a gradient of concentration is expected from central to peripheral sites. Use of CRH increases the sensitivity of the test:

- a basal central-to-peripheral adrenocorticotrophic hormone gradient of >2:1 or a CRH-stimulated gradient of >3:1 is indicative of Cushing's disease
- there is a false-negative rate of ≈5% in Cushing's disease; correcting the values of adrenocorticotrophic hormone by assay of prolactin may improve sensitivity.

Imaging

Most corticotroph adenomas are <1 cm and give a hypointense signal on MRI that fails to enhance with gadolinium. Using standard MRI protocols, 40% of corticotroph microadenomas are not visualized and 'incidentalomas' are found in 10% of the healthy population, emphasizing the importance of biochemical assessment.

Management

Surgery

Trans-sphenoidal surgery

Selective microadenomectomy by an experienced surgeon is the treatment of choice in most patients with Cushing's disease. Long-lasting remission without other pituitary hormonal deficiency is achieved in 60%–70% of cases.

Adrenal surgery

Laparoscopic bilateral adrenalectomy may be required to control cortisol levels. Nelson's syndrome (development of a locally aggressive pituitary tumour secreting high levels of adrenocorticotrophic hormone, resulting in pigmentation) is a major concern following bilateral adrenalectomy in patients with refractory Cushing's disease. The tumour may be treated with further surgery and radiotherapy, but these seldom cure the disease.

Medical therapy

Medical therapy to lower cortisol may be used in preparation for surgery or after unsuccessful surgery. It is seldom a long-term solution, and is mainly used as an adjunctive treatment with other modalities such as pituitary radiotherapy. Associated conditions such as hypertension and diabetes mellitus must also be treated (see Chapter 20, Sections 20.8–20.10), although there may be rapid improvement with control of cortisol levels. Thromboprophylaxis is becoming increasing routine, usually with heparin, but the duration of treatment remains controversial.

Adrenal steroidogenesis inhibitors

The following adrenal steroidogenesis inhibitors may be used:

- metyrapone at doses 500–1000 mg orally, three or four times per day, increasing every 72 hours.
- ketoconazole, 200–400 mg orally, three times per day, increasing every 3–4 days

The dose is titrated against clinical response and biochemistry with an aim for a mean serum cortisol level of 150–300 mmol/L (5.4–10.9 µg/dL) or normalization of elevated UFC levels, but ketoconazole also lowers testosterone levels. Stomach acid is needed for absorption of ketoconazole, and liver function tests require close monitoring. A new non-racemic formulation is currently under trial. Metyrapone causes an increase in steroid androgenic precursors, and hirsutism is a major adverse effect in women; this does not occur with ketoconazole. Metyrapone causes a rapid increase in 11-deoxycortisol, measured as cortisol in many immunoassays, and caution is needed in the interpretation of biochemical results to avoid overzealous treatment and adrenal insufficiency.

Other medical treatments

- o,p'-DDD (mitotane) is usually reserved for the treatment of adrenocortical carcinoma, but can be used a lower doses in Cushing's disease.
- Pasireotide, a multireceptor somatostatin analogue, reduces adrenocorticotrophic hormone and is effective in approximately 25%–40% of patients with Cushing's disease, but hyperglycaemia is a major side effect.
- Mifepristone, a glucocorticoid receptor antagonist is also effective for treatment, but no biochemical monitoring is possible and it can be a challenge to use.
- High-dose dopamine agonists (cabergoline) can be effective in some cases.
- Gefitinib, an EGFR inhibitor, has been suggested for patients with resistant tumours.
- Osilodrostat, a novel 11-hydroxylase inhibitor, is currently under trial.
- In an acute emergency setting, intravenous etomidate blocks 11-beta-hydroxylation and may be life-saving.

Associated conditions such as hypertension and diabetes mellitus must also be treated (see Chapter 20, Sections 20.8–20.10), although there may be rapid improvement with control of cortisol levels.

Pituitary radiotherapy

Following transsphenoidal surgery, persisting hypercortisolaemia may be treated with pituitary radiotherapy, or gamma-knife radiosurgery. Progressive anterior pituitary failure is the major side effect; growth hormone deficiency is present in almost all patients 10 years after treatment, and gonadotrophin deficiency in about 15%. About 4 years after treatment, 80% of patients are in remission with respect to circulating plasma cortisol levels. It is important to demonstrate that hypercortisolaemia can be controlled with medical therapy prior to administering radiotherapy.

Prognosis

Inadequately treated Cushing's syndrome has a fivefold standardized mortality rate, but this normalizes with timely control of hypercortisolaemia, although some cardiovascular risk remains, especially if patients are not cured with initial surgery. Depression often persists for years after cure, and patients should be warned that they are likely to feel worse for the first 1–2 years after effective intervention. Relapse may occur in 30% of cases up to 30 years later, and long-term follow up is strongly recommended.

Conclusion

It would seem reasonable to follow up all patients for life in view of the chance of long-term recurrence and the secondary complications which may persist.

Patient support groups

The Pituitary Foundation: http://www.pituitary.org

Further reading

Biller BM, Grossman AB, Stewart PM, et al. Treatment of ACTH-dependent Cushing's syndrome: A consensus statement. *J Clin Endocrinol Metab* 2008; 93: 2454–62.

Clayton RN, Jones PW, Reulen RC, et al. Mortality in patients with Cushing's disease more than 10 years after remission: a multicentre, multinational, retrospective cohort study. *Lancet Diabetes Endocrinol* 2016; 4(7): 569–76.

Newell-Price J, Bertagna X, Grossman AB, et al. Cushing's syndrome. *Lancet* 2006; 367: 1605–17.

Nieman LK, Biller BM, Findling JW, et al. Treatment of Cushing's syndrome: An Endocrine Society clinical practice guideline. *J Clin Endocrinol Metab* 2015;100: 2807–31.

Tritos NA and Biller BM. Medical management of Cushing's disease. *J Neuro-oncol* 2014; 117: 407–14.

3.8 Non-functioning pituitary tumours

Introduction

Non-functioning pituitary tumours do not secrete hormones in quantities sufficient to produce a discrete clinical syndrome. Hence, patients usually present with local mass effects or hypopituitarism. Increasingly, non-functioning pituitary tumours are discovered incidentally on cranial imaging performed for non-endocrine indications.

Pathology

Histologically, there are several subgroups. The largest comprises tumours of gonadotroph origin which contain scattered cells, or groups of cells, showing positive immunostaining for FSH, LH, or their subunits. In vitro, non-functioning pituitary tumour cells frequently secrete small amounts of these hormones. Another group (null cell tumours and oncocytomas) fail to immunostain for any anterior pituitary hormones or their subunits. Finally, about 15% of non-functioning pituitary tumours are 'silent adenomas' with uniform immunostaining for anterior pituitary hormones (most commonly adrenocorticotrophic hormone) but without the clinical effects of hypersecretion [1]. Preliminary whole-exome sequencing studies of sporadic non-functioning pituitary tumours have not revealed mutations previously associated with pituitary tumourigenesis, a finding consistent with their low proliferation rates and generally benign behaviour [2]. The molecular pathogenesis of non-functioning pituitary tumours remains unknown.

Epidemiology

Non-functioning pituitary tumours are the second most common pituitary adenoma after prolactinoma, with an estimated population prevalence of 1:4500 [3]. Two-thirds are diagnosed in men during the sixth decade when they present typically with pressure symptoms, especially visual failure. Non-functioning pituitary tumours comprise approximately 50% of tumours in large surgical series.

Natural history

In a meta-analysis of studies including a total of 865 patients with non-functioning pituitary incidentalomas, lesions ≥10 mm in diameter (macrolesions) were four times more likely to increase in size during follow-up than were those <10 mm in diameter (microlesions) [4]. Karavitaki et al. reported 40 patients with non-operated non-functioning pituitary tumours; 16 with microadenomas and 24 with macroadenomas were followed for a mean of 42 months (range 8–128). The 48-month probability of radiological enlargement was 19% for microadenomas but no patient developed optic chiasmal compression. By contrast, 44% of macroadenomas showed enlargement on MRI, and two-thirds of these patients developed new or worsened visual field defects [5].

Clinical presentation

An expanding sella mass causes headache in about one-quarter of patients, and acute pituitary apoplexy within a previously unsuspected non-functioning pituitary tumour sometimes occurs. Suprasellar extension of the tumour may cause optic chiasmal compression, typically producing a bitemporal hemianopia, and visual field defects are found in over 50% of patients with macroadenomas.

Cranial nerve symptoms due to cavernous sinus invasion are unusual in the absence of apoplexy.

Hypopituitarism is common. Non-functioning pituitary tumours may first be suspected from a routine thyroid profile showing secondary hypothyroidism. Similarly, pituitary pathology should be considered in a man with reduced libido and erectile dysfunction and who has low serum testosterone in association with low-normal gonadotrophins.

Disconnection hyperprolactinaemia occurs in around half of patients with non-functioning macroadenomas, although serum prolactin is rarely higher than 2000 mU/L in the absence of prolactin-elevating medications (normal ranges: <600, women and <300, men) [6].

Differential diagnosis

It is important to remember that not all macrolesions in the sella region are pituitary macroadenomas. There may be clinical, endocrine, and radiological pointers to alternative diagnoses, as listed in Box 3.2. As a further pitfall for the unwary, these lesions can also produce disconnection hyperprolactinaemia. It should emphasized that diabetes insipidus is not a presenting feature of a primary pituitary tumour.

Management

Observation

Most patients with NF macroadenomas require active treatment, usually with primary surgery. However, old age frailty, absence of visual pathway compression, significant co-morbidities, or patient reluctance for surgery sometimes make a period of 'watching waiting' reasonable. Such patients should have repeat MRI after 6 months and annually thereafter if the situation remains stable, together with visual field assessments at similar intervals. As noted in 'Natural history', macroadenomas frequently enlarge over time, at which point the need for active intervention should be readdressed.

Surgery

If the tumour displaces or abuts the optic structures, there is a clear need for surgical decompression. There is no rapidly-acting medical option for non-functioning pituitary tumours, such as there is for macroprolactinoma. Surgery is mostly possible via the trans-sphenoidal route, nowadays often assisted by direct endoscopic vision. Surgery has the advantage of both decompressing the lesion and providing tissue for definitive histological diagnosis (Box 3.2). If the preoperative serum prolactin is >2000 mU/L a carefully supervised trial of dopamine agonist therapy may be advised, just in case the lesion proves to be a macroprolactinoma associated with an unusually low serum prolactin level. However, if the mass fails to shrink (even if serum prolactin becomes undetectable), surgical exploration is advisable.

Following trans-sphenoidal decompression, impaired vision improves in the majority of patients (often during the first few days) and normalizes in some. Mild impairments of anterior pituitary function may improve after surgical decompression but major preoperative deficits usually persist. Trans-sphenoidal surgery performed by a specialist pituitary surgeon is a safe procedure with acceptably low complication rates (i.e. CSF leakage, meningitis, and loss of pituitary function). Patient-rated

---

Box 3.2 Indicators of a diagnosis other than non-functioning pituitary tumour in a patient with a non-functioning pituitary 'macro-lesion'

Craniopharyngioma
Cystic change and calcification on CT, diabetes insipidus, hypothalamic dysfunction

Meningioma
Increased and homogeneous signal on MRI (pre- and post-gadolinium), dural 'tail', adjacent hyperostosis, epicentre often suprasellar

Metastasis
Unusual irregular shape, compression/invasion of internal carotid artery in cavernous sinus, diabetes insipidus, other indicators of malignancy (weight loss, breast lump, smoker, abnormal chest X-ray)

Hypophysitis
Increased and homogeneous gadolinium enhancement on MRI, female (especially peripartum), personal/family history of autoimmune disease

Carotid artery aneurysm
Markedly increased and homogeneous gadolinium enhancement on MRI

---

quality of life appears to be normal or near-normal in patients with non-functioning pituitary tumours after modern tumour management and with good endocrine aftercare [7].

Management after surgery
MRI surveillance
The first surveillance MRI scan should be performed at least 3–4 months after surgery, to minimize uncertainty due to resolving haemorrhage, surgical artefact, and tissue swelling. Greenman et al. showed the best predictors of regrowth for non-functioning pituitary tumours after surgical decompression were the presence of cavernous sinus invasion on the preoperative MRI, and the presence of a tumour remnant on the post-operative MRI [8]. If the early post-operative MRI showed no residual tumour, 60% of patients remained in radiological remission after 10 years. However, of those with a tumour remnant, 30% had tumour regrowth after 2 years and 70% after 5 years. From these and similar data from other centres, it appears reasonable to perform MRI at annual intervals for at least 5 years after the baseline post-operative scan, if early radiotherapy is not applied.

Should radiotherapy be used for all non-functioning pituitary tumour remnants, or is there a medical option?
In the past, pituitary radiotherapy was given routinely to all patients with non-functioning pituitary tumours after surgical decompression. This approach was very effective in reducing tumour recurrence, as shown in Figure 3.12a [9]. However, not all patients with a post-operative non-functioning pituitary tumour remnant will experience a clinically relevant recurrence. Furthermore, pituitary radiotherapy usually causes permanent hypopituitarism in the longer term, and there are other concerns about second tumour formation (rare), cognitive changes, and increased cerebrovascular risk. It would, therefore, be highly desirable to be able to select non-functioning pituitary tumour patients for whom radiotherapy is essential for tumour growth control.

It has been recognized for many years that approximately two-thirds of non-functioning pituitary tumours express D2 dopamine receptors, albeit in smaller numbers than those found in prolactinomas.

The dramatic tumour shrinkage seen in patients with macroprolactinoma following dopamine-agonist therapy was not observed in patients with non-functioning pituitary tumours. However, in an early review, Bevan et al. reported that only 1% of non-functioning pituitary tumours *increased* in size following long-term dopamine agonist therapy, whereas 91% remained static, and 8% shrank [10]. Interest in the use of dopamine agonists for non-functioning pituitary tumours was revived by studies using cabergoline; these showed tumour remnant stabilization, and even shrinkage, in tumours expressing D2 receptors [11]. Recent evidence suggests cabergoline may reduce cell viability in non-functioning pituitary tumours by inhibiting local vascular endothelial growth factor (VEGF) secretion [12]. These observations have the potential to alter the traditional management algorithm for non-functioning pituitary tumours—if a post-operative remnant is not causing local pressure problems, simple growth restraint (and not necessarily tumour shrinkage) is all that is required. 'Proof-of-concept' clinical studies have been reported by Greenman et al., albeit with relatively small groups of patients, but the results were encouraging (Figure 3.12b) [13].

Management pathway after debulking surgery
The management pathway in Figure 3.13 incorporates the possibility of using a trial of cabergoline for tumour remnants not causing pressure effects and for which ongoing MRI surveillance (rather than early radiotherapy) is deemed to be reasonable. Although the evidence is limited, my present practice is to use a cabergoline dose higher than is typically required in prolactinoma treatment but unlikely (on present evidence) to cause cardiac adverse effects.

It should be recognized that some non-functioning pituitary tumours behave aggressively from the outset and require early radiotherapy and sometimes multiple surgical debulkings. These tumours have extensive extrasellar invasion but are, fortunately, relatively rare. Some may be suitable for treatment with temozolomide, and the 50% with low *MGMT* expression may have the best potential for response to this chemotherapy [14].

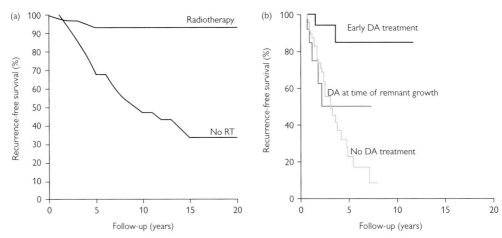

RT = radiotherapy, DA = dopamine agonist (mainly bromocriptine, some cabergoline or quinagolide)

Fig 3.12 Effects of adjunctive treatments after primary surgery for non-functioning pituitary tumour (NFPT). (a) Pituitary radiotherapy within 12 months of surgery reduces NFPT regrowth. (b) Dopamine agonist therapy after surgery (without radiotherapy) reduces NFPT remnant growth in a significant proportion.
Panel a: Reproduced with permission from Gittoes NJ et al., Radiotherapy for non-functioning pituitary tumours, *Clinical Endocrinology*, Volume 48, pp. 331–337, Copyright © 1998 John Wiley and Sons Ltd. Panel b: Reproduced with permission from Greenman Y et al., Postoperative treatment of clinically non-functioning pituitary adenomas with dopamine agonists decreases tumour remnant growth, *Clinical Endocrinology*, Volume 63, pp. 39–44, Copyright © 2005 John Wiley and Sons Ltd.

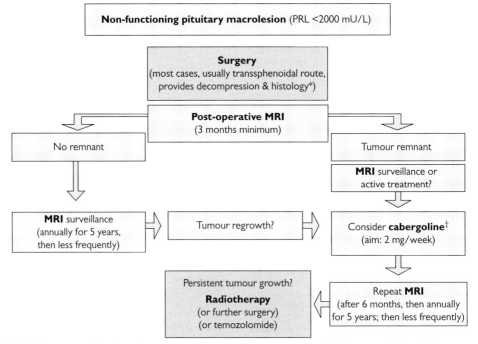

Fig 3.13 Management pathway for patients with non-functioning pituitary tumours, after debulking surgery; PRL, prolactin.
* Future prospects: tumour receptor analysis may guide appropriate medical therapy.
† Future prospects: chimeric dopamine agonist/somatostatin analogue or multifunctional somatostatin analogue compounds may have a role.

Silent adrenocorticotrophic-hormone tumours

It has been suggested that silent adrenocorticotrophic-hormone tumours behave more aggressively than other types of non-functioning pituitary tumour. The Oxford group reported 28 patients followed for a mean of 7.5 years [15]. The recurrence rate was no higher in this group compared to those with adrenocorticotrophic-hormone-negative tumours, although two of the recurrences were extremely aggressive tumours requiring multimodal therapies to control. A recent review of silent tumours advocates rigorous post-operative surveillance in order to diagnose and treat recurrences at the earliest opportunity [16].

Future developments

Further exploration of medical treatments for non-functioning pituitary tumours is urgently needed. A UK prospective, placebo-controlled, trial of cabergoline treatment for remnants of non-functioning pituitary tumours is currently being planned and Greenman has recently amplified and conformed her earlier study [17]. Routine assessment of dopamine-receptor status in non-functioning pituitary tumours by immunohistochemistry would guide the rational use of dopamine-agonist therapy in patients with post-operative remnants [18].

Non-functioning pituitary tumours variably express somatostatin receptors, predominantly subtypes SSTR2 and 3. Several short-term studies of octreotide have been reported in patients with non-functioning pituitary tumours but the results have been variable and there is no present justification to support the routine use of relatively expensive and SSTR2-focused somatostatin analogues [1]. However, the recently available multiligand somatostatin analogue pasireotide does possess SSTR3 activity and is worthy of investigation in patients with non-functioning pituitary tumours. Similarly, future chimeric agents with *combined* D2 dopamine and broad-spectrum somatostatin receptor activities would also be attractive candidates for medical therapy for non-functioning pituitary tumours.

References and further reading

1. Greenman Y and Stern N. Non-functioning pituitary adenomas. *Best Pract Res Clin Endocrinol Metab* 2009; 23: 625–8.
2. Newey PJ, Nesbit MA, Rimmer AJ, et al. Whole-exome sequencing studies of non-functioning pituitary adenomas. *J Clin Endocrinol Metab* 2013; 98: E796–800.
3. Fernandez A, Karavitaki N, and Wass JAH. Prevalence of pituitary adenomas: a community-based, cross-sectional study in Banbury (Oxfordshire, UK). *Clin Endocrinol* 2010; 72: 377–82.
4. Fernández-Balsells MM, Murad MH, Barwise A, et al. Natural history of non-functioning pituitary adenomas and incidentalomas: A systematic review and metaanalysis. *J Clin Endocrinol Metab* 2011; 96: 905–12.
5. Karavitaki N, Collison K, Halliday J, et al. What is the natural history of nonoperated non-functioning pituitary adenomas? *Clin Endocrinol* 2007; 67: 938–43.
6. Karavitaki N, Thanabalasingham G, Shore HC, et al. Do the limits of serum prolactin in disconnection hyperprolactinaemia need re-definition? A study of 226 patients with histologically verified non-functioning pituitary macroadenoma. *Clin Endocrinol* 2006; 65: 524–9.
7. Capatina C, Christodoulides C, Fernandez A, et al. Current treatment protocols can offer a normal or near-normal quality of life in the majority of patients with non-functioning pituitary adenomas. *Clin Endocrinol* 2013; 78: 86–93.
8. Greenman Y, Ouaknine G, Veshchev I, et al. Postoperative surveillance of clinically non-functioning pituitary macroadenomas: Markers of tumour quiescence and regrowth. *Clin Endocrinol* 2003; 58: 763–9.
9. Gittoes NJ, Bates AS, Tse W, et al. Radiotherapy for non-functioning pituitary tumours. *Clin Endocrinol* 1998; 48: 331–7.
10. Bevan JS, Webster J, Burke CW, et al. Dopamine agonists and pituitary tumor shrinkage. *Endocrine Rev* 1992; 13: 220–40.
11. Pivonello R, Matrone C, Filippella M, et al. Dopamine receptor expression and function in clinically non-functioning pituitary tumors: Comparison with the effectiveness of cabergoline treatment. *J Clin Endocrinol Metab* 2004; 89: 1674–83.
12. Gagliano T, Filieri C, Minoia M, et al. Cabergoline reduces cell viability in non-functioning pituitary adenomas by inhibiting vascular endothelial growth factor secretion. *Pituitary* 2013; 16: 91–100.
13. Greenman Y, Tordjman K, Osher E, et al. Postoperative treatment of clinically non-functioning pituitary adenomas with dopamine agonists decreases tumour remnant growth. *Clin Endocrinol* 2005; 63: 39–44.
14. Widhalm G, Wolfsberger S, Preusser M, et al. O(6)-methylguanine DNA methyltransferase immunoexpression in non-functioning pituitary adenomas: Are progressive tumors potential candidates for temozolomide treatment? *Cancer* 2009; 115: 1070–80.
15. Bradley KJ, Wass JA, and Turner HE. Non-functioning pituitary adenomas with positive immunoreactivity for ACTH behave more aggressively than ACTH immunonegative tumours but do not recur more frequently. *Clin Endocrinol* 2003; 58: 59–64.
16. Cooper O and Melmed S. Subclinical hyperfunctioning pituitary adenomas: the silent tumors. *Best Pract Res Clin Endocrinol Metab* 2012; 26: 447–60.
17. Greenman Y, Cooper O, Yaish I, et al. Treatment of clinically nonfunctioning pituitary adenomas with dopamine agonists. *Eur J Endocrinol* 2016; 175(1): 63–72.
18. Vieira Neto L, Wildemberg LE, Moraes AB, et al. Dopamine receptor subtype 2 expression profile in non-functioning pituitary adenomas and *in vivo* response to cabergoline therapy. *Clin Endocrinol* 2015; 82: 739–46.

3.9 Gonadotroph adenomas

Introduction

Gonadotroph adenomas are benign clonal neuroendocrine proliferations arising from adenohypophysial gonadotroph cells.

Epidemiology

Nearly 30% of all clinically diagnosed pituitary adenomas are gonadotroph adenomas, representing about two-thirds of surgically treated non-functioning sellar lesions [1]. Gonadotroph adenomas are more frequent in males, with a mean age of presentation of 55 years.

Clinical features

Gonadotroph adenomas usually manifest as macroadenomas. They present as incidentalomas but much more frequently with compressive symptoms, the most common being visual field defects, headache, and anterior pituitary deficiency. Rarely, patients develop ophthalmoplegia or apoplexy.

Pituitary function evaluation reveals evidence of hypogonadism and/or growth-hormone deficiency in more than half of all patients at presentation. Hyperprolactinaemia (usually <100 ng/mL (2000 mIU/L) and due to a stalk effect), secondary adrenal insufficiency, and hypothyroidism are less common. A detailed clinical history and physical exam will elicit loss of libido in a great proportion of male individuals, and up to a third may have testicular atrophy [2]. More than 50% of postmenopausal women will have inappropriately low gonadotrophins.

Imaging features

Magnetic resonance is the optimal imaging modality. Such studies should carefully be evaluated for non-adenomatous lesion characteristics such as predominantly cystic content, or calcification suggestive of a Rathke's cleft cyst or a craniopharyngioma. On T1-weighted images, pituitary adenomas may be hypointense or isointense relative to normal pituitary tissue before and after gadolinium administration. T2-weighted images of pituitary macroadenomas may be especially heterogeneous, reflecting cystic or necrotic areas. Gonadotroph adenomas range from neoplasms that invade bone, cavernous sinuses, and brain to large tumours that grow upwards and compress the optic chiasm. Nevertheless, when compared to other non-functioning pituitary adenomas that are recognized for their more aggressive clinical course, such as silent corticotroph adenomas and silent subtype 3 adenomas, gonadotroph adenomas tend to be less often >4 cm and have less cavernous sinus invasion and less lobulation [3].

Natural history

If left untreated, up to 50% of non-functioning pituitary macroadenomas grow after a 5-year follow-up [4]. There might also be spontaneous regression of tumour volume in about 10% of cases, possibly due to ischaemia or haemorrhage. In contrast, non-functioning pituitary microadenomas show significant growth in only approximately 10% of cases [5].

Biochemical diagnosis

Gonadotroph adenomas are considered clinically non-functioning, but hypersecretion of gonadotrophins or, more frequently, of their free subunits, occurs in up to half of the cases, especially FSH in men, and the free alpha subunit in premenopausal women. The biochemical diagnosis of gonadotroph adenomas in postmenopausal women can be particularly problematic due to physiological gonadotrophin elevation. Dynamic testing is rarely utilized to diagnose gonadotroph adenomas but, when available, a TRH stimulation test may be done to demonstrate a paradoxical response of LH, FSH, alpha subunits, and beta-LH. Significant increases in serum beta-LH or, less commonly, FSH and LH, are considered diagnostic.

Pathogenesis

Gonadal steroids participate in the negative-feedback regulation of the secretion of pituitary gonadotrophins. There are a few case reports of gonadotroph adenomas in patients with prolonged untreated primary hypogonadism. However, there is still no convincing experimental evidence linking the loss of negative feedback to the pathogenesis of these adenomas. On the other hand, the biological behaviour of gonadotroph adenomas may be influenced by their differential pattern of oestrogen-receptor expression. For instance, invasive non-functioning pituitary adenomas have higher expression of oestrogen receptor alpha than non-invasive ones do, and this is seen more often in women than in men. The expression of oestrogen receptor beta is reduced in invasive non-functioning pituitary adenomas in both women and men.

Activin stimulates gonadotrophin secretion, and its effects are modulated by activin receptors and follistatin. Follistatin binds activin and downregulates its activity. Enhanced activin signalling is a possible pathogenic mechanism in gonadotroph adenomas, as they express activin receptors, and follistatin expression is reduced or diminished [6].

Several tumour-suppressor genes have been implicated in the pathogenesis of non-functioning pituitary adenomas. Examples of such genes include MEG3, RB1, and CDKN2A. MEG3 functions as a non-coding tumour-suppressor gene, and its expression is diminished in gonadotroph adenomas [7]. Silencing of RB1 and CDKN2A genes through promoter hypermethylation has also been reported in non-functioning pituitary adenomas.

Fibroblast growth factor receptor 4 (FGFR4) is overexpressed in several tumours. Pituitary-tumour-derived FGFR4 (ptd-FGFR4) is a truncated kinase-encoding variant that has been found in different pituitary adenoma subtypes including gonadotroph adenomas. It results in abnormal cell adhesiveness by displacing N-cadherin from the cell membrane [8].

Genetic susceptibility

There are several syndromes where the development of pituitary tumours is common. In the majority of patients with multiple endocrine neoplasia type 1, multiple endocrine neoplasia type 4, and familial isolated pituitary adenoma, these tumours are functional, but non-functioning pituitary adenomas have also been described.

Pathological features

Positivity for steroidogenic factor 1 (SF-1), the principal gonadotroph lineage specific transcription factor, and/

or oestrogen receptor alpha in a hormone-negative pituitary adenoma is diagnostic of a gonadotroph adenoma, regardless of gonadotrophin expression [9]. These tumours exhibit variable and often only focal immunoreactivity for the alpha subunit, beta-FSH, and beta-LH. Grossly, gonadotroph adenomas are large, well-vascularized, soft, tan-to-brown-coloured tumours. They frequently exhibit areas of haemorrhage or necrosis.

Prognosis and treatment

In the hands of experienced neurosurgeons, transsphenoidal surgery can result in gross total removal of macroadenomas. Transfrontal approaches may (rarely) be required for very large tumours with complex suprasellar extension.

Surgical removal of suspected gonadotroph adenomas is indicated when visual field defects are present; these typically improves following surgery. The correction of hypopituitarism, in contrast, is less consistent.

Since gonadotroph adenomas have a propensity to grow, periodic imaging of the pituitary sella as well as evaluation of pituitary function is warranted in individuals in whom a conservative approach is considered.

After surgery alone, about 30% of patients relapse within 5–10 years. Monitoring pituitary tumour remnants with serial imaging is required in order to identify disease recurrence. The decision on timing of adjunctive treatment rests on the demonstration of disease progression or evidence of residual disease. Radiotherapy has been shown to reduce recurrence rates, so diverse forms of it may be indicated for situations in which surgical removal is incomplete or not possible. Radiosurgery is usually reserved for smaller lesions that are more than 3–5 mm from the chiasm and optic nerves [10]. Fractionated radiotherapy is a better option for larger tumours that are close to the optic apparatus.

Medical therapy has, thus far, proven to be ineffective in the management of gonadotroph adenomas. Dopamine agonists may contribute to tumour stabilization or reduction of burden. Somatostatin analogues have not been proven to be efficacious except in a few reported cases. Temozolomide, an alkylating agent that has been used for several types of brain tumours, is a new therapeutic option for recurrent aggressive non-functional pituitary tumours.

References and further reading

1. Yamada S, Ohyama K, Taguchi M, et al. A study of the correlation between morphological findings and biological activities in clinically nonfunctioning pituitary adenomas. Neurosurgery 2007; 61: 580–4; discussion 4–5.
2. Young WF Jr, Scheithauer BW, Kovacs KT, et al. Gonadotroph adenoma of the pituitary gland: A clinicopathologic analysis of 100 cases. Mayo Clin Proc 1996; 71: 649–56.
3. Nishioka H, Inoshita N, Sano T, et al. Correlation between histological subtypes and MRI findings in clinically nonfunctioning pituitary adenomas. Endocr Pathol 2012; 23: 151–6.
4. Dekkers OM, Pereira AM, and Romijn JA. Treatment and follow-up of clinically nonfunctioning pituitary macroadenomas. J Clin Endocrinol Metab 2008; 93: 3717–26.
5. Molitch ME. Management of incidentally found nonfunctional pituitary tumors. Neurosurg Clin N Am 2012; 23: 543–53.
6. Asa SL and Ezzat S. The pathogenesis of pituitary tumors. Annu Rev Pathol 2009; 4: 97–126.
7. Cheunsuchon P, Zhou Y, Zhang X, et al. Silencing of the imprinted DLK1-MEG3 locus in human clinically nonfunctioning pituitary adenomas. Am J Pathol 2011; 179: 2120–30.
8. Ezzat S, Zheng L, Winer D, et al. Targeting N-cadherin through fibroblast growth factor receptor-4: Distinct pathogenetic and therapeutic implications. Mol Endocrinol 2006; 20: 2965–75.
9. Mete O and Asa SL. Clinicopathological correlations in pituitary adenomas. Brain Pathol 2012; 22: 443–53.
10. Kanner AA, Corn BW, and Greenman Y. Radiotherapy of nonfunctioning and gonadotroph adenomas. Pituitary 2009; 12: 15–22.
11. Ntali G, Capatina C, Grossman A, et al. Clinical review: Functioning gonadotroph adenomas. J Clin Endocrinol Metab 2014; 12: 4423–33.

3.10 Thyrotrophinomas

Introduction

Hyperthyroidism resulting from excessive thyroid stimulation by thyrotrophin (TSH) is rare. However, since the advent of ultrasensitive TSH immunometric assays as the first-line test for thyroid function, an increased number of patients with normal or elevated levels of TSH in the presence of high thyroid-hormone concentrations have been recognized.

Although central hyperthyroidism is mainly due to a pituitary TSH-secreting adenoma (TSH-oma), biochemical findings similar to those found in TSH-omas may be recorded in some patients affected with resistance to thyroid hormones (see Chapter 13, Section 13.6). Failure to recognize these different diseases may result in dramatic consequences, such as improper thyroid ablation in patients with central hyperthyroidism, or unnecessary pituitary surgery in patients who are resistant to thyroid hormones. Conversely, early diagnosis and correct treatment of TSH-omas may prevent the occurrence of neurological complications, such as visual defects by compression of the optic chiasm, or hypopituitarism, and should improve the rate of cure.

Epidemiology

TSH-producing adenoma is a rare disorder, accounting for about 0.5% to 2.0% of all pituitary adenomas, the prevalence in the general population being 1–2 cases per million.

However, this figure is probably underestimated, as the number of reported cases of TSH-omas tripled in the last decade. The increased incidence of TSH-omas has been further confirmed by recent data which was obtained from the Swedish Pituitary Registry and demonstrates an increased incidence of TSH-omas over time (0.05 per 1 million per year in 1990–4 to 0.26 per 1 million per year in 2005–9), the national prevalence in 2010 being 2.8 per 1 million inhabitants.

Pathophysiology

None of the large number of candidate genes, including common proto-oncogenes and tumour-suppressor genes as well as pituitary specific genes, was found mutated and thus able to confer growth advantage to thyrotropes. Mutation in thyroid hormone receptor beta was recently shown be a potential mechanism for impaired T3-dependent negative regulation of both TSH and its subunits. Moreover, TSH-omas may be found in the setting of multiple endocrine neoplasia type 1. Nonetheless, molecular mechanisms leading to the formation of TSH-omas are presently unknown, as is true for the large majority of pituitary adenomas.

Clinical features

Patients with TSH-oma present with signs and symptoms of hyperthyroidism that are frequently associated with those related to the pressure effects of an expanding pituitary adenoma, such as headache and visual field defects. Clinical features of hyperthyroidism are sometimes milder than expected on the basis of circulating free thyroid hormone levels, likely due to the slowly progressive onset of hyperthyroidism. In several mixed growth-hormone/TSH adenomas, signs and symptoms of hyperthyroidism may be clinically missed, as they are overshadowed by those of acromegaly.

The presence of a goitre is the rule. Partial or total hypopituitarism is seen in about 25% of cases. Unilateral exophthalmos due to orbital invasion by pituitary tumour was reported in three patients with TSH-omas.

Investigations

- Serum TSH levels in the patients with TSH-oma are normal or slightly high, whereas free thyroid-hormone levels are definitely elevated. Variations of the biological activity of secreted TSH molecules most likely account for the findings of normal TSH in the presence of high thyroid-hormone levels.

- Particular clinical situations and possible laboratory artefacts may cause a biochemical profile similar to that present in central hyperthyroidism. Since these situations and artefacts are relatively common, they should be excluded before performing an extensive evaluation of the pituitary–thyroid axis. Circulating anti-T4 and/or anti-T3 antibodies, as well as abnormal forms of albumin or transthyretin, can interfere in the immunometric assay based on 'analogue' or 'one-step' methods, leading to an overestimation of hormone levels. Possible interfering factors in TSH measurement are heterophilic antibodies directed against or cross-reacting with mouse IgG (i.e. the monoclonal antibodies used in the immunometric assays) (see Chapter 1, Section 1.2).

- The measurement of glycoprotein hormone alpha subunit and some in vivo or in vitro parameters of peripheral thyroid-hormone action are additional useful parameters for the diagnosis of TSH-omas. In our hands, the finding of elevated serum SHBG, as it occurs in the common forms of hyperthyroidism, was able to differentiate hyperthyroid patients with TSH-oma from those with resistance to thyroid hormones.

- Both stimulatory and inhibitory tests have been proposed for the diagnosis of TSH-oma. Classically, the T3 suppression test has been used to assess the presence of a TSH-oma. A complete inhibition of TSH secretion after T3 suppression test (80–100 µg/day per 8–10 days) has never been recorded in TSH-oma. Obviously, this test is strictly contraindicated in elderly patients or those with coronary heart disease. The TRH test has been widely used to investigate the presence of a TSH-oma. In 83% of patients, TSH levels do not increase after TRH injection. As 95% of TSH-omas maintain sensitivity to somatostatin, the administration of long-acting somatostatin analogues for 2–3 months may help in differentiating TSH-oma from resistance to thyroid hormones. Only patients with TSH-oma are responsive in term of reduction/normalization of TSH and free thyroid hormone.

- As with other tumours of the region of the sella turcica, MRI or CT scan must be carried out in order to visualize the tumour. Microadenomas are today reported with increasing frequency.

Differential diagnosis

When the existence of central hyperthyroidism is confirmed, several diagnostic steps have to be carried out to differentiate a TSH-oma from resistance to thyroid hormones. Indeed, the presence of neurological signs and symptoms of an expanding intracranial mass or clinical features of concomitant hypersecretion of other pituitary hormones (acromegaly, galactorrhea, amenorrhea) points to the presence of a TSH-oma. Radiological evidence of a pituitary tumour strongly supports the diagnosis of TSH-oma. However, the possible presence of pituitary incidentalomas should always be considered, due to their frequent occurrence. TSH unresponsiveness to TRH stimulation and/or to T3 suppression tests favours the presence of a TSH-oma. Indexes of thyroid hormone action at the tissue level (such as SHBG levels) are in the hyperthyroid range in patients with TSH-oma, whilst they are normal/low in resistance to thyroid hormones.

Treatment and outcome

Surgical resection is the recommended therapy for TSH-secreting pituitary tumours, with the aim of removing neoplastic tissues and restoring normal pituitary/thyroid function. However, a radical removal of large tumours, which still represent the majority of TSH-omas, is particularly difficult because of the marked fibrosis of these tumours and the local invasion involving the cavernous sinus, the internal carotid artery, or the optic chiasm. Particular attention has to be paid to presurgical preparation of the patient: anti-thyroid drugs or somatostatin analogues along with propranolol should be used aiming the restoration of the euthyroidism. After surgery, partial or complete hypopituitarism may result. Evaluation of pituitary functions, particularly adrenocorticotrophic hormone secretion, should be carefully undertaken soon after surgery, and hormone replacement therapy initiated if needed (see Chapter 3, Section 3.3).

If surgery is contraindicated or declined, as well as in the case of surgical failure, pituitary radiotherapy may be considered, the recommended dose being no less than 45 Gy fractionated at 2 Gy per day or 10–25 Gy in a single dose if a stereotactic gamma unit is available.

Several patients require medical therapy in order to control the hyperthyroidism. Today, the medical treatment of TSH-omas rests on long-acting somatostatin analogues, such as octreotide and lanreotide. Treatment with these analogues leads to a reduction of TSH secretion in almost all cases, with restoration of the euthyroid state in the majority of them. During octreotide therapy, tumour shrinkage occurs in about half of patients, and vision improvement in 75%. Resistance to octreotide treatment has been documented in only 4% of cases. Patients on somatostatin analogues have to be carefully monitored, as untoward side effects, such as cholelithiasis and carbohydrate intolerance, may become manifest.

No data on the recurrence rates of TSH-oma in patients judged cured after surgery or radiotherapy have been reported. However, the recurrence of the adenoma does not appear to be frequent, at least in the first years after successful surgery. In general, the patient should be evaluated clinically and biochemically two or three times the first year post-operatively, and then every year. Pituitary imaging should be performed every 2 or 3 years, but should be promptly done whenever an increase in TSH and thyroid-hormone levels, or clinical symptoms, occur. In the case of persistent macroadenoma, a close visual fields follow-up is required, as the visual function is threatened.

Further reading

Beck-Peccoz P, Lania A, and Persani L. 'TSH-producing adenomas', in Jameson JL, and DeGroot LJ, eds, *Endocrinology, Adult and Pediatric* (7th edition), 2016. Vol. 1. Elsevier, pp. 266–90.

Gurnell M, Visser TJ, Beck-Peccoz P, et al. 'Resistance to thyroid hormone', in Jameson JL and DeGroot LJ, eds, *Endocrinology, Adult and Pediatric* (7th edition), 2016. Vol. 2. Elsevier, pp. 1648–67.

Losa M, Giovanelli M, Persani L, et al. Criteria of cure and follow-up of central hyperthyroidism due to thyrotropin-secreting pituitary adenomas. *J Clin Endocrinol Metab* 1996; 81: 3086–90.

Mannavola D, Persani L, Vannucchi G, et al. Different response to chronic somatostatin analogues in patients with central hyperthyroidism. *Clin Endocrinol (Oxf)* 2005; 62: 176–81.

Socin HV, Chanson P, Delemer B, et al. The changing spectrum of TSH-secreting pituitary adenomas: diagnosis and management in 43 patients. *Eur J Endocrinol* 2003; 148: 433–42.

3.11 Pituitary incidentalomas

Introduction

Clinically non-functioning adenomas range from being completely asymptomatic, and therefore detected either at autopsy or as incidental findings on head MRI or CT scans performed for other reasons, to causing significant hypothalamic/pituitary dysfunction and visual symptoms due to their large size. About three-quarters of clinically non-functioning adenomas are actually gonadotroph adenomas. Less commonly, clinically non-functioning adenomas stain positively for adrenocorticotrophic hormone, growth hormone, prolactin, or TSH but do not secrete these hormones in sufficient quantities so as to cause clinical syndromes; such tumours are referred to as 'silent' corticotroph, somatotroph, lactotroph, or thyrotroph adenomas. A number of other lesions may also be found in the sella, including aneurysms, craniopharyngiomas, Rathke's cleft cysts, meningiomas, and metastases.

Pituitary adenomas have been found at autopsy in about 10% of subjects not suspected of having pituitary disease whilst alive, with about 40% staining positively for prolactin and <0.1% being macroadenomas. CT and MRI scans of the sella in normal subjects show lesions compatible with pituitary adenomas in frequencies ranging from 4% to 40%, emphasizing the difficulty in distinguishing small lesions from artefacts. As in the autopsy data, macroadenomas have been found very uncommonly in such studies.

In series of patients reported with pituitary incidentalomas, 304 of the 454 patients (67%) had macroadenomas, a proportion much greater than would be expected based on the autopsy findings, suggesting that the mass effects of such tumours may have caused some of the symptomatology causing the patients to have the scans in the first place.

Endocrinologic evaluation of the asymptomatic incidental mass

Many of the changes occurring with hormone oversecretion syndromes may be quite subtle and only slowly progressive; therefore, screening for hormonal oversecretion even in asymptomatic patients is warranted. It is not clear whether patients with minimal clinical evidence of hormone oversecretion are free from the increased risk for the more subtle cardiovascular, bone, oncological, and possibly other adverse effects we usually associated with Cushing's disease or acromegaly. Screening tests should include a serum prolactin, IGF-1, and either a midnight salivary cortisol or an overnight DST. For very large tumours, the prolactin sample should be diluted 1:100 to avoid the 'hook effect'. (see also Chapter 1, Section 1.2). All patients should be assessed for hypopituitarism, as even those with microadenomas have sometimes been found to have hypopituitarism.

Natural history and follow-up of incidental clinically non-functioning adenomas

In 11 series totalling 522 patients with pituitary clinically non-functioning adenomas that were not treated either surgically or medically, thereby giving an indication of their natural history, of the 166 patients with microadenomas, 17 (10%) experienced tumour growth, 11 (7%) showed evidence of a decrease in tumour size, and 138 (83%) remained unchanged in size in follow-up MRI scans over periods of up to 8 years. Of the 356 patients with macroadenomas, 86 (24%) showed evidence of tumour enlargement, 45 (13%) showed evidence of a decrease in tumour size, and 225 (63%) remained unchanged in size on follow-up MRI scans. In 7 of the 86 macroadenomas with tumour size increase, the increase was due to tumour haemorrhage. Growth rates are highly variable, with some patients showing tumour growth by 2 years but others not showing growth until 20 years. Thus, at least for patients with macroadenomas, surveillance MRI scans should be carried out for at least 20 years, although the frequency of scanning can be reduced after the first few years if there is no evidence of tumour growth.

Management of incidental clinically non-functioning adenomas

Therapy is indicated for tumours that are hypersecreting. For patients with incidental non-functioning adenomas, significant tumour enlargement appears to occur in only 10% of those with microadenomas and 24% of those with macroadenomas. If there are visual field defects, surgery is indicated. If a tumour abuts the optic chiasm, even though visual fields are normal, consideration should be given to surgery; if surgery is not done, then visual fields should be tested at 6–12 monthly intervals. Because hypopituitarism is potentially correctable with tumour resection, this is also a relative indication for surgery. Tumours >2 cm should also be considered for surgery simply because of their already demonstrated propensity for growth. A completely asymptomatic tumour could simply be followed with repeat scans, initially yearly and later less often; surgery would be deferred until there is evidence of tumour growth. Haemorrhage into such tumours is uncommon but anticoagulation may predispose to this complication; surgery would prevent such a complication. An attempt at medical therapy with a dopamine agonist or octreotide is reasonable for macroadenomas, realizing that only about 10%–20% of such patients will respond with a decrease in tumour size.

Overall, the decision to proceed with surgery for adenomas is affected by the rate and extent of growth and any clinical consequences, such as the development of visual field defects or pituitary hormone deficiencies, as well as the patient's co-morbidities and risks for surgery (see Figure 3.14).

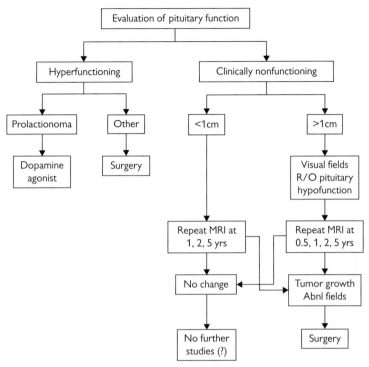

Fig 3.14 Flow diagram indicating the approach that should be taken with patients found to have a pituitary incidentaloma. The first step is to evaluate patients for pituitary hyperfunction and then treat those found to be hyperfunctioning. Of patients with tumours that are clinically non-functioning, those with macroadenomas are evaluated further for evidence of chiasmal compression and hypopituitarism. Scans are then repeated at progressively longer intervals to assess for enlargement of the tumours; Abnl, abnormal; R/O, rule out.

Reprinted from *Endocrinology and Metabolism Clinics of North America*, Volume 37, Issue 1, Molitch ME, Nonsecreting tumors and pituitary incidentalomas, pp. 151–171, Copyright © 2008, with permission from Elsevier.

Further reading

Buurman H and Saeger W. Subclinical adenomas in postmortem pituitaries: Classification and correlations to clinical data. *Eur J Endocrinol* 2006;154:753–8.

Colao A, DiSomma C, Pivonello R, et al. Medical therapy for clinically non-functioning pituitary adenomas. *Endocr Relat Cancer* 2008; 15: 905–15.

Dekkers OM, Hammer S, de Keizer RJW, et al. The natural course of non-functioning pituitary macroadenomas. *Eur J Endocrinol* 2007; 156: 217–24.

Fernandez-Balsells MM, Murad MH, Barwise A, et al. Natural history of nonfunctioning pituitary adenomas and incidentalomas: A systematic review and metaanalysis. *J Clin Endocrinol Metab* 2011; 96: 905–12.

Freda PU, Beckers M, Katznelson L, et al. Pituitary incidentaloma: An Endocrine Society clinical practice guideline. *J Clin Endocrinol Metab* 2011; 96: 894–904.

Molitch ME. Pituitary incidentalomas. *Best Pract Res Clin Endocrinol Metab* 2009; 23: 667–75.

3.12 Pituitary carcinoma

Definition
The diagnosis of pituitary carcinoma requires the documented presence of craniospinal and/or systemic metastases arising from a tumour originating in the adenohypophysis.

Pathogenesis
Pituitary carcinomas are thought to arise from an accumulation of genetic and epigenetic events occurring in an adenoma–carcinoma sequence [1]. Loss of cellular senescence or proliferation arrest, characteristic of benign pituitary adenomas, has been suggested to underlie the transformation into a malignant tumour [2], but this remains uncertain [3]. Common cancer-related genetic mutations, such as in p53, are rare in pituitary carcinoma, although HRAS mutations have been described in metastatic deposits [4]. Genetic aberrations involved in pituitary carcinogenesis include loss of expression of cell-cycle inhibitors (p21, retinoblastoma protein, p27), increased telomerase activity, HER2/neu gene amplification, and overexpression of galectin-3 [1, 5].

Epidemiology
Pituitary carcinomas account for 0.2% of all pituitary tumours [6]. The majority of cases present in the third to fifth decades, with an equal occurrence in both sexes [7]. Pituitary tumours destined to become pituitary carcinomas begin as macroadenomas with a mean latency period until development of metastases of 7 years [5].

Clinical features
Most commonly, pituitary carcinomas produce either prolactin or adrenocorticotrophic hormone with an initial clinical presentation indistinguishable from their benign counterparts. Non-functioning pituitary carcinomas occur less frequently, whilst growth hormone and TSH-secreting carcinomas are rare. The emergence of an aggressive pituitary tumour demonstrating resistance to standard therapies and rapid regrowth after surgery or radiotherapy should alert to the possible diagnosis of a pituitary carcinoma. Direct effects of the primary sellar tumour cause most of the morbidity and mortality associated with pituitary carcinoma, particularly visual loss, cranial nerve palsies, and hormone hypersecretion [4]. Systemic metastases occur more frequently than craniospinal metastases (47% and 40%, respectively), with a minority of cases (13%) exhibiting both. Metastases can occur anywhere within the cranial nervous system, and other described sites include cervical lymph nodes, bone, lung, liver, kidney, and ovary [7].

Investigations
Functioning pituitary carcinomas typically exhibit high hormone levels, but there is significant overlap with levels found among adenomas. A progressive increase in hormone levels in the presence of minimal or stable tumour within the sella should raise the clinical suspicion of metastatic deposits. Pituitary carcinomas appear as invasive macroadenomas on pituitary imaging: non-contiguous tumour deposits may represent intracranial metastases. Imaging of spine, chest, and abdomen could reveal other sites of metastasis. There are no histopathological,

immunohistochemical, or ultrastructural features to reliably distinguish a pituitary carcinoma from an adenoma. The WHO criteria to denote an 'atypical pituitary adenoma' (Ki67 >3%, p53 immunopositivity >3%, and increased mitotic rate) may indicate a tumour with malignant potential requiring close follow-up [8].

Management
Pituitary carcinomas are challenging to manage and require a multimodal treatment approach, often with palliative intent. Repeated debulking surgery of sellar or metastatic tumours can relieve compressive symptoms, whilst radiotherapy is frequently employed to stall tumour regrowth. Medical therapies such as dopamine agonists in prolactin-secreting pituitary carcinoma are often used at maximal doses if tolerated. The oral alkylating chemotherapeutic agent temozolomide is the first chemotherapeutic to show substantial activity against pituitary carcinomas. Response to temozolomide may be dramatic and prolonged: its use should be considered early in the treatment course of pituitary carcinomas. 06-Methylguanine-DNA methyltransferase (MGMT), a DNA repair protein, has been proposed as a predictor of response to temozolomide [9].

Prognosis
The prognosis for patients with pituitary carcinoma is poor. The mean survival is less than 4 years and may be less than 1 year in cases of adrenocorticotrophic hormone carcinomas, although occasional long-term survival has been reported [4]. Early application of chemotherapy may be associated with longer survival [10].

Future developments
New targeted therapeutics such as multikinase inhibitors and VEGF inhibitors (e.g. bevacizumab), alone or in combination with PI3K/mTOR inhibitors (such as everolimus) may prove useful in the management of pituitary carcinomas [7]. There is emerging interest in the use of the oral alkylating agent temozolomide in combination with targeted therapies and the broad-spectrum somatostatin analogue pasireotide. The clinical application of treatment response biomarkers might also guide more effective use of medical therapies in the management of pituitary carcinoma. Guidelines summarizing the current state of management have recently been published [11].

References and further reading
1. Scheithauer BW, Kurtkaya-Yapicier O, Kovacs KT, et al. Pituitary carcinoma: A clinicopathological review. Neurosurgery 2005; 56: 1066–74.
2. Melmed S. Pathogenesis of pituitary tumors. Nat Rev Endocrinol 2011; 7: 257–66.
3. Alexandraki KI, Khan MM, Chahal HS, et al. Oncogene-induced senescence in pituitary adenomas and carcinomas. Hormones 2012; 11: 297–307.
4. Pei L, Melmed S, Scheithauer B, et al. H-ras mutations in human pituitary carcinoma metastases. J Clin Endocrinol Metab 1994; 78: 842–6.
5. Kaltsas GA, Nomikos P, Kontogeorgos G, et al. Clinical review: Diagnosis and management of pituitary carcinomas. J Clin Endocrinol Metab 2005; 90: 3089–99.

6. Pernicone PJ, Scheithauer BW, Sebo TJ, et al. Pituitary carcinoma: A clinicopathological study of 15 cases. *Cancer* 1997; 79: 804–12.

7. Heaney AP. Clinical review: Pituitary carcinoma: Difficult diagnosis and treatment. *J Clin Endocrinol Metab* 2011; 96: 3649–60.

8. Lloyd RV, Kovacs K, and Young WF. *Pituitary Tumors*, 2004. IARC Press.

9. McCormack AI, Wass JA, and Grossman AB. Aggressive pituitary tumours: The role of temozolomide and the assessment of MGMT status. *Eur J Clin Invest* 2011; 41: 1133–48.

10. Kaltsas GA, Mukherjee JJ, Plowman PN, et al. The role of cytotoxic chemotherapy in the management of aggressive and malignant pituitary tumors. *J Clin Endocrinol Metab* 1998; 83: 4233–8.

11. Raverot G, Burman P, McCormack A, et al. ESE Clinical practice guidelines for the management of aggressive pituitary tumours and carcinomas. *Eur J Endocrinol* 2018; 178: G1–24.

3.13 Craniopharyngioma and parasellar cysts

Craniopharyngioma

Definition and epidemiology

Craniopharyngiomas are rare epithelial tumours arising along the path of the craniopharyngeal duct. They account for 2%–5% of all the primary intracranial neoplasms and for up to 15% of the intracranial tumours in children. Their incidence is reported as 0.13 per 100,000 person-years. They may be detected at any age, even in the prenatal and neonatal periods, with a bimodal age distribution, and peak incidence rates of ages 5–14 and 50–74 years have been proposed.

Pathology

Craniopharyngiomas are WHO Grade 1 tumours. Rare cases of malignant transformation (possibly triggered by previous irradiation) have been described. Their pathogenesis has not been clarified. However, the majority, if not all, of the adamantinomatous subtype have beta-catenin mutations, whilst the papillary subtype seem to specifically show *BRAF* mutations; the latter may be therapeutically relevant.

Histologically, two primary subtypes have been recognized, the adamantinomatous and the papillary, but transitional or mixed forms have also been described. The adamantinomatous subtype macroscopically shows cystic and/or solid components, necrotic debris, fibrous tissue, and calcification (especially common in children). The cyst contains liquid ranging from 'machinery oil' to shimmering cholesterol-laden fluid, and their margins are sharp and irregular, often making the identification of the surgical planes difficult. The epithelium is composed of a palisaded basal layer of small cells; above this, there is an intermediate layer of variable thickness composed of loose aggregates of stellate cells ('stellate reticulum') and a top layer facing into the cyst lumen with abruptly enlarged, flattened, and keratinized to flat plate-like squamous cells. The flat squames are desquamated singly or in distinctive stacked clusters forming nodules of 'wet' keratin. The papillary variety has almost exclusively been described in adults. Macroscopically, it tends to be solid or mixed with cystic and solid components, calcification is rare, and the cyst content is usually viscous and yellow. It is generally well circumscribed, and infiltration of adjacent brain tissue by neoplastic epithelium is less frequent than in the adamantinomatous type, or even absent. Microscopically, it is composed of mature squamous epithelium forming pseudopapillae and of an anastomosing fibrovascular stroma without the presence of peripheral palisading of cells or stellate reticuli.

Clinical, hormonal, and imaging features at presentation

Craniopharyngiomas may exert pressure effects to various brain structures (visual pathways, brain parenchyma, the ventricular system, major blood vessels, and the hypothalamo-pituitary system) resulting in multiple clinical features (neurological, visual, hypothalamo-pituitary); headaches, nausea/vomiting, visual disturbances, growth failure (in children), and hypogonadism (in adults) are the most frequently described. A substantial number of patients present with compromised hypothalamo-pituitary function; reported rates for pituitary hormone deficits are 35%–95% for growth hormone, 38%–82% for FSH/LH, 21%–62% for adrenocorticotrophic hormone, 21%–42% for TSH, and 6%–38% for vasopressin.

Most of the craniopharyngiomas are detected in the sellar/parasellar region; rare ectopic locations have also been described. A suprasellar component has been reported in 94%–95% of the cases. The size of craniopharyngiomas has been reported >4 cm in 14%–20% of the cases and <2 cm in 4%–28%. Their consistency is purely or predominantly cystic in 46%–64%, purely or predominantly solid in 18%–39%, and mixed in 8%–36%. Calcification has been shown in 45%–57% (probably more common in children), and hydrocephalus in 20%–38% (also more frequent in childhood populations). Plain skull X-rays may show calcification and abnormal sella. CT is helpful for the evaluation of the bony anatomy, the identification of calcification, and the discrimination of the solid and the cystic components (the cystic fluid is hypodense and the solid portions, as well as the cyst capsule show enhancement following contrast administration). MRI is particularly important for the topographic and structural analysis of the tumour (see also Chapter 3, Section 3.3). A solid lesion appears as iso- or hypo-intense relative to the brain on pre-contrast T1-weighted images, shows enhancement following gadolinium administration, and is usually of mixed hypo- or hyperintensity on T2-weighted sequences (see Figure 3.15). A cystic element is usually hypo-intense on T1- and hyperintense on T2-weighted sequences. On T1-weighted images, a thin, peripheral, contrast-enhancing rim of the cyst is demonstrated. Protein, cholesterol, and methaemoglobin may cause high signal on T1-weighted images. The differential diagnosis includes Rathke's cleft cyst, dermoid cyst, epidermoid cyst, pituitary adenoma, germinoma, hamartoma, suprasellar aneurysm, arachnoid cyst, suprasellar abscess, glioma, meningioma, sacroidosis, TB, and Langerhans cell histiocytosis.

Treatment options

Surgery combined or not with adjuvant external irradiation is the most widely used first therapeutic approach. (Figure 3.16). The extent of resection depends mainly on the size and location (particularly difficult for retrochiasmatic sites or sites within the third ventricle) of the tumour, as well as the presence of brain invasion. The mean interval for the diagnosis of recurrent tumours following various primary treatment modalities ranges between 1.0 and 4.3 years and relapses as late as 30 years after initial therapy have been reported. Based on retrospective, non-randomized series with radiological confirmation of the radicality of resection, the recurrence rates following gross total removal range between 0% and 62% at 10 years follow-up. These are significantly lower than those reported after partial or subtotal resection (25%–100% at 10 years). In cases of limited surgery, adjuvant radiotherapy improves significantly the local control rates (recurrence rates 10%–63% at 10 years). Finally, radiotherapy alone provides 10 years recurrence rates ranging between 0%–23%. The growth rate of craniopharyngiomas varies considerably, and reliable clinical, radiological, and pathological criteria predicting their behaviour are lacking. The management of recurrent tumours remains difficult, as scarring/adhesions from previous operations or irradiation make successful removal difficult. The beneficial effect of radiotherapy (preceded or not by second surgery) in recurrent lesions has been clearly shown.

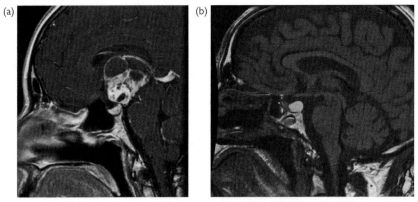

Fig 3.15 (a) Pituitary MRI of a craniopharyngioma: a sagittal T1-weighted image with a superiorly lobulated shape and mixed solid and cystic characteristics. (b) Pituitary MRI of a Rathke's cleft cyst: the sagittal T1-weighted image shows hyperintense signal.

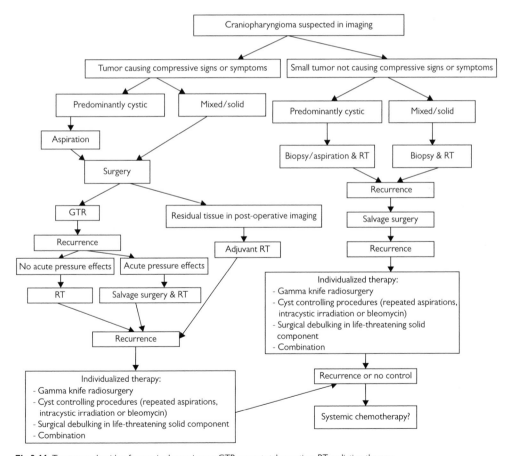

Fig 3.16 Treatment algorithm for craniopharyngiomas; GTR, gross total resection; RT, radiation therapy.
Reproduced from Karavitaki N and Cudlip S, Craniopharyngiomas, *Endocrine Reviews*, Volume 27, Issue 4, pp. 371–397, https://doi.org/10.1210/er.2006-0002. Copyright (2006) with permission of Oxford University Press on behalf of the Endocrine Society.

Intracavitary irradiation (brachytherapy) delivers a higher radiation dose to the cyst lining than irradiation via external radiotherapy and results in damage of the secretory epithelial lining, elimination of the fluid production, and cyst shrinkage. The efficacy of various beta- and gamma-emitting isotopes (mainly ^{32}phosphate, ^{90}yttrium, ^{186}rhenium, and ^{198}gold) has been assessed in a number of studies but, given that none of them has the ideal physical and biological profile, there is no consensus on which is the most suitable therapeutic agent. In several studies with a mean or median follow-up between 3.1 and 11.9 years, intracavitary irradiation (mainly with ^{90}yttrium or ^{32}phosphorus providing radiation doses of 200–267 Gy), complete or partial cyst resolution was seen in 71%–88% of the cases, stabilization in 3%–19% and an increase in 5%–10%. New cyst formation or increase in the solid component of the tumour was observed in 6.5%–20% of the cases. Although beta emitters have short-range tissue penetrance, lesions in close proximity to the optic apparatus should be approached with caution.

A small number of reports have shown that the intracystic installation of the antineoplasmatic agent bleomycin may be an effective therapy for some cystic tumours. Direct leakage of the drug to surrounding tissues during the installation procedure, diffusion although the cyst wall, or high drug dose has been associated with various toxic or even fatal effects. The value of this treatment option in tumour control or even in the delaying of potentially harmful surgery and/or radiotherapy, as well as the optimal protocol and the clear-cut criteria predicting the long-term outcome, remain to be established in large series with appropriate follow-up.

Stereotactic radiosurgery achieves tumour control in a substantial number of patients with small volume lesions. Tumour volume and close attachment to critical structures, as the optic apparatus, are limiting factors for its application. It may be particularly useful for well-defined residual disease following surgery or for the treatment of small solid recurrent tumours, particularly after failure of conventional radiotherapy.

Long-term morbidity and mortality

Craniopharyngiomas are associated with significant long-term morbidity (mainly involving endocrine, visual, hypothalamic, neurobehavioural, and cognitive sequelae) attributed to the damage of critical structures by the primary or recurrent tumour and/or to the adverse effects of the therapeutic interventions. The rates of individual hormone deficits range between 88% and 100% for growth hormone, 80%–95% for FSH/LH, 55%–88% for adrenocorticotrophic hormone, 39%–95% for TSH, and 25%–86% for vasopressin. Compromised vision has been reported in up to 63% of the patients treated by surgery combined or not with radiotherapy during an observation period of 10 years. Hypothalamic damage may result in hyperphagia and uncontrollable obesity; disorders of thirst and water/electrolyte balance; behavioural and cognitive impairment; loss of temperature control; and disorders in the sleep pattern. Of those, obesity is the most frequent (reported in 26%–61% of the patients treated by surgery combined or not with radiotherapy) and is a consequence of the disruption of the mechanisms controlling satiety, hunger, and energy balance. Compromised neuropsychological and cognitive function in patients with craniopharyngioma after surgery and radiation therapy contributes significantly to poor academic and work performance, disrupted family and social relationships, and impaired quality of life. The mortality rates of patients with craniopharyngioma have been reported to be 3–6 times higher than that of the general population and the 10-year survival rates range between 83% and 93%. Apart from the deaths directly attributed to the tumour (pressure effects to critical structures) and to the surgical interventions, the risk of cardio-/cerebrovascular and respiratory mortality is increased. It has also been suggested that, in childhood populations, the hypoadrenalism and the associated hypoglycaemia, as well as the metabolic consequences of vasopressin deficiency and absent thirst may contribute to the excessive mortality. The impact of tumour recurrence on the long-term mortality is widely accepted, and the 10-year survival rates in such cases range between 29% and 70%.

Rathke's cleft cysts

Rathke's cleft cysts are benign sellar and/or suprasellar lesions found in 13%–33% of routine autopsies and arising from remnants of the Rathke's pouch. Their contents vary from clear CSF-like fluid to thick mucoid material. They are lined by single or pseudostratified cuboidal or columnar epithelium with or without cilia and with goblet cells.

Symptomatic cases are rare. The presenting manifestations are the result of compression to adjacent structures, and the most common ones are headaches, hypopituitarism of varying degrees (approximately 50%), hyperprolactinaemia, visual disturbance, and diabetes insipidus.

Their imaging features are variable. Forty per cent are completely intrasellar, whereas 60% have some suprasellar extension. On CT, the cyst density ranges from hypodense, to isodense, to mixed. On MRI they have a variable T1 signal (hyper-, hypo-, or isointense), depending on their content. Small intracystic nodules corresponding to proteinaceous concentrations may be demonstrated, presenting with lower T2- and higher T1- signal intensity than the rest of the cyst. The nodules do not enhance and are virtually pathognomonic for the Rathke's cleft cysts.

Symptomatic cases are managed by surgery. The risk of recurrence following evacuation and biopsy ranges between 8% and 33%, with a relapse-free rate of 88% at 24 months, and 52% at 48 months. Although not widely accepted, the extent of removal may predict relapse.

Mucoceles of sphenoid sinus

Mucoceles of the sphenoid sinus are very rare, benign, cystic lesions lined by a secretory pseudostratified columnar epithelium. They result from chronic obstruction of the sinus; prior sinus disease, allergic history, trauma, and surgery of the sphenoid sinus have been implicated in their pathogenesis. Their clinical manifestations depend on the degree of involvement of the adjacent structures and include headache, decrease in visual acuity, oculomotor palsies, exophthalmos, trigeminal nerve hypoesthesia, and pituitary insufficiency. On CT, they appear as well-encapsulated, non-enhancing cystic masses. On MRI, they are expansive, well-delineated masses with a homogeneously hyperintense T1 and T2 signals. They show no enhancement. Marsupialization by partial removal of the anterior and inferior walls of the mucocele with an endoscopic endonasal approach is probably the treatment of choice, preventing relapse and complications in most of the cases.

Arachnoid cysts

Arachnoid cysts are benign, intra-arachnoidal, space-occupying lesions filled with clear CSF and not communicating with the ventricular system. Five to sixty per cent are found in the middle cranial fossa. They are usually congenital. Microscopically, the cyst wall consists of vascular collagenous membrane lined by flattened arachnoid cells. Symptomatic patients present with hydrocephalus, visual impairment, endocrine dysfunction, and syndromes resulting from brain stem compression. On imaging, they typically appear as sharply demarcated extra-axial cysts, with no identifiable internal architecture and no enhancing. The cyst has the same signal intensity as CSF in all sequences. Symptomatic patients have been treated with stereotactic aspiration, cyst fenestration, cystoperitoneal shunting, microsurgical excision, and endoscopic ventriculocystostomy or ventriculocisternostomy. Stereotactic intracavitary irradiation has been applied in a limited number of cases, leading to cyst regression and symptomatic improvement without reported complications.

Dermoid cysts

Dermoid cysts are rare benign lesions most commonly found in the midline sellar, parasellar, or frontonasal areas. They arise from the inclusion of ectodermally committed cells at the time of neural tube closure. The cyst is a well-defined, lobulated, 'pearly' mass containing thick, foul-smelling, yellow material. Hair or teeth may also be present. The capsule consists of keratinized squamous epithelium supported by collagen and often has plaques of calcification. In thicker parts, the lining is supplemented with dermis containing hair follicles and sebaceous and apocrine glands. The presenting manifestations are attributed to local mass effect. They may rarely rupture spontaneously in the subarachnoid space. Malignant transformation has also been reported, with poor prognosis. On CT imaging, dermoid cysts are usually rounded, well-circumscribed, extremely hypodense lesions. Peripheral capsular calcification is frequent. Enhancement after contrast administration is rare. On T1 images, non-ruptured cysts appear hyperintense with no enhancement. On T2 images, the signal intensity is heterogeneous, varying from hypo- to hyperintense. Radical surgical resection, when possible to be achieved, is generally curative.

Epidermoid cysts

Epidermoid cysts are benign, cystic lesions representing 0.2%–1.8% of all primary intracranial tumours. They arise from the inclusion of ectodermal epithelial tissue into the neural tube, and 10%–15% of the cases have been found in the sellar/parasellar regions. Macroscopically, they have an irregular, cauliflower-like outer surface that grows to encase vessels and nerves. The cyst content includes a soft, waxy, or flaky keratohyalin material resulting from the desquamation of its wall. They are lined by squamous epithelium with a linear keratohyalin granule layer. They are slow growing lesions, with most of them being asymptomatic. Occasionally, they may be associated with mass effects, cranial neuropathy, seizures, or (in the case of rupture) granulomatous meningitis. Malignant transformation has also been reported, with poor prognosis. On CT scans, they appear as well-defined hypo-attenuated masses resembling CSF and not enhancing. Calcification may be detected in 10%–25% of cases. On T1- and T2-weighted MRI sections, they are typically isointense or slightly hyperintense to CSF. Most do not enhance. Surgical treatment offers good results.

Further reading

Buchinsky FJ, Gennarelli TA, Strome SE, eat al. Sphenoid sinus mucocele: A rare complication of transsphenoidal hypophysectomy. *Ear Nose Throat J* 2001; 80: 886–8.

Caldarelli M, Massimi L, Kondageski C, et al. Intracranial midline dermoid and epidermoid cysts in children. *J Neurosurg* 2004; 100: 473–80.

Karavitaki N, Cudlip S, Adams CBT, et al. Craniopharyngiomas. *Endocr Rev* 2006; 27: 371–97.

Karavitaki N, Wass JAH. Non-adenomatous pituitary tumours. *Best Pract Res Clin Endocrinol Metab* 2009; 23: 651–65.

Karavitaki N. Radiotherapy of other sellar lesions. *Pituitary* 2009; 12: 23–9.

Larkin S, Karavitaki N, and Ansorge O. Rathke cleft cyst. *Handb Clin Neurol* 2014; 124: 255–69.

Mohn A, Schoof E, Fahlbusch R, et al. The endocrine spectrum of arachnoid cysts in childhood. *Pediatr Neurosurg* 1999; 31: 316–21.

Muller HL. Craniopharyngioma. *Endocr Rev* 2014; 35: 514–43.

Trifanescu R, Ansorge O, Wass JA, et al. Rathke's cleft cysts. *Clin Endocrinol* 2012; 76: 151–60.

Trifanescu R, Ansorge O, Wass JA, Grossman AB, Karavitaki N. Rathke's cleft cysts. *Clin Endocrinol (Oxf)* 2012; 76: 151–60.

3.14 Pituitary apoplexy

Introduction

Classical pituitary apoplexy (derived from Greek word apoplēxia meaning 'striking away') is a potentially life-threatening condition due to acute ischaemic infarction or haemorrhage of the pituitary gland and is characterized by sudden onset headache, vomiting, visual impairment, ophthalmoplegia, and altered consciousness. Apoplexy often results in hypopituitarism, causing haemodynamic instability, mainly due to adrenocorticotroph deficiency.

Subclinical pituitary apoplexy is radiological or histo-pathological detection of asymptomatic pituitary infarction or haemorrhage, whereas classical pituitary apoplexy is a clinical diagnosis.

Incidence

The incidence of classical pituitary apoplexy is 2%–7%, and is often the first presentation of underlying pituitary tumour [1]. Most cases present in the fifth or sixth decades and have a slight male preponderance (1.5–2.0:1.0) [1–3].

Aetiology

The pituitary has a rich vascular supply: the anterior pituitary is supplied by the superior hypophyseal artery, the posterior pituitary is supplied by the inferior hypophyseal artery, and portal vessels originate from capillaries of median eminence and anastomose with hypophyseal circulation, supplying about 70% of the pituitary. Venous drainage is into the adjacent venous sinus and subsequently into jugular veins. This complex and rich vascular system in bony sella turcica, coupled with an expanding tumour, highly predisposes to bleeding. Another theory is that the pituitary tumour outgrows the blood supply, causing ischaemic necrosis followed by haemorrhagic conversion of the infarcted area. However, these theories fail to explain the presence of pituitary apoplexy in small tumours. Although the exact mechanism remains unclear, several risk factors are identified in about one-third of cases, as illustrated in Box 3.3.

Clinical features

A sudden increase in intrasellar contents causes increased intrasellar pressure resulting in various clinical manifestations. The most common and an early symptom is

---

Box 3.3 Precipitating factors

Systemic hypertension (26%–33%)
   Coagulopathies: sickle cell anaemia, disseminated intravascular coagulation, etc.
   Pregnancy and post-partum state
   Major trauma: head trauma, road traffic accidents causing multiple fractures
   Major surgery: coronary artery bypass graft, abdominal surgery, hip replacement, etc.
   Medications: antiplatelet agents (9%), dopamine agonists, clomiphene, oestrogen therapy, isosorbide mononitrate, chlorpromazine, GnRH agonists, withdrawal of octreotide
   Dynamic pituitary function tests (<1%): TRH (70%), CRH, GnRH, metyrapone, etc.
   Radiation therapy and gamma-knife therapy

Abbreviations: CRH, corticotrophin-releasing hormone; GnRH, gonadotrophin-releasing hormone; TRH, thyrotrophin-releasing hormone.

---

sudden-onset severe headache (89%–95%), followed by nausea and vomiting (43%–80%) caused by a combination of meningeal irritation, dura matter compression, and enlargement of sellar walls. Altered visual acuity and visual field defects (85%), classically bitemporal, are due to suprasellar extension involving the optic apparatus: the optic nerve, the optic chiasma, and/or the optic tracts. Diplopia (>50%) results from compression of the third, fourth, and sixth nerves, due to lateral compression of the contents of the cavernous sinus. The third nerve is the most common cranial nerve affected and its involvement can lead to ipsilateral ptosis and mydriasis. It is reported that ophthalmoplegia is more common than chiasmal involvement, and blindness can develop in one or both eyes [4]. Various clinical manifestations secondary to compression of surrounding anatomical structures are illustrated in Table 3.8.

Table 3.8 Clinical features of pituitary apoplexy in relation to compression of surrounding anatomical structures

Symptoms	Anatomical structures compressed	Direction of tumour expansion
Visual field defect	Optic apparatus	Superior
Blindness	Optic nerve	Superior
Anosmia/hyposmia	Hypothalamus	Superior
Proptosis	Cavernous sinus	Lateral
Diplopia, mydriasis, ptosis	Third cranial nerve	Lateral
Diplopia secondary to ophthalmoplegia	Third, fourth, and sixth cranial nerves (cavernous sinus)	Lateral
Facial pain, corneal anaesthesia	Fifth cranial nerve	Lateral
Hemiplegia	Internal carotid artery	Lateral
Epistaxis, CSF rhinorrhoea	Sphenoid sinus	Downward

This table is adapted from *Endocrinology and Metabolic Clinics of North America*, Volume 22, Rolih CA and Ober KP., Pituitary apoplexy, pp. 291–302, Copyright © Elsevier, 1993.

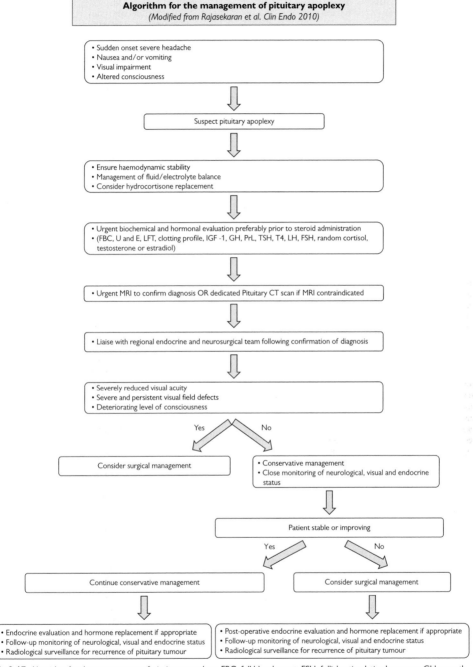

Fig 3.17 Algorithm for the management of pituitary apoplexy; FBC, full blood count; FSH, follicle-stimulating hormone; GH, growth hormone; LFT, liver function test; LH, luteinizing hormone; PrL, prolactin; T4, thyroxine; TSH, thyroid-stimulating hormone; U and E, urea and electrolytes.
Adapted with permission from Rajasekaran S. et al., UK guidelines for the management of pituitary apoplexy, *Clinical Endocrinology*, Volume 74, Issue 1, pp. 9–20, Copyright © 2010 John Wiley and Sons Ltd.

The majority of patients (nearly 80%) demonstrate partial or complete hypopituitarism at the time of presentation: adrenocorticotroph (70%), thyrotroph (50%), somatotroph (60%), gonadotroph (75%), and hyperprolactinaemia (6%) [1, 5]. About 20%–30% of these patients may have had pre-existing endocrine dysfunction, due to the underlying macroadenoma. The most important endocrine dysfunction is hypocortisolaemia from adrenocorticotrophic-hormone deficiency, resulting in hypotension (70%) and requiring urgent resuscitation with intravenous fluids and parenteral steroids. Hyponatraemia (about 40%) is due to hypocortisolaemia and/or inappropriate vasopressin secretion. Rare instances of resolution of hypersecretory tumours, specifically in acromegaly, have been reported.

Management

For a diagram showing an algorithm for the management of pituitary apoplexy, see Figure 3.17. The radiological investigation of choice is MRI, which is shown to confirm the diagnosis in about 88% of patients, in contrast to 21% with CT [1]. Urgent biochemical evaluation for electrolytes, renal function and liver function, together with a clotting screen, a full blood count, and a biochemical pituitary profile (random cortisol, IGF-1, growth hormone, prolactin, TSH, T4, LH, FSH, and testosterone or estradiol), along with formal visual acuity, eye movements, and visual field assessment need to be done in all patients suspected of pituitary apoplexy.

Acute severe hypocortisolaemia is present in about two-thirds of patients with pituitary apoplexy and is an important cause of mortality. Prompt corticosteroid replacement is vital along with intravenous fluids to treat haemodynamic instability following endocrine evaluation. Hydrocortisone 100–200 mg intravenous bolus followed by 50–100 mg 6-hourly by intramuscular injection is given until the acute episode resolves and is then switched to oral hydrocortisone 20–30 mg per day in three divided doses. Following stabilization of the patient, preferably in a high-dependency unit, prompt referral to a regional specialist endocrine/neurosurgical team is made.

Surgery versus conservative management

The role of acute neurosurgical intervention remains a key controversy in the management of pituitary apoplexy. The rarity of the condition renders it difficult to undertake randomized controlled trials, and the evidence for definitive management is derived largely from retrospective case series. Early surgical intervention (<8 days) was noted to have better visual and endocrine outcomes than expectant management did [1, 7]. Recent observational retrospective studies suggest no difference in visual and endocrine outcomes in both categories [5, 8]. There is general consensus for decompression in persistent, deteriorating neuro-ophthalmic signs and reduced level of consciousness.

However, there is a lack of defined criteria for assessing neuro-ophthalmic deficits with respect to favouring surgical intervention over conservative management. Conservatively managed patients need close monitoring of neurological and visual status, and surgical decompression is to be considered if neuro-ophthalmic signs persist or worsen.

Prognosis and follow-up

Overall, mortality is 1.6%– 2.0%, with a marginal tendency towards surgically treated rather than conservatively managed patients. Ocular involvement is noted in 50% of the cases, 80% of which resolve by the end of 1 year. Reduced visual acuity and ocular palsies resolve fully, and residual visual field defects are noted in about v20%– 30% [9].

The majority of the treated patients require long-term hormonal replacement, irrespective of conservative or surgical approaches: corticosteroids 60%–80%, thyroid hormone 50%–60%, testosterone 60%–80%, and desmopressin 10%–25% [1, 5, 8]. Recurrence of pituitary apoplexy is rare, but recurrence of the tumour is common and hence annual radiological surveillance is undertaken for first 5 years and 2-yearly thereafter. Patients are preferably followed up in a joint endocrine/neurosurgical clinic with input from a pituitary multidisciplinary team. Redo surgery and/or radiotherapy should be considered if recurrence is noted.

References and further reading

1. Randeva HS, Schoebel J, Byrne J, et al. Classical pituitary apoplexy: Clinical features, management and outcome. *Clin Endocrinol (Oxf)* 1999; 51: 181–8.
2. Dubuisson AS, Beckers A, and Stevenaert A. Classical pituitary tumour apoplexy: Clinical features, management and outcomes in a series of 24 patients. *Clin Neurol Neurosurg* 2007; 109: 63–70.
3. Woo HJ, Hwang JH, Hwang SK, et al. Clinical outcome of cranial neuropathy in patients with pituitary apoplexy. *J Korean Neurosurg Soc* 2010; 48: 213–8.
4. Milazzo S, Toussaint P, Proust F, et al. Ophthalmologic aspects of pituitary apoplexy. *Eur J Ophthalmol* 1996; 6: 69–73.
5. Ayuk J, McGregor EJ, Mitchell RD, et al. Acute management of pituitary apoplexy: Surgery or conservative management? *Clin Endocrinol (Oxf)* 2004; 61: 747–52.
6. Rolih CA and Ober KP Pituitary apoplexy. *Endocrinol Metab Clin North Am* 1993; 22: 291–302.
7. Bills DC, Meyer FB, Laws ER Jr, et al. A retrospective analysis of pituitary apoplexy. *Neurosurgery* 1993; 33: 602–8; discussion, 608–9.
8. Gruber A, Clayton J, Kumar S, et al. Pituitary apoplexy: Retrospective review of 30 patients: Is surgical intervention always necessary? *Br J Neurosurg* 2006; 20: 379–85.
9. Simon S, Torpy D, Brophy B, et al. Neuro-ophthalmic manifestations and outcomes of pituitary apoplexy: A life and sight-threatening emergency. *N Z Med J* 2011; 124: 52–9.
10. Rajasekaran S, Vanderpump M, Baldeweg S, et al. UK guidelines for the management of pituitary apoplexy. *Clin Endocrinol (Oxf)* 2011; 74: 9–20.

3.15 Surgical treatment

Introduction

The first description of surgery to the pituitary gland was by Canton and Paul in 1893; then, in 1906, Sir Victor Horsley describes the transcranial approach to a pituitary tumour. Craniotomy remained a dangerous procedure with a reported mortality of 50%–80%. The trans-sphenoidal technique was developed and refined between 1910 and 1950 by Hirsch and Cushing. This was further developed by Guiot in Paris and Hardy in Montreal, whilst most recently the endoscope has become increasingly used.

Surgical technique

There are two routes of access to the pituitary gland: trans-sphenoidal and transcranial. The trans-sphenoidal route is by far the most common route of access; it is unusual to approach a pituitary tumour transcranially but there are sound indications for doing so, although they are becoming less frequent as a result of the improved access and visualization that endoscopic techniques now permit. All pituitary surgery is carried out under oro-tracheal intubation general anaesthesia.

Endoscopic endonasal trans-sphenoidal surgery utilizes rigid endoscopes with 0°-, 30°-, or 45°-angled lenses. Angled endoscopes provide the ability to look laterally or into the suprasellar spaces. The use of the endoscope avoids the need to use a nasal retraction system and post-operative nasal packs. Increasingly, the use of the endoscope allows the surgeon to apply the technique to resect larger more complex lesions and to access regions of the skull base such as the anterior cranial fossa floor and the parasellar regions, which previously would have been approached from a transcranial route. The endoscopic endonasal approach also permits the construction of vascularized nasoseptal mucosal flaps, which facilitate the repair of significant dural breaches. Endoscopic surgery allows management of other pathologies such as CSF leak, meningioma, chordoma, craniopharyngioma, and cholesteatoma through an endonasal route, as opposed to transcranial route, in selected cases.

In the majority of trans-sphenoidal pituitary surgery cases, the patient is mobilized from bed on Day 1 and able to be discharged on the second post-operative day. If the procedure is more complex and requires a lumbar drain, it is common for the patient to be discharged on Post-operative day 4. The patient returns to the endocrine outpatient unit for further endocrine tests and baseline visual field tests the week following surgery.

Indications for surgery

Indications for surgery are as follows:

- pituitary apoplexy:
  - evidence of cranial nerve palsy or acute visual failure
  - surgery is aimed at reducing mass effect by removing the haemorrhage and the associated necrotic pituitary tumour

- in many cases, a more conservative approach can be pursued with correction of endocrine and electrolyte disturbances and monitoring of vision

- progressive mass effect of tumour:
  - correction or prevention of visual deficits; this generally forms the largest single group of patients requiring surgical treatment
  - prolactin-secreting tumours are better managed with dopamine agonists in the first instance; a small proportion of these patients may need surgery if there is drug intolerance or the tumour does not respond to drug treatment
  - other lesions in this category include craniopharyngioma, Rathke's cleft cyst, pituitary metastasis, intrasellar meningioma, and upper third clivus lesions such as chordoma

- normalization of pituitary hypersecretion:
  - the primary treatment of choice in acromegaly and Cushing's disease is trans-sphenoidal surgery
  - in many cases, the tumour is a microadenoma (<1 cm) and thus a surgical 'cure' is possible
  - in cases of secretory macroadenomas (which are typically somatotroph adenomas), additional medical therapy or radiotherapy may be required after surgery in order to adequately control hormone levels after surgery
  - microprolactinomas causing infertility, amenorrhoea, and altered bone density, and not suitable for medical therapy, should also be considered suitable for trans-sphenoidal surgery
  - rare tumours, include those producing TSH and LH/ FSH

- biopsy of sellar/suprasellar lesions:
  - when doubt over the origin of a pituitary lesion and further treatment hinges on histological diagnosis, a biopsy may be performed
  - one such example is the enhancing suprasellar lesion seen on MRI with a normal serum tumour and inflammatory markers

Contraindications to surgery

Contraindications to surgery are rare, and virtually never absolute. In cases where a trans-sphenoidal operation is deemed not appropriate, the pituitary tumour is best approached via a craniotomy. The contraindications are as follows:

- absolute contraindications:
  - ectatic carotid artery or unprotected aneurysm lying within or anterior to the pituitary fossa

- relative contraindications:
  - non-pneumatized sphenoid sinus; can now be overcome with neuronavigation and high-speed drill technique
  - severe systemic disease, making general anaesthesia more risky
  - disorders of coagulation

- severe acromegaly with coexistent hypertension, diabetes, cardiomyopathy, pulmonary disease, and airway obstruction; in these cases, pretreatment of the acromegaly with somatostatin analogues, and treatment of the other systemic manifestations of acromegaly, reduce perioperative complications
- florid Cushing's disease, in which case pretreatment (see Chapter 3, Section 3.7) may reduce complications
- profound hypopituitarism should also be corrected prior to proceeding with surgery; although cortisol and thyroid replacement leads to only a temporary and short delay, correction of abnormalities of sodium may take slightly longer to correct

Preoperative investigations: General principles

- Ascertain the endocrine diagnosis with full endocrine assessment.
- Ascertain the anatomical diagnosis with MRI, preferably with gadolinium enhancement (see Figures 3.18 and 3.19). Identification of microadenoma is key in terms of confirming the diagnosis, allowing a more selective adenomectomy, and can help predict the likelihood of a surgical 'cure' (see Figure 3.20). In cases of a macroadenoma, ascertain the relationship of the tumour to surrounding structures, including the optic nerves and chiasm, the cavernous sinus, and the sphenoid and clival bones, as well as the degree of suprasellar extension (see Figure 3.21). Other tumours such as craniopharyngiomas may also have specific characteristics (Figure 3.22).

Aims of treatment

The aims of treatment are as follows:
- reduction/elimination of the mass effect of the tumour, in particular compression of the optic pathways
- control of hormone overproduction by a pituitary adenoma
- minimization of the risk of tumour recurrence

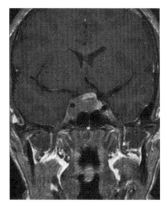

Fig 3.19 Coronal MRI demonstrating a macroadenoma which fills the pituitary fossa but extends into the right cavernous sinus.

- preservation of normal pituitary function
- obtaining tissue for a definitive histopathological diagnosis

Complications of pituitary surgery

In general, pituitary surgery is well tolerated and safe. However, all surgery has associated complications.

Intra-operative and early post-operative complications
Concerning complications which are the result of injury to structures in the path of the nasal approach or surrounding the surgical target of the pituitary gland, there is little evidence to suggest that either the endoscopic technique or the microscopic technique is superior in terms of tumour resection but the microscopic technique has been associated with a lower incidence of vascular injury. The endoscopic technique gives excellent access to the pituitary fossa and facilitates techniques such as nasoseptal flaps, extended trans-sphenoidal surgery and access to other compartments of the skull base that the microscopic technique cannot access (see Table 3.9).

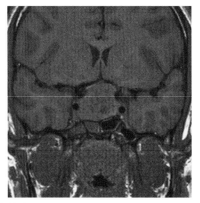

Fig 3.18 Coronal MRI demonstrating a typical pituitary macroadenoma. The tumour is seen to be invading the right cavernous sinus and distorting the optic chiasm.

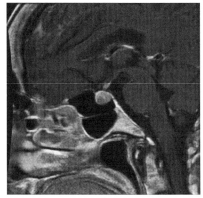

Fig 3.20 Sagittal MRI with contrast, demonstrating a low-signal microadenoma within the enhancing pituitary gland.

(a)

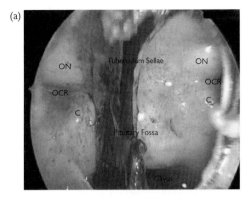

(b)

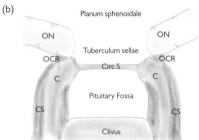

Fig 3.21 (a) Operative image and (b) schematic demonstrating the relationships between the optic nerves, the carotid arteries, and the pituitary gland within the sphenoid sinus; C, carotid artery; OCR, optico-carotid recess; ON, optic nerve.

Delayed complications
Delayed complications associated with endonasal trans-sphenoidal surgery mostly pertain to nasal complications: sinusitis, synechiae, and nasal crusting. Persistent pain is not a complication that is associated with the endoscopic endonasal trans-sphenoidal approach for pituitary surgery (see Table 3.10).

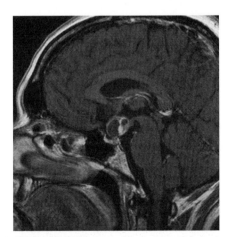

Fig 3.22 Sagittal MRI demonstrating a cystic craniopharyngioma extending into the suprasellar cistern. The tumour displaces the pituitary stalk posteriorly.

Table 3.9 Summary of the main complications of trans-sphenoidal pituitary surgery calculated from pooled data in a large meta-analysis

Complication	Microscopic (%)	Endoscopic (%)
Death	0.23	0.49
CSF leak	6.34	7.00
Meningitis	2.08	1.11
Vascular injury	0.50	1.58
Visual loss	0.60	0.72
Diabetes insipidus (temporary)	10.23	9.10
Diabetes insipidus (permanent)	4.25	2.31
Hypopituitarism	11.64	8.50
Complete resection	64.40	68.70
Nerve injury	0.53	0.28
Epistaxis	—	2.00

Data from Ammirati M, Wei L, Ciric I. Short-term outcome of endoscopic versus microscopic pituitary adenoma surgery: a systematic review and meta-analysis. *Journal of Neurology, Neurosurgery, and Psychiatry.* 2012 Dec 15.

Outcomes of trans-sphenoidal pituitary surgery
Vision
If visual function is compromised due to the tumour, it will improve following surgery in around 90% of patients, with occasional patients showing deterioration. Factors predicting a lack of visual recovery are preoperative evidence of optic atrophy; severity of visual field deficit; poor visual acuity; duration of symptoms; and increasing age of the patient.

Visual outcome in pituitary apoplexy
Visual acuity improves in almost all patients, especially if surgery is carried out within a week of the onset of symptoms. In surgically decompressed cases, visual field and ocular paresis will improve in 95% and 100%, respectively, with approximately 50% and 65%, respectively, achieving full recovery.

Headache
Headache is a symptom of both macro- and microadenomas, with an up to 90% chance of resolution or improvement following surgery for a non-functioning macroadenoma or Rathke's cleft cyst, but only in half of patients with hypersecreting adenomas.

Table 3.10 Delayed complications of endonasal trans-sphenoidal surgery

Complication	Rate (%)
Acute sinusitis	2.2
Chronic sinusitis	1.5
Synechiae	8.8
Prolonged nasal crusting	10.4
Nasal septum deviation	3.7

Data from Kilty SJ, McLaughlin N, Bojanowski MW, Lavigne F. Extracranial Complications of endoscopic transsphenoidal sellar surgery. *Journal of Otolaryngology-Head & Neck Surgery.* 2010 Jun; Volume 39, Issue 3, pp. 309–314.

Cushing's disease

Trans-sphenoidal surgery is accepted as the first line treatment in Cushing's disease, but often no tumour is seen radiologically. Remission rates are highly variable, but in the best centres a 'cure' rate of 75%–85% should be attainable, although for revision surgery this falls to 50%. Features predicting long-term remission include positive histology for tumour obtained, microadenoma, no cavernous sinus invasion, and undetectable early postoperative cortisol levels. Tumour recurrence remains a problem even many years after surgery, with long-term remission figures falling to 60%–70%; for this reason, follow-up is required for many years. Adjuvant radiotherapy, given as either conventional or stereotactic radiotherapy, results in remission in 60%–83% of patients at the expense of other endocrinopathies, but there can be a delay in normalization of cortisol levels of 3 years or more.

Prolactinoma

In prolactinoma, patients will require surgery in 15%–30% of cases, with a remission rate of up to 90% with surgery. Recurrence rates are estimated at 17%–50% for microprolactinomas, and 20%–80% for macroprolactinomas, despite initially successful surgery. Radiotherapy may be required for patients with residual tumours, and has been shown to be effective in many cases. This is dependent upon residual tumour volume and serum prolactin levels.

Primary radiotherapy using stereotactic techniques has been advocated for microadenomas by some workers: this can result in a cure in up to 50%, and an improvement in serum prolactin in 30%.

Acromegaly

A number of tumour features are known to predict the likelihood of remission, including tumour size, preoperative IGF-1 level, and invasion into the cavernous sinus, which is graded using the Knosp system. Once the tumour has invaded past the lateral border of the carotid artery, the chance of surgical remission falls to 30%. If the tumour is confined to the sella or is medial to the midpoint of the carotid artery, then there is an 80% chance of surgical remission. Macroadenomas treated with surgery have a cure rate of around 50%. Patients who continue to have active acromegaly despite surgery can be managed with somatostatin analogues, and subsequent radiotherapy if medical management fails to reduce the growth hormone to a level not associated with increased morbidity and mortality.

Non-functioning macroadenoma

The primary indication for surgery in this group of tumours is to decompress the optic apparatus and facilitate recovery of visual function. Surgical decompression facilitates an improvement in visual function in 80%–90% of patients. Improvement in endocrine function has been described following surgery; however, the outcome studies have shown conflicting results. Surgery is not currently indicated in an attempt to improve pituitary function. The chances of complete surgical resection are predicted by the size of the tumour and the degree of invasion into the cavernous sinus, with complete surgical resection achievable in approximately 60% of all non-functioning macroadenomas. Recurrence rates

in patients in whom radiotherapy is withheld can be as high as 50% at 10 years, whilst radiotherapy can reduce this rate to 2%–3%. Due to the complications of radiotherapy, many physicians will now defer radiotherapy if a post-operative MRI scan demonstrates a complete tumour resection. Continued surveillance with MRI can pick up early tumour recurrence before symptoms arise, and based on this either further surgery and/or radiotherapy can be given. Up to 95% of patients retain normal pituitary function after trans-sphenoidal surgery. However, only 10%–16% of patients with established endocrine deficiencies preoperatively have partial or complete restoration of pituitary function after surgery.

Advances in pituitary surgery

Advances in pituitary surgery include the following:
- endoscopic pituitary surgery
- image-guided neurosurgery, otherwise called neuronavigation:
  - has become widespread in neurosurgical practice
  - allows identification and confirmation of anatomy during pituitary surgery and is useful in revision surgery
- intra-operative MRI:
  - increasingly, higher-field scanners are being used to improve the resolution of the images obtained during surgery
  - whilst this development has much promise, as yet only modest improvements in tumour removal have been obtained in experienced surgical hands
- stereotactic radiotherapy techniques, such as gamma knife

Further reading

Ammirati M, Wei L, and Ciric I. Short-term outcome of endoscopic versus microscopic pituitary adenoma surgery: A systematic review and meta-analysis. *J Neurol Neurosurg Psychiatry* 2013; 84: 843–9.

Dekkers OM, Pereira AM, and Romijn JA. Treatment and follow-up of clinically nonfunctioning pituitary macroadenomas. *J Clin Endocrinol Metab* 2008; 93: 3717–26.

Ebersold MJ, Quast LM, Laws ER Jr, et al. Long-term results in transsphenoidal removal of nonfunctioning pituitary adenomas. *J Neurosurg* 1986; 64: 713–19.

Giustina A, Chanson P, Bronstein MD, et al. A consensus on criteria for cure of acromegaly. *J Clin Endocrinol Metab* 2010; 95: 3141–8.

Jane JA Jr, Starke RM, Elzoghby MA, et al. Endoscopic transsphenoidal surgery for acromegaly: Remission using modern criteria, complications, and predictors of outcome. *J Clin Endocrinol Metab* 201; 96: 2732–40.

Kilty SJ, McLaughlin N, Bojanowski MW, et al. Extracranial complications of endoscopic transsphenoidal sellar surgery. *J Otolaryngol Head Neck Surg* 2010; 39: 309–14.

Losa M, Mortini P, Barzaghi R, et al. Early results of surgery in patients with nonfunctioning pituitary adenoma and analysis of the risk of tumor recurrence. *J Neurosurg* 2008; 108: 525–32.

Turner HE, Adams CB, and Wass JA. Trans-sphenoidal surgery for microprolactinoma: An acceptable alternative to dopamine agonists? *Eur J Endocrinol* 1999; 140: 43–7.

Turner HE, Stratton IM, Byrne JV, et al. Audit of selected patients with nonfunctioning pituitary adenomas treated without irradiation: A follow-up study. *Clin Endocrinol (Oxf)* 1999; 51: 281–4.

3.16 Pituitary radiotherapy

Introduction

External beam radiotherapy remains an important component of the management of patients with pituitary adenoma and is effective at controlling the growth of progressive tumours and normalizing elevated hormone levels in secreting tumours.

Traditionally, all patients with residual non-functioning pituitary adenoma received post-operative radiotherapy, as the majority of tumours were considered to progress. This approach resulted in a tumour-control rate in excess of 90% at 10 years, and 85%–92% in 20 years. With improvement in surgical techniques and routine use of MRI, radiotherapy is reserved for progressive tumours based on the perceived threat to function, particularly vision.

The factors associated with a higher risk of recurrences following surgery include younger age, the presence of extrasellar extension, cavernous sinus invasion, and presence of macroscopic residual disease. In functioning pituitary adenoma, immunohistochemical staining for p16, retinoblastoma protein, cyclin D1, MIB-1 antigen, and p53 are risk factors for recurrence. However, currently it is not clear whether the presence of these risk factors warrants immediate post-operative radiotherapy.

Indications for post-operative radiotherapy

Radiotherapy in the management of non-functioning pituitary adenoma

The majority of patients with residual non-functioning pituitary adenoma are managed by surveillance with regular, usually annual MRI imaging. Radiotherapy is considered at the time of progressive disease, which in more than half of the progressors occurs beyond 10 years after surgery. Immediate post-operative radiotherapy may be appropriate if there is considerable residual tumour or progression is likely to be of threat to vision or other functional deficit, and the tumour is not amenable to surgery.

Functioning pituitary adenoma
Acromegaly

Surgery remains the first-line treatment, followed by somatostatin analogues in patients who fail to achieve a biochemical remission after surgery or those in whom tumours recur. Subsequent management is not fully defined. The options are continuing systemic therapy with somatostatin analogues or radiotherapy to allow for their withdrawal. Radiotherapy is also recommended in case of poor tolerance and resistance to somatostatin analogues and in patients with progressive tumour mass.

Cushing's disease

Patients with persistent Cushing's disease after surgery are considered for early radiotherapy. It is also recommended as prevention of Nelson's syndrome after adrenalectomy.

Prolactinoma

As medical management is highly effective in prolactinoma, radiotherapy is reserved for the few patients who fail medical management or recur after successful primary treatment.

Principles of radiotherapy

Radiotherapy is aimed at delivering a uniform radiation dose to the residual pituitary adenoma, with least possible radiation to surrounding structures, to minimize the risk of side effects. High precision is achieved by increased accuracy of tumour delineation using high-quality MRI, by improved immobilization during planning and treatment, and by intensive quality assurance using on-treatment imaging.

The traditional view of the biological effect of radiation demonstrated in malignant disease is the inhibition of proliferation. At a molecular level, radiation causes DNA damage, which leads to cell attrition either as programmed cell death (apoptosis) or reproductive cell death. The time taken to manifest the therapeutic effect of radiotherapy at cellular and tissue levels depends on the rate of proliferation of the tumour. The theory is that, as pituitary adenomas are slow-growing, the effect may take months or years to manifest. In practice, appreciable tumour shrinkage, if any, is uncommon.

Conventional radiotherapy is given at a dose of 1.8 Gy per fraction once a day 5 days per week, up to a total dose of 45–50 Gy. This dose is below the tolerance of the brain and, therefore, the risk of structural damage is <1%.

Radiotherapy can also be given as a single large fraction (a technique called radiosurgery; see 'Radiosurgery') or as few large fractions (hypofractionated radiotherapy).

Radiotherapy techniques

Conformal radiotherapy

Three-dimensional conformal radiotherapy is the standard of care. The steps in radiotherapy planning include non-invasive immobilization, usually in a lightweight thermoplastic mask; high-quality MRI co-registered with 3D CT; and computerized 3D planning using multiple shaped fixed or rotating beams. During the delivery of treatment, accuracy is ensured with on-treatment imaging.

Stereotactic radiotherapy

The term 'stereotactic' was introduced at the time of employment of surgical stereotactic techniques for tumour localization and this was linked with immobilization in a fixed or relocatable non-invasive stereotactic frame. Stereotactic radiotherapy given in a single fraction was termed 'radiosurgery' and that given in multiple fractions as 'fractionated stereotactic radiotherapy'. With modern imaging and image co-registration, there is no longer the need to use stereotactic fiducial systems and frames and, in its fractionated form, the technique is appropriately named 'high-precision conformal radiotherapy'.

Radiosurgery

Radiosurgery can be delivered using a multiheaded cobalt unit known as the gamma knife, with a conventional linear accelerator (linac) capable of high-precision treatment or with a robotic, mounted small-size linac (cyberknife). The gamma-knife technique results in an inhomogeneous dose to the tumour, and small areas of high radiation dose (hotspots).

Efficacy and toxicity of radiotherapy

Conventional radiotherapy

The actuarial local control expressed as progression-free survival is following conventional radiotherapy in the region of 90% at 10 years and 70%–85% at 20 years.

In patients with acromegaly, the time to achieve a 50% reduction in growth hormone is in the region of 2 years. Higher levels of growth hormone and IGF-I take longer time to normalize, and normalization is achieved in 30%–50% at 5–10 years and in 75% at 15 years. The reported 8-year hormonal control rate in Cushing's disease is 74% with conventional radiotherapy; in some series, all patients achieve normalization, albeit this may occur slowly. The median time for achieving normal cortisol level is approximately 2 years.

Radiation side effects
The commonest late toxicity of radiotherapy is hypopituitarism, occurring in 30%–60% of patients 10 years after treatment. Growth hormone secretion is most frequently affected, followed by gonadotrophin, adrenocorticotrophic-hormone, and TSH secretions. The incidence of radiation optic neuropathy with conventional radiotherapy is 1%–3%, and the risk of brain necrosis is 0.2%.

Patients with pituitary adenoma treated with surgery and radiotherapy have an increased incidence of cerebrovascular accidents attributable to multiple factors, including metabolic and cardiovascular consequences of hypopituitarism, the effects of individual endocrine syndrome, surgical intervention, and the vascular effects of radiotherapy. Currently, it remains unclear whether patients with pituitary adenoma per se have an increased incidence of stroke compared with general population.

Radiotherapy is associated with a small risk of developing a second radiation-induced brain tumour, and the reported cumulative incidence is 2% at 20 years. It also remains unclear whether patients with pituitary adenoma have a predisposition to brain tumours.

Fractionated stereotactic radiotherapy and high-precision conformal radiotherapy
The results of fractionated stereotactic radiotherapy and high-precision 3D conformal radiotherapy are similar to those obtained via conventional radiotherapy, with a 5-year actuarial progression-free survival in the region of 97%. The rate of normalization of elevated hormones in secreting tumours is the same as that achieved with conventional radiotherapy. The incidence of hypopituitarism for high-precision radiotherapy compared to conventional radiotherapy is reported to be lower. The incidence of other late effects is likely to be similar to that for conventional radiotherapy, although long-term studies on this are not available.

Gamma-knife radiosurgery
There are no reliable 10-year actuarial progression-free survival data for radiosurgery. A systematic review reported 5-year progression-free survival of 94% for non-functioning pituitary adenoma. As the tumours treated with gamma-knife stereotactic radiosurgery are smaller than those treated with fractionated radiotherapy, the efficacy of gamma-knife stereotactic radiosurgery in terms of tumour control is considered worse than that achieved with fractionated treatment.

In patients with acromegaly, the time to achieve a 50% reduction in growth hormone levels is no faster and remains in the region of 2 years. Fifty-one per cent of patients with Cushing's disease achieve biochemical remission at a median of 2 years, with no evidence of faster decline in hormone levels than obtained with fractionated treatment.

Long-term tumour control in secreting tumours treated with gamma-knife stereotactic radiosurgery is not clear and, in some instances, inferior. The most common complication after stereotactic radiosurgery remains hypopituitarism, and the reported incidence ranges from 0% to 66%. Optic nerve and cranial complications are reported in up to 11% of cases. There are no long-term studies to reliably assess the risk of cerebrovascular events and incidence of second tumours.

Factors affecting the efficacy of radiation
With conventional radiotherapy, there is no advantage in terms of local control for radiotherapy doses higher than 45–50 Gy. A higher-margin dose in gamma-knife stereotactic radiotherapy does not improve the chance or speed of achieving endocrine remission and control of tumour growth.

Pre-radiotherapy hormonal levels correlate with the time taken for normalization. Both with conventional radiotherapy and with stereotactic radiosurgery, with lower initial hormonal levels, normalization occur earlier and this is seen both following fractionated radiotherapy and single-fraction stereotactic radiosurgery.

There is no evidence to suggest that the use of systemic treatment to reduce hormone secretion alters the efficacy of radiotherapy.

Whilst radiosurgery has been used for small residual tumours away from critical structures, the evidence suggests that it is less effective in terms of tumour control, with no advantage in achieving a faster hormonal normalization and is associated with greater risk if involving critical structures. There is currently little justification for its use, particularly as small non-functioning residual tumours may not require any further treatment. Fractionated high-precision conformal radiotherapy remains the standard of care in patients with pituitary adenoma requiring pituitary radiotherapy.

Further reading
Ajithkumar T and Brada M. 'Pituitary radiotherapy', in Wass JAH, Stewart PM, Amiel SA, et al. *Oxford Textbook of Endocrinology and Diabetes*, 2011. Oxford University Press, pp. 176–86.

Reddy R, Cudlip S, Byrne JV, et al. Can we ever stop imaging in surgically treated and radiotherapy-naive patients with non-functioning pituitary adenoma? *Eur J Endocrinol* 2011; 165: 739–44.

Sattler MG, Vroomen PC, Sluiter WJ, et al. Incidence, causative mechanisms, and anatomic localization of stroke in pituitary adenoma patients treated with postoperative radiation therapy versus surgery alone. *Int J Radiat Oncol Biol Phys* 2013; 87: 53–9.

3.17 Parasellar pituitary conditions

Introduction

Approximately 10% of all neurological tumours arise from the pituitary region, an anatomically complex area composed of various structures [1]. Although the sellar region has specific landmarks, the parasellar region is not clearly delineated and includes structures such as brain tissue, meninges, visual pathways, and other cranial nerves, along with major blood vessels, the hypothalamo-pituitary system, and bony structures (Figure 3.23). A diversity of clinical symptoms/signs can develop from a number of lesions originating from these structures according to their location, size, and growth potential, as well as the subsequent damage to adjacent vital organs [2].

Although pituitary adenomas are the most common lesions extending to the parasellar region, two large studies have revealed that a different aetiology, mainly other tumours and cystic lesions, is found in 8%–9% of cases [2, 3] (Table 3.11). As cystic parasellar lesions, mainly Rathke's cysts and craniopharyngiomas, are covered elsewhere (see Section 3.13), this section will mainly concentrate on other parasellar tumours and parasellar inflammatory/infective conditions. Due to the relative rarity of parasellar lesions, there are currently no specific guidelines regarding their diagnosis and management. Most recommendations are based on previously published extensive personal experience and availability of local expertise, as there are many similarities in clinical presentation, diagnosis, and overall management of different parasellar lesions.

Clinical presentation

Non-pituitary adenomatous parasellar lesions present mainly with symptoms attributed to deficient pituitary function or mass effect due to compression of nearby vital structures (Figure 3.23). Involvement of the hypothalamo-pituitary system causes partial or complete hormonal deficiencies, hyperprolactinaemia due to stalk compression, and, rarely, hypothalamic syndrome [2, 3] (Table 3.12). In contrast to pituitary adenomas, diabetes insipidus can occur in the absence of the identification of a specific aetiology [3]. Symptoms of mass effect are not unique to specific parasellar lesions and can vary according to the location, size, and extension of the lesion. Headache is a common presenting symptom that develops either as a result of increased intracranial pressure, distortion of the diaphragm, or irritation of the parasellar dura [1, 2]. Visual complaints (visual loss or constriction of visual fields) are also common due to the proximity of parasellar lesions to the optic nerves, the optic chiasm, and the optic tracts [1, 2]. In addition, abnormalities of the cranial nerves traversing through the cavernous sinus can be found in up to 20% [1].

Diagnostic approach: Therapeutic considerations

Radiological imaging currently represents the best means to establish the diagnosis of parasellar lesion; both thin-sectioned CT and MRI facilitate the anatomical delineation of parasellar lesions, although distinguishing between different aetiologies is not always possible. MRI is the modality of choice, providing multiplanar high-contrast images, whereas CT has a complementary role in identifying bony destruction. Histological confirmation is usually obtained through surgical specimens commonly performed for debulking purposes [4]; open skull biopsy or image-guided needle biopsy are used when surgery is precluded. Surgery is performed either by craniotomy or trans-sphenoidally; for massive lesions, a two-stage procedure may be required. Trans-sphenoidal surgery can also be used for midline lesions without significant lateral extension [4]. Radiotherapy, conventional or

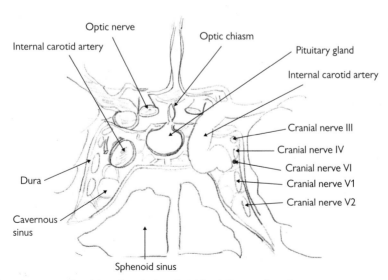

Fig 3.23 Schematic representation of the various structures that delineate the parasellar region.

Optic nerve

Internal carotid artery

Optic chiasm

Pituitary gland

Internal carotid artery

Cranial nerve III

Cranial nerve IV

Cranial nerve VI

Cranial nerve V1

Cranial nerve V2

Dura

Cavernous sinus

Sphenoid sinus

Table 3.11 Lesions of different aetiologies that can present as parasellar pathology; tumours are graded according to WHO classification

Malignant lesions* (tumours)	Low-grade malignant lesions (tumours/cysts)	Benign lesions (tumours/cysts)	Inflammatory/ infective lesions	Other pathology
Gliomas (WHO I-IV)	Craniopharyngiomas	Meningiomas (WHO I)	Pituitary abscess	Vascular lesions:
	Chrordomas		TB	• aneurysms
Germ-cell tumours	Chordosarcomas	Rathke's cysts	Hypophysitis	• cavernous sinus thrombosis
Primary lymphomas	Hemangiopericytomas	Hamartomas	Sarcoidosis	Miscellaneous:
Metastases	Langerhans cell	Paragangliomas	Wegener's granulomatosis	• suprasellar arachnoiditis
Ependymoblastomas	histiocytosis**	Lipomas		
		Neurinomas	Granulomatous diseases	
		Schwannomas		
		Parasellar granular cell tumours		
		Arachnoid cysts		

Based on data from 199 patients with parasellar lesions; the most common pathology was Rathke's cyst (28%–42%) followed by craniopharyngiomas (12%–14%), benign tumours (10% meningiomas), and malignant tumours (12%–25% metastases). Inflammatory lesions were the least common pathologies, being encountered in 5%–9%; the most common was lymphocytic hypophysitis.

*The malignant potential of a parasellar tumour is defined according to the WHO classification and relies on histological criteria as follows: WHO Grade I (tumours of low proliferative potential and the possibility of being cured following surgical resection), WHO Grade II (infiltrative tumours with low mitotic activity that can recur and progress to higher grade malignancies), WHO Grade III (tumours with histological evidence of malignancy), and WHO Grade IV (mitotically active tumours with rapid evolution of disease).

** Langerhans cell histiocytosis is currently considered a neoplastic disease.

Data from Freda, P.U. et al. (1996) Unusual causes of sellar/parasellar masses in a large transsphenoidal surgical series. *Journal of Clinical Endocrinoly and Metabolism*, 81, 3455–3459; Valassi, E. et al. (2010) Clinical features of nonpituitary sellar lesions in a large surgical series. *Clinical Endocrinology.* (Oxf) 73, 798–807.

stereotactic, can be used either as primary treatment or to prevent further tumour growth or recurrence, albeit with potential adverse effects to nearby tissues and the hypothalamo-pituitary system [1]. Chemotherapy is used for responsive malignant tumours, such as germ-cell tumours, and when other modalities have failed, whereas

Table 3.12 Clinical features and endocrine abnormalities in patients with parasellar lesions other than pituitary adenomas, derived from the two largest studies published[2, 3] (n = 199)

Presenting symptoms	%
Headache	34
Dizziness	8
Hearing loss	4
Cognitive complaints	3
Blurred vision/visual loss	22
Cranial nerve palsy	9
Visual field impairment	51
Fatigue/weakness	10
Galactorrhoea	13
Anterior pituitary hormonal deficit	37
Hyperprolactinaemia	28
Diabetes insipidus	6

Data from Freda, PU et al. (1996) Unusual causes of sellar/parasellar masses in a large transsphenoidal surgical series. *Journal of Clinical Endocrinology and Metabolism*, 81, 3455–3459; Valassi E et al. (2010) Clinical features of nonpituitary sellar lesions in a large surgical series. *Clinical Endocrinology.* (Oxf) 73, 798–807.

disease-directed treatment is currently limited. Optimum hormonal replacement therapy is offered in all patients with hypothalamo-pituitary involvement.

The two largest series published to date have shown that the majority of parasellar lesions are cystic (mainly Rathke's cysts and craniopharyngiomas), followed by benign tumours and malignant tumours, and a minority are of inflammatory/infective origin [2, 3] (Table 3.11).

Parasellar tumours

Chordomas and chondrosarcomas

These cartilaginous tumours account for approximately 10% of parasellar lesions and originate from the primitive notochord in the skull base [1]. Both tumours are positive for S-100 protein but, unlike chordomas, chondrosarcomas are negative for cytokeratin markers [1]. Chordomas are slow-growing, mainly arising from the clivus in the midline, and can reach a considerable size, extending along the entire skull base and causing destruction of the sella (Figure 3.24 and 3.25), with relatively limited pituitary hormonal deficiency [2]; some may progress to malignant transformation. Chondrosarcomas arise off the midline at the suture line and are considered malignant tumours (WHO Grades II–III, Table 3.11), although they rarely metastasize outside the skull. Both tumours cause bone destruction and variable degrees of calcification on CT, show neural and vascular involvement on MRI, and are mostly hypovascular. The molecular basis of chordoma, involves the expression of brachyury, a transcription factor whose gene is located on 6q27 and influences cell differentiation, as well as other candidates, is under investigation [5]. Surgery is the treatment of choice, although radical excision is rarely achieved due to bone invasiveness. Other forms of therapy such as radiotherapy, and chemotherapy for recurrent lesions,

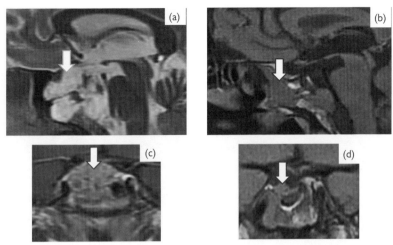

Fig 3.24 MRI of a patient with a chordoma, preoperatively (a, c) and post-operatively (b, d).

have not produced consistent results, but radiosurgery can be helpful.

Meningiomas

Meningiomas (WHO Grade I, Table 3.11) are a diverse group of tumours that arise from the arachnoid 'cap' cells of the arachnoid villi in the meninges and account for one-third of primary brain tumours. Approximately 10%–15% of these tumours arise from the parasellar region (Figure 3.26 and Figure 3.27), rarely occupying the whole sella, and mimicking pituitary adenomas; in contrast to other parasellar lesions, they can encase and cause narrowing of blood vessels. They usually present with visual problems and occasionally endocrine dysfunction with mildly raised prolactin levels; symptoms may worsen during pregnancy. Although malignant transformation may occur, it is relatively rare. It has recently been shown that *NF2* gene alterations are found in 50% of patients. Other rare mutations include those in *TRAF7*, *KLF4*, *AKT1*, and *SMO* in benign meningiomas, whilst progression to a clinically aggressive meningioma is linked to inactivation of *CDKN2A* and *CDKN2B*, as well as involving other signalling-molecule genes [6]. Imaging characteristics allow preoperative diagnosis,

as lesions arise from the dura, having a broad attachment and a linear, enhancing dural tail extending along the dura away from the lesion, with occasional areas of calcification, and with occasional bone thickening and sclerosis [1, 7]. Surgical excision is the treatment of choice (Figure 3.28 Figure 3.29) but recurrences are seen in 7%–20% of Grade I lesions, and in 39%–40% of atypical lesions defined as WHO Grade II and characterized by aggressive histologic features (increased mitotic activity, nuclear atypia, and necroses) [1, 6]. A combination of surgery and radiotherapy is used for recurrent lesions. Although prognosis is overall good, it is worse in patients with incomplete resections and potentially malignant histology.

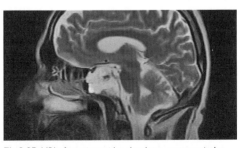

Fig 3.25 MRI of a patient with a chordoma, preoperatively (sagittal T2 image).

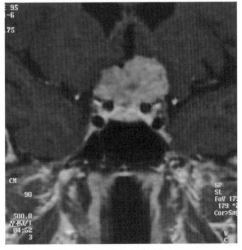

Fig 3.26 MRI of a patient with a suprasellar meningioma, preoperatively (coronal T1 post-contrast image).

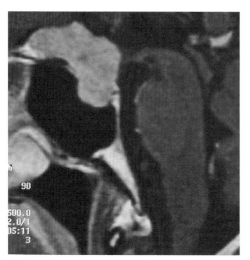

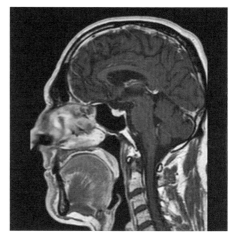

Fig 3.29 MRI of a patient with a meningioma, post-operatively (completely resected: sagittal T1 post-contrast image).

Fig 3.27 MRI of a patient with a suprasellar meningioma, preoperatively (sagittal T1 image).

Gliomas

Gliomas arise in the hypothalamus, the optic nerve, and the optic tract, with the main histopathologic subtype being pilocytic astrocytoma, a low-grade malignant lesion occasionally associated with neurofibromatosis type 1. Five glioma molecular groups have been defined with the use of three alterations: mutations in the *TERT* promoter, mutations in *IDH*, and co-deletion of chromosome arms 1p and 19q (1p/19q co-deletion). Different ages at onset, overall survival, and associations with germ-line variants have been recognized, implying distinct mechanisms of pathogenesis [8]. The remainder hypothalamic/optic chiasm lesions are diffuse *astrocytomas* that can progress to an anaplastic astrocytoma or glioblastoma [1, 2]. They present as large suprasellar masses

with homogenous enhancement and occasional necrosis [7]. Approximately 10% can occur in the brainstem, extending to the parasellar region, and, in 30%, can become purely malignant. The median survival of low-grade gliomas is 7.3 years, whereas that of high-grade tumours is 11.2 months. For aggressive subtypes, temozolomide, an oral derivative of dacarbazine, has achieved 51% clinical and 31% radiological improvement [1].

Ependymomas are tumours arising from the radial glia and are composed of cells that form gland-like structures directed towards the vessel walls. They usually arise from the floor of the fourth ventricle, causing symptoms due to hydrocephalus; few cases involving the sella/parasellar region have been described up to now. The majority are low-grade tumours, although some can become anaplastic, resembling medulloblastomas and necessitating treatment with radiotherapy and chemotherapy [9].

Other tumours and malignant lesions

Hamartomas are congenital heterotopias of neuronal origin located within the tuber cinereum, mostly affecting children and causing precocious puberty, epilepsy (classical gelastic or laughing) and symptoms of mass effects [1]. Hypothalamic hamartomas are found in 33% of patients with true precocious puberty [1, 10] and contain GnRH neurons. MRI is the primary diagnostic imaging modality utilized, with the lesion being isointense to grey matter and non-enhancing with contrast [1, 2]. Hormonal therapy with GnRH agonists along with the surgery are used to treat precocious puberty and also the epileptic component. Surgery is offered when medical therapy fails or in cases of rapid tumour growth, and the outcome is better when the seizure focus has been found by EEG to originate in or near the mass. Other less common benign lesions are *dermoids, paragangliomas, lipomas,* and *neurinomas*.

Germinomatous germ-cell tumours and non-germinomatous germ-cell tumours (choriocarcinoma, teratoma, embryonal sinus tumours, and embryonal carcinoma) are mostly found in the first two decades of life and can be diagnosed by histology or on the basis

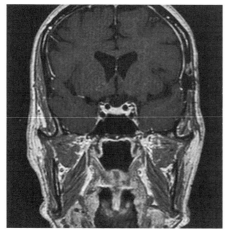

Fig 3.28 MRI of a patient with a meningioma, post-operatively (coronal T1 post-contrast image).

of elevation of specific tumour markers (beta-human chorionic gonadotrophin, alpha-fetoprotein) or typical CT/MRI findings [1]. When a preoperative diagnosis is available, surgical exploration is not necessary, as these tumours are sensitive to platinum-based chemotherapy and radiotherapy [1]. Other malignant tumours of the parasellar region are lymphomas and metastases from other primary tumours [1]; metastases are usually found in the presence of an obvious primary such as a lung or breast carcinoma.

Parasellar inflammatory/infective conditions

A number of infectious and granulomatous processes can present as parasellar lesions. *Abscesses* of the region can develop from direct extension from the sphenoid sinus, the cavernous sinus, CSF, or secondary bacteraemia; a mass may also develop due to secondary infections [2]. An abscess should always be suspected in the setting of a mass in a patient with meningitis. *TB* can produce basilar meningitis and findings suggestive of a parasellar lesion with or without hypopituitarism, usually accompanied by evidence of TB elsewhere [2, 11] (Figure 3.30). Only a few cases have been described, most of which were documented after surgery, characterized by an encapsulated lesion with a contrast-enhancing wall [7]. A high clinical suspicion, timely intervention, and anti-tuberculous therapy may help in alleviation of commonly encountered symptoms such as visual disturbances, headache, and hormonal abnormality [11]. Fungal infection of the pituitary can also occur and include aspergillosis and coccidioidomycosis [11].

Sarcoidosis

Sarcoidosis can present with a mass, diabetes insipidus, cranial neuropathy, and varying degrees of hypopituitarism [2]. Sarcoidosis of the hypothalamo-pituitary system is usually accompanied by other evidence of neurosarcoidosis and/or systemic sarcoidosis although this is not always the case. In a recent review of 24 patients, 22 had pituitary dysfunction, the most common being gonadotrophin deficiency, and 12 had diabetes insipidus; MRI abnormalities were found in all 24 patients [12] (Figure 3.31). Although all patients were treated with prednisolone, only two recovered their pituitary function after 4 years [11].

Granulomatous hypophysitis

Granulomatous hypophysitis is extremely rare and is mostly found in middle-aged women; diabetes insipidus is not a common finding [11]. Other rare granulomatous diseases that may present as parasellar lesions include *Wegener's granulomatosis, Takayasu's disease, Crohn's disease,* and *Cogan's syndrome* [11] (rare inflammatory condition of ears and eyes).

Lymphocytic hypophysitis

Lymphocytic hypophysitis is the result of an autoimmune process with focal or diffuse inflammatory infiltration and varying degrees of pituitary gland destruction [11, 13]. A presumptive clinical diagnosis can be made based on a history of gestational or post-partum hypopituitarism, a contrast-enhancing mass with imaging features characteristic of lymphocytic hypophysitis, a pattern of pituitary hormone deficiency with early loss of ACTH and TSH, relatively rapid development of hypopituitarism, and a degree of pituitary failure disproportionate to the size of the mass. Symptoms resulting from partial hypopituitarism or pan-hypopituitarism occur in approximately 80% of cases, and multiple deficiencies are found in approximately 75% of cases [7, 11, 13]. Although appropriate therapy remains controversial, glucocorticoids and azathioprine in 44 treated patients reduced the mass in 84% of them and improved anterior and posterior pituitary function in 45% and 41%, respectively [13] (Figure 3.32).

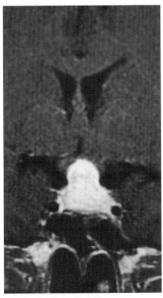

Fig 3.30 MRI of a patient with TB (coronal T1 post-contrast image).

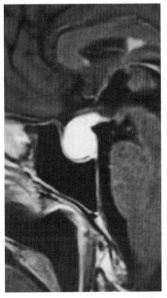

Fig 3.31 MRI of a patient with neurosarcoidosis (sagittal T1 post-contrast image).

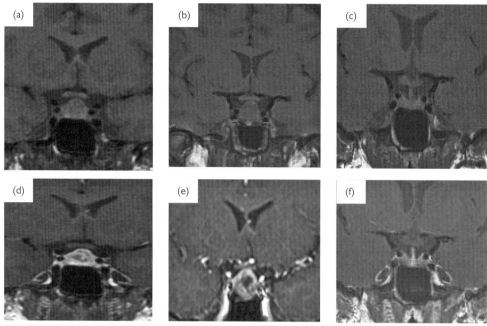

Fig 3.32 A 38-year-old woman with amenorrhoea, bilateral galactorrhoea, temporal headaches, polyuria, and polydipsia. (a, d) MRI before any treatment, showing the increased size of the pituitary gland. (b, e) MRI one month later, after carbergoline 0.25 mg twice weekly, showing no change in size. (c, f) MRI taken after cabergoline discontinuation and following treatment with prednisolone 40 mg/day reveals a substantial improvement. Imaging findings that have been reported to be useful for distinguishing pituitary adenoma from lymphocytic hypophysitis include a pre-contrast homogeneous signal intensity; an intact sella floor; suprasellar extension; a loss of high signal intensity in the posterior pituitary on T1-weighed MRI; stalk thickening; mass symmetry; homogeneous enhancement; and an adjacent dural enhancement (dural tail).

Immunomodulatory hypophysitis

Novel immunotherapies are increasingly used in advanced malignancies, and hypophysitis is now being recognized after such immunomodulatory therapies such as CTLA-4 blockers (e.g. ipilimumab) and less commonly anti-PD1 immunotherapy (pembrolizumab). This is characterized by pituitary enlargement (usually mild), associated with pan-/isolated pituitary hormone deficiencies, especially ACTH deficiency. Management is appropriate with anterior pituitary hormone replacement. Many endocrinologists would advise continuing immunomodulatory treatment with adequate hormone replacement therapy. Follow-up and repeat MRI is essential, as there may be recovery of pituitary function (rarely for ACTH). However, if there are symptoms of an enlarging pituitary mass, immunomodulatory drugs may be omitted, and high-dose glucocorticoids administered, tapered over several weeks.

Langerhans cell histiocytosis

Langerhans cell histiocytosis is characterized by the clonal proliferation of specific dendritic cells and, in this manner, represents a neoplastic rather than an inflammatory disease; this view was reinforced further by the finding of specific *BRAF* mutations in a significant number of such patients [1]. Langerhans cell histiocytosis is relatively rare, showing a predilection for the hypothalamo-pituitary region and leading to diabetes insipidus and anterior pituitary involvement in up to 20% [14]. Making an early and

accurate diagnosis is important, as mortality can be up to 20% in patients with multisystem disease, and 50% of patients develop permanent sequelae. MRI is the best means of assessing hypothalamo-pituitary involvement and, in addition to a mass lesion, characteristic thickening of the pituitary stalk is also found [14]. Vinblastine together with steroids is the most frequently used therapy but the purine analogue cladribine has shown efficacy in patients with recurrent and disseminated disease [1]. However, molecular targeted therapies based on specific genetic aberrations are evolving as promising therapies.

IgG4-related hypophysitis

IgG4-related hypophysitis has been recently recognized in the context of IgG4-related disease, a systemic fibro-inflammatory disorder characterized by extensive infiltration of IgG4-positive plasma cells leading to storiform fibrosis into various organs with or without elevated serum IgG4 levels [15]. In order to design a proper follow-up plan, Leporati suggested some diagnostic criteria for IgG4-related hypophysitis; these include a wide spectrum of endocrine manifestations ranging from normal pituitary function to panhypopituitarism [16]. These criteria are (1) histopathological presence of mononuclear infiltrate of the pituitary gland, rich in lymphocytes and plasma cells, with more than 10 IgG4-positive cells per high-power field, (2) a sellar mass and/or thickened pituitary stalk on pituitary MRI when pituitary histopathology is unavailable, (3) biopsy-proven IgG4-positive lesions in other organs, (4) increased serum IgG4 level (>140 mg/dL), and (5) shrinkage of the pituitary mass and symptom improvement with steroids. The diagnosis is regarded as possible when only the first criterion is met, when both the second and the third criteria are met or when the second criterion together with both the fourth and the fifth criteria are present. Although histological confirmation remains the gold standard, the diagnosis was made with biopsy-proven pituitary involvement in only six cases. Despite the central role of IgG4-positive plasma cells in the pathogenesis of this disease, the trigger for IgG4 overproduction has not been clearly defined.

References and further reading

1. Kaltsas GA, Evanson J, Chrisoulidou A, et al. The diagnosis and management of parasellar tumours of the pituitary. *Endocr Relat Cancer* 2008; 15: 885–903.

2. Freda PU, Wardlaw SL, and Post KD. Unusual causes of sellar/parasellar masses in a large transsphenoidal surgical series. *J Clin Endocrinol Metab* 1996; 81: 3455–9.

3. Valassi E, Biller BM, Klibanski A, et al. Clinical features of nonpituitary sellar lesions in a large surgical series. *Clin Endocrinol (Oxf)* 2010; 73, 798–807.

4. Jagannathan J, Kanter AS, Sheehan JP, et al. Benign brain tumors: Sellar/parasellar tumors. *Neurol Clin* 2007; 25, 1231–49, xi.

5. Scheil-Bertram S, Kappler R, Von Baer A, et al. Molecular profiling of chordoma. *Int J Oncol* 2014; 44: 1041–55.

6. Mawrin C, Chung C, and Preusser M. Biology and clinical management challenges in meningioma. *Am Soc Clin Oncol Educ Book* 2015; 35: e106–15.

7. Famini P, Maya MM, and Melmed S. Pituitary magnetic resonance imaging for sellar and parasellar masses: Ten-year experience in 2598 patients. *J Clin Endocrinol Metab* 2011; 96: 1633–41.

8. Eckel-Passow JE, Lachance DH, Molinaro AM, et al. Glioma groups based on 1p/19q, IDH, and TERT promoter mutations in tumors. *N Engl J Med* 2015; 372: 2499–508.

9. Belcher R, Chahal HS, Evanson J, et al. Recurrent pituitary ependymoma: A complex clinical problem. *Pituitary* 2010; 13: 176–82.

10. Judge DM, Kulin HE, Page R, et al. Hypothalamic hamartoma: A source of luteinizing-hormone-releasing factor in precocious puberty. *N Engl J Med* 1977; 296: 7–10.

11. Carpinteri R, Patelli I, Casanueva FF, et al. Pituitary tumours: Inflammatory and granulomatous expansive lesions of the pituitary. *Best Pract Res Clin Endocrinol Metab* 2009; 23: 639–50.

12. Langrand C, Bihan H, Raverot G, et al. Hypothalamo-pituitary sarcoidosis: A multicenter study of 24 patients. *QJM* 2012; 105: 981–95.

13. Lupi I, Manetti L, Raffaelli V, et al. Diagnosis and treatment of autoimmune hypophysitis: A short review. *J Endocrinol Invest* 2011; 34: e245–52.

14. Makras P, Samara C, Antoniou M, et al. Evolving radiological features of hypothalamo-pituitary lesions in adult patients with Langerhans cell histiocytosis (LCH). *Neuroradiology* 2006; 48: 37–44.

15. Stone JH, Zen Y, and Deshpande V. IgG4-related disease. *N Engl J Med* 2012; 366: 539–51.

16. Batista RL, Borba CG, Machado VC, et al. IgG4-related hypophysitis: A new addition to the hypophysitis spectrum. *J Clin Endocrinol Metab* 2011; 96: 1971–80.

Chapter 4

Posterior pituitary gland

Chapter contents

4.1 Diabetes insipidus

Definition and presentation
Diabetes insipidus is the excess production of dilute urine:
- adults: >40 mL/kg in 24 hours (>~3 L in 24 hours)
- children: >100 mL/kg in 24 hours

Patients present with polyuria, nocturia, and polydipsia.

Epidemiology
Diabetes insipidus is rare. The prevalence of adult hypothalamic/cranial diabetes insipidus (see 'Classification of diabetes insipidus') is 1/25,000. There is no gender bias.

Pathophysiology
Vasopressin and renal water loss
Renal water loss is regulated by the action of the nine-amino acid peptide hormone vasopressin on the cells lining the collecting duct of distal nephron. Vasopressin is synthesized within magnocellular neurons in the hypothalamus, and is stored within nerve terminals in the posterior pituitary gland. Vasopressin acts on type 2 vasopressin receptors on the cell surfaces of collecting duct cells to increase the production of the vasopressin-dependent water channel aquaporin 2, which facilitates the reabsorption of water from the tubular lumen along a concentration gradient. There is a linear relationship between plasma vasopressin and plasma osmolality. Vasopressin synthesis and release is linked to plasma osmolality through osmosensitive sensory neurones within the circumventricular region; these neurons are close to but separate from the magnocellular neurones making vasopressin. Thirst regulation is in parallel with that of vasopressin, using pathways that are closely linked but functionally discrete.

Classification of diabetes insipidus
Three types of diabetes insipidus are recognized (see Table 4.1).

Aetiology
Hypothalamic/cranial diabetes insipidus secondary to pituitary adenoma is unusual (see Table 4.2). The presence of diabetes insipidus together with a pituitary mass should raise suspicion of an alternative diagnosis. The most common cause of nephrogenic diabetes insipidus is a tubulopathy secondary to metabolic toxicity or drug effects (see Box 4.1)

Inherited forms of diabetes insipidus are rare and normally present in childhood. Loss-of-function mutations have been implicated in the following genes:
- AVP (encodes vasopressin): autosomal dominant hypothalamic/cranial diabetes insipidus

- AVPR2 (encodes the vasopressin type 2 receptor): X-linked nephrogenic diabetes insipidus
- AQP2 (encodes aquaporin 2): autosomal recessive and autosomal dominant nephrogenic diabetes insipidus

Primary polydipsia is associated with excessive drinking and causes low plasma vasopressin and low plasma and urinary osmolality, and may also produce nephrogenic diabetes insipidus due to impaired concentrating ability due to solute washout.

Investigations
The aims of investigations in diabetes insipidus are to confirm the diagnosis and to establish the aetiology. Serum potassium, calcium, and blood glucose should always be checked first, and a baseline serum and urinary osmolality; in severe cases, this may be sufficient to make a diagnosis of diabetes insipidus.

The water deprivation test
The water deprivation test is an indirect test of the functional integrity of the vasopressin axis. Vasopressin-dependent urine concentrating capacity is evaluated during the osmotic stress of dehydration produced through prolonged (8 hours) water deprivation. Following confirmation of the diagnosis in the initial phase, renal sensitivity to exogenous vasopressin analogue (desmopressin) subsequently classifies the problem as hypothalamic/cranial diabetes insipidus or nephrogenic diabetes insipidus. Indeterminate results are not uncommon, especially in mild forms of diabetes insipidus. See Table 4.3.

Hypothalamic/cranial diabetes insipidus can be confirmed and classified by direct measurement of vasopressin or co-peptin (a peptide fragment of the large vasopressin precursor, produced in equimolar amounts to vasopressin) during graded osmotic stress, produced by infusion of hypertonic saline (0.05 mL/kg per minute

Table 4.2 Aetiology of hypothalamic/cranial diabetes insipidus

Primary	
Genetic	Autosomal dominant
	Autosomal recessive
	Wolfram syndrome (also called DIDMOAD (for diabetes insipidus, diabetes mellitus, optic atrophy, and deafness))
Developmental	Septo-optic dysplasia
Idiopathic	—
Acquired	
Trauma	Head injury
	Post neuro- or pituitary surgery
Tumour	Craniopharyngioma
	Germinoma
	Metastasis
Inflammatory	Neurohypophysitis
	Sarcoidosis
	Histiocytosis

Table 4.1 Classification of diabetes insipidus

Classification	Pathophysiology
Hypothalamic/cranial diabetes insipidus	Relative or absolute lack of vasopressin
Nephrogenic diabetes insipidus	Partial or complete resistance to renal effects of vasopressin
Dipsogenic diabetes insipidus	Primary polydipsia leading to appropriate diuresis

Data from Ball, SG, 2010, Hyponatraemia, *Journal of the Royal College of Physicians of Edinburgh*, 40, pp. 240–245.

Box 4.1 Aetiology of nephrogenic diabetes insipidus

Inherited
Mutations in *AVPR2* (X-linked recessive)
   Mutations in *AQP2* (both autosomal recessive and autosomal dominant)

Acquired
Drugs:
- lithium
- demeclocycline

Metabolic:
- hypercalcaemia
- hypokalaemia
- hyperglycaemia

Chronic renal disease
Post-obstructive uropathy

Data from Ball SG., 'The neurohypophysis', edited by Wass AH, Stewart PM, Amiel SA. et al., *Oxford Textbook of Endocrinology and Diabetes*, Second Edition, 2011.

Table 4.3 Water deprivation test: Interpretation of urine osmolality results

Diagnosis	Urine osmolality post water deprivation (mOsm/kg)	Urine osmolality post desmopressin (mOsm/kg)
Hypothalamic/ cranial diabetes insipidus	<300	>750
Nephrogenic diabetes insipidus	<300	<300
Dipsogenic diabetes insipidus	>750	>750

Data from Ball SG., 'The neurohypophysis', edited by Wass AH, Stewart PM, Amiel SA. et al., *Oxford Textbook of Endocrinology and Diabetes*, Second Edition, 2011.

of 5% hypertonic saline for 2 hours). In hypothalamic/ cranial diabetes insipidus, vasopressin or co-peptin levels are undetectable or show a subnormal response. In contrast, they are inappropriately raised in nephrogenic diabetes insipidus.

A therapeutic trial of exogenous desmopressin is an alternative diagnostic test when water deprivation proves non-diagnostic. Plasma sodium levels need to be closely monitored. Patients with primary polydipsia show progressive dilutional hyponatraemia; those with nephrogenic diabetes insipidus remain unaffected, whilst hypothalamic diabetes insipidus patients report symptomatic improvement but remain normonatraemic.

Pituitary function tests and MRI
All patients with hypothalamic/cranial diabetes insipidus should undergo pituitary function tests to exclude a wider problem with endocrine function. Importantly, an underlying tumour should be excluded with neuroimaging of the pituitary and parapituitary region.

Management
Treatment of patients with hypothalamic/cranial diabetes insipidus associated with significant symptoms is with the synthetic vasopressin analogue desmopressin.

This can be administered through parenteral, nasal, oral, or buccal routes in divided doses. The aim of therapy should be to reduce symptoms without producing hyponatraemia. Usual starting doses (100–200 μg orally or 5–10 μg through the nasal route) are prescribed at bedtime. The usual maintenance dose by mouth is 100–600 μg daily in divided doses or 10–40 μg daily in divided doses via the nasal route. Plasma sodium levels should be monitored 1–2 days after initiation of therapy. Once the patient has been established on a stable dose, 6-monthly or annual monitoring is recommended.

Nephrogenic diabetes insipidus is managed by removing the cause, where possible. For persistent severe symptoms, high-dose parenteral desmopressin can be used. This rarely reduces urine volume by more than 50%. Thiazide diuretics and NSAIDs can be considered as an alternative, alone or in combination.

Dipsogenic diabetes insipidus is managed by reducing fluid intake.

Further reading

Ball S. Diabetes insipidus. *Medicine* 2013; 41: 519–21.

Ball SG, Baylis PH. Normal and abnormal physiology of the hypothalamus-posterior pituitary, 2013. Available at http://web.archive.org/web/20130706083414/http://www.endotext.org/neuroendo/neuroendo2/neuroendoframe2.htm (accessed 23 Dec 2017).

Babey M, Kopp P, and Robertson GL. Familial forms of diabetes insipidus: Clinical and molecular characteristics. *Nat Rev Endocrinol* 2011; 7: 701–14.

Hannon MJ, Sherlock M, and Thompson CJ. 2011. Pituitary dysfunction following traumatic brain injury or subarachnoid haemorrhage. *Best Pract Res Clin Endocrinol Metab* 2011; 25: 783–98.

4.2 Hyponatraemia

Definition and classification

Hyponatraemia is defined as a plasma sodium below the lower limit of the normal reference range, commonly less than 134 mmol/L. Hyponatraemia can be classified on the basis of biochemistry, rate of development, or scale of symptoms. See Tables 4.4–4.6.

Epidemiology and clinical presentation

Hyponatraemia is the commonest electrolyte disturbance in hospital-based patients, seen in some 15%–20% of non-selected emergency admissions. It is associated with increased morbidity and mortality across a range of clinical conditions. Whether this relationship is causal or a reflection of two independent variables, linked through disease severity, remains unclear.

Symptoms directly associated with hyponatraemia are largely neurological. As plasma osmolality falls in line with falling sodium concentration, CNS neuronal function is disturbed and cerebral oedema develops within a constrained skull compartment, raising intracranial pressure. Over time, efflux of cellular inorganic and organic osmolytes into the extracellular fluid within the CNS serves to reduce osmotic and volume shifts. However, this CNS adaptation requires time and has a limited capacity.

The degree of biochemical hyponatraemia and severity of symptoms may be discordant. This reflects a number of factors:

- the rate of development of hyponatraemia: a rapid fall in plasma sodium does not allow adequate time for CNS adaptation and is more likely to result in cerebral oedema and neurological dysfunction
- the intrinsic CNS-adaptive capacity to osmolar stress/ hyponatraemia
- the range and degree of co-morbidity

Aetiology and approach to differential diagnosis

Hypotonic hyponatraemia

The plasma sodium concentration reflects the balance of plasma water and sodium content. Whilst hyponatraemia can be the result of imbalance in either component, in most circumstances it is the result of excess in plasma water. This may be the result of excess water intake (voluntary or iatrogenic) or reduced renal free water clearance. Importantly, the latter can be produced through a primary problem with excess or inappropriate production of the anti-diuretic hormone vasopressin or, secondarily, baro-stimulated production of vasopressin triggered by reduced effective circulating volume. This latter mechanism underpins the hyponatraemia seen in hypovolaemia. Thus, even in the context of a primary renal sodium leak (from diuretics or glucocorticoid deficiency), baro-stimulated vasopressin production contributes to the clinical picture.

Non-hypotonic hyponatraemia

Non-hypotonic hyponatraemia describes a range of clinical situations in which the measured plasma sodium concentration is low, but the plasma is not hypotonic. Pseudohyponatraemia is a laboratory artefact produced when high levels of lipids or protein effectively reduce the volume of the aqueous phase of plasma. Direct potentiometric methods (such as those used in blood gas analysers) produce a true measurement of sodium concentration in this context.

Other causes of non-hypotonic hyponatraemia include hyperglycaemia and elevated urea (see Table 4.7).

An approach to the investigation and differential diagnosis of hyponatraemia is outlined in Figure 4.1.

Syndrome of inappropriate anti-diuretic hormone secretion

See also Section 4.3. Syndrome of inappropriate anti-diuretic hormone secretion (often abbreviated as SIADH) is a common cause of hyponatraemia. Diagnostic criteria and the range of more common clinical presentations are outlined in Box 4.2 and Table 4.8.

Management of hyponatraemia

Patients with moderate or severe symptoms require close clinical and biochemical monitoring in a high-dependency setting (see Figure 4.2). Hypertonic saline

Table 4.4 Classification based on sodium

Classification	Plasma sodium (mmoles/L)
Mild	130–4
Moderate	125–9
Profound	<125

Table 4.5 Classification based on rate of development

Classification	Timescale
Acute	<48 hours (evidenced)
Chronic	>48 hours (evidenced)
Uncertain	Absence of biochemical or clinical evidence to support classification

Table 4.6 Classification based on symptoms

Classification	Symptoms
Moderate	Nausea
	Confusion
	Headache
Severe	Vomiting
	Cardiorespiratory distress
	Seizures
	Glasgow Coma Scale <8

Table 4.7 Non-hypotonic hyponatraemia

Classification	Examples
Pseudohyponatraemia	Dyslipidaemia
	Hyperproteinaemia
Isotonic hyponatraemia	Hyperglycaemia
	Irrigant fluids used in urological surgery
Hypertonic hyponatraemia	Elevated urea (renal impairment)

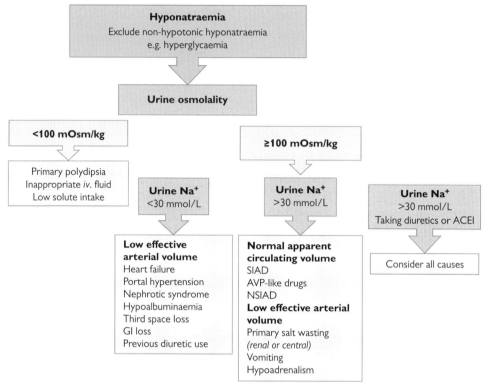

Fig 4.1 Diagnostic algorithm for patients presenting with hyponotraemia; ACEI, angiotensin-converting-enzyme inhibitor; AVP, arginine vasopressin; GI, gastrointestinal; *iv.*, intravenous; NSIAD, nephrogenic syndrome of inappropriate anti-diuresis; SIAD, syndrome of inappropriate anti-diuresis.
Reproduced from *Endocrine Connections*, 5, 5, Ball S, Barth J, Levy M. and the Society for Endocrinology Clinical Committee, Society For Endocrinology Endocrine Emergency Guidance: Emergency management of severe symptomatic hyponatraemia in adult patients. © 2016 The authors.

may be indicated and can be administered as intravenous 150 mL boluses of 3% NaCl or equivalent, aiming to raise the serum sodium by 5 mmol/L within 1–2 hours and reduce cerebral oedema. The rise in serum sodium must be limited to 8–10 mmol/L in the first 24 hours, and no more than 8 mmol/L per 24 hours thereafter. Overcorrection should be actively managed and requires expert advice.

Patients presenting with mild symptoms should undergo investigations to establish aetiology, followed by consideration of cause-specific treatment. Intervention aimed solely at raising the serum sodium may not be recommended. If treatment is initiated, the principles of rate of change of sodium remain common: limit to 8 mmol/L in the first 24 hours and no more than 8 mmol/L per 24 hours thereafter. It is important to note that autocorrection of hyponatreamia after fluid overload or adrenal crisis may exceed this rate if not managed appropriately.

Table 4.8 Common causes of syndrome of inappropriate anti-diuretic hormone secretion

Cause	Examples
Drugs	Anticonvulsants
	Antidepressants
Chest disease	Infection
	Tumour
	COPD
CNS disease	Tumour
	Infection
	Haemorrhage

Data from Ball SG., 'The neurohypophysis', edited by Wass AH, Stewart PM, Amiel SA. et al., *Oxford Textbook of Endocrinology and Diabetes*, Second Edition, 2011.

Box 4.2 Diagnostic criteria for syndrome of inappropriate anti-diuretic hormone secretion

Hyposmolality (<275 mOsm/kg)
Urine osmolality >100 mOsm/kg
Urine sodium concentration >30 mmol/L
Normal adrenal and thyroid function
Absence of oedema

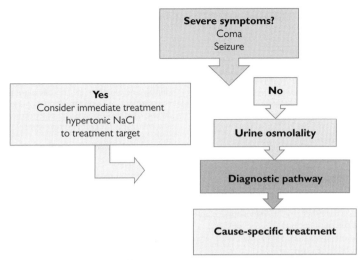

Fig 4.2 Management algorithm for the treatment of hyponotraemia.
Reproduced from *Endocrine Connections*, 5, 5, Ball S, Barth J, Levy M. and the Society for Endocrinology Clinical Committee, Society For Endocrinology Endocrine Emergency Guidance: Emergency management of severe symptomatic hyponatraemia in adult patients. © 2016 The authors.

Table 4.9 Cause-specific treatment of hyponatraemia

Cause	Recommended treatment
Reduced effective arterial volume (hypovolaemia)	Intravenous 0.9% saline or balanced crystalloid solution 0.5–1.0 mL/kg per hour
Syndrome of inappropriate anti-diuretic hormone secretion	Fluid restriction 750–1 L per 24 hours or fluid restriction with increased solute intake

In patients with hyponatraemia due to reduced effective arterial volume and who are haemodynamically unstable, the need for rapid resuscitation overrides the risk of over-rapid correction of serum sodium. In other patients with reduced effective arterial volume (e.g. heart failure or cirrhosis with portal hypertension) clinicians must balance the benefits and risks of withdrawing the causative drug or recommending fluid resuscitation, based on the overall clinical picture (see Table 4.9). In some patients with syndrome of inappropriate anti-diuretic hormone secretion, treatment of the underlying infection or withdrawal of the causative drug (where possible) may resolve the problem. Others may require a more active approach.

Further reading

Grant P, Ayuk J, Bouloux PM, et al. The diagnosis and management of inpatient hyponatraemia and SIADH. *Eur J Clin Invest* 2015; 45: 888–94.

Mohmand HK, Issa D, Ahmad Z, et al. Hypertonic saline for hyponatraemia: Risk of inadvertent overcorrection. *Clin J Am Soc Nephrol* 2007; 2: 1110–17.

Spasovski G, Vanholder R, Allolio B, et al. Clinical practice guideline on diagnosis and treatment of hyponatraemia. *Eur J Endocrinol* 2014; 170: G1–47; erratum, *Eur J Endocrinol* 2014; 171: X1.

Sterns RH, Nigwekar SU, and Hix JK. The treatment of hyponatremia. *Semin Nephrol* 2009; 29: 282–99.

Upadhyay A, Jaber BL, and Madias NE. Epidemiology of hyponatraemia. *Semin Nephrol* 2009; 29: 227–38.

Verbalis JG, Goldsmith SR, Greenberg A, et al. Hyponatraemia treatment guidelines 2007: Expert panel recommendations. *Am J Med* 2007; 120: S1–21.

4.3 Syndrome of inappropriate anti-diuretic hormone secretion

Introduction

Syndrome of inappropriate anti-diuretic hormone secretion (commonly abbreviated as SIADH) is a common cause of hyponatraemia resulting from failure to suppress vasopressin release in face of low plasma osmolality. The ensuing obligate antidiuresis together with persisting fluid intake produces dilutional hyponatraemia.

Causes

For causes of syndrome of inappropriate anti-diuretic hormone secretion, see Box 4.3.

Clinical assessment and diagnosis

Most patients with syndrome of inappropriate anti-diuretic hormone secretion are clinically euvolemic.

Diagnostic criteria for syndrome of inappropriate anti-diuretic hormone secretion include:

- hyponatraemia with low serum osmolality
- urine osmolality >100 mOsm/kg
- urine sodium > 30 mmol/L

Box 4.3 Causes of syndrome of inappropriate anti-diuretic hormone secretion

Drugs:
- antidepressants (tricyclics, SSRIs)
- dopamine agonists
- anticonvulsants (carbamazepine, phenytoin, sodium valproate)
- opiates

CNS disturbances:
- stroke
- haemorrhage
- infection
- trauma
- Guillain–Barré syndrome

Malignancies:
- small-cell lung cancer
- pancreatic cancer
- duodenal cancer
- head and neck cancers

Surgery:
- abdominal surgery
- thoracic surgery
- pituitary surgery

Pulmonary disease:
- pneumonia
- pneumothorax

Idiopathic disease

Metabolic porphyrias

- absence of hypovolaemic and hypervolemic states
- normal renal and adrenal function

Management

Identify and treat the cause where possible. Principles of management of hyponatraemia in general apply for syndrome of inappropriate anti-diuretic hormone secretion. The following interventions are specific for managing this syndrome:

- fluid restriction
- demeclocycline
- vasopressin receptor anatgonists

Fluid restriction

The mainstay of treatment when the clinical condition is stable is restriction of fluid intake to 0.5–1.0 L/day. The sodium level rise may be very gradual (over days) or partial. Restriction must include all fluids.

Demeclocycline

Demeclocycline improves hyponatraemia by producing a form of diabetes insipidus and thus increasing renal water loss. It is used at a dose of 600–1200 mg/day.

Vasopressin receptor antagonists

Vasopressin receptor antagonists (known as vaptans) increase renal water excretion without affecting electrolyte excretion and are tolerated well. They are available in both oral (tolvaptan) and intravenous forms (conivaptan) and can be used for asymptomatic or mildly symptomatic patients. Vaptans increase thirst, thus limiting the plasma sodium rise; hence, they should not be used as a first-line treatment option. While there is evidence of efficacy, a precise role for vaptans in the management of SIADH remains to be defined. They may have a role in specific situations: such as where hyponatraemia due to SIADH limits treatment with chemotherapy agents that require high, nephro-protective fluid loads. They should not be used in SIADH producing severe hyponatraemia, where they are associated with an increased risk of over-correction.

Further reading

Schrier RW, Gross P, Gheorghiade M, et al. Tolvaptan, a selective oral vasopressin V2-receptor antagonist, for hyponatraemia. N Engl J Med 2006; 355:2099.

Berl T, Quittnat-Pelletier F, Verbalis JG et al. Oral Tolvaptan is safe and effective in chronic hyponatraemia. J Am Soc Nephrol 2010; 21: 705–712, 2010. doi: 10.1681/ASN.2009080857

Review and analysis of differing regulatory indications and expert panel guidelines for the treatment of hyponatremia. Verbalis JG, Grossman A, Höybye C, Runkle I. Curr Med Res Opin. 2014 Jul;30(7):1201–7.

Diagnosis, evaluation, and treatment of hyponatremia: expert panel recommendations. Verbalis JG, Goldsmith SR, Greenberg A, Korzelius C, Schrier RW, Sterns RH, Thompson CJ. Am J Med. 2013 Oct;126(10 Suppl 1):S1–42.

4.4 Disorders of hypothalamic dysfunction

Introduction

Hypothalamic tumours arise in the midline distally from the third ventricle:

- craniopharyngiomas; arise from remnants of Rathke's pouch (see also Chapter 3, Section 3.13)
- epidermoid cysts
- ependymomas
- geminomas; atypical teratomas, pinealomas
- infundibulomas
- hamartomas
- gangliocytomas

Other hypothalamic disorders include (see also Chapter 3, Section 3.17):

- granulomatous disorders
- histiocytosis X (Langerhans cell histiocytosis)
- sarcoidosis
- basilar meningitis
- disorders caused by radiation therapy (for nasopharyngeal or intracranial tumours)
- disorders caused by trauma (head injury)

Syndromes associated with hypothalamic dysfunction include:

- septo-optic dysplasia
- Laurence–Moon–Biedl syndrome
- Prader–Willi syndrome

Manifestations of hypothalamic dysfunction

Endocrine manifestations of hypothalamic disorders include:

- hypopituitarism caused by deficiencies of hypothalamic trophic factors
- isolated deficiencies:
  - isolated GHRH deficiency
  - deregulation of GnRH: precocious puberty, delayed puberty, amenorrhea
  - deregulation of prolactin secretion
  - deregulation of adrenocorticotrophic hormone secretion
  - vasopressin deficiency (diabetes insipidus)

Neurologic manifestations of hypothalamic disorders include:

- disorders of food intake:
  - hyperphagia
  - anorexia
- disorders of fluid intake:
  - adipsia
  - psychogenic water drinking
  - chronic hyponatraemia
  - essential hyponatraemia
- disorders of temperature regulation:
  - hyperthermia
  - hypothermia
  - temperature fluctuations
- disorders of mood and memory:
  - rage
  - apathy
  - memory loss
  - excessive sexuality
  - hallucinations
- disorders of sleep and consciousness:
  - disturbed sleep
  - somnolence
  - coma
- disorders of autonomic regulation:
  - sweating
  - cardiac arrhythmias
- periodicity syndromes:
  - epilepsy

Therapies of hypothalamic dysfunction

Endocrine management of hypothalamic disorders is as follows:

- replacement therapy of hormonal deficiencies (see Chapter 3, Section 3.4)
- surgical removal of tumours (see Chapter 3, Section 3.15)
- radiotherapy

Further reading

Giustina A and Braunstein GD. 'Hypothalamic syndromes', in Jameson JL and L. De Groot L, eds, *Endocrinology: Adult and Pediatric* (7th edition), 2016. Elsevier, 174–87.

Chapter 5

Pineal gland

Chapter contents

5.1 Melatonin and pineal tumours

Pineal structure

The pineal gland (epiphysis cerebri; see Figure 5.1) is a small (100–150 mg in humans), unpaired central structure. The mammalian pineal is a secretory organ, whereas in fish and amphibians it is directly photoreceptive (the 'third eye') and, in reptiles and birds, it has a mixed photoreceptor and secretory function. The main mammalian cell type is the pinealocyte, considered to have evolved from photoreceptor cells. In humans and some other species, the gland usually shows a degree of calcification after puberty and, as a result, it has been used as a neuroradiological marker. Calcification may not be associated with a decline in metabolic activity, except that activity declines in general with ageing. The main secretory product is the hormone melatonin (N-acetyl-5-methoxytryptamine). Pinealectomy removes detectable circulating melatonin, and the gland is the main source of this hormone in the periphery. Other sites of synthesis exist, notably the retina, but without contributing to blood levels. The principal innervation is sympathetic, arising from the superior cervical ganglion.

Melatonin

Melatonin is synthesized within the pinealocytes, from tryptophan. The activity of serotonin-N-acetyltransferase (also known as arylalkylamine N-acetyl transferase) is usually rate limiting in melatonin production. The pineal secretes melatonin with a marked circadian rhythm, normally at night, in all species, whether they are nocturnal or diurnal. The rhythm is endogenous, being generated by interacting networks of clock genes in the suprachiasmatic nuclei, which is the major central rhythm-generating system or 'clock' in mammals (the pineal itself is a self-sustaining 'clock' in some, if not all, lower vertebrates). The rhythm is synchronized to the 24-hour day, primarily by the alternation of light and darkness. Ocular light of suitable intensity, timing, and spectral composition will shift the rhythm to earlier or later times and suppress melatonin secretion at night. A novel non-image-forming

photoreceptor system with a maximum response to blue light (~480 nm) is implicated, with a pivotal role for a new opsin: melanopsin. In humans and rodents, melatonin is metabolized to 6-sulphatoxymelatonin, primarily within the liver, by 6-hydroxylation, followed by sulphate conjugation. Both melatonin and 6-sulphatoxymelatonin in body fluids are used extensively to determine the state of the circadian system and are used as rhythm markers for research and the diagnosis of circadian rhythm disorders. Melatonin declines with age, and there is evidence for slightly higher levels and earlier timing in women.

Pineal function: Seasonal rhythms

The primary function of the pineal gland is to convey information concerning daylength for the organization of daylength-dependent functions in photoperiodic species (see Figure 5.1). These include reproduction, appetite, bodyweight, and timing of pubertal development. An intact innervated pineal gland is essential for the perception of photoperiod change and it is the secretion profile of melatonin, long in short days and short in long days, which provides seasonal timing information. The interpretation of the signal, as with daylength, depends on the physiology (e.g. long- or short-day breeder) of the species in question. In sheep, melatonin can time the whole seasonal cycle, at least of reproduction, acting as a seasonal *zeitgeber* for a presumed endogenous circannual rhythm. The circannual rhythm of prolactin secretion (synchronized by photoperiod) is dependent on the melatonin signal acting via the pars tuberalis.

Reproduction in domestic ruminants and the winter coat of animals such as mink, arctic foxes, and cashmere goats has commercial significance, and can be manipulated by photoperiod and melatonin administration. Implanted melatonin induces short-day effects, and a number of commercial preparations of melatonin have been developed to this end.

Human reproduction

In humans, usually seasonal changes are modest, given the lighting environment of our 24-hour society. Later melatonin secretion in winter than in summer is sometimes reported, and changes in melatonin duration are seen if long or short completely dark nights are artificially imposed for several weeks. Initial interest in the human pineal gland as an endocrine organ was concerned with a possible inhibitory effect on pubertal development. There is no consensus as to whether or not it influences the timing of human puberty. However, in general, evidence suggests that exogenous melatonin is inhibitory to human reproductive function at high levels. Attempts to develop melatonin as a contraceptive pill in combination with a synthetic progestin 'minipill' have not been successful. In the author's opinion, low, timed doses of melatonin used to reinforce circadian organization are likely to improve fertility in humans. Acute oral doses of melatonin stimulate prolactin secretion. Acute effects on other pituitary hormones are somewhat inconsistent, although a relationship between melatonin and vasopressin may exist.

Pineal function: Circadian rhythms

The pineal appears to have a quite modest physiological role in the circadian system of humans. This is essentially

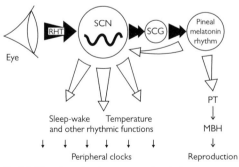

Fig 5.1 The relationships between circadian rhythm generation, pineal melatonin, and downstream effects; MBH, medio-basal hypothalamus; PT, pars tuberalis; RHT, retino-hypothalamic tract; SCG, superior cervical ganglion; SCN, suprachiasmatic nucleus.
Reproduced with permission from Arendt J. Melatonin and the Mammalian Pineal Gland. Chapman Hall © 1995.

the reinforcement of 'night-time physiology'. The evidence mostly concerns lowered core body temperature and enhanced sleep quality and timing. We can sleep without melatonin—although we sleep better when the timing of the melatonin rhythm (as a surrogate for the whole circadian system) is in the correct phase with respect to desired sleep time. Melatonin is also implicated in circadian thermoregulation, blood pressure regulation, and the immune system.

Therapeutic use of melatonin

The actions of exogenous melatonin within the circadian system have received a great deal of attention in the last two decades. Timed melatonin is able to shift all measured circadian rhythms and induce sleepiness during the daytime, initially observed in the 1970s and 1980s. These effects are time and dose dependent but sufficiently robust to show that melatonin has clear therapeutic effects in circadian rhythm disorders. It is recommended for use in jet lag, delayed sleep phase disorder, free-running sleep disorder of the blind, shift work, and irregular sleep–wake cycles in neurological disabilities. Its use in the blind is of particular interest: light is the main factor maintaining circadian rhythms on a 24-hour cycle. With no light perception at all, the rhythms of many blind people drift away from 24 hours, a condition akin to a lifetime's intermittent jet lag. Melatonin, in low (0.5–5.0 mg usually) daily doses, correctly timed, can replace the light–dark time cue and restore good quality sleep and daytime alertness. It has proved useful for sleep problems in children with neurological/developmental disorders and is registered for use in insomnia of the over-50s in Europe. Several commercial preparations and analogues now exist, as well as a slow-release preparation, and can be prescribed for various sleep problems in Europe and a number of other countries. Recently the European Food Safety Authority has concluded that, to reduce sleep onset latency, 1 mg of melatonin should be consumed close to bedtime. The target population is the general population. However, the dose and timing may well be inappropriate for many people. In the US, melatonin is freely available as a nutritional supplement. However, correct timing of treatment, especially in jet lag and shift work, is not simple. Melatonin has largely been developed as a 'sleep hormone' but this is a misnomer; it is a 'darkness hormone'.

In adult mammals, melatonin serves to modulate circadian phase and strengthen coupling. Since optimal circadian phase is important to health, this is clearly a very significant function. In fetal and neonatal mammals, it may help to programme the circadian system and to determine the timing of developmental stages, especially puberty.

Metabolism

Pinealectomy in rats was reported to induce insulin resistance many years ago. Only recently it was found that *MTNR1B*, the gene that encodes melatonin receptor 1B, possessed variants that were closely associated with fasting glucose, reduced beta-cell function, and an increased risk of type 2 diabetes in humans. The risk genotype predicts the future development of type 2 diabetes. Given that this is an ever-increasing problem in the developed world, the scope for therapeutic interventions is clearly to be explored. Circadian control of metabolism means that there is much scope for the effects of melatonin in this area.

Cancer

The WHO recently concluded in a monograph (produced by the International Agency for Research on Cancer) summarized in *The Lancet* that there was good evidence for the beneficial effects of melatonin on cancer in animals, but insufficient as yet for efficacy in humans. For many years now, a hypothesis concerning the increased incidence of breast cancer in the developed world related this to the suppression of melatonin by artificial light at night, notably during shift work. It is more likely due to the entire circadian system being disrupted.

Pineal tumours

Tumours of the pineal region in children are frequently associated with abnormal pubertal development. In precocious puberty it was thought that the capacity of the pineal to inhibit sexual development was impaired. Much evidence now suggests that precocity is due to the production of beta-hCG by germ-cell tumours of the pineal. Delayed puberty has also been associated with pineal tumours. Pineal tumours are heterogeneous and may arise from germ cells (teratomas, germinomas, choriocarcinomas, endodermal sinus tumours, mixed germ-cell tumours), pineal parenchymal cells (pineoblastoma and pineocytoma), and the supporting stroma (gliomas). All are rare (less than 1% of intracranial space-occupying lesions) and tend to occur below 20 years of age with the exception of parenchymal cell tumours, which occur equally in adults and children. Germinomas respond well to radiation therapy, although many now use chemotherapy followed by cerebrospinal radiotherapy, whereas primary surgery is more frequently the treatment of choice in other types. Tumour markers in CSF, alpha-fetoprotein and beta-hCG, together with CSF cytology and imaging (CT or MRI), aid in the differential diagnosis. The most common symptoms are secondary to hydrocephalus (headache, vomiting, and drowsiness) together with the triad of visual problems, diabetes insipidus, and reproductive abnormalities. Germinomas and teratomas occur predominantly in males. Precocious puberty is more commonly associated with teratoma. As beta-hCG is identical to beta-LH, pubertal development can be directly attributed to ectopic beta-hCG production in many cases. Moreover, the predominance in boys may be explained on the basis that LH alone can stimulate testosterone production, whereas in girls both LH and FSH are required for ovarian follicular development and oestrogen production. A 5-year survival of 62% was quoted for germinomas, but only 14% for other malignant tumours.

Classification of pineal parenchymal tumours is complicated by the presence of mixed pineocytoma–pineoblastoma types, some with intermediate differentiation. A new classification has been proposed based on histological features, which is closely related to patient survival. A new type of pineal tumour was described in 2003—the pineal papillary tumour. These tumours of the pineal region are similar to those described for ependymal cells of the subcommissural organ, and may be derived from these specialized ependymocytes.

There is no consistent information on overproduction or underproduction of melatonin with specific types of tumour. Some work suggests that melatonin is absent or very low in treated or untreated pineal germinomas, but the consequences remain to be defined.

Many clinical attempts have been made to relate circulating melatonin to endocrine and other pathology. The results on the whole are difficult to interpret and inconsistent.[1]

Miscellaneous

The numerous reports of various effects of melatonin, not obviously endocrine related, in animals and in vitro are beyond the scope of this article. Many of these concern 'protective' effects attributed to antioxidant activity. There is some evidence for anti-cancer and cardioprotective activity. Melatonin has been described as a pleiotrophic hormone.

Mechanisms of action of melatonin

High-affinity saturable, specific, and reversible melatonin binding to cell membranes is most prominent in the suprachiasmatic nuclei and the pars tuberalis of the pituitary, but has also been found in many brain and other areas, including the retina, cells of the immune system, a number of cancer cell lines, the gonads, the kidney, the skin, and the cardiovascular system.

Melatonin membrane receptors have been cloned and three initial subtypes (Mel 1a, Mel 1b, and Mel 1c) were renamed MT1, MT2, and MT3. They are a new family of G-protein-coupled receptors, have high affinity (Kd 20–160 picomolar) and inhibit forskolin-stimulated cAMP formation. Within the suprachiasmatic nuclei, the phase shifting receptor appears to be MT2, whilst MT1 is associated with acute suppression of electrical activity in the suprachiasmatic nuclei. There is redundancy between the subtypes.

Within the pars tuberalis of the pituitary gland, melatonin has multiple effects on the expression of clock genes via the MT1 receptor. Melatonin acts in the pars tuberalis to control thyroid hormone action in the medio-basal hypothalamus. Long-day-induced TSH beta in the pars tuberalis leads to changes in seasonal reproductive function via the induction of type 2 deiodinase, the reduction of type 3 deiodinase, and subsequent local T3 activation of GnRH in long-day breeders, whilst it terminates reproductive activity in short-day breeders. In the pars tuberalis, melatonin sets the phase of Eya3 and its synergistic partner(s), which activate TSH beta. Subsequently, melatonin suppresses Eya3.

Numerous other physiological responses have been ascribed to MT1 and MT2 receptors. A third putative mammalian melatonin receptor, MT3, has been identified as the enzyme quinone reductase.

Further reading

Arendt J. Melatonin: Characteristics, concerns and prospects. *J Biol Rhythms* 2005; 20: 291–303.

Arendt J. The pineal gland and pineal tumours. Available at http://www.ncbi.nlm.nih.gov/books/NBK279108/ (accessed 23 Dec 2017).

Dubocovich ML. Melatonin receptors: Role in sleep and circadian rhythm regulation. *Sleep Med* 2007; 8: 34–42.

García JJ, López-Pingarrón L, Almeida-Souza P, et al. Protective effects of melatonin in reducing oxidative stress and in preserving the fluidity of biological membranes: A review. *J Pineal Res* 2014; 56: 225–37.

Hazlerigg D. The evolutionary physiology of photoperiodism in vertebrates. *Prog Brain Res* 2012; 199: 413–22.

Hut RA. Photoperiodism: Shall EYA compare thee to a summer's day? *Curr Biol* 2011; 11: R22–25.

Morgenthaler TI, Lee-Chiong T, Alessi C, et al. Practice parameters for the clinical evaluation and treatment of circadian rhythm sleep disorders. An American Academy of Sleep Medicine Report. *Sleep* 2007; 30: 1445–59.

---

[1] Adapted from Endotext.org, Arendt J., Chapter 15, The Pineal Gland and Pineal Tumours. Copyright © 2000–2017, MDText.com, Inc.

Chapter 6

Adrenal gland

Chapter contents

6.1 Adrenal anatomy and physiology

Introduction

The adrenal gland is a vital mediator of an organism's response to stress, and is a critical regulator of immune function, blood pressure, and energy homeostasis. It focuses multiple endocrine systems—the hypothalamo-pituitary–adrenal axis, the renin–angiotensin–aldosterone system, the sympatho-adrenal axis—within one organ. This close anatomical proximity is no coincidence, and over recent times the manner in which these systems communicate within the gland has become clearer.

Adrenal embryology

The adrenal cortex arises from cells of the intermediate mesoderm. A distinct adrenal primordium is apparent from 33 days post conception, and by 50 days these cells have begun to take on the ultrastructural appearance of steroidogenic cells. During the eighth week of gestation, the adrenal cortex becomes divided into two rudimentary zones by a mechanism that remains unknown, and by the ninth week a mesenchymal capsule has formed around the gland. The zones of this fetal cortex are the inner fetal zone and the subcapsular definitive zone. The fetal zone cells are larger, and this zone takes up most of the fetal adrenal, in a histological pattern similar to that of the adult zona reticularis. The definitive zone comes to resemble the adult zona glomerulosa early in the third trimester, whilst a transitional zone between the fetal zone and the definitive zone similarly resembles the adult zona fasciculata.

The adrenal medulla develops from invasion of the fetal cortex by cells derived from the neural crest. These sympathogonia migrate in nerves from the sympathetic chain, and along blood vessels penetrating the fetal cortex. They are scattered within the cortex initially, and can differentiate into ganglion cells or chromaffin cells. Cortisol from the transitional zone induces the enzyme phenylethanolamine N-methyltransferase (PNMT) and directs the majority of chromaffin cells to become adrenergic. The islands of medullary tissue coalesce into the adult medulla only in the second year of postnatal life, whilst small islets remain scattered throughout the cortex. Extra-adrenal chromaffin cells have a more significant physiological role in fetal life than in the adult, when their pathological development into paragangliomas is their most important clinical consequence. In contrast to mainly noradrenergic paragangliomas, phaeochromocytomas tend to secrete primarily adrenaline, for the reasons outlined above.

The fetal adrenal develops an extensive vascular supply by the eighth week of gestation. Adrenal arteries supply blood to a subcapsular arteriolar plexus, and these give rise to capsular capillaries that feed thin walled venous sinusoids and traverse the cortex. In the adult adrenal, these coalesce into another plexus in the zona reticularis and venules pass between the chromaffin cells to enter the adrenal vein. When the medullary islands combine, they are also supplied by branches that come directly from the subcapsular plexus and bypass the zona reticularis. In this way, most cells in the adrenal are only 1–2 cells away from a vascular endothelial cell. The arterial supply in the adult adrenal is in multiple branches derived from the aorta, the renal artery, and the inferior phrenic arteries, whilst the venous drainage is usually a single vein, direct to the inferior vena cava or the renal vein, on the left and right, respectively. In addition, subcapsular and medullary lymphatic plexus drain to lumbar and para-aortic lymph nodes.

Relative to its size, the adrenal gland receives the largest autonomic nerve supply of any organ. Myelinated sympathetic preganglionic fibres from the interomediolateral cell column or the lateral horn in vertebral levels T10–11 synapse on the medullary chromaffin cells. The cortex receives an afferent nerve supply from the medulla, with sympathetic fibres that travel along the blood vessels.

Steroid production from the fetal adrenal is involved in maintaining intrauterine homeostasis and in the maturation of fetal organ systems (including the adrenal itself) in preparation for extrauterine life. The fetal zone produces large amounts of the adrenal androgen DHEA and its sulphate DHEAS, which are largely converted to oestrogens by placental aromatase. The transitional zone produces cortisol, with a peak immediately before birth, and this is at least partly regulated by adrenocorticotrophic hormone from the fetal pituitary. The definitive zone acquires the capacity for aldosterone synthesis late in gestation, and forms the zona glomerulosa in the adult. Soon after birth, the fetal zone rapidly disappears, and androgen secretion decreases. It is only with the maturation of the zona reticularis during adrenarche in the child that this returns. The maintenance of zonation in the adrenal cortex is an area of intense interest, with one of the most widely held views being that a common pool of precursors in the periphery of the gland migrate centripetally and differentiate, with signalling through the sonic hedgehog and Wnt pathways thought to be significant.

The adult adrenal gland comes to lie anterior and superior to the upper kidney in its own fascial compartment, and weighs 4–5 g, 90% of which is cortical.

Adrenocortical physiology

Functional zonation of the adrenal cortex allows mineralocorticoid, glucocorticoid, and adrenal androgen secretion to be regulated independently of each other. This is achieved in part through the differential expression of steroidogenic enzymes and cofactors, and distinct cell surface receptors in the different zones. The layout of these zones can be seen in Figure 6.1.

In all cortical cells, steroid production begins with cholesterol uptake and then trafficking to the inner mitochondrial membrane and conversion to pregnenolone by the cytochrome p450 enzyme p450scc (for side-chain cleavage). The main source of cholesterol is plasma LDL, with a lesser contribution from intracellular acetyl CoA. In a zone-dependent manner, adrenocorticotrophic hormone, angiotensin 2, and increasing potassium ion concentrations all increase cholesterol availability by increasing the expression and activity of LDL receptors, thus stimulating beta-hydroxy beta-methylglutaryl (HMG)-CoA reductase and hormone-sensitive lipase. The steroidogenic acute regulatory protein StAR controls the trafficking of cholesterol to the inner mitochondrial membrane, and this too is upregulated and phosphorylated by adrenocorticotrophic hormone and via stimulation by angiotensin 2 and potassium ions. In this way, steroid-hormone secretion can be induced within minutes.

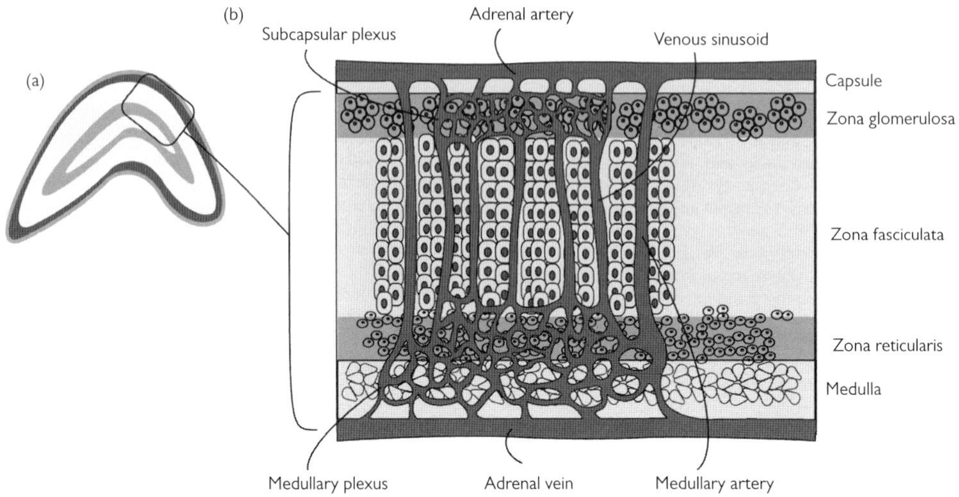

Fig 6.1 Zonation of the adrenal gland. (a) A schematic diagram of the whole adrenal gland. (b) Adrenal zonation and the blood supply.

The steroidogenic enzyme pathway is illustrated in Figure 6.2. The enzymes are divided into cytochrome p450 enzymes and hydroxysteroid dehydrogenases. Cytochrome p450 enzymes use electrons derived from NADPH to facilitate their catalytic actions. Type 1 p450 enzymes are mitochondrial and use ferredoxin reductase (a flavoprotein) and ferredoxin (a protein containing iron and sulphur) as cofactors; type 2 enzymes are microsomal, and use the enzymes p450 oxidoreductase and cytochrome b5 as their cofactors. Hydroxysteroid dehydrogenases convert hydroxysteroids to ketosteroids using nicotinamide cofactors without intermediary protein, but, unlike the p450 enzymes, different isoforms may catalyse the reverse reaction.

Cytochrome p450 enzymes
The enzyme p450scc (encoded by *CYP11A1*) controls the rate-limiting step in steroidogenesis and is present in all three zones. It catalyses three reactions: hydroxylation at C20, hydroxylation at C22, and cleavage of the amine side chain. The pregnenolone generated is trafficked back out of the mitochondria.

The enzyme p450c17 (encoded by *CYP17A1*) catalyses two reactions: 17-alpha-hydroxylation, and 17,20 lyase, which were originally thought to be the actions of two distinct enzymes. The two activities can be controlled separately to a degree by availability of cofactors. Higher levels of p450 oxidoreductase and cytochrome b5 in the zona reticularis favour the 17,20-lyase activity, and increase the level of androgen secretion from this zone.

The enzyme p450c21 (encoded by *CYP21A1*) is the 21-alpha-hydroxylase enzyme that generates 11-deoxycorticosterone from progesterone, and 11-deoxycortisol from 17-alpha-hydroxyprogesterone. The gene locus is highly recombinogenic, making congenital adrenal hyperplasia due to 21-hydroxylase deficiency one of the most common autosomal recessive disorders (1 in 20,000 live births). In the absence of enzyme activity, the inability to convert progesterone to 11-deoxycorticosterone results in aldosterone deficiency, and

the inability to convert 17-alpha-hydroxyprogesterone to 11-deoxycortisol results in cortisol deficiency. At its most severe, this causes hypoglycaemia, hyponatraemia, hyperkalaemia, and acidosis, with hypotension and cardiovascular collapse. The absence of cortisol delivery to the medulla results in lower adrenaline levels, compounding the hypotension and hypoglycaemia. Increased shuttling of intermediates to adrenal androgens causes variable amounts of virilization depending on the specific abnormality.

The enzymes p450c11 beta (encoded by *CYP11B1*) and p450c11AS (encoded by CYP11B2), which are closely related, catalyse the final steps in the synthesis of glucocorticoids and mineralocorticoids, following trafficking of 11-deoxycorticosterone or deoxycortisol back to the inner mitochondrial membrane. The enzyme p450c11 beta has a single 11-hydroxylation activity and is expressed in the zona fasciculata; p450c11AS can also catalyse 18-hydroxylation and 18-methyl-oxidation and its expression only in the zona glomerulosa results in aldosterone production in this layer alone. An unequal crossing over of these genes can result in glucocorticoid-remediable hyperaldosteronism, when a hybrid gene allows aldosterone synthesis in the zona fasciculata when stimulated by adrenocorticotrophic hormone.

Hydroxysteroid dehydrogenase enzymes
3-Beta-hydroxysteroid dehydrogenase is common to all of the steroidogenic cells. It converts the C3 hydroxyl to a keto group, and isomerizes the double bond from the B to the A ring. The type 2 isoform is predominant in the adrenal glands and the gonads. Low levels in the zona reticularis ensure that DHEA is the most abundant adrenal androgen.

17-Beta-hydroxysteroid dehydrogenase isoforms are important in the gonads and the periphery in generating testosterone and interconverting oestrogens. Small amounts of testosterone in the zona reticularis are probably a result of local production of 17-beta-hydroxysteroid dehydrogenase type 5.

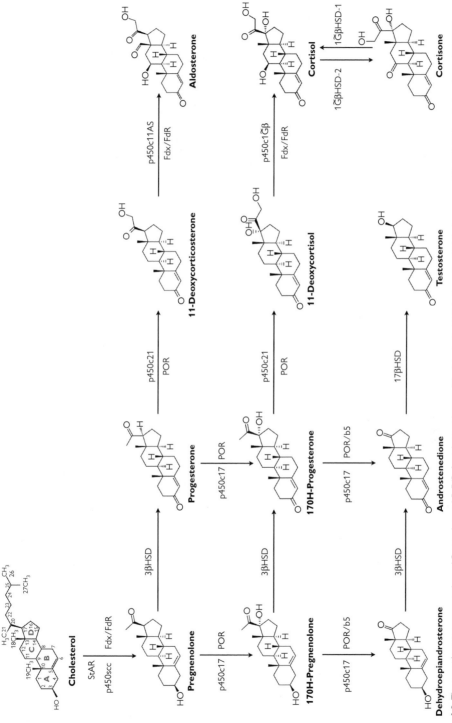

Fig 6.2 The steroidogenic enzyme pathway; b5, cytochrome b5; FdR, ferredoxin reductase; Fdx, ferredoxin; HSD, hydroxysteroid dehydrogenase; p450c11β, 11-beta-hydroxylase; p450c11AS, aldosterone synthase; p450c17, 17-alpha-hydroxylase and 17.20 lyase; p450c21; 21-hydroxylase; p450scc, side chain cleavage; POR, cytochrome p450 oxidoreductase.

Although 11-beta-hydroxysteroid dehydrogenase is not expressed in the adrenal glands, the ability of the two isoforms of this enzyme to interconvert cortisol and its inactive metabolite cortisone is vital to regulating the actions of both cortisol and aldosterone. 11-Beta-hydroxysteroid dehydrogenase type 2 prevents cortisol from activating the mineralocorticoid receptor in the kidney, whilst 11-beta-hydroxysteroid dehydrogenase type 1 serves to amplify the cortisol signal in the liver, muscle, and nervous tissue.

Mineralocorticoids

The principal mineralocorticoid is aldosterone, and this is secreted in amounts three orders of magnitude less than cortisol. 11-Deoxycorticosterone has mineralocorticoid activity but this is not physiologically significant. In the zona glomerulosa, cells are small, and arranged in rounded clusters in a subcapsular layer making up around 15% of the cortex, depending on serum sodium levels. An aldosterone-secreting Conn's adenoma does not usually have a typical zona glomerulosa appearance, suggesting that a functional description may be more appropriate. Cells in the zona glomerulosa are distinguished by expression of the type 1 angiotensin 2 receptor AT1, aldosterone synthase, low levels of p450c17, and no expression of p450c11 beta.

Cells in the zona glomerulosa express receptors for adrenocorticotrophic hormone but the main regulators of secretion are angiotensin 2 and small increases in the extracellular potassium concentration. Angiotensin 2 levels increase because of volume depletion causing renin release in the kidney, but sodium depletion does not seem to cause aldosterone release through this mechanism. Aldosterone release is inhibited by somatostatin, heparin, atrial natriuretic peptide, and dopamine.

Binding of angiotensin 2 to the G-protein-coupled AT1 receptor activates multiple downstream signalling pathways. Phospholipase C is the best characterized second messenger, causing an increase in intracellular calcium. Increasing potassium concentration depolarizes the zona glomerulosa cell membrane, also leading to calcium influx. In the short term (minutes to hours), this increases the activity of StAR, whilst in the longer term (hours to days) it upregulates CYP11B2. Angiotensin 2 upregulation of the mitogen-activated protein kinase pathway stimulates zona glomerulosa cell proliferation.

The classical effects of aldosterone are mediated by binding to the mineralocorticoid receptor in the cytosol. These receptors are distributed widely across a range of tissues, including the kidneys, cardiomyocytes, and the vascular endothelium. The mineralocorticoid receptor is a member of a steroid-receptor superfamily that includes the glucocorticoid receptor and the androgen receptor. Ligand binding induces dimerization and dissociation from chaperone proteins, including Hsp90. The bound receptor then translocates to the nucleus and is recruited to target genes by direct DNA binding or by associating with other DNA-bound transcription factors. There are also more rapid effects of aldosterone mediated by fast-acting signalling cascades, but no distinct receptor has been identified to account for these. It is possible that the mineralocorticoid receptor is also responsible for these non-genomic effects, perhaps by binding additional receptors itself.

The mineralocorticoid receptor binds cortisol and aldosterone with equal affinity, and it is widely held that cortisol, present in 100-fold excess of aldosterone, is inactivated by the action of 11-beta-hydroxysteroid dehydrogenase type 2 in the kidney. However, even in tissues with a plentiful supply of this enzyme, clearance of active cortisol is rarely complete, remaining at ten times the level of aldosterone. The mechanism by which the mineralocorticoid receptor occupied by cortisol is held inactive is yet to be fully elucidated.

Aldosterone induces renal retention of sodium, by upregulating epithelial sodium channels (ENaCs) in the distal tubules. This is probably not the mechanism whereby hyperaldosteronism increases blood pressure; this is, instead, proposed to be the result of a direct aldosterone action on the vasculature and the CNS. Oxidative stress upregulates the expression of the mineralocorticoid receptor in cardiac cells, where it induces cardiac remodelling and fibrosis. Aldosterone itself can promote inflammation and oxidative stress, and contribute to impaired insulin signalling, whilst it induces swelling and stiffening of vascular epithelial cells and counteracts their ability to trigger vasodilatation. This pro-inflammatory role is in contrast to the anti-inflammatory effects of glucocorticoid signalling.

Glucocorticoids

Cortisol is the principal glucocorticoid secreted from the adrenal cortex. Most comes from the zona fasciculata, although the zona reticularis secretes smaller amounts. The zona fasciculata cells are broader than those in the zona glomerulosa and arranged in columns two cells wide, in parallel to the fenestrated sinusoids. Adrenocorticotrophic hormone binds to the type 2 melanocortin receptor (MC2R) and activates a cAMP-mediated downstream signalling pathway. The rapid effects of adrenocorticotrophic hormone receptor binding have been described already in terms of cholesterol import and trafficking. Chronically (hours to days), there is increased expression of p450scc, p450c17, p450c21, p450c11 beta, and ferredoxin. Adrenal blood flow increases, and the zona fasciculata layer hypertrophies. Adrenocorticotrophic hormone fails to induce high levels of DHEA secretion from the zona fasciculata due to the low levels of cytochrome b5 in this zone. The role for cytokines derived from immune cells within both the cortex and the medulla in modulating steroid production is increasingly recognized as important.

The glucocorticoid receptor is found in almost all cell types, and ligand binding is essentially identical to the for the mineralocorticoid receptor. Receptor activation generally results in an inhibition of DNA synthesis. The effects of cortisol excess are well characterized, but the actual physiological role for the hormone is less clear-cut.

Glucocorticoids are named for their effect to modify glucose metabolism—they stimulate gluconeogenesis and antagonize insulin—but whether this is an important homeostatic mechanism in normal individuals is debated. A role for inhibiting inflammation through negatively regulating signalling pathways controlled by the nuclear factor kappa B and AP-1 transacting factors and by upregulating anti-inflammatory cytokine gene expression is hypothesized to be more significant. The pro-inflammatory effects of mineralocorticoid-receptor activation, which can be stimulated by cortisol, would appear to support this contention. Cortisol levels are increased in line with the circadian rhythm of pituitary adrenocorticotrophic hormone secretion, and in response to physical stresses such as hypotension, hypoglycaemia, and fever. The CNS effects of increasing appetite and paranoia under stress have a theoretical evolutionary benefit, and are commonly observed in cortisol excess.

Adrenal androgens

Adrenal androgens are the most abundant steroids secreted from the adrenal gland (>20 mg/day). The principal androgens secreted are DHEA, its sulphate DHEAS, androstenedione, and very small amounts of testosterone. As the fetal zone regresses in the neonate, very little androgen secretion takes place until adrenarche. The adult zona reticularis is a network of smaller, more compact cells than the zona fasciculata.

The stimulus for zona reticularis maturation at adrenarche is unknown. Adrenocorticotrophic hormone plays a permissive role, whilst a cortical androgen-stimulating factor has long been sought. Roles for the growth hormone/IGF-1 axis, or oestrogens produced by aromatase in the medulla, have been suggested. The physical consequences of zona reticularis maturation at adrenarche are the development of pubic hair, with a possible CNS role for DHEA in fine-tuning the GnRH pulse generator to signal puberty. Pubertal development per se is not affected, nor is the individual's final height, but premature adrenarche is associated with later metabolic disease and polycystic ovarian syndrome.

The enzyme p450c17, and the cofactors p450 oxidoreductase and cytochrome b5 are upregulated at adrenarche, favouring 17,20-lyase activity and therefore androgen production. Levels of 3-beta-hydroxysteroid dehydrogenase type 1 decrease, so more DHEA is produced than androstenedione. Although MC2R is expressed, cortisol production is restricted by low levels of p450c21 and p450c11 beta 1. As DHEA accumulates, there is conversion to androstenedione, and to testosterone in very small amounts. SULT2A1, the sulphotransferase which produces DHEAS, is upregulated at adrenarche, but whether DHEAS is an active endocrine hormone is not clear. The affinity of DHEA for the androgen receptor is low until peripheral conversion to testosterone and dihydrotestosterone.

Adrenal medulla and catecholamines

Adrenal medulla chromaffin cells are larger than cortical cells. Most secrete adrenaline (80%), with the remainder secreting noradrenaline or, in a minority of cases, dopamine. They are functionally equivalent to postganglionic sympathetic nerves, with the terminal on the opposite side to the endothelium of wide venous sinusoids. Catecholamines are packaged with chromogranins and a variety of neuropeptides within dense granules. The chromogranins have a role in processing, storage, and release of the contents of the granules.

Tyrosine is converted to dopamine by the actions of tyrosine hydroxylase and DOPA decarboxylase.

Dopamine beta-hydroxylase converts this to noradrenaline, and this is converted in the cytoplasm to adrenaline under the action of PNMT in adrenergic chromaffin cells, before being taken up into another storage vesicle. Catecholamine has a half-life in the circulation of only 10–100 seconds before being recovered by sympathetic nerves and chromaffin cells and metabolized to metanephrines by the action of catechol-O-methyltransferase.

Catecholamine release is stimulated by acetylcholine release from the preganglionic sympathetic nerves, but there is a basal secretion even without neural input. The pathways inducing adrenaline and noradrenaline release are different, demonstrated by the manner in which haemorrhage causes preferential noradrenaline release, and hypoglycaemia causes adrenaline release. The 'fight-or-flight' response to severe stress is due to a 60-fold increase in catecholamine secretion and is associated with increases in heart rate, metabolic rate, and blood pressure, glucose mobilized from liver and muscle, and dilatation of bronchioles and pupils. Compounds released in anaphylaxis (bradykinin, histamine, angiotensin 2) can also stimulate catecholamine release, whilst mast cell degranulation can itself be stimulated by adrenocorticotrophic hormone. Medullary peptides including neuropeptide Y and adrenomedullin have regulatory roles in catecholamine biosynthesis and release, but they may exert their own endocrine effects. Adrenomedullin can elicit vasodilatation and natriuresis, for instance, whilst neuropeptide Y causes vasoconstriction, and local production of CRH and adrenocorticotrophic hormone modulates the function of the adrenal cortex.

Conclusion

The commonly held view of the adrenal gland with its anatomically and functionally distinct regions must be updated in light of an emerging understanding of the co-ordination between them. The clinical significance of the endocrine, paracrine, and neuronal interactions between the medulla, the cortex, and the immune system is likely to become more apparent in the years ahead.

Further reading

Ehrhart-Bornstein M and Bornstein SR. Cross-talk between adrenal medulla and adrenal cortex in stress. *Ann NY Acad Sci* 2008; 1148: 112–17.

Funder JW. Aldosterone and mineralocorticoid receptors: Past, present, and future. *Endocrinology* 2010; 151: 5098–102.

Ishimoto H and Jaffe RB. Development and function of the human fetal adrenal cortex: A key component in the fetoplacental unit. *Endocr Rev* 2011; 32: 317–55.

Vinson GP. The adrenal cortex and life. *Mol Cell Endocrinol* 2009; 300: 2–6.

Yates R, Katugampola H, Cavlan D, et al. Adrenocortical development, maintenance, and disease. *Curr Top Dev Biol* 2013; 106: 239–312.

6.2 Laboratory investigation of adrenal disease

Introduction

The initial step in the laboratory investigation of adrenal disease is establishing inappropriately low cortisol secretion, with the most commonly used tests being an early morning cortisol and a short Synacthen® test (Figure 6.3). Both a standard high-dose (250 µg) and a standard low-dose (1 µg) short Synacthen® test are available, with neither test showing clear superiority over the other. Once cortisol deficiency has been identified, further investigations are necessary to determine whether the cause is primary or secondary (due to adrenocorticotrophic hormone deficiency) adrenal insufficiency. Assessment of adrenocorticotrophic hormone status, mineralocorticoid status, and/or other pituitary hormone levels is usually most helpful. Other tests of cortisol reserve used to diagnose secondary adrenal insufficiency are the insulin tolerance and metyrapone tests (see Chapter 3, Section 3.4). Once the type of disorder has been elucidated, the underlying cause should then be established (e.g. a pituitary adenoma causing adrenocorticotrophic hormone deficiency). In primary adrenal failure, hyponatraemia and hyperkalaemia are frequently, but not invariably, present.

- A short Synacthen® test is not recommended for diagnosis of acute cortisol insufficiency (e.g. within 4–6 weeks of pituitary surgery).
- A morning plasma cortisol <100 nmol/L (3.6 µg/dL) is consistent with cortisol deficiency, and further testing is rarely necessary.
- A morning cortisol >350 nmol/L (13 µg/dL) excludes significant cortisol deficiency, with 95% sensitivity.
- Abnormalities of CBG can give misleading results, for example with cirrhosis, nephrotic syndrome, or oestrogen therapy (falsely raised plasma cortisol level with oestrogen). Where available, direct assay of plasma free cortisol or alternatively salivary cortisol during Synacthen® testing may overcome this.

Primary adrenal failure (Addison's disease)

See also Section 6.11. Consider patient age and gender, as well as any other clinical disorders (e.g. autoimmune conditions, TB). In addition, the following investigations should be performed:

- testing for adrenal autoantibodies: antibodies to the adrenal cortex, and particularly 21-hydroxylase, are

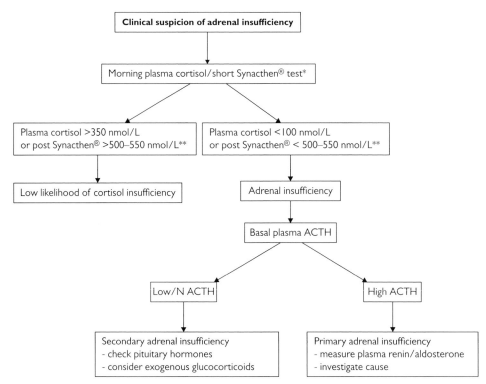

Fig 6.3 Algorithm for investigation of adrenal insufficiency; ACTH, adrenocorticotrophic hormone; N, normal.
* If high index of suspicion for primary adrenal failure, check adrenocorticotrophic hormone, renin, and aldosterone with basal cortisol and do not delay treatment.
** Cut-off values will be laboratory/assay dependant.

present in 60%–80% of autoimmune Addison's disease early after presentation

- long-chain fatty-acid measurement: as a marker of X-linked adrenoleukodystrophy, particularly for males with no evidence of autoimmunity
- adrenal imaging: may be helpful, e.g. for TB or haemorrhage (see also Section 6.3).
- genetic testing: if primary adrenal failure is associated with hypogonadotrophic hypogonadism in a male, then a mutation in DAX (dosage-sensitive sex-reversal gene) should be considered and genetic testing performed

Secondary adrenal failure (adrenocorticotrophic hormone deficiency)

See also Chapter 3, Section 3.4. In pituitary/hypothalamic disease, assess for signs of a mass lesion (headache, peripheral visual field defect). Check anterior pituitary hormones (T4, TSH, prolactin, IGF-1, LH, FSH, and testosterone/estradiol) and consider pituitary imaging (see Chapter 3, Section 3.3).

Cortisol excess (Cushing's syndrome)

See also Chapter 3, Section 3.7, and Section 6.8. The three recommended screening tests to assess for cortisol excess are:

- 24-hour UFC excretion
- low-dose (1 mg overnight, or standard 2-day) DST
- late-night salivary cortisol measurement

Generally, two abnormal tests are desirable to establish the diagnosis. Once cortisol excess has been confirmed, a plasma adrenocorticotrophic hormone level should be measured. A suppressed adrenocorticotrophic hormone level indicates an adrenal cause, and imaging of the adrenal glands should then be performed (see Section 6.3). If the adrenocorticotrophic hormone level is normal or raised, then adrenocorticotrophic-hormone-dependent Cushing's syndrome is present. Further biochemical testing is required to distinguish between a pituitary source (Cushing's disease) and ectopic adrenocorticotrophic hormone (see Section 6.8).

Primary aldosteronism

See also Section 6.4. Screening for aldosterone excess is usually recommended for patients with the following conditions:

- hypertension and spontaneous or drug-induced hypokalaemia (note that hypokalaemia is only present in 30%–50% of patients with confirmed primary aldosteronism)
- severe or resistant hypertension
- hypertension and/or stroke at a young age (<20 years old)
- hypertension with adrenal 'incidentaloma'

Screening for primary aldosteronism:
The aldosterone-to-renin ratio

- Initial testing involves measuring a morning (after patient has been up for >2 hours and seated for >5 minutes) *plasma renin* (plasma renin activity or plasma renin concentration) and *plasma aldosterone*.
- Most antihypertensive agents can be continued although mineralocorticoid receptor antagonists (spironolactone and eplerenone) are best avoided and should be ceased at least 4 weeks prior (see Table 6.1).
- An elevated plasma aldosterone-to-renin ratio is supportive of the diagnosis. See Figure 6.4 for a suggested algorithm.
- Plasma renin is usually very low or undetectable in primary aldosteronism
- Plasma aldosterone is usually >416 pmol/L (15 ng/dL) ('grey zone' 250–416 pmol/L (9–15 ng/dL)). A plasma aldosterone <250 pmol/L (9 ng/dL) excludes primary aldosteronism.
- Cut-off criteria will be laboratory/assay dependent.
- As hypokalaemia may suppress aldosterone secretion, ideally the plasma potassium should be normalized by supplementation.
- If plasma aldosterone and renin are both elevated, consider secondary hyperaldosteronism (e.g. renovascular disease).
- If renin and aldosterone are both reduced, consider other mineralocorticoid excess syndromes (e.g. liquorice, cortisol, or deoxycorticosterone excess).

Many antihypertensive agents can alter measurements of renin and aldosterone (Table 6.1). Thus, for equivocal cases, repeated measurements are recommended on non-interfering antihypertensive agents such as selective alpha-1 adrenoceptor blockers (e.g. doxazosin, prazosin) and/or non-dihydropyridine calcium channel blockers

Table 6.1 Effect of antihypertensive medication on measurements

	Plasma renin activity	Plasma aldosterone concentration	Ratio of plasma aldosterone concentration to plasma renin activity
Spironolactone/eplerenone	↑	↑	↓
Diuretics	↑	→ ↑	↓
ACE inhibitors	↑	↓	↓
Angiotensin 2 receptor blockers	↑	↓	↓
Calcium blockers (dihydropyridine)	↑	↓	↓
Beta blockers	↓	↓	↑
Central alpha 2 agonists (clonidine/methyldopa)	↓	↓	↓

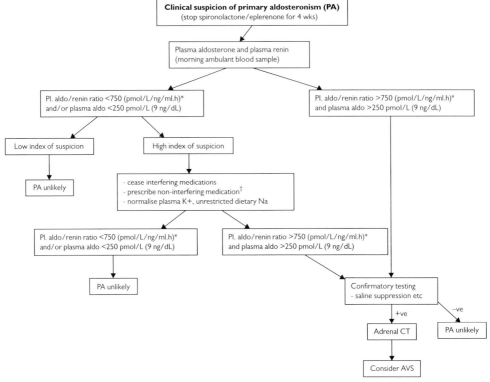

Fig 6.4 Algorithm for investigation of primary aldosteronism; +ve, positive; –ve, negative; aldo, aldosterone; AvS, adrenal vein sampling; pl., plasma.
* For plasma aldosterone measured in nanograms per decilitre, plasma aldosterone:renin ratio >20.
† Non-interfering antihypertensive agents: dozaxosin/prazosin, verapamil, hydralazine.

(e.g. verapamil). The use of beta blockers can cause false-positive results, whilst ACE inhibitors or angiotensin inhibitors can cause false-negative results, and withdrawal for 3–4 weeks has been recommended. However, if there is autonomous aldosterone secretion, many would consider that a readily detectable renin on any drug combination would exclude a diagnosis of primary hyperaldosteronism.

Confirming primary aldosteronism
The goal in confirming primary aldosteronism is to demonstrate failure to suppress aldosterone despite fluid/salt loading. The choice of test depends on laboratory and local expertise. Tests that can be used include:
- plasma aldosterone: a plasma aldosterone level >277 pmol/L (10 ng/dL) following the intervention supports primary aldosteronism, with indeterminate results between 139 and 277 pmol/L (5–10 ng/dL)
- saline infusion test: intravenous saline, 2 L over 4 hours; measure plasma aldosterone at baseline and at 4 hours
- oral sodium loading: oral sodium chloride (300 mmol of sodium daily) and potassium supplementation for 3 days; measure 24-hour urine aldosterone on the

third day (positive test: aldosterone >33 nmol/24 hours, sodium excretion >200 mmol/24 hours)
- fludrocortisone suppression test: fludrocortisone 100 μg four times daily for 4 days; measure plasma aldosterone at baseline and on the fourth day

Identifying the cause of primary aldosteronism
The challenge is to differentiate a *unilateral adrenal source of aldosterone excess*, usually an aldosterone-secreting adenoma, where surgery may be curative, from *bilateral adrenal hyperplasia*.
Tests for this include the following:
- imaging of the adrenal glands:
  - CT/MRI may identify a unilateral adenoma; however, adrenal incidentalomas are often found in patients >50 years old. The adrenal imaging may show no obvious lesion
  - recent research has suggested that ^{11}C-metomidate-PET scanning may be very helpful, but currently this remains a research technique
- bilateral adrenal vein sampling:
  - currently considered the 'gold standard' test for differentiating a unilateral source of aldosterone production from bilateral adrenal secretion.

- should only be considered if surgical management would be pursued
- a skilled interventional radiologist is required, and sampling under continuous adrenocorticotrophic hormone stimulation may be preferable

Technique for bilateral adrenal vein sampling
In bilateral adrenal vein sampling, the femoral vein is catheterized, and samples from the inferior vena cava (peripheral sample), and both adrenal veins are assayed for aldosterone and cortisol. A raised central to peripheral cortisol ratio >2–3:1 is necessary to confirm successful cannulation (>5:1 under adrenocorticotrophic hormone stimulation). As the right adrenal vein is often difficult to cannulate, samples taken from above and below the vein may be helpful. All aldosterone measurements should be normalized for cortisol secretion (aldosterone-to-cortisol ratio). Complications of the procedure occur in 2% of patients and include groin haematoma, adrenal haemorrhage, and dissection of the adrenal vein.

Interpretation of test results for bilateral adrenal vein sampling
- The best evidence to support a unilateral source of aldosterone is a suppressed contralateral aldosterone-to-cortisol ratio of <1 (aldosterone-to-cortisol ratio low-side to peripheral).
- A lateralized ratio (aldosterone-to-cortisol ratio high-side to low-side) of >4 indicates a unilateral aldosterone source; a ratio <3 is suggestive of bilateral adrenal hyperplasia. Ratios between 3 and 4 fall into the 'grey zone'.

Genetics of primary aldosteronism
If primary aldosteronism is confirmed in a patient <20 years old, or there is a family history of primary aldosteronism or haemorrhagic strokes in those <40 years old, genetic testing for glucocorticoid-remediable aldosteronism (also known as familial hyperaldosteronism type 1) is recommended.

Germ-line mutations in *KCNJ5* have been associated with familial bilateral adrenal hyperplasia, and somatic mutations in *KCNJ5* and other genes are described in 50% of aldosterone-secreting adenomas, However, such mutations do not affect diagnosis or treatment.

Phaeochromocytoma
See also Section 6.14. Screening for phaeochromocytoma should be considered in patients with:
- paroxysmal symptoms (episodic headache, sweating, palpitations)
- familial disease (multiple endocrine neoplasia type 2, Von Hippel–Lindau disease, *SDH* mutations, neurofibromatosis)
- resistant hypertension
- hypertension at a young age (<20 years old)
- an adrenal incidentaloma

Investigations are focused on demonstrating catecholamine hypersecretion, which is best achieved by measuring their metabolites (metanephrine and normetanephrine) in urine or plasma (see Figure 6.5).

Testing for phaeochromocytoma is as follows.
- There is no consensus on whether plasma or urinary measurement of fractionated metanephrines (metanephrine and normetanephrine measured separately) should be the preferred test, with important

considerations being local test availability and the pre-test likelihood of a phaeochromocytoma.
- Measurement of plasma metanephrines or urinary metanephrines is highly sensitive (95%–100%); however, the specificity of plasma metanephrines is lower at around 85%, resulting in a higher rate of false-positive tests. Some experts recommend screening individuals with a low index of suspicion with 24-hour urinary metanephrines, with measurement of plasma metanephrines preferable when phaeochromocytoma is more likely (e.g. familial syndrome, previous phaeochromocytoma, adrenal mass characteristic for a phaeochromocytoma; see Section 6.14).
- There is no role for the measurement of plasma catecholamines: however, urinary catecholamines may be useful.
- Certain medications such as tricyclic and serotonin–norepinephrine reuptake inhibitors, and increased sympathetic activity (e.g. significant physical stress/illness, panic attacks, autonomic dysfunction with spinal cord injury), can increase metanephrine measurements (see Table 6.2). Medications which have negligible effect on measurements of metanephrines include diuretics, ACE inhibitors, angiotensin 2 receptor blockers, and SSRI antidepressants.

Plasma metanephrines
- Plasma metanephrines preferably should be measured after 20 minutes of supine resting.
- It is an easier test, particularly for children.
- Beware of false-positive results, particularly in older individuals.
- The test can be used in patients with renal failure.
- Normal plasma metanephrines essentially excludes a phaeochromocytoma.

Twenty-four-hour urinary metanephrines
- Twenty-four-hour collection can be inconvenient and may be incomplete.
- Urinary creatinine is recommended to verify adequate collection.
- This test is not useful in patients with renal failure.
- If catecholamines also being measured, an acid collection will be required.

A clonidine suppression test is rarely necessary to distinguish between phaeochromocytoma and a false-positive result. Clonidine 0.3 mg is given orally and plasma normetanephrine measured before and 3 hours following the dose. Phaeochromocytoma is associated with failure of suppression of plasma normetanephrine (3-hour value fails to fall by >40% and remains above the normal range).

If phaeochromocytoma is confirmed biochemically, adrenal imaging should then be performed (see Section 6.3)

Genetics of phaeochromocytoma
Up to 30% of patients diagnosed with a phaeochromocytoma will have an associated familial disorder. Universal screening for a genetic condition is recommended by some, but should be considered mandatory for patients with the following:
- phaeochromocytoma diagnosed at <45 years old
- a family history of phaeochromocytoma/paraganglioma
- bilateral adrenal phaeochromocytoma
- paraganglioma
- malignant phaeochromocytoma

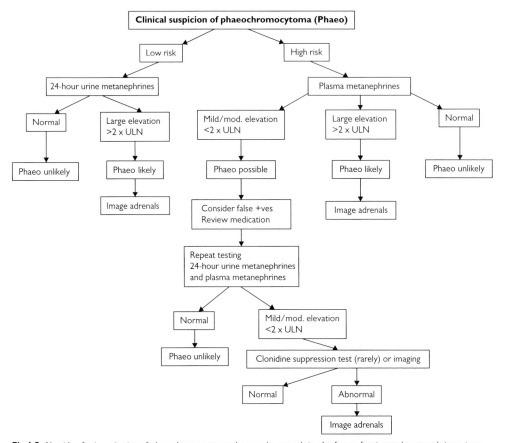

Fig 6.5 Algorithm for investigation of phaeochromocytoma; the term 'metanephrines' refers to fractionated metanephrines; +ves, positives; mod., moderate; ULN, upper limit of normal range.

Table 6.2 Effect of medication on measurements

	Urine				Plasma			
	E	NE	MN	NMN	E	NE	MN	NMN
Phenoxybenzamine	—	↑	—	↑	—	↑	—	↑
Selective alpha blockers (e.g. doxazosin)	—	↑	—	—	—	—	—	—
Beta blockers (e.g. metoprolol)	↑	↑	↑	↑	—	—	↑	—
Labetolol	↑	↑	↑	↑	—	—	↑	—
Calcium channel blockers	↑	↑	—	—	—	↑	—	—
Tricyclic antidepressants		↑		↑		↑		↑
SNRIs (e.g. venlafaxine)				↑				↑
MAOIs and phenothiazines			↑				↑	
Paracetamol	↑	↑	↑	↑		↑		↑

Abbreviations: E, epinephrine; NE, norepinephrine; MAOI, monoamine oxidase inhibitor; MN, metanephrine; NMN, normetanephrine; SNRI, serotonin and norepinephrine reuptake inhibitor.

Note: Other agents associated with false-positive results include atypical antipsychotics, sympathomimetics, amphetamines, prochlorperazine, caffeine (high intake), and nicotine (high intake).

Genetic testing is available for mutations in *VHL*, *RET*, *SDHA*, *SDHB*, *SDHC*, *SDHD*, *SDHAF2*, *TMEM127*, and *MAX*. Other rare susceptibility genes have been recently reported. For neurofibromatosis type 1, the diagnosis is usually made on the basis of clinical features rather than genetic testing. Genetic testing should be performed sequentially, based on clinical characteristics (see Section 6.14).

Adrenal incidentalomas

See also Section 6.9. The key diagnoses not to miss are adrenal cancer and phaeochromocytomas. All patients with an adrenal incidentaloma should be screened for *phaeochromocytoma* and *cortisol excess*. If there are clinical features of Cushing's syndrome, investigate as for cortisol excess (see Section 6.8). Autonomous cortisol secretion without clinical features (subclinical Cushing's syndrome) is described in 5%–20% of adrenal incidentalomas.

Tests include:

- plasma metanephrines or 24-hour urine metanephrines
- overnight 1 mg DST

The cut-off criteria for an abnormal overnight DST are variably quoted. Many consider a plasma cortisol >138 nmol/L (5.0 µg/dL) consistent with autonomy of cortisol secretion, compared to the more stringent criteria of plasma cortisol >50 nmol/L (1.8 µg/dL) used in most clinical settings to screen for Cushing's syndrome. Thus, levels between 50 and 138 nmol/L can be considered indeterminate.

If cortisol fails to suppress (i.e. >50–138 nmol/L) after 1 mg dexamethasone, then measure:

- morning plasma adrenocorticotrophic hormone level
- 24-hour UFC excretion

Abnormality in two or more tests is considered necessary to diagnose subclinical Cushing's syndrome. Basal adrenocorticotrophic hormone levels are assay dependent, with adrenal cortisol excess associated with a suppressed level <2.2 pmol/L (<10 ng/L). Commonly, the 24-hour UFC is normal.

If hypertension or hypokalaemia is present, screening for primary aldosteronism with aldosterone-to-renin ratio is recommended.

In females with hyperandrogenism (hirsutism/acne), plasma DHEAS and testosterone should be measured.

If bilateral adrenal masses or clinical features suggesting congenital adrenal hyperplasia, are present, consider screening with 17-hydroxyprogesterone levels.

Congenital adrenal hyperplasia

See also Chapter 7, Section 7.5. Over 90% of cases of congenital adrenal hyperplasia are due to 21-hydroxylase (p450c21) deficiency, with elevation of the normal substrate for 21-hydroxylase, plasma 17-hydroxyprogesterone, being the key to diagnosis.

Routine neonatal screening is performed in many countries at 2–4 days after birth. False-positive results are described in premature and sick infants, and false-negative results are occasionally seen. A very high level of 17-hydroxyprogesterone is usually found in affected neonates (>105 nmol/L (3500 ng/mL)).

In older children and adults, an initial measurement of plasma 17-hydroxyprogesterone is recommended, preferably measured in the morning, and for menstruating females in the follicular phase. The interpretation of this test is as follows.

- Basal 17-hydroxyprogesterone >45 nmol/L (1487 ng/dL) is consistent with congenital adrenal hyperplasia; 17-hydroxyprogesterone <6 nmol/L (198 ng/dL) excludes congenital adrenal hyperplasia
- For 17-hydroxyprogesterone >6 nmol/L, a short Synacthen® test should be performed with 17-hydroxyprogesterone measured at 60 minutes after 250 µg of Synacthen®
- A stimulated 17-hydroxyprogesterone >45 nmol/L confirms the diagnosis; 17-hydroxyprogesterone <35 nmol/L (1156 ng/dL) excludes congenital adrenal hyperplasia
- For equivocal stimulated values between 35 and 45 nmol/L, liquid chromatography followed by tandem mass spectrometry or genetic testing maybe helpful

Once a diagnosis of classic congenital adrenal hyperplasia has been made, other laboratory testing should include the cortisol response to Synacthen® and assessment of the mineralocorticoid axis (plasma renin activity and aldosterone).

Measurement of plasma androgens (testosterone/androstenedione) is helpful in both classic and non-classic congenital adrenal hyperplasia, and can guide therapy.

Other forms of congenital adrenal hyperplasia may need to be considered, particularly in the childhood period, with elevated 17-hydroxyprogesterone levels also being seen in 11-beta-hydroxylase and p450 oxidoreductase deficiencies. Associated clinical features should direct investigations (see Table 6.3) with consideration of deoxycorticosterone, 11-deoxycortisol, 17-hydroxypregnenolone, DHEAS, and androstenedione measurements after adrenocorticotrophic hormone stimulation. Steroid profiling by liquid chromatography with tandem mass spectrometry may replace these tests, where available.

Genetics of adrenal hyperplasia

Mutations in *CYP21A2* are detected in up to 95% of patients with congenital adrenal hyperplasia due to 21-hydroxylase deficiency and may be useful adjuncts for equivocal hormonal measurements, and for genetic counselling.

Renal tubular abnormalities

See also Sections 6.6 and 6.7. These are rare conditions that should also be considered when hypokalaemia is associated with metabolic alkalosis. In Bartter syndrome and Gitelman syndrome, the blood pressure is normal or low despite activation of the renin/angiotensin system. Measurement of urine calcium excretion and plasma magnesium are helpful in differentiating between the two disorders (see Table 6.4). Excessive vomiting or surreptitious diuretic use should also be considered in the differential diagnosis.

Table 6.3 Uncommon causes of congenital adrenal hyperplasia

Affected enzyme	Clinical features
11-beta-hydroxylase	Ambiguous genitalia, virilization, usually also hypertension, hypokalaemia
3-beta-hydroxysteroid dehydrogenase	Ambiguous genitalia/mild virilization
17-alpha-hydroxylase	Often pubertal presentation with hypogonadism, hypertension, hypokalaemia

Table 6.4 Features associated with renal tubular abnormalities

	Blood pressure	Plasma renin	Plasma aldosterone	Plasma magnesium	Urine calcium
Bartter syndrome	N/↓	↑	↑	N	↑/N
Gitelman syndrome	N/↓	↑	↑	↓	↓
Liddle syndrome	↑	↓	↓	N	N

In Liddle syndrome, hypertension is present with suppression of renin and aldosterone levels (see Table 6.4).

Genetics of renal tubular abnormalities

There are a number of recognized mutations in these tubular conditions: however, genetic analysis is usually not undertaken.

Non-aldosterone mineralocorticoid excess

See also Section 6.5. Non-aldosterone mineralocorticoid excess is a rare condition which presents like primary aldosteronism, with hypertension and hypokalaemia; however, low renin and aldosterone levels are found, as another mineralocorticoid or mineralocorticoid-like effect is present. The genetic condition *apparent mineralocorticoid excess* is due to an inactivating mutation in the gene for 11-beta-hydroxysteroid dehydrogenase type 2, *HSA11B2*, and has a similar biochemical profile to that seen with *chronic liquorice consumption*, with a raised ratio of free cortisol to cortisone. Raised levels of deoxycorticosterone may be seen with *rare forms of* congenital adrenal hyperplasia, particularly 11-beta-hydroxylase deficiency (see Chapter 7, Section 7.5), or a *deoxycorticosterone-secreting adrenal tumour*.

Genetic testing for mutations in *HSA11B2* is available for apparent mineralocorticoid excess.

Further reading

Eisenhofer G, Goldstein DS, Walther MM. Biochemical diagnosis of phaeochromocytoma: How to distinguish true from false positive test results. *J Clin Endocrinol Metab* 2003; 88: 2656–66.

Funder JW, Carey RM, Fardella C, et al. Case detection, diagnosis and treatment of patients with primary aldosteronism: An Endocrine Society clinical practice guideline. *J Clin Endocrinol Metab* 2008; 93: 3266–81.

Funder JW, Carey RM, Mantero F, et al. The management of primary aldosteronism: case detection, diagnosis, and treatment: An Endocrine Society clinical practice guideline. *J Clin Endocrinol Metab* 2016; 101: 1889–1916.

Galan SR and Kann PH. Genetic and molecular pathogenesis of phaeochromocytoma and paraganglioma. *Clin Endo* 2013; 78: 165–75.

Inder WJ and Hunt PJ, Glucocorticoid replacement in pituitary surgery: Guidelines for perioperative assessment and management. *J Clin Endocrinol Metab* 2002; 87: 2745–50.

Kaltsas G, Chrisoulidou A, Piaditis G, et al. Current status and controversies in adrenal incidentalomas. *Trends in Endocrinol Metabol* 2013; 23: 602–9.

Lenders JW, Eisenhofer G, Mannelli M, et al. Phaeochromocytoma. *Lancet* 2005; 366: 665–75.

Pacak K, Eisenhofer G, Ahlman H, et al. Pheochromocytoma: Re commendations for clinical practice from the First International Symposium. *Nat Clin Pract Endocrinol Metab* 2007; 3: 92–102.

Speiser PW, Azziz R, Baskin LS, et al. Congenital adrenal hyperplasia due to steroid 21-hydroxylase deficiency; An Endocrine Society clinical practice guideline. *J Clin Endocrinol Metab* 2010; 95: 4133–60.

Terzolo M, Stigliano A, Chiodini I, et al. AME position statement on adrenal incidentaloma. *Eur J Endocrinol* 2011; 164: 851–70.

Young WF. Primary aldosteronism: Renaissance of a syndrome. *Clin Endocrinol* 2007; 66: 607–18.

Zeiger M, Thompson G, Duh QY, et al. American Association of Clinical Endocrinologists and American Association of Endocrine Surgeons medical guidelines for the management of adrenal incidentalomas. *Endocrine Pract* 2009 15(Suppl. 1): 1–20.

6.3 Imaging the adrenal glands

Introduction

Adrenal lesions are frequently identified in routine clinical practice, and pathognomonic imaging features have been established for many of these lesions, including myelolipomas, adenomas, haematomas, and cysts. The majority of adrenal lesions are benign. However, as the adrenal gland is also a frequent site for metastastic disease, distinguishing between benign and malignant masses on imaging is essential. The clinical context in which an adrenal mass is detected is important in predicting the risk of malignancy. Based on pathological studies, about 6% of patients over 60 years of age harbour an adrenal adenoma. Of these, 80% of are benign. Adrenal masses are also frequently discovered during imaging performed for staging of patients with cancer. The incidence of adrenal masses increases to 9%–13% in patients with a known underlying malignancy. The adrenal gland is a relatively frequent site for metastatic disease but, even in patients with a known carcinoma, only 26%–36% of adrenal masses are metastatic. This incidence of metastatic adrenal lesions increases to 71% if the adrenal mass is larger than 4 cm and demonstrates an increase in size on follow-up imaging within 1 year.

CT and MRI have a pivotal role in both detection and characterization of adrenal lesions. In functional adrenal disease, clinical and biochemical findings are vital for interpreting the imaging findings. This section describes characteristic imaging features of common adrenal lesions and the application of modern imaging techniques in evaluating adrenal masses.

Incidentally detected adrenal mass

See also Section 6.9. Incidentally detected adrenal masses in patients with no known malignancy occur in 6% of all abdominal CT examinations.

The important questions to answer before a suitable management plan can be made is whether the lesion is functioning or non-functioning and whether it is benign or malignant. Function is clinically and biochemically established, whilst benign adrenal masses such as lipid-rich adenomas, myelolipomas, adrenal cysts, and adrenal haemorrhage have pathognomonic cross-sectional imaging appearances (see Figures 6.6–6.9).

The nature of incidentally detected adrenal masses can be determined with a high degree of accuracy using CT and MRI alone. FDG PET is also increasingly used in clinical practice, for characterizing incidentally detected lesions. CT and MRI techniques are optimized to maximize specificity for benign adrenal adenomas whilst still maintaining an acceptable sensitivity. Conversely, PET techniques are optimized for detection of malignant disease.

A small minority of adrenal masses elude precise characterization on cross-sectional imaging and remain indeterminate. These are usually some lipid-poor adenomas, adrenal metastases, adrenal carcinomas, and phaeochromocytomas.

CT

Lesion size and contour

On non-enhanced CT, the likelihood of malignancy increases with lesion size, irregular lesion margins and appearance, and a temporal increase in size. Lesions greater than 4 cm in diameter have a higher likelihood of being either metastases or primary adrenal carcinomas. Rapid change in size raises the suspicion of malignancy, as adenomas are slow-growing lesions.

Guidelines published by the American College of Radiology (the Incidentally Detected Abdominal and Pelvic Lesions Committee) suggest that, for lesions that are >4 cm in size and do not have typical imaging features, such as those seen in benign lesions, adrenal resection without any other additional imaging workup should be considered, once biochemical evaluation to exclude phaeochromocytomas has been performed. The same guidelines also controversially suggest that, in patients who have no history of prior malignancy and present with a <4 cm adrenal mass with benign imaging features, a follow-up in 6–12 months is adequate, and no additional imaging is required. In the author's experience, other confirmatory features of a benign lesion are needed before this guideline can always be safely applied.

Intracellular lipid content of the adrenal mass

The majority (>70%) of adenomas have a high intracellular lipid content which lowers their non-contrast CT

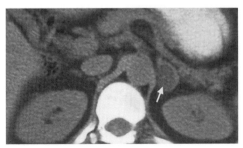

Fig 6.6 Lipid-rich adenoma. Non-contrast CT image. An incidentally detected, left-sided, homogenous adrenal mass is arrowed. The attenuation value of the non-contrast image is 5 HU, in keeping with a benign, lipid-rich adrenal adenoma.

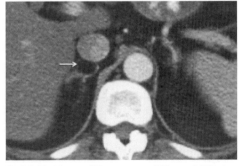

Fig 6.7 Myelolipoma. CT image acquired 60 seconds following intravenous contrast media injection. A homogenous, right-sided adrenal mass with a fat density similar to that of retroperitoneal fat, and an attenuation value of −25 HU, in keeping with a myelolipoma (arrowed).

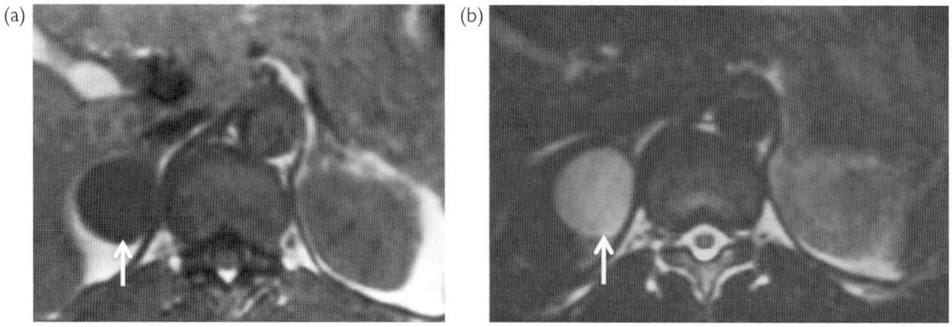

(a)

(b)

Fig 6.8 Adrenal cyst. (a) Axial T1-weighted MRI. A well-defined, low-signal, homogenous right adrenal mass is demonstrated (arrow). The signal intensity is similar to that of cerebrospinal fluid, in keeping with a fluid-filled mass. (b) Axial T2-weighted MRI. The mass (arrowed) has a uniform, featureless, high-T2 signal intensity. No internal architecture is present. The appearances are typical for an adrenal cyst.

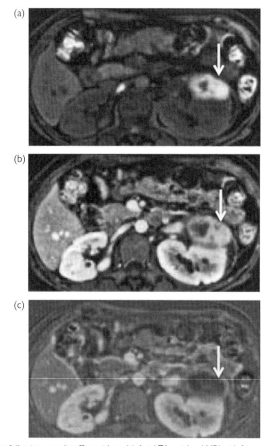

(a)

(b)

(c)

Fig 6.9 Adrenal haemorrhage following a road traffic accident. (a) Axial T1-weighted MRI with fat saturation. A left adrenal mass with high signal intensity indicating blood is shown by the arrow. The blood may indicate haemorrhage related to trauma alone or within an underlying mass. To distinguish between these, post contrast enhanced images are acquired. (b) Axial T1-weighted MRI with fat saturation and gadolinium enhancement: the lesion is indicated with an arrow. (c) An axial subtracted image: the lesion is indicated with an arrow. Subtraction images of post and pre-gadolinium images are required to identify areas of enhancing solid tissue. In this patient, no underlying enhancing tissue is seen. The blood is therefore secondary to trauma alone. Follow-up in 3 months showed resolution of the haemorrhage.

density and hence their Hounsfield attenuation value. If an adrenal mass measures 0 HU or less, the specificity of the mass being a benign lipid-rich adenoma is 100% but the sensitivity is only an unacceptable 47%. If a threshold attenuation value of 10 HU is adopted, specificity is 98% and sensitivity increases to a clinically acceptable 71%. Therefore, 10 HU is the most widely used threshold value for the diagnosis of a lipid-rich adrenal adenoma.

Lesions with a non-contrast CT attenuation greater than 10 HU require further evaluation with contrast-washout CT, MRI, or scintigraphy.

Contrast-enhancement and contrast-washout characteristics
On non-contrast enhanced CT, up to 12%–30% of benign adenomas have an attenuation value of greater than 10 HU and are considered lipid poor. Malignant lesions and phaeochromocytomas are also lipid poor. Characterization of adrenal masses using contrast-enhanced CT relies on the unique physiological perfusion patterns of adenomas. Adenomas enhance rapidly after intravenous iodine-based contrast administration and demonstrate a rapid washout of contrast medium—a phenomenon termed contrast-enhancement washout. Both lipid-rich and lipid-poor adenomas behave similarly, as this property of adenomas is independent of their lipid content (see Figure 6.10). Malignant lesions and phaeochromocytomas enhance rapidly but demonstrate a slower washout of contrast medium (see Figure 6.11).

These contrast-medium enhancement-washout values are only applicable to relatively homogeneous masses without large areas of necrosis or haemorrhage.

The percentage of absolute contrast-enhancement washout (ACEW) can be calculated thus:

$$ACEW = \frac{CECT - DCT}{CT - NCCT} \times 100,$$

where CT is the CT attenuation value of the mass, in Hounsfield units, 60 seconds after commencement of intravenous contrast administration; CECT is the contrast-enhanced CT attenuation value of the mass, in Hounsfield units, 60 seconds after commencement of intravenous contrast administration; DCT is the delayed attenuation value, which is the attenuation value of the mass, in Hounsfield units, 15 minutes after the commencement of contrast administration; and NCCT is the non-contrast CT attenuation, that is, the attenuation value of the mass prior to administration of contrast media.

An absolute contrast-enhancement washout of 60% or higher has a sensitivity of 86%–88% and a specificity of 92%–96% for the diagnosis of an adenoma.

A non-contrast CT attenuation value of 0 HU or lower is specific for adenomas and supersedes the contrast washout characteristics. Phaeochromocytomas may cause confusion as they may rarely be of sufficiently low attenuation (1.8–42.0 HU) on non-contrast-enhanced CT to be mistaken for adenomas and show contrast washout profiles similar to adenomas. Therefore, if there is doubt, a phaeochromocytoma should be excluded by clinical and biochemical evaluation.

MRI
On conventional T1 and T2 images, MRI may allow differentiation of benign from malignant adrenal masses on the basis of signal intensity differences. Metastases and carcinomas in general have higher fluid content due to necrosis than adenomas do and therefore are of higher

(a)
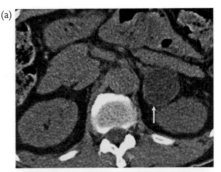

(b)
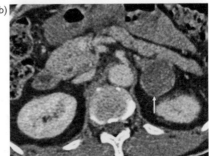

(c)
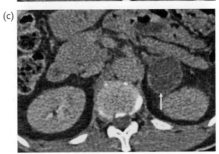

Fig 6.10 Adrenal adenoma contrast washout properties. (a) Non-contrast CT image showing a left adrenal mass (arrowed). (b) Post-contrast CT image 60 seconds following contrast administration; the mass is arrowed. (c) Post-contrast CT image 15 minutes following contrast administration; the mass (arrowed) has a non-contrast attenuation of 15 HU. This mass requires contrast washout characterization. At 60 seconds, the attenuation value was 75 HU and, at 15 minutes, it was 22 HU. This provides an absolute washout of 88% consistent with a benign, lipid-poor adenoma.

signal intensity on T2-weighted images than the surrounding normal adrenal gland. Adenomas are homogeneously iso- or hypo-intense compared with the normal adrenal gland. However, considerable overlap exists between the signal intensities of adenomas and metastases, and up to a third of lesions remain indeterminate.

The accuracy in differentiating benign from malignant masses can be improved by using intravenous gadolinium injection and T1-weighted sequences. After gadolinium enhancement, 90% of adenomas demonstrate homogeneous or ring enhancement, while 60% of malignant masses have heterogeneous enhancement. However,

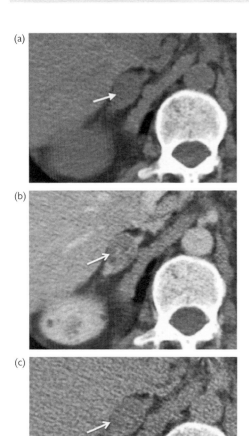

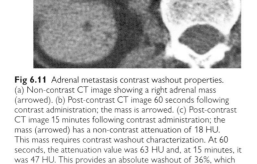

Fig 6.11 Adrenal metastasis contrast washout properties. (a) Non-contrast CT image showing a right adrenal mass (arrowed). (b) Post-contrast CT image 60 seconds following contrast administration; the mass is arrowed. (c) Post-contrast CT image 15 minutes following contrast administration; the mass (arrowed) has a non-contrast attenuation of 18 HU. This mass requires contrast washout characterization. At 60 seconds, the attenuation value was 63 HU and, at 15 minutes, it was 47 HU. This provides an absolute washout of 36%, which is consistent with a non-adenomatous mass. The mass was present in a patient with renal cell carcinoma and preoperatively characterized as a metastasis. The assessment was histologically confirmed after resection.

as with signal characteristics alone, there is considerable overlap in enhancement characteristics of benign and malignant masses, limiting its clinical application.

Chemical-shift imaging

Chemical-shift imaging relies on the fact that, within a magnetic field, protons in water molecules oscillate or precess at a slightly different frequency than the protons

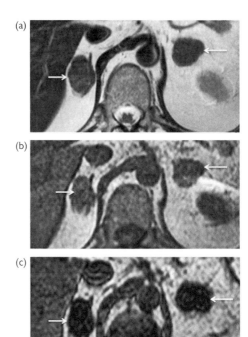

Fig 6.12 Chemical shift imaging in a benign adenoma. (a) Axial T2 MRI. Bilateral adrenal masses are arrowed. Both have a homogenous, low T2 signal intensity suggestive of adenomas. (b) Axial T1 in-phase MRI. The bilateral adrenal masses are arrowed. (c) Axial T1 out-phase MRI; the bilateral adrenal masses are arrowed. The in-phase and out-phase images demonstrate visual loss-of-signal intensity in both adrenal masses. The homogenous loss-of-signal intensity is consistent with benign adrenal adenomas.

in lipid molecules do. By selecting appropriate sequencing parameters, separate images can be acquired with the water and fat protons oscillating in phase and out of phase to each other. On in-phase images, the signal of water plus fat protons is additive. On out-of-phase images, the image is derived from the difference of the signal intensities of water and fat protons. Therefore, adenomas which contain intracellular lipid lose signal intensity on out-of-phase images compared to in-phase images, whereas malignant lesions and pheochromocytomas which lack intracellular lipid remain unchanged.

Simple visual assessment of signal loss is accurate and diagnostically sufficient in most cases but quantitative methods to evaluate the signal loss may be useful in equivocal cases (Figure 6.12).

There are several quantitative ways of assessing the degree of loss of signal intensity including the adrenal-to-splenic ratio and signal-intensity index.

PET

Whole-body FDG PET improves the characterization of malignant adrenal lesions with a high sensitivity in detecting malignant lesions but a specificity ranging between 87%–97%. This loss of specificity is attributable to a small number of adenomas and other benign lesions that mimic high metabolic activity of malignant lesions.

When compared to FDG uptake in the liver, benign adenomas have been shown to have FDG uptake less than, equal to, or more than the liver in 51%, 38%, and 10%, respectively (see Figure 6.13). Non-adenomas have FDG uptake equal to, or more than the liver in 25% and 75%, respectively. However, as 48% of adenomas demonstrate moderate and high FDG, they mimic malignant masses, thereby limiting the role of FDG PET in clinical practice.

Quantitative evaluation using standardized uptake values with a cut-off value of 2.68–3.00 separates malignant from benign adrenal masses with high sensitivity (99%), specificity (92%), positive predictive value (89%), and negative predictive value (99%). When combined, FDG PET and CT data, including contrast-washout characteristics, are analysed, the sensitivity, specificity, positive predictive value, and negative predictive value for malignant adrenal masses improve to 100%, 98%, 97%, and 100%, respectively. False-positive lesions for malignancy encountered at integrated PET–CT include adrenal adenomas, phaeochromocytomas, adrenal endothelial cysts, and inflammatory and infectious lesions. False negatives for malignancy have been reported in adrenal metastases with haemorrhage or necrosis, small (<10 mm) metastatic nodules, and metastases from pulmonary bronchioalveolar carcinoma or carcinoid tumours.

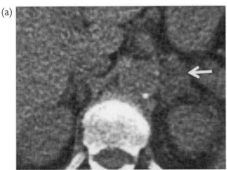

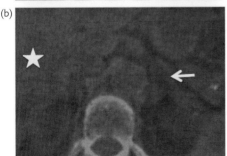

Fig 6.13 PET–CT adenoma. (a) Non-contrast CT image. An enlarged left adrenal gland is arrowed in a patient undergoing staging investigations for oesophageal cancer. The non-contrast CT attenuation was 16 HU. (b) Fused PET–CT image. The ^{18}F-fluorodeoxyglucose-PET tracer uptake in the left adrenal gland (arrowed) is similar to the background uptake of the liver (indicated by the star), consistent with an adenoma.

The specificity of PET can be improved with the use of ^{11}C-metomidate, a marker of 11-beta-hydroxylase, as a tracer for adrenocortical tissue. With this tracer, pheochromocytomas, metastases to the adrenal gland, and non-adrenal cortical masses are all ^{11}C-metomidate-uptake negative. However, the tracer has an increased uptake in both adenomas and adrenocortical carcinomas; hence, it cannot be used to distinguish between these lesions.

Imaging functional disorders of the adrenal gland

In diseases of adrenal dysfunctional, imaging is an adjunct to clinical and biochemical findings. It can be used to identify the lesion site, determine whether lesions are unilateral or bilateral, plan surgical or medical management, and characterize lesions as far as possible. Table 6.5 summarizes the imaging features of common adrenal functional disorders.

Adrenocorticotrophic-hormone-independent Cushing's syndrome
See also Section 6.8.

Adenomas
Hyperfunctioning adrenocorticotrophic-hormone-secreting adenomas, which account for most of the cases of adrenocorticotrophic-hormone-independent Cushing's syndrome, have imaging features similar to other benign adrenal adenomas.

Adrenal carcinoma
Functioning carcinomas are more common in women and children, with resultant Cushing's syndrome or virilization. In adults, 30%–40% of adrenal carcinomas are hyperfunctioning. Carcinomas are highly necrotic and, commonly, adrenal vein invasion, vena cava invasion, adjacent kidney invasion, and/or retroperitoneal invasion is frequently present at the time of presentation. However, incidental carcinomas are detected early, and venous invasion may not be present (see Figure 6.14).

Multiplanar imaging using multidetector CT and MRI allows better assessment of invasion into adjacent structures, which is important for surgical planning. A large mass, high suspicion of malignancy, and surrounding invasion preclude laproscopic adrenelectomy, which may be suitable for benign adenomas.

Adrenocorticotrophic-hormone-dependent Cushing's syndrome
See also Chapter 3, Section 3.7. The majority of cases of adrenocorticotrophic-hormone-dependent Cushing's syndrome are due to a small pituitary adenoma, which can be seen on gadolinium-enhaced MRI. In negative or inconclusive MRI, petrosal venous sampling is necessary to localize the adenoma.

In ectopic production of adrenocorticotrophic hormone, the role of imaging is to locate the source. In approximately 12%–20% of patients, despite repeated biochemical and radiological investigations, the source of the ectopic production may not be identified.

CT of the chest, the abdomen, and the pelvis, with intravenous contrast enhancement, is the most sensitive imaging modality for identifying ectopic sources of adrenocorticotrophic-hormone production and detecting liver and nodal metastases. MRI is useful in resolving equivocal CT findings or where CT is negative

Table 6.5 Common functional adrenal disorders and imaging findings

Condition		Imaging findings
Cushing's syndrome	ACTH: independent: • 95% due to adenoma or carcinoma • large adenomas may be indistinguishable from carcinomas • rarely, primary pigmented nodular hyperplasia or • ACTH-indepenedent macronodular hyperplasia ACTH dependent: • Cushing's disease • ectopic ACTH production	Adenomas are usually lipid rich, have features that are similar to those of other adenomas, and are generally between 2 and 7 cm.
		Carcinomas are unilateral masses, usually >6 cm in size, with necrosis, haemorrhage, fibrosis, and calcification
		On imaging, adrenal glands in PPNAD may be normal or minimally hyperplastic with multiple, cortical nodules. Secondary to pigmentation, the nodules demonstrate lower T1- and T2-signal intensity on MRI, compared to the surrounding atrophic cortical tissue. The nodules do not normally exceed 5 mm but in older patients may be 1–3 cm. Bilateral uptake of ^{131}I-cholesosterol scinitigraphy confirms an adrenal source of cortisol production.
		There is massive bilateral adrenal enlargement, nodularity, and distortion of the adrenal contour, due to the presence of multiple lipid-rich adenomas. Nodules vary in size from 1 cm to 5.5 cm.
		Adrenals usually exhibit nodular or diffuse hyperplasia affecting the entire adrenal gland. The largest glands, usually lobular and nodular, occur when there is an ectopic source.
		Pituitary adenoma on MRI of the pituitary may be seen.
		Carcinoid tumours and small-cell carcinomas of the lung and thymus, medullary carcinoma of the thyroid, pancreatic neuroendocrine neoplasms, neuroblastoma pheochromocytomas, and some benign ovarian tumors may also be seen.
Conn's syndrome	Aldosterone-producing adenoma (aldosteronoma)	Imaging features similar to those of other lipid-rich adenomas may be seen. Size ranges between 1.6 and 5cm, with a median size of 2 cm.
	Bilateral adrenal hyperplasia	Enlargement of the adrenal glands on CT, with the adrenal limb width > 5mm and the adrenal body >1.2 cm, may be seen.
Virilization	Congenital adrenal hyperplasia in children	Gross enlargement of both adrenal glands may be seen on CT and MRI as diffuse or nodular enlargement with preservation of normal adreniform configuration.
	Adenomas and carcinomas in adults	Imaging features similar to those of all other adenomas and carcinomas may be seen.
Medullary hyperfunction	Medullary hyperplasia	On imaging, adrenal glands may be normal or may demonstrate unilateral or bilateral involvement with diffuse or nodular disease. The body of the adrenal glands are most frequently enlarged, with relative preservation of the limbs. Bilateral adrenal MIBG uptake may be present.
	Phaeochromocytoma	Sporadic phaeochromocytomas are large at the time of diagnosis (90% larger than 2 cm), whilst screened lesions are smaller.
		On unenhanced CT, the tumours are soft-tissue masses, are rarely calcified, and demonstrate intense contrast enhancement. Variable degrees of necrosis are present, and the tumours may appear cystic. A peripheral rim of intensely enhancing soft tissue can still be demonstrated in cystic lesions.
		On MRI, most are iso- or hypo-intense compared to the liver on T1-weighted imaging. High T1-weighted signal intensity corresponding to areas of haemorrhage is seen in up to 20% of lesions. On CSI, typical phaeochromocytomas do not show signal-intensity loss on opposed-phase images.
		MIBG uptake is present in most lesions.

Abbreviations: ACTH, adrenocorticotrophic hormone; CSI, chemical-shift imaging; MIBG, metaiodobenzylguanidine; PPNAD, primary pigmented nodular adrenocortical disease.

but a high index of suspicion persists, particularly in the abdomen. In the pancreas, MRI may identify small islet-cell tumours not seen on CT. Overall, two large studies have found ^{111}In-octreotide scintigraphy and whole-body venous sampling generally unhelpful in localizing sources of ectopic adrenocorticotrophic-hormone production. FDG PET has been evaluated and shown to be inferior to CT and MRI in the detection of ectopic sources of adrenocorticotrophic hormone.

Primary hyperaldosteronism (Conn's syndrome)
See also Section 6.4. The causal distinction between an aldosteronoma and bilateral adrenal hyperplasia is crucial, as management of the two causes differs entirely.

CT and MRI are used to differentiate between the two causes after clinical and biochemical confirmation of Conn's syndrome. The small size of aldosteronomas makes their detection challenging. CT has a sensitivity and specificity varying between 88% and 100%, and 33% and 100%, respectively. On CT, if the adrenal-limb width is 5 mm or greater, sensitivity for diagnosing bilateral adrenal hyperplasia is 100% and the specificity is close to 100% (see Figures 6.15 and 6.16).

CT and MRI have a comparative performance in the detection of aldosterone-producing adenomas, with a sensitivity and specificity of 87%–93% and 82%–85% for CT, and 83% and 92% for MRI, respectively. The poor specificity in detection of aldosterone-producing

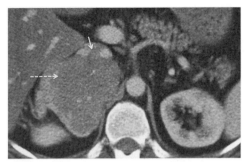

Fig 6.14 Large adrenal carcinoma with vascular invasion. Contrast-enhanced CT image. A large, right, adrenal heterogeneous mass with internal vascularity is seen in this patient with Cushing's syndrome (dashed arrow). The mass demonstrates invasion of the inferior vena cava (arrow), a feature strongly suggestive of a malignant adrenal mass.

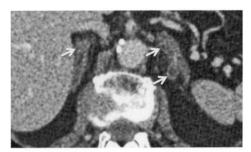

Fig 6.16 Bilateral adrenal hyperplasia. Contrast-enhanced CT image. Both adrenal glands have nodular enlargement (arrows). As the changes are bilateral, the cause of the Conn's is likely to be adrenal hyperplasia.

adenomas is due to concomitant contralateral non-functioning nodules masking small functional adenomas, the presence of unilateral dominant nodules in bilateral adrenal hyperplasia simulating an aldosterone-producing adenoma, and increasing bilateral nodularity with age and hypertension. The sensitivity is limited by small size of aldosterone-producing adenomas, although this should improve with increasing use of thinner adrenal sections (1–2 mm) acquired by multidetector CT. Overall, a high specificity for the detection of aldosterone-producing adenomas is desirable to avert unsuccessful surgery in patients with bilateral adrenal hyperplasia.

Adrenal venous sampling for aldosterone levels is very accurate in preoperative assessment of Conn's syndrome. The accuracy of adrenal venous sampling in lateralizing an aldosterone-producing adenoma exceeds 95% when the procedure is technically successful. As adrenal venous sampling is not without risks, it is used selectively and reserved for patients with:
- normal or equivocal adrenal glands
- the presence of bilateral adrenal nodules, which may either be macronodules of adrenal hyperplasia or mask a unilateral aldosteroma

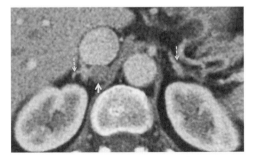

Fig 6.15 Aldosteronoma. Contrast-enhanced CT image from a 45-year-old man presenting with Conn's syndrome. A 1 cm adenoma is seen in the right adrenal medial limb (arrow). The remainder of the right adrenal gland and the left adrenal are normal. The appearances are characteristic of an aldosteronoma.

- there is disagreement between CT and MRI findings or between imaging and biochemical findings

Adrenal venous sampling is essential in these patients, to avoid unnecessary and inappropriate adrenalectomy.

Virilization

The role of imaging lies in detection of surgically resectable sources of androgen excess in the adrenal glands, ovaries, or testes. In young patients, MRI or ultrasound are modalities of choice to avoid ionizing radiation from CT. Adrenal and pelvic venous catherization is reserved for patients in whom uncertainty remains as to the presence of small tumours which cannot be excluded biochemically or on imaging.

Hyperfunctioning adrenomedullary disorders
See also Section 6.14.

Phaeochromocytomas

Once a clinical and biochemical diagnosis of phaeochromocytoma has been made, imaging studies are performed to localize the tumour and to aid surgical planning for resection. Contrast-enhanced CT and MRI are highly accurate in the detection of adrenal phaeochromocytomas, with reported sensitivities of between 93% and 100%, and a positive predictive value exceeding 90% (see Figures 6.17 and 6.18).

The tracer agent metaiodobenzylguanidine (MIBG) is most commonly labelled with [123]iodine (for diagnosis) or [131]iodine (for treatment) for whole-body scintigraphy in the detection and localization of primary and metastatic paragangliomas. The sensitivity of MIBG scintigraphy is reported to be between 87% and 90%, lower than both CT and MRI, as the detection of lesions depends on the ability of the tumours to take up the tracer. However, the strength of MIBG is its high specificity, which exceeds 90%.

Patients with a phaeochromocytoma may have more than one tumour in the adrenal glands or in ectopic locations. The commonest sites of extra-adrenal paragangliomas are the para-aortic region at the level of the renal hila (46%), the organ of Zuckerkandl (29%), the thoracic paraspinal region (10%), the bladder (10%) and the head and neck (2%–4%). Owing to the superior tissue contrast and tissue characterization obtained with MRI, the sensitivity of MRI has been shown to be equivalent or better than CT in the demonstration of extra-adrenal paragangliomas. In addition to tissue characterization, MRI

(a)

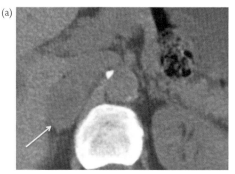

(b)

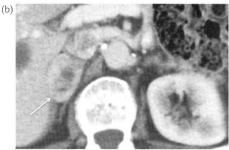

Fig 6.17 Phaeochromocytoma. (a) Non-contrast CT image demonstrating a right adrenal mass (arrowed) with an attenuation value of 20 HU. (b) Contrast-enhanced CT image showing the right adrenal mass (arrowed) enhancing avidly and heterogeneously with areas of necrosis. These appearances, in the presence of a biochemically suspected phaeochromocytoma, would be confirmatory.

(a)

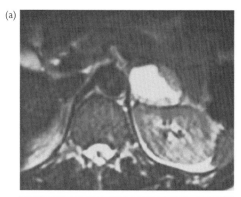

(b)

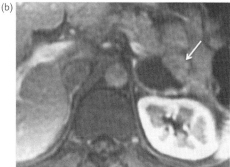

(c)

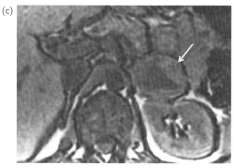

Fig 6.18 Phaeochromocytoma. (a) Axial T2-weighted MRI showing a partly solid cystic mass. There is cystic, high T2 signal intensity centrally and solid, peripheral intermediate-signal-intensity tissue. (b) Post-gadolinium-enhanced T1-weighted image with fat saturation. The peripheral areas of solid tissue (arrowed) demonstrate enhancement, distinguishing the mass from a simple cyst. Phaeochromocytomas retain at least some solid tissue. (c) Out-phase T1-weighted image showing no loss of signal intensity in the solid areas (arrowed), excluding an adenoma and consistent with a phaeochromocytoma.

is useful in problem areas such as the spinal cord and the bladder wall, for intra-cardiac tumours, and for tumours adjacent to the inferior vena cava, the internal jugular vein, and the carotid arteries. MRI shows excellent natural contrast on T2-weighted images between the hyperintense paraganglioma and the hypo-intense flowing blood.

The choice of initial imaging modality in a patient suspected of having a phaeochromocytoma depends on the institutional expertise with CT, MRI, and MIBG scintigraphy. Unlike CT and MRI, MIBG scintigraphy is inherently a whole-body imaging modality with the advantage of simultaneously detecting extra-adrenal locations of tracer uptake in metastasis or extra-adrenal paragangliomas. CT and MRI have similar levels of sensitivity and specificity. They have the advantage of concurrently detecting associated tumours (pancreatic tumours, renal cell carcinoma, neurofibromata, thyroid carcinoma, extra-adrenal paragangliomas) in patients with neuroendocrine syndromes. The multiplanar abilities of MRI and multidetector CT imaging are very useful in the surgical planning for resection of phaeochromocytomas and extra-adrenal paragangliomas.

PET–CT has been evaluated in localizing phaeochromocytomas, when cross-sectional imaging and MIBG scintigraphy are negative but a phaeochromocytoma is biochemically suspected. Different PET tracers have been used, including ^{11}C-hydroxyephedrine, ^{11}C-epinephrine, ^{18}F-fluorodopamine (FDA), and ^{18}F-fluorodihydroxyphenylalanine. The most reliable has

been shown to be FDA, which can localize adrenal and extraadrenal lesions, including metastatic lesions. FDG PET displays a relatively low sensitivity (70%) and therefore is not recommended for the initial diagnostic evaluation. Nonetheless, it can be useful for a metastatic lesions.

Despite encouraging data, the cost and availability of PET, particularly FDA PET, limits its application to specialized centres only.

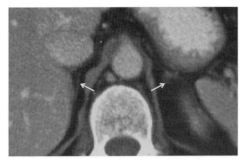

Fig 6.19 Autoimmune adrenal atrophy. Contrast-enhanced CT image. Both adrenal glands (arrowed) are small and barely visible on thin-slice CT imaging. These appearances are typical for chronic adrenal atrophy, of which autoimmune atrophy is the commonest cause in the Western world.

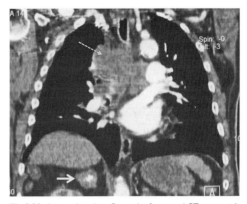

Fig 6.20 Acute adrenalitis. Coronal reformatted CT image with contrast enhancement. A large mediastinal and right hilar nodal mass is demonstrated by the dashed arrow. The right adrenal gland (block arrow) is enlarged with calcification but maintains the adreniform contour. These appearances are suggestive of an acute adrenalitis. In the patient, TB was confirmed in the mediastinal nodes, and the adrenal enlargement resolved following treatment for TB.

Adrenal hypofunction (Addison's disease)

See also Section 6.11.

Primary adrenal hypofunction

Primary adrenal hypofunction can either be the result of Addison's disease (primary adrenal insufficiency) or be secondary to hypothalamo-pituitary adrenocorticotrophic-hormone deficiency. The acquired causes of primary adrenal hypofunction include autoimmune disease, infection (e.g. TB, AIDS, cytomegalovirus, histoplasmosis), drugs, adrenal haemorrhage, Waterhouse–Friderichsen syndrome, metastatic disease, sarcoidosis, amyloidosis, and haemochromatosis. Autoimmune disease is the most common cause in the Western countries, accounting for 68%–94% of primary adrenocortical failure. Worldwide, TB of the adrenal glands remains the commonest cause of adrenal insufficiency.

On imaging, autoimmune adrenal disease results in often barely discernable, atrophic, non-calcified adrenal glands (see Figure 6.19).

Adrenal hypofunction present for less than 2 years is defined as subacute Addison's disease and is usually a result of adrenalitis. Imaging plays an important role in evaluating these cases. Typically, in untreated adrenalitis the adrenal glands are enlarged and may demonstrate central necrosis and rim enhancement. These features are not typical of any one pathogen, and adrenal biopsy may be required to distinguish between the causes of adrenalitis (e.g. TB, histoplasmosis, and other fungal infections). In acute adrenal TB, bilateral adrenal enlargement is seen in 91% of cases. This can be mass-like, and calcification is seen in up to 59%. Peripheral rim enhancement is seen in 47% of patients (see Figure 6.20). After successful treatment, 88% of enlarged glands decrease or return to normal size and configuration. Calcification in atrophic adrenal glands is most often seen in granulomatous diseases (TB, histoplasmosis, and sarcoidosis). However, calcification in adrenal glands is not pathognomonic for granulomatous adrenalitis and is indistinguishable from calcification due to previous haemorrhage.

Conclusion

Adrenal imaging has become increasingly important in the assessment of incidental adrenal masses and is an essential adjunct to clinical and biochemical findings in the evaluation and management of adrenal dysfunction. CT remains the mainstay of cross-sectional adrenal imaging. MRI is increasingly favoured in patients unable to undergo CT, in children, and in patients being screened for adrenal tumours. The majority of adrenal pathologies have characteristic imaging features. However, in a small number of masses, there is an overlap of benign and malignant disease. Emerging technologies such as PET CT add to the radiologist's armamentarium to distinguishing between benign and malignant masses. Close collaboration is required between the endocrinologists and radiologist to obtain the correct diagnosis and to select the most appropriate imaging strategy.

Further reading

Bhatia KS, Ismail MM, Sahdev A, et al. 123 I-metaiodobenzylguanidine (MIBG) scintigraphy for the detection of adrenal and extra-adrenal phaeochromocytomas: CT and MRI correlation. *Clin Endocrinol* 2008; 69: 181–8.

Boland GW, Blake MA, Holalkere NS, et al. PET/CT for the characterization of adrenal masses in patients with cancer: Qualitative versus quantitative accuracy in 150 consecutive patients. *Am J Roentgenol* 2009; 192: 956–62.

Boland GW, Lee MJ, Gazelle GS, et al. Characterization of adrenal masses using unenhanced CT: An analysis of the CT literature. *Am J Roentgenol* 1998; 171: 201–4.

Bovio S, Cataldi A, Reimondo G, et al. Prevalence of adrenal incidentaloma in a contemporary computerized tomography series. *J Endocrinol Invest* 2006; 29: 298–302.

Francis IR, Casalino DD, Arellano RS, et al. ACR appropriateness criteria: Incidentally discovered adrenal mass. Available at http://www.acr.org/SecondaryMainMenuCategories/quality_safety/app_criteria/pdf/ExpertPanelonUrologicImaging/IncidentallyDiscoveredAdrenalMassDoc7.aspx (accessed 20 Feb 2012).

Frilling A, Tecklenborg K, Weber F, et al. Importance of adrenal incidentaloma in patients with a history of malignancy. *Surgery* 2004; 136: 1289–96.

Hennings J, Lindhe O, Bergstrom M, et al. [11C]metomidate positron emission tomography of adrenocortical tumors in correlation with histopathological findings. *J Clin Endocrinol Metab* 2006; 91: 1410–4.

Kaltsas GA, Mukherjee JJ, Kola B, et al. Is ovarian and adrenal venous catheterization and sampling helpful in the investigation of hyperandrogenic women? *Clin Endocrinol (Oxf)* 2003; 59: 34–43.

Lingam RK, Sohaib SA, Rockall AG, et al. Diagnostic performance of CT versus MR in detecting aldosterone-producing adenoma in primary hyperaldosteronism (Conn's syndrome). *Eur Radiol* 2004; 14: 1787–92.

Pena CS, Boland GW, Hahn PF, et al. Characterization of indeterminate (lipid-poor) adrenal masses: Use of washout characteristics at contrast-enhanced CT. *Radiology* 2000; 217: 798–802.

Sahdev A, Sohaib A, Monson JP, et al. CT and MR imaging of unusual locations of extra-adrenal paragangliomas. *Eur Radiol* 2005; 15: 85–92.

Sohaib SA, Peppercorn PD, Allan C, et al. Primary hyperaldosteronism (Conn syndrome): MR imaging findings. *Radiology* 2000; 214: 527–31.

Vincent JM, Trainer PJ, Reznek RH, et al. The radiological investigation of occult ectopic ACTH-dependent Cushing's syndrome. *Clin Radiol* 1993; 48: 11–17.

Yang ZG, Guo YK, Li Y, et al. Differentiation between tuberculosis and primary tumors in the adrenal gland: Evaluation with contrast-enhanced CT. *Eur Radiol* 2006; 16: 2031–6.

6.4 Primary aldosteronism

Definition

Mineralocorticoid hypertension is characterized by an excess mineralocorticoid activity, which in the presence of high sodium intake (e.g. greater than 6.3 g (133 mEq) NaCl per day) induces sodium retention, water retention, and potassium loss, with ensuing high blood pressure, blunting of renin secretion, and hypokalaemia. Mineralocorticoid hypertension is a highly prevalent form of high blood pressure and can be due to several causes, some of which are rare and some, such as primary aldosteronism, much more common (Box 6.1). This section is meant to provide updated information on the diagnosis and treatment of mineralocorticoid hypertension, with particular emphasis on the most common cause of primary aldosteronism.

Pathophysiology

Due to the underlying pathophysiology, a low or undetectable plasma renin is the hallmark of mineralocorticoid hypertension (see Figure 6.21). In primary aldosteronism, there is increased aldosterone secretion, which is held to be autonomous of the renin–angiotensin system. In the other forms of aldosteronism, excess activation of the mineralocorticoid receptor leads, via aldosterone-independent mechanisms, to the suppression of renin and blunted aldosterone secretion.

Regardless of the cause, excess activation of the mineralocorticoid receptor, along with high blood pressure, damages the cardiovascular system. This damage can ultimately cause atrial fibrillation, ischaemic and/or haemorrhagic stroke, 'flash' pulmonary oedema, myocardial infarction, and heart failure.

Early identification of mineralocorticoid hypertension, followed by diagnosis of its subtypes and treatment with surgery and/or specific medical treatment (Box 6.1), is, therefore, of paramount importance to avoid these harmful consequences to the heart, arterial wall, and kidneys, which can ultimately translate into cardiovascular events.

Prevalence

Data on the prevalence of mineralocorticoid hypertension are scant, mainly because the border between mineralocorticoid hypertension and low-renin essential hypertension is uncertain, prospective studies are lacking, and evidence is therefore, at best, anecdotal. By contrast, data on prevalence of primary aldosteronism are more abundant and altogether show that (i) primary aldosteronism is much more common than usually held, and (ii) most cases are found in normokalaemic patients. This implies that hypokalaemia is not a *sine qua non* of the disease; thus, if the search strategy for primary aldosteronism is limited to hypertensive patients who are hypokalaemic, the diagnosis may be missed in many patients. This might explain why primary aldosteronism has been considerably under-diagnosed, and therefore its prevalence underestimated in patients with hypertension (Rossi, 2011).

The first large prospective survey designed to provide solid data on the prevalence of primary aldosteronism showed that primary aldosteronism is involved in more than 11% of consecutive patients newly diagnosed with hypertension and referred to hypertension centres. About half of these patients were found to have a surgically curable subtype (Box 6.1), which renders primary aldosteronism the most common curable endocrine form of hypertension in referred patients with hypertension.

Clinical features and investigations

According to the 2008 Endocrine Society guidelines, screening for primary aldosteronism is mandatory in the categories of patients (Box 6.2), because they have a higher pretest probability of primary aldosteronism, particularly if they have resistant hypertension and are candidates for adrenalectomy, as these patients can benefit most (Funder et al., 2008). However, the more recently released Endocrine Society practice guidelines and most experts favour a wide screening strategy for primary aldosteronism, such as testing all newly presenting patients with hypertension. This proposal stands on the high prevalence of primary aldosteronism, and on the beneficial effects of an early diagnosis followed by specific treatment. Implementation of this broad strategy is, however, controversial, because many feel that it could be too challenging for the healthcare systems of many countries.

Box 6.1 Mineralocorticoid hypertension

Primary aldosteronism

Surgically not curable:
- bilateral adrenal hyperplasia
- unilateral aldosterone-producing adenoma with bilateral adrenal hyperplasia
- familial types (see Chapter 6, Section 6.5), including type 1 hyperaldosteronism (also known as glucocorticoid-remediable aldosteronism)

Surgically curable:
- aldosterone-producing adenoma (aldosteronoma)
  unilateral
  bilateral
- primary unilateral adrenal hyperplasia
- multinodular unilateral adrenocortical hyperplasia
- ovary aldosterone-secreting tumour
- familial type 2 hyperaldosteronism
- familial type 3 hyperaldosteronism (*KCNJ5* potassium channel germinal mutations)
- aldosterone-producing adenoma or bilateral adrenal hyperplasia with concomitant phaeochromocytoma
- aldosterone-producing carcinoma

Apparent mineralocorticoid excess

- loss-of-function genetic variants of beta-hydroxysteroid dehydrogenase type 2
- chronic abuse of liquorice, glycerrithinic acid, carbenoxolone
- use of topic preparations containing alpha-F-steroids

Liddle syndrome

- Beta or gamma mutations in epithelial sodium channels

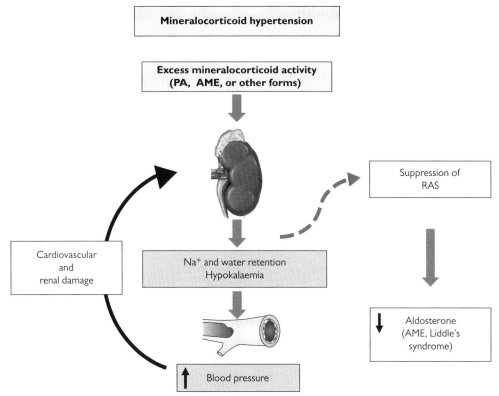

Fig 6.21 Pathophysiology of mineralocorticoid hypertension; AME, apparent mineralocorticoid excess; PA, primary aldosteronism; RAS, renin–angiotensin system.

The first step for diagnosing mineralocorticoid hypertension requires the demonstration of a plasma renin level (measured as plasma renin activity or direct active renin concentration, DRC) that is disproportionately low in relation to sodium intake and does not respond to stimulation (see Figure 6.22). The second step is to measure the plasma aldosterone concentration, which is crucial to differentiate primary aldosteronism from apparent mineralocorticoid excess: excess aldosterone levels with low renin strongly suggest primary aldosteronism, whilst a low plasma aldosterone concentration indicates apparent mineralocorticoid excess or Liddle syndrome.

On the basis of this premise, use of the aldosterone-to-renin ratio has been introduced as a simplified approach to the detection of primary aldosteronism. The proper use of this ratio requires consideration of a range of issues (Table 6.6): the aldosterone-to-renin ratio value depends on the plasma aldosterone concentration and levels of renin, which means that very different plasma aldosterone concentrations and renin values can produce the same ratio. Moreover, even when the plasma aldosterone concentration is normal, a suppressed renin value will increase the aldosterone-to-renin ratio. Both the plasma renin activity and direct active renin concentration assay lose their precision when the levels of renin are low. Because of this, the

---

Box 6.2 Clinical features associated with an increased likelihood of primary aldosteronism

The following clinical features are associated with an increased likelihood of primary aldosteronism:
- resistant hypertension
- Grade 2 or 3 hypertension
- spontaneous or diuretic-induced hypokalaemia
- incidentally discovered, apparently non-functioning adrenal mass (incidentaloma)
- early onset (juvenile) hypertension and/or stroke (occurring at <50 years of age)

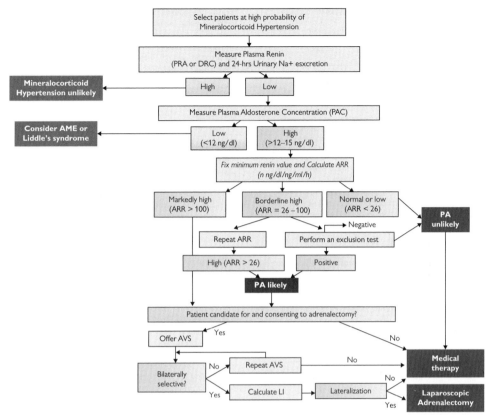

Fig 6.22 Diagnostic workup of mineralocorticoid hypertension (MH) and primary aldosteronism. The discovery of a low renin level, which does not respond to stimulation, is a strong clue to the presence of a form of MH. The finding of low plasma aldosterone is a hint to the presence of apparent mineralocorticoid excess syndrome or a genetic tubular defect, such as Liddle's syndrome, causing excess tubular sodium reabsorption. Clinical prescreening to identify patients with a high pretest probability of primary aldosteronism should be followed by tests to identify excess aldosterone secretion and to determine the cause (unilateral or bilateral). The screening tests carry a high false-positive rate. Tests aimed at identification of instances of false-positive results are useful to exclude, the diagnosis of primary aldosteronism. Because such tests have limitations, which follow from the existence of many patients with angiotensin II-dependent idiopathic hyperaldosteronism and aldosterone-producing adenoma, in patients with a considerably increased ARR, we repeat the ARR and/or perform a captopril test after sodium repletion. We then proceed to subtyping only if the ARR is confirmed to be raised. AVS, adrenal venous sampling; DRC, direct active renin concentration; LI, lateralized index; PA, primary aldosteronism; PRA, plasma renin activity. Adapted from *Endocrinology and Metabolism Clinics of North America*, Volume 40, Issue 2, Rossi GP, Diagnosis and Treatment of Primary Aldosteronism, pp. 313–332, Copyright (2011) with permission from Elsevier.

lowest renin value to be included in the calculation of the ratio should be fixed at a minimum (which is 0.2 ng/mL per hour for plasma renin activity and 0.36 ng/mL for direct active renin; Rossi, 2011). This precaution avoids over inflating the aldosterone-to-renin ratio when levels of renin are very low, as in the elderly and in people of African origin. The combination of an increased aldosterone-to-renin ratio and a plasma aldosterone concentration >15 ng/dL (416 pmol/L), rather than the aldosterone-to-renin ratio alone, should therefore be used to detect patients with primary aldosteronism.

In the PAPY study, the optimal cut-off for the aldosterone-to-renin ratio, corresponding to a sensitivity of 81% and a specificity of 85%, was found to be 26 ((ng/dL)/(ng/mL per hour)). However, the aldosterone-to-renin ratio carries quantitative information: a markedly

high value, for example, one greater than 100, is a strong indication that the patient has primary aldosteronism and an exclusion test adds nothing in terms of diagnostic accuracy; as recently shown for the captopril test (Maiolino, et al. 2017). Values of the aldosterone-to-renin ratio that are less raised (e.g. between 26 and 100) should be confirmed at retesting, and also regarded as a clue of the presence of primary aldosteronism.

The most crucial step in screening for primary aldosteronism is a careful preparation of the patient, both in terms of drugs and in terms of conditions for the testing (Table 6.7). Most antihypertensive drugs affect plasma aldosterone concentration, renin values, or both, and thereby the aldosterone-to-renin ratio. Therefore, treatment must be properly modified before measuring the levels of aldosterone and renin. The alpha-1-receptor

Table 6.6 Suggestions for the correct use of the aldosterone-to-renin ratio as a screening test

Factors affecting the aldosterone-to-renin ratio	Suggestion
Serum levels of potassium	Correct hypokalaemia, if present, before performing the test.
PAC	A high PAC might originate from low salt intake or use of diuretics. Thus, prepare the patient with adequate salt intake and measure the 24-hour urinary sodium excretion to estimate sodium intake. Withdraw diuretics at least 3–4 weeks (and mineralocorticoid-receptor antagonists at least 6 weeks) before testing.
Renin assay	Because of the low precision of the PRA or DRC assay for low renin values, fix the lowest level of renin to be used in the aldosterone-to-renin ratio.
Patient position and blood sampling	Standardize the position of the patient and sampling conditions at your centre.
Handling of the samples	Handling and storage of plasma samples differ for PRA and DRC assays.
Drugs	The alpha-1-receptor blocker doxazosin and long-acting calcium channel blockers are allowed.
Accuracy of the aldosterone-to-renin ratio	The cut-off value that provides the best combination of sensitivity and specificity should be identified at each centre by ROC curves and Youden index analysis.

Abbreviations: PAC, plasma aldosterone concentration; PRA, plasma renin activity; DRC, direct active renin concentration; ROC, receiver operating characteristic.

blocker doxazosin and the long-acting calcium channel blockers have negligible effects on the aldosterone-to-renin ratio, and therefore can be used alone or in combination to control blood pressure during screening in patients in whom interrupting antihypertensive treatment could be harmful, such as in those with severe and/or resistant hypertension, and/or with evidence of target organ damage or previous cardiovascular events. When the patient needs a stronger treatment than these agents, knowledge of the effects of the different drugs on the aldosterone-to-renin ratio and its components can enable a clinician to confirm or exclude the diagnosis of primary aldosteronism.

As regards the conditions for testing, the patients should be investigated in the morning after they have being resting supine, or sitting quietly, for 1 hour. Prior or concomitant measurement of the serum levels of potassium is helpful to exclude hypokalaemia, which, if present, reduces aldosterone secretion and can lead to false-negative results. A 24-hour collection of urine to measure urinary sodium excretion provides an assessment of the electrolyte intake, which is essential for a correct interpretation of renin and aldosterone values, given the well-known inverse relationship between plasma renin, or aldosterone, and sodium intake.

Exclusion of primary aldosteronism

The screening tests often give false positive results that must be identified and excluded before selecting the patient for adrenal vein sampling (Figure 6.21). To identify such false-positive cases, the guidelines recommend performing a 'confirmatory' test, which includes the oral sodium-loading test, the saline-infusion test, the

Table 6.7 Effects of drugs and conditions

Factor	PAC	Renin	ARR	False-positive rate	False-negative rate
Medications					
Beta blockers	↓	↓↓	↑	↑↑	↓
Central alpha-2 agonists	↓	↓↓	↑	↑	↓
NSAIDs	↓	↓↓	↑	↑	↓
Potassium-losing diuretics	↑	↑↑	↓	↓	↑
Potassium-sparing diuretics	↑	↑↑	↓	↓	↑
Angiotensin-converting enzyme inhibitors	↓	↑↑	↓	↓	↑
Angiotensin 2-receptor blockers	↓	↑↑	↓	↓	↑
Long-acting calcium channel blockers	→↓	→	↓	→↓	→↑
Renin inhibitors	↓	↓↑*	↓*↑*	↓*↑*	↓*↑*
Potassium status					
Hypokalaemia	↓	→↑	↓	↓	↑
Potassium loading	↑	→↑	↑	↑	↓
Sodium status					
Sodium depletion	↑	↑↑	↓	↓	↑
Sodium loading	↓	↓↓	↑	↑	↓
Ageing	↓	↓↓	↑	↑	↓

Abbreviations: ARR, aldosterone-to-renin ratio; DRC, direct active renin concentration; PAC, plasma aldosterone concentration; plasma renin activity, plasma renin activity.

Note: Beta blockers reduce levels of renin but affect PAC relatively less, thus raising the ARR; therefore, it is better to stop administering them at least 3–4 weeks before the assay, as failure to do so increases the false-positive rate. Drugs that raise the PRA more than PAC, such as diuretics and mineralocorticoid receptor antagonists, should be withdrawn (at least 3–4 and 6 weeks before, respectively), to reduce the rate of false-negative diagnoses. Angiotensin-converting enzyme inhibitors, angiotensin 2-receptor blockers, and renin inhibitors raise renin and reduce aldosterone secretion. Therefore, they reduce the ARR and markedly increase the false-negative rate. Because of this, they also should be withdrawn at least 3–4 weeks before performing the ARR.

*Renin inhibitors lower PRA but raise DRC. This effect would be expected to increase false positives when renin is measured as PRA, and false negatives for renin measured as DRC.

captopril-challenge test, and the fludrocortisone-with-salt-loading test. Unfortunately, aldosterone secretion is dependent on angiotensin in many patients with primary aldosteronism, who show suppression of aldosterone after blunting the levels of renin. Therefore, relying on these tests can lead to missing the diagnosis in several patients with primary aldosteronism; because of this limitation, once a markedly raised aldosterone-to-renin ratio (e.g. >100) has been found, we prefer to proceed directly with adrenal vein sampling if the patient is willing to pursue a surgical cure and is a reasonable candidate for general anaesthesia and surgery. This strategy is supported by results of a very large study by Maiolino et al. Therefore, it can be wise to confirm the raised value by performing a second aldosterone-to-renin ratio under more carefully controlled conditions, before proposing adrenal vein sampling to patients with an aldosterone-to-renin ratio that is raised, but not markedly so (Figure 6.21).

The most popular 'confirmatory' tests are the saline infusion test and the captopril test. At a low sodium intake, the saline infusion test is more accurate than the captopril test, but both tests have moderate sensitivity and high specificity in patients on an adequate sodium intake, for example >133 mmol/L per day (6.3 g NaCl per day). At their optimal cut-off values, which is a plasma aldosterone concentration of 7.5 ng/dL (207 pmol/L) for the saline-infusion test, and 10 ng/dL (277 pmol/L) for the captopril test, the negative predictive value exceeds the positive predictive value for both tests. This feature means that these tests are more useful to exclude, rather than to confirm, the presence of primary aldosteronism. Therefore, they should be regarded as exclusion rather than confirmatory tests.

Imaging of primary aldosteronism

A high-resolution CT scan with 2–3 mm cuts represents the best available technique for identifying adrenal nodules. According to the 2016 Endocrine Society Guidelines (Funder et al., 2016), MRI or CT should be performed in patients with primary aldosteronism to identify the aldosterone-producing carcinomas that are large but (fortunately) rare. The far more common aldosterone-producing adenomas are often <20 mm of maximum diameter, and the other surgically curable subtypes of primary aldosteronism, including primary unilateral adrenal hyperplasia or multinodular unilateral adrenocortical hyperplasia, entail lesions that are tiny, and thus hardly detectable on CT or MRI. In addition, a non-functioning adrenal mass (incidentaloma) can be found in a patient with primary aldosteronism and concur with a small aldosterone-producing adenoma or with unilateral adrenocortical hyperplasia, both of which are undetectable on CT. Moreover, in a patient with primary aldosteronism, an adrenal nodule can be an aldosterone-producing adenoma or a macronodule of hyperplasia attributable to idiopathic hyperaldosteronism or to primary unilateral adrenal hyperplasia. Only less than 2% of incidentalomas, which are common at autopsy regardless of the presence of hypertension, are aldosterone-producing adenomas. These considerations explain why, overall, the results of CT scans can be misleading in about half of patients, and might lead to useless and/or inappropriate adrenalectomy in one-quarter of the patients and to exclusion from adrenalectomy of about another quarter

of those potentially curable with this procedure. This implies that an imaging-guided strategy for subtype differentiation of primary aldosteronism is inadequate to achieve discrimination between surgically curable and not curable subtypes of primary aldosteronism.

Subtype differentiation by adrenal vein sampling

All guidelines agree that adrenal vein sampling is the standard test for differentiating unilateral from bilateral causes of primary aldosteronism and therefore should be offered to all patients before adrenalectomy. However, adrenal vein sampling is expensive, technically demanding, and carries a tiny risk of adrenal vein rupture (Funder et al., 2008). As an indication for adrenalectomy, adrenal vein sampling should only be used in patients for whom there is unequivocal biochemical evidence of primary aldosteronism and in whom the surgically incurable forms of mineralocorticoid excess have been excluded (Rossi, 2011). In addition, the patients should be candidates for general anaesthesia and surgery and must be willing to achieve long-term cure of primary aldosteronism with adrenalectomy. By contrast, some centres contend that adrenal vein sampling can be omitted in patients <35 years old with solitary unilateral apparent adenoma on CT scan, because incidentalomas are rare in young patients and, therefore, an adrenal mass in a young patient with primary aldosteronism 'must be an aldosterone-producing adenoma' (Rossi, 2011). This proposition is based on a Mayo Clinic study where, however, there were only 6 patients younger than 35 years of age. The logical ground of this reasoning is, however, weak because the hyperaldosteronism and the incidentaloma are independent occurrences, which means that the rarity of incidentaloma before the age of 35 by no means implies that an adrenal node in a patient with primary aldosteronism is automatically an aldosterone-producing adenoma. Moreover, primary aldosteronism can be due to micronodular bilateral adrenal hyperplasia or to a small aldosterone-producing adenoma that is invisible on CT and is contralateral to the identified node.

Undoubtedly, the performance and interpretation of adrenal vein sampling require considerable expertise; therefore, this test should only be performed in experienced tertiary referral centres. For these reasons only the essential information that will enable practising endocrinologists to prepare their patients for adrenal vein sampling and to select appropriate referral centres for their patients with primary aldosteronism is provided here. For more detailed information the reader is referred to a recently published review (Rossi, 2018). First, adrenal vein sampling should be undertaken after the withdrawal, if feasible, of all confounding drugs or tapering treatment, particularly those drugs that reduce the levels of aldosterone as indicated for the screening test (Table 6.7). Second, it should only be performed after correction of hypokalaemia, if present, as hypokalaemia reduces aldosterone secretion and, therefore, can minimize lateralization. Third, a major source of variation in the interpretation of adrenal vein sampling results is the difficulty of catheterizing the right adrenal vein, which is short and in 15% of the cases shares an egress with inferior accessory hepatic veins. The latter situation results in mixing of adrenal blood with liver blood, which dilutes the plasma cortisol concentration and plasma aldosterone concentration, owing to the liver's metabolism of the steroids

(Rossi, 2011). The measurement of the plasma cortisol concentration in adrenal vein blood is to confirm correct catheter placement, which is essential for calculation of the selectivity index, and to correct for dilution during sampling. Super-selective catheterization of the right adrenal vein after prior identification of the hepatic vein by CT, or rapid measurement of cortisol levels in the adrenal vein during adrenal vein sampling can obviate these problems. Finally, use of bilaterally simultaneous catheterization during adrenal vein sampling is essential when adrenal vein sampling is performed without adrenocorticotrophic hormone stimulation, because it avoids generating artificial differences between the adrenal glands owing to the different timing of the blood sampling during adrenal vein sampling, which is a stressful situation (Seccia et al., 2009). Cosyntrophin (adrenocorticotrophic hormone) stimulation is used to abolish the stress-related differences between the adrenal glands, but is unnecessary when bilateral simultaneous adrenal vein sampling is used (Seccia et al., 2012). Moreover, this stimulation has a confounding effect on the lateralization index (see the next paragraph) and, therefore, should not be used before or during adrenal vein sampling (Seccia et al., 2009).

Calculating the lateralization index, which is done by dividing the ratio of the plasma aldosterone concentration to the plasma cortisol concentration on the dominant side by the ratio of the plasma aldosterone concentration to the plasma cortisol concentration on the contralateral side of the adrenal gland, is necessary to make an accurate diagnosis (Rossi, 2011). However, assessment of the results of adrenal vein sampling by the lateralization index ignores the fact that the secretion of hormones from the contralateral adrenal gland is seldom suppressed to levels similar to peripheral values and is most often higher than the peripheral values, especially when stimulated with adrenocorticotrophic hormone. To address some of the yet controversial and/or unresolved issues concerning the interpretation of results from adrenal vein sampling an international multicentre study, the Adrenal Vein Sampling International Study (http://clinicaltrials.gov/ct2/show/NCT01234220), has been launched. The Phase II of this study has recently been completed and the analysis of results is currently ongoing. The data gathered so far on a very large number of adrenal vein sampling studies carried out at centres scattered over Europe, Asia, and North America have shown an extremely low rate of major complications (0.57%), thus dispelling the idea that adrenal vein sampling is dangerous (Seccia et al., 2012).

C^{11}-Metomidate PET could be an alternative approach for the demonstration of lateralized aldosterone excess, but this technique requires a facility with a cyclotron for the preparation of the tracer and, therefore, could only be developed at large tertiary referral centres. Whether ^{11}C-metomidate PET could identify the majority of aldosterone-producing adenomas remains to be proven.

Management

Both the 2008 and the 2016 Endocrine Society Guidelines state that lateralized aldosterone secretion should be demonstrated before undertaking surgery in patients who are candidates for general anaesthesia and wish to achieve long-term cure (Funder et al., 2008 and 2016). Laparoscopic adrenalectomy is currently the best treatment, as it can be performed during a short hospital stay at a very low operative risk (Rossi, 2011).

Overall, surgery cured primary aldosteronism in 33%–72% of patients and resulted in marked improvements in 40%–50% of patients. This wide variation of results is explained by the fact that, at some centres, adrenalectomy is performed on the basis of imaging alone, which can be misleading in a substantial proportion of patients. When performed after demonstration of lateralized aldosterone excess, adrenalectomy cured or led to a marked improvement of hypertension in ~82% of the patients, practically all of the patients were cured from the hyperaldosteronism, and there was a significant decrease of left ventricular mass, mainly through a decrease of left ventricular cavity diameter. Even when antihypertensive treatment cannot be withdrawn after adrenalectomy, the number and/or the doses of antihypertensive drugs could be markedly decreased and/or resistant hypertension was resolved in the long term. This can lead to a considerable improvement in several indexes of quality of life.

The outcome for blood pressure was found to be predicted by the duration of hypertension and by the extent of vascular remodelling, both of which are caused by a delayed diagnosis. Overall, available evidence supports the concept that, the sooner the diagnosis is made and adrenalectomy performed, the better the outcome. Failure to cure primary aldosteronism can occur because of an inaccurate diagnosis (adrenal vein sampling not performed or results incorrectly interpreted) or, more frequently, from the concurrence of essential hypertension. Due to the high prevalence of both primary aldosteronism and primary (essential) hypertension, up to one-third of patients with primary aldosteronism would be expected to have concurrent primary hypertension. In these patients, adrenalectomy can cure primary aldosteronism but not hypertension.

On the whole accumulating evidence points to the superiority of adrenalectomy over long-term medical treatment for the prevention of cardiovascular events. In fact, at least two retrospective surveys (Wu et al., 2016; Hundemer et al., 2017) support this view. Moreover, the results of the first prospective study, the longitudinal phase of the PAPY Study, showed that adrenalectomy was clearly superior in preventing incident atrial fibrillation at long-term, (Rossi et al., 2018) thus emphasizing again the key importance of achieving a timely diagnosis of lateralized primary aldosteronism.

A treatment based on mineralocorticoid receptor antagonists, such as spironolactone, canrenone, potassium canrenoate, and eplerenone (which is more selective, but is also more expensive, weaker, and shorter acting than the other antagonists and is not generally available), is a reasonable alternative to adrenalectomy for patients who are not candidates for surgery or do not show lateralized aldosterone excess. The occurrence of gynaecomastia and impotence, which are the more annoying side effects of the mineralocorticoid receptor antagonists, is dose dependent, which suggests the use of reduced doses in combination, if necessary, with other agents, such as long-acting calcium channel blockers, ACE inhibitors, or angiotensin-receptor blockers. ACE inhibitors and angiotensin-receptor blockers can be particularly useful, as they effectively control the counter-regulatory stimulation of the renin–angiotensin system triggered by the diuretic action of the mineralocorticoid receptor antagonists. Aldosterone synthase inhibitors are also being developed and tested in Phase 3 trials as an effective strategy to control hyperaldosteronism.

Acknowledgements
The author's work was supported by research grants from FORICA (The Foundation for Advanced Research in Hypertension and Cardiovascular Diseases), the Società Italiana dell'Ipertensione Arteriosa, and grants from the Ministry of University and Scientific Research (MIUR) and the University of Padova.

References and further reading
Amar L, Azizi M, Menard J, et al. Aldosterone synthase inhibition with LCI699: A proof-of-concept study in patients with primary aldosteronism. *Hypertension* 2010; 56: 831–8.

Funder JW, Carey RM, Fardella C, et al. Case detection, diagnosis, and treatment of patients with primary aldosteronism: An Endocrine Society clinical practice guideline. *J Clin Endocrinol Metab* 2008; 93: 3266–81.

Funder JW, Carey RM, Mantero F, et al. The Management of Primary Aldosteronism: Case Detection, Diagnosis, and Treatment: An Endocrine Society Clinical Practice Guideline. *J Clin Endocrinol Metab* 2016; 101: 1889–1916.

Hundemer GL, Curhan GC, Yozamp N, et al. Cardiometabolic outcomes and mortality in medically treated primary aldosteronism: a retrospective cohort study. *Lancet Diabetes Endocrinol* 2018; 6(1): 51–59.

Kempers MJ, Lenders JW, van Outheusden L, et al. Systematic review: Diagnostic procedures to differentiate unilateral from bilateral adrenal abnormality in primary aldosteronism. *Ann Intern Med* 2009; 151: 329–37.

Maiolino G, Rossitto G, Bisogni V, et al. Quantitative value of aldosterone-renin ratio for detection of aldosterone-producing adenoma: the aldosterone-renin ratio for primary aldosteronism (AQUARR) study. *J Am Heart Assoc* 2017; 6(5): e005574. doi: 10.1161/JAHA.117.005574.

Milliez P, Girerd X, Plouin PF, et al. Evidence for an increased rate of cardiovascular events in patients with primary aldosteronism. *J Am Coll Cardiol* 2005; 45: 1243–8.

Rossi GP. Update in adrenal venous sampling for primary aldosteronism. *Curr Opin Endocrinol Diabetes Obes* 2018. doi: 10.1097/MED.0000000000000407. [Epub ahead of print]

Rossi GP. A comprehensive review of the clinical aspects of primary aldosteronism. *Nat Rev Endocrinol* 2011; 7: 485–95.

Rossi GP, Barisa M, Allolio B, et al. 2012 The Adrenal Vein Sampling International Study (AVIS) for identifying the major subtypes of primary aldosteronism. *J Clin Endocrinol Metab* 2012; 97:1606–14.

Rossi GP, Belfiore A, Bernini G, et al. Comparison of the captopril and the saline infusion test for excluding aldosterone-producing adenoma. *Hypertension* 2007; 50: 424–31.

Rossi GP, Bernini G, Caliumi C, et al. A prospective study of the prevalence of primary aldosteronism in 1,125 hypertensive patients. *J Am Coll Cardiol* 2006; 48: 2293–300.

Rossi GP, Bolognesi M, Rizzoni D, et al. Vascular remodeling and duration of hypertension predict outcome of adrenalectomy in primary aldosteronism patients. *Hypertension* 2008; 51: 1366–71.

Rossi GP, Maiolino G, Flego A, et al. Adrenalectomy Lowers Incident Atrial Fibrillation in Primary Aldosteronism Patients at Long Term. *Hypertension* 2018; 71(4): 585–91.

Rossi GP, Rossi E, Pavan E, et al. Screening for primary aldosteronism with a logistic multivariate discriminant analysis. *Clin Endocrinol (Oxf)* 1998; 49: 713–23.

Rossi GP, Sacchetto A, Pavan E, et al. Remodeling of the left ventricle in primary aldosteronism due to Conn's adenoma. *Circulation* 1997; 95: 1471–8.

Rossi GP, Sechi LA, Giacchetti G, et al. Primary aldosteronism: Cardiovascular, renal and metabolic implications. *Trends Endocrinol Metab* 2008; 19: 88–90.

Seccia TM, Miotto D, Battistel M, et al. A stress reaction affects assessment of selectivity of adrenal venous sampling and of lateralization of aldosterone excess in primary aldostronism. *Eur J Endocrinol* 2012; 166: 1–8.

Seccia TM, Miotto D, De Tonil R, et al. Adrenocorticotrophic hormone stimulation during adrenal vein sampling for identifying surgically curable subtypes of primary aldosteronism: Comparison of three different protocols. *Hypertension* 2009; 53: 761–6.

Wu VC, Wang SM, Chang CH, et al. Long term outcome of Aldosteronism after target treatments. *Sci Rep* 2016; 6: 32103. doi: 10.1038/srep32103.

6.5 Mineralocorticoid hypertension

Other forms of mineralocorticoid hypertension

The forms of hypertension described in this section need to be considered and excluded in patients with a putative form of surgically curable primary aldosteronism, because they require a targeted medical treatment rather than surgery. There have been several major discoveries in the field of the familial forms of primary aldosteronism due to germ-line mutations, which have led to an altogether new classification of these forms (Table 6.8).

Familial hyperaldosteronism type 1 (FH-1)

Familial hyperaldosteronism type 1 (also known as glucocorticoid-remediable aldosteronism) is an autosomal-dominant, monogenic form of hypertension that accounts for less than 1% of cases of primary aldosteronism. Clinically, it features an early onset of moderate-to-severe hypertension, a high incidence of premature stroke, hyperaldosteronism with low renin values, and, most importantly, the correction of both hypertension and hyperaldosteronism by exogenous glucocorticoids. The underlying genetic defect is unequal recombination between the genes CYP11B1 (which encodes 11-beta-hydroxylase) and CYP11B2 (which encodes aldosterone synthase), resulting in a chimeric (hybrid) gene that contains CYP11B1 sequence (including the promoter) at its 5′ end, and CYP11B2 sequence at its 3′ end. The resulting chimeric enzyme has an adrenocorticotrophic-hormone-dependent aldosterone-synthase activity and is expressed throughout the adrenal cortex. This results in ectopic synthesis of the aldosterone synthase in the adrenal zona fasciculata, leading to adrenocorticotrophic-hormone-dependent aldosterone overproduction and increased levels of the cortisol derivatives 18-hydroxycortisol and 18-oxocortisol. This dependency from adrenocorticotrophic hormone also explains why in affected individuals, treatment with low-dose dexamethasone usually normalizes blood pressure and corrects completely the hyperaldosteronism, a clear cut example of molecularly targeted Precision Medicine.

The presence of the chimeric gene can be documented by the long-template PCR method, which has superseded the Southern blot method, and is 100% sensitive, specific, and cheap.

Screening

Children or young hypertensives who have low plasma renin activity and/or an increased aldosterone-to-renin ratio and are relatives of patients with familial hyperaldosteronism type 1 or patients with primary aldosteronism but have no evidence of an adrenal mass should be screened for the chimeric gene.

Familial hyperaldosteronism type 2 (FH-2)

Familial cases of PA that do not respond to dexamethasone treatment were known for years, but only the availability of the genetic test for FH-1 allowed to establish that they did not have the chimeric gene. These cases were, therefore, by exclusion defined as familial hyperaldosteronism type 2 (FH-2) (OMIM: 605635). They comprise both adrenocortical hyperplasia and/or APA and are clinically undistinguishable from sporadic PA except than for the familial occurrence (Torpy et al. 1998; Stowasser et al. 1992).

Linkage analysis identified a quantitative trait locus (QTL) on chromosome 7p22, the responsible gene(s) remain unknown until very recently when Lifton's laboratory starting from a multiplex kindred featuring autosomal dominant FH-2 originally reported by Stowasser et al. in 1992, identified a recurrent functional variant (R172Q) in the CLCN2 gene in 8 of the probands with early onset primary aldosteronism. Such gene encodes the chloride channel ClC-2, which is expressed in many tissues, including brain, kidney, lung, intestine, and the adrenal gland. Using exomes sequencing in 80 additional probands with unsolved early onset PA, two de novo mutations (M22K and R172Q) and four independent occurrences of the R172Q were identified (Scholl et al. 2018). When tested in vitro in zona glomerulosa cells (H295R) these germline mutations showed gain of function, e.g. enhanced chloride efflux at physiological membrane potentials, as compared to wild type channel, and therefore caused membrane depolarization, increased CYP11B2 expression and aldosterone over-production. Along the same line, by analysing 12 patients with young onset hypertension and hyperaldosteronism diagnosed by age 25, Zennaro's group reported an additional de novo germline CLCN2 variant (G24N) in a highly conserved inactivation site of the N-terminal cytoplasmic domain (Fernandes-Rosa et al. 2018). They explored the impact of the G24N variant on the membrane potential of H295R cells transfected with this mutation under basal and Ang II- and K⁺-stimulated conditions. They found that the mutation conferred a higher aldosterone production under all the conditions; they also showed that aldosterone synthesis in mutated cells involved calcium influx via both L-type and T-type calcium channels (Fernandes-Rosa et al. 2018). Thus, CLCN2 variants result in a strong gain of function, in line with the dominant clinical phenotype caused by the mutations even if present only in the heterozygous state.

Noteworthy, the identification of these chloride channel mutations pointed for the first time to a role of anion channels in the regulation of cell membrane potential and aldosterone biosynthesis in adrenal zona glomerulosa. Thus, these seminal discoveries will likely generate new possibilities for the diagnosis and, possibly, treatment of early onset PA cases.

Familial hyperaldosteronism type 3 (FH-3)

In 2011, alongside the identification of somatic mutations in aldosterone producing adenoma (APA) in the KCNJ5 gene encoding the Kir3.4 K⁺ channel (OMIM: 600734), new forms of familial hyperaldosteronism were discovered (Choi et al. 2011) and defined as FH-3. A novel clinical molecular classification was then proposed (Lenzini and Rossi, 2015), which defines FH-3 as a genetic disease made of two distinct subtypes, one severe (Type A) requiring bilateral laparoscopic adrenalectomy and one milder (Type B) usually responding well to antihypertensive therapy (Table 6.8).

FH-3 type A

Choi et al. (2011) examined a pedigree characterized by drug-resistant hypertension due to severe aldosteronism and bilateral adrenal hyperplasia, which required bilateral adrenalectomy. The index case and his two daughters had a mutation (T158A) in the KCNJ5 gene,

Table 6.8 Clinical and molecular classification of Familial Hyperaldosteronism (FH)

Type	Subtypes	Transmission	Gene Mutation	Adrenal CT Findings	Extra-Adrenal Abnormalities	Drug-resistant hypertension	Treatment
FH-1		Autosomal Dominant	*CYP11B2/CYP11B1* Chimeric	BAH or APA	No	No	Low-dose Dexamethasone
FH-2		Autosomal Dominant	*CLCN2* (R172Q, M22K, R172Q, G24N)	None	No	No	MRA
FH-3	Type A	Autosomal Dominant	*KCNJ5* (T158A, I157S, E145Q)	BAH	No	Yes	Bilateral adrenalectomy
	Type B	Autosomal Dominant	*KCNJ5* (G151E, Y152C)	None	No	No	MRA + other antihypertensive Drugs if needed
FH-4		Autosomal Dominant	*CACNA1H* (M1549V, S196L, P2083L, V1951E)	Little or none	Mental retardation, social and development disorders	No	MRA + other antihypertensive Drugs if needed
FH-5 (PASNA)		Autosomal Dominant	*CACNA1D* (I770M, G403D)	None	Seizures and neurologic abnormalities	No	Calcium channel blockers

Abbreviations: BAH, Bilateral Adrenal Hyperplasia; APA, Aldosterone Producing Adenoma; MRA, Mineralocorticoid Receptor Antagonist; PASNA, primary aldosteronism with seizures and neurologic abnormalities.

mapping close to the Kir3.4 selectivity filter, which causes a threonine (Thr)-to-alanine (Ala) substitution at codon 158 resulting in reduced K^+ selectivity, increased Na^+ conductance, and cell membrane depolarization.

Another heterozygous mutation at position 470, resulting in isoleucine (I, Ile) to serine (S, Ser) substitution at amino acid 157 (I157S) was thereafter found in a mother and daughter, who presented with severe PA, bilateral massive adrenal hyperplasia and early-onset drug-resistant hypertension (Charmandari et al. 2012).

A further E145Q germline mutation previously known to occur in APA was reported in a 2 year-old Caucasian girl presenting with polydipsia, polyuria, failure to thrive, profound hypokalemia, severe hyperaldosteronism with renin suppression, and arterial hypertension resistant to treatment, which led to bilateral laparoscopic adrenalectomy in spite of negative CT and MR imaging (Akerstrom et al. 2012; Cheng et al. 2014). Like for other KCNJ5 mutations, functional characterization of this mutation showed Na^+-dependent cell membrane depolarization, and increased intracellular Ca2+ concentration causing high CYP11B2 expression (Monticone 2013).

FH-3 type B

In 2012 two studies independently reported the G151E germline mutation in patients with milder form of hyperaldosteronism (Scholl et al. 2012; Mulatero 2012). These patients had no evidence of adrenal hyperplasia and their hypertension could be easily controlled with drugs (Scholl et al. 2012). In vitro the mutation showed very prominent effects featuring a very large Na^+ conductance with rapid Na^+-dependent cell lethality. These paradoxical findings could be accounted for by the fact that the Na^+ influx-dependent cell death can limit the expansion of zona glomerulosa cell mass, thus preventing the development of hyperplasia with ensuing less prominent PA. Hence, the over-production of aldosterone in the surviving zona glomerulosa cells can be sufficient to raise blood pressure, but not high enough to render hypertension resistant to drug treatment.

Another germline mutation (Y152C) was detected in a patient with mild form of hyperaldosteronism due to an adrenal adenoma, but it remains unclear if this is another familial form or a sporadic de novo mutation as no information on other family members were given (Monticone 2013).

Familial hyperaldosteronism type 4 (FH-4)

A recurrent germline gain of function mutation in CACNA1H gene (M1549V) was identified in 5 children with PA before age 10 as the cause of FH-4 (Table 6.8). The mutation was inherited in 3 of the cases and occurred de novo in two (Scholl 2015). All patients showed hyperaldosteronism with low plasma renin activity, but no evidence of mass or hyperplasia on adrenal imaging at the time of presentation. There were no recurrent or distinctive features in the index cases, e.g. history of seizures or neurologic or neuromuscular disorders.

The CACNA1H gene on chromosome 16p13 encodes the pore-forming α1 subunit of the T-type voltage-dependent calcium channel Cav3.2 and is highly expressed in the adrenal zona glomerulosa and is activated at slightly depolarized potentials.

Whole-cell patch clamp experiments in human embryonic kidney (HEK)-293 cells showed that the M1549V CACNA1H channel exhibited activation to less depolarized potentials and very slow inactivation, two features held to cause enhanced Ca^{2+} influx in adrenal glomerulosa cells. The over-expression of M1549V in HAC15 adrenocortical cells mutant channel increased CYP11B2 gene expression and aldosterone production in basal conditions, while co-treatment with the T-type calcium channel blocker mibefradil abolished aldosterone production, indicating that M1549V CACNA1H mutation induces autonomous aldosterone production via T-type calcium channels.

Four additional germline CACNA1H mutations in patients with PA and different clinical features were identified by Zennaro's group (Daniil 2016). A M1549I de novo mutation occurred in the same position of M1549V and caused hypertension and hyperaldosteronism alongside mild mental retardation, social skills alterations, learning disabilities and development disorders. The S196L and P2083L were identified in two families affected by hypertension and primary aldosteronism. The V1951E germline variant was also identified in a patient with APA, cured by unilateral adrenalectomy.

In vitro electrophysiological experiments demonstrated that these new CACNA1H mutations changed the electrophysiological properties of the channel similar to M1549V (Scholl 2015). Furthermore, transfections of mutant in H295R-S2 cells induced high aldosterone levels and overexpression of genes coding for steroidogenic enzymes after K^+ stimulation.

PASNA Syndrome

The Primary Aldosteronism with Seizures and Neurologic Abnormalities syndrome (PASNA, OMIM #615474) phenotype (Table 6.8) was the first calcium channel mutation found to be associated with also extra-adrenal symptoms (Scholl 2013). Two de novo germline mutations (I770M, G403D) in the CACNA1D gene were detected in two children with severe hypertension diagnosed at birth, hypokalaemia and neurological manifestations, including seizures and cerebral palsy (Scholl 2013). This gene, located on chromosome 3p14.3, encodes for Cav1.3, the α subunit of the L-type voltage gated calcium channel. Both are gain of function mutations and had already been found in sporadic forms of APA (Scholl 2013; Azizan 2013). They cause channel activation at membrane potentials close to the resting of the zona glomerulosa cells (-80mV), increase Ca^{2+} influx and stimulation of aldosterone production.

Apparent mineralocorticoid excess

Apparent mineralocorticoid excess is a rare monogenic form hypertension caused by a loss of activity of 11-beta-hydroxysteroid dehydrogenase type 2. In the target tissues of aldosterone, this enzyme inactivates cortisol to cortisone and co-localizes with the mineralocorticoid receptor. Under normal conditions, the inactivation protects the receptor from cortisol, thus allowing aldosterone to gain access to its receptor. Several mutations in HSD11B2 were found to lead to a blunted enzyme activity, which results in cortisol-induced activation of the mineralocorticoid receptor, thus mimicking primary aldosteronism despite the lack of aldosterone excess.

Apparent mineralocorticoid excess is inherited as an autosomal recessive trait and is characterized by a close genotype–phenotype correlation: homozygous patients usually present all the associated clinical signs (classic apparent mineralocorticoid excess), whilst heterozygous patients show only mild hypertension and a moderately abnormal ratio of tetrahydrocortisol and allotetrahydrocortisol to tetrahydrocortisone, or cortisol to cortisone, in the urine, or even a normal phenotype, which make them hardly distinguishable from those with low-renin essential hypertension. Homozygous apparent mineralocorticoid excess usually presents early in life, with severe hypertension, hypokalaemia, metabolic alkalosis, and low levels of renin and aldosterone. The biochemical diagnosis can be made by the demonstration of an increased (up to 33) ratio of tetrahydrocortisol and allotetrahydrocortisol to tetrahydrocortisone, or cortisol to cortisone (normal values about 1), in a 24-hour urine collection.

Subjects ingesting large amount of liquorice or carbenoxolone can present with a condition that mimics apparent mineralocorticoid excess, because of the inhibiting effect of these substances on 11-beta-hydroxysteroid dehydrogenase type 2, and their (weak) mineralocorticoid activity. It is conceivable that some of the patients developing liquorice- or carbenoxolone-associated apparent mineralocorticoid excess are heterozygous for one or more of the numerous mutations of *HSD11B2*, although this possibility has not been explored thus far.

Liddle syndrome

See also Section 6.6. Although, strictly speaking, Liddle syndrome is not a form of mineralocorticoid hypertension, it will be briefly mentioned here because it enters in the differential diagnosis with apparent mineralocorticoid excess. Liddle syndrome is an autosomal-dominant form of hypertension and is induced by a point mutation in the genes coding for the beta or gamma subunits of the eNaC in the distal renal tubule. These mutations cause an alteration or deletion in a conserved proline-rich PY motif in the cytoplasmic tails corresponding to the C-terminal ends of either subunits. Disruption of this motif prevents inactivation of the channel, which remains constitutively (permanently) activated, with ensuing excess tubular reabsorption of sodium, consequent salt-sensitive hypertension, and suppression of renin and aldosterone. Thus, clinically, the syndrome closely resembles apparent mineralocorticoid excess in that both conditions do not show excess aldosterone, although the aldosterone-to-renin ratio can be elevated because of renin suppression.

As the ENaC is amiloride and triamterene sensitive, these drugs are particularly effective in curing Liddle syndrome. Nonetheless, only the demonstration of the mutations in the beta or gamma subunits of the ENaC allows an unequivocal diagnosis of Liddle syndrome.

Future developments

The identification of mutations in the selectivity filter of potassium channels of the KCNJ5 type was rapidly followed by that of mutations in other genes such as *ATP1A1*, *ATP2B3*, and *CACNA1D*, which play a role in the regulation of aldosterone secretion. These discoveries have triggered enormous investigative efforts, whose results are difficult to anticipate at this time but are expected to change our understanding of and diagnostic and therapeutic approach to primary aldosteronism and possibly to mineralocorticoid hypertension.

For the time being, by following a few simple rules and a streamlined approach, physicians can successfully and cost-effectively identify and treat many patients with so-called essential hypertension but whose high blood pressure is caused by hyperaldosteronism. In these patients, the clue to mineralocorticoid hypertension is a low plasma renin, which responds little or not at all to stimulatory manoeuvres. Identification of mineralocorticoid hypertension and primary aldosteronism is particularly beneficial when hypertension is severe and/or resistant to treatment, because specific treatment can bring the blood pressure under control despite withdrawal, or a prominent reduction in the number and dosage, of antihypertensive medications.

References and further reading

Akerstrom T, Crona J, Delgado Verdugo A, et al. Comprehensive re-sequencing of adrenal aldosterone producing lesions reveal three somatic mutations near the KCNJ5 potassium channel selectivity filter. *PLoS One*. 2012; 7: e41926. doi: 10.1371/journal.pone.0041926.

Azizan EA, Poulsen H, Tuluc P, et al. Somatic mutations in ATP1A1 and CACNA1D underlie a common subtype of adrenal hypertension. *Nat Genet* 2013; 45:1055–60.

Beuschlein F, Boulkroun S, Osswald A, et al. Somatic mutations in ATP1A1 and ATP2B3 lead to aldosterone-producing adenomas and secondary hypertension. *Nat Genet* 2013; 45: 440–4, 444e1–2.

Boulkroun S, Beuschlein F, Rossi GP, et al. Prevalence, clinical, and molecular correlates of KCNJ5 mutations in primary aldosteronism. Hypertension 2012; 59: 592–8.

Charmandari E, Sertedaki A, Kino T, et al. A novel point mutation in the KCNJ5 gene causing primary hyperaldosteronism and early-onset autosomal dominant hypertension. *J Clin Endocrinol Metab.* 2012; 97:E1532-9. doi:10.1210/jc.2012-1334.

Cheng CJ, Sung CC, Wu ST, et al. Novel KCNJ5 Mutations in Sporadic Aldosterone-producing Adenoma Reduce Kir3.4 Membrane Abundance. *J Clin Endocrinol Metab.* 2014: jc20143009. doi:10.1210/jc.2014-3009.

Choi M, Scholl UI, Yue P, et al. K+ channel mutations in adrenal aldosterone-producing adenomas and hereditary hypertension. *Science* 2011; 331: 768–72.

Daniil G, Fernandes-Rosa FL, Chemin J, et al. CACNA1H Mutations Are Associated With Different Forms of Primary Aldosteronism. *EBioMedicine.* 2016;13:225–36. doi:10.1016/j.ebiom.2016.10.002.

Fernandes-Rosa FL, Daniil G, Orozco IJ, et al. A gain-of-function mutation in the CLCN2 chloride channel gene causes primary aldosteronism. *Nat Genet.* 2018. doi:10.1038/s41588-018-0053-8.

Lenzini L and Rossi GP. The molecular basis of primary aldosteronism: From chimeric gene to channelopathy. *Curr Opin Pharmacol* 2015; 21: 35–42.

Monticone S, Hattangady NG, Penton D, et al. a Novel Y152C KCNJ5 mutation responsible for familial hyperaldosteronism type III. *J Clin Endocrinol Metab.* 2013; 98: E1861-5. doi:10.1210/jc.2013-2428.

Mulatero P, Tauber P, Zennaro MC, et al. KCNJ5 mutations in European families with nonglucocorticoid remediable familial hyperaldosteronism. *Hypertension.* 2012; 59: 235–40. doi:10.1161/HYPERTENSIONAHA.111.183996.

Scholl UI, Goh G, Stölting G, et al. Somatic and germline CACNA1D calcium channel mutations in aldosterone-producing adenomas and primary aldosteronism. *Nat Genet* 2013; 45: 1050–4.

Scholl UI, Nelson-Williams C, Yue P, et al. Hypertension with or without adrenal hyperplasia due to different inherited mutations in the potassium channel KCNJ5. *Proc Natl Acad Sci USA.* 2012; 109: 2533–8. doi:10.1073/pnas.1121407109; 10.1073/pnas.1121407109.

Scholl UI, Stölting G, Nelson-Williams C, et al. Recurrent gain of function mutation in calcium channel CACNA1H causes early-onset hypertension with primary aldosteronism. *Elife*. 2015. doi:10.7554/eLife.06315.001.

Scholl UI, Stölting G, Schewe J, et al. CLCN2 chloride channel mutations in familial hyperaldosteronism type II. *Nat Genet*. 2018. doi:10.1038/s41588-018-0048-5.

Stowasser M, Gordon RD, Tunny TJ, et al. Familial hyperaldosteronism type II: five families with a new variety of primary aldosteronism. *Clin Exp Pharmacol Physiol*. 1992; 19:319–22.

Torpy DJ, Gordon RD, Lin JP, et al. Familial hyperaldosteronism type II: description of a large kindred and exclusion of the aldosterone synthase (CYP11B2) gene. *J Clin Endocrinol Metab*. 1998; 83:3214–18. doi:10.1210/jcem.83.9.5086.

6.6 Liddle syndrome

Definition and epidemiology
Liddle syndrome is a rare form of hypertension with autosomal-dominant inheritance and characterized by severe early onset hypertension associated with decreased plasma levels of potassium, renin, and aldosterone. Its prevalence is unknown. About 80 cases have been reported to date.

Pathophysiology
Liddle syndrome (OMIM 177200) is due to gain-of-function mutations in the genes encoding for two subunits of the ENaC, which is involved in sodium reabsorption from the distal nephron to the late portion of the distal convoluted tubule, the connecting tubule, and the collecting duct (see Figure 6.23). The ENaC comprises three subunits (alpha, beta, and gamma), and the mutations occur on the C-terminus of the beta and gamma subunits, encoded by *SCNN1B* and *SCNN1G* (chromosomal location 16p13–p12), respectively, in a proline-rich region called the PY motif. This motif is highly conserved in the C-termini of all ENaC subunits and serves as a binding site for the Nedd4 family of ubiquitin ligases. Mutations impair the interaction of the ENaC with Nedd4 and the subsequent degradation of the ENaC by the ubiquitin proteasome system. This results in the constitutive expression of ENaCs in the membrane, thus inducing sodium reabsorption, secondary potassium and proton secretion, and, ultimately, volume-expanded hypertension. Recently, another mechanism has been described; an intrinsic increase of the ENaC activity was observed for a mutant located in the extracellular domain of the alpha subunit, implicating the *SCNN1A* gene in this disease.

Clinical features
Severe hypertension is found in young patients, from infancy to young adulthood (before 35 years of age). Children are usually asymptomatic. Adults can present with symptoms of hypokalaemia such as weakness, fatigue, myalgia, constipation, or palpitations. A family history of hypertension across several generations is often present.

Investigations
Diagnosis is suspected by the fortuitous detection of early onset hypertension, especially in the presence of family history. It is then confirmed by blood and urinary electrolyte tests which show hypokalaemia, decreased or normal plasma levels of renin and aldosterone, metabolic alkalosis with high sodium plasma levels, and low rates of urinary excretion of sodium and aldosterone, with high rates of urinary potassium excretion. Some cases with normal potassium levels have been described. The diagnosis is confirmed by genetic testing.

Management
Treatment is based on administration of potassium-sparing diuretics, such as amiloride (up to 40 mg/day) or triamterene, which act by blocking ENaC activity. This results in reduction of blood pressure and correction of hypokalaemia and metabolic alkalosis. Conventional antihypertensive therapies are not effective (including spironolactone, as it acts via the mineralocorticoid receptor). Patients must also follow a low-sodium diet.

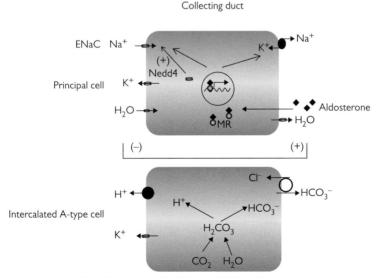

Fig 6.23 Schematic representation of principal and intercalated A-type cells in the collecting duct, showing the proteins implicated in sodium reabsorption and proton and potassium secretion, as well as regulation by aldosterone and Nedd4; ENaC, epithelial sodium channel; MR, mineralocorticoid receptor.

Complications and prognosis

With treatment, prognosis is good. Without treatment, cardiovascular (premature stroke or sudden death) and renal complications (end-stage renal disease) usually occur.

Further reading

Hansson JH, Nelson-Williams C, Suzuki H, et al. Hypertension caused by a truncated epithelial sodium channel gamma sub-unit: Genetic heterogeneity of Liddle syndrome. *Nat Genet* 1995; 11: 76–82.

Jeunemaitre X, Bassilana F, Persu A, et al. Genotype–phenotype analysis of a newly discovered family with Liddle's syndrome. *J Hypertens* 1997; 15: 1091–100.

Rossi E, Farnetti E, Nicoli D, et al. A clinical phenotype mimicking essential hypertension in a newly discovered family with Liddle's syndrome. *Am J Hypertens* 2011; 24: 930–5.

Rotin D. Role of the UPS in Liddle syndrome. *BMC Biochem* 2008; 21; 9: S51.

Salih M, Gautschi I, van Bemmelen MX, et al. A missense mutation in the extracellular domain of αENaC causes Liddle Syndrome. *J Am Soc Nephrol* 2017; 28: 3291–99.

Shimkets RA, Warnock DG, Bositis CM, et al. Liddle's syndrome: Heritable human hypertension caused by mutations in the beta subunit of the epithelial sodium channel. *Cell* 1994; 79: 407–14.

Staub O, Gautschi I, Ishikawa T, et al. Regulation of stability and function of the epithelial Na+ channel (ENaC) by ubiquitination. *Embo J* 1997; 16: 6325–64.

Warnock DG. Liddle syndrome: An autosomal dominant form of human hypertension. *Kidney Int* 1998; 53: 18–24.

6.7 Bartter and Gitelman syndromes

Definition and epidemiology

Bartter syndrome and Gitelman syndrome are rare salt-losing renal tubulopathies with autosomal-recessive inheritance. They are caused by loss-of-function mutations in genes encoding for proteins participating in NaCl reabsorption in the thick ascending limb of Henle's loop and in the distal convoluted tubule, which reabsorb about 20% and 7%, respectively. In addition, a transient form of antenatal Bartter syndrome linked to chromosome X has recently been described.

Their estimated prevalence is 1:1,000,000 and 1:40,000, respectively.

Genetic classification

Bartter syndrome has been classified into four genetic subtypes: type 1 is caused by mutations in *SLC12A1*, which encodes the furosemide-sensitive sodium–potassium–chloride cotransporter of the apical membrane of the epithelium in the thick ascending limb of Henle's loop; type 2 is caused by mutations in *KCNJ1*, which encodes for the apical potassium channel Kir1.1 (or ROMK); type 3 is related to mutations in *CLCNKB*, which encodes the chloride channel ClC-Kb, which is expressed in the basolateral side of the distal convoluted tubule and the thick ascending limb of Henle's loop; type 4a is caused by mutations in *BSND*, which encodes the protein barttin (an accessory beta subunit of the ClC-Kb and ClC-Ka channels); and type 4b is a digenic disease caused by loss-of-function mutations in *CLCNKA* and *CLCNKB*. Finally, type 5 is related to mutations in *MAGED2* gene, which encodes for a nuclear protein that affects the expression and function of at least of two sodium-chloride cotransporters. Most of the cases of Gitelman syndrome are due to mutations in *SLC12A3*, which encodes the thiazide-sensitive NaCl cotransporter expressed in the apical membrane of the epithelium of the distal convoluted tubule. In about 3% of cases, Gitelman syndrome is caused by mutations in *CLCNKB*. Recently, the genetic basis of a new syndrome known as EAST syndrome, which is characterized by epilepsy, ataxia, sensorineural deafness, and a tubulopathy with the same characteristics as Gitelman syndrome, has been identified. EAST is also a rare autosomal-recessive disease caused by mutations in *KCNJ10*, which encodes the potassium channel Kir4.1, which is expressed in glial cells in the cerebral and cerebellar cortex; in the stria vascularis; and in the distal convoluted tubule. The location of the different proteins and their genetic classification are summarized in Figure 6.24.

Pathophysiology

Salt losing generates a hypovolaemic status with a secondary activation of the renin–angiotensin–aldosterone system and normal or low blood pressure; the compensatory increase in NaCl reabsorption, and in potassium ion and hydrogen ion secretion in the collecting duct, due to aldosterone action, is responsible for the hypokalaemic metabolic alkalosis detected in patients with these two syndromes. But they also have different clinical and biological characteristics explained by the functions and regulation of implicated nephron segment and/or the presence and function of the specific proteins in other organs. These differences are described in 'Clinical presentation'.

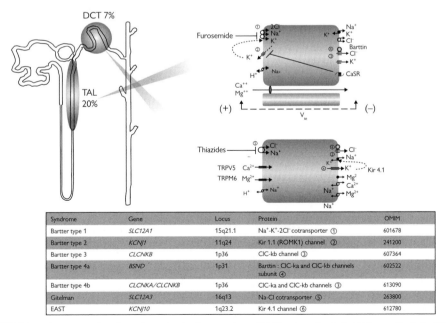

Syndrome	Gene	Locus	Protein	OMIM
Bartter type 1	*SLC12A1*	15q21.1	Na⁺-K⁺-2Cl⁻ cotransporter ①	601678
Bartter type 2	*KCNJ1*	11q24	Kir 1.1 (ROMK1) channel ②	241200
Bartter type 3	*CLCNKB*	1p36	ClC-kb channel ③	607364
Bartter type 4a	*BSND*	1p31	Barttin : ClC-ka and ClC-kb channels subunit ④	602522
Bartter type 4b	*CLCNKA/CLCNKB*	1p36	ClC-ka and ClC-kb channels ③	613090
Gitelman	*SLC12A3*	16q13	Na-Cl cotransporter ⑤	263800
EAST	*KCNJ10*	1q23.2	Kir 4.1 channel ⑥	612780

Fig 6.24 Schematic representation of a nephron, showing the percentage of NaCl reabsorption in the thick ascending limb of Henle's loop (TAL) and the distal convoluted tubule (DCT), as well as the cells of these segments, with the location of proteins implicated in Bartter, Gitelman, and EAST syndromes. The table summarizes the genetic classification.

Clinical presentation

Bartter syndrome

There are two distinct presentations of Bartter syndrome: antenatal and 'classical'. The most severe presentation is antenatal Bartter syndrome, sometimes referred to 'hyperprostaglandin E syndrome'; however, hyperprostaglandinuria is secondary to hypovolaemia and is not specific to Bartter syndrome. Antenatal Bartter syndrome corresponds to Bartter syndrome types 1, 2, 4, and some cases of type 3 and associates with maternal polyhydramnios; premature birth; intrauterine and postnatal polyuria complicated by severe dehydration episodes; recurrent vomiting; failure to thrive; and growth retardation. These symptoms are related to the important role of the thick ascending limb of Henle's loop in NaCl reabsorption, as well as the generation of the corticopapillary osmolar gradient necessary for urinary concentration. As paracellular calcium reabsorption in this segment is passive and dependent on NaCl reabsorption, hypercalciuria and nephrocalcinosis are frequent. Type 2 antenatal Bartter syndrome presents with transitory neonatal hyperkalaemia in about 75% of the cases, which is attributed to the involvement of the Kir1.1 channel in the secretion of potassium in the collecting duct, as well as to the immaturity of the Na–K–ATPase pump and other potassium channels expressed in the collecting duct in the preterm infant. Type 4 antenatal Bartter syndrome is associated with deafness, as ClC-Ka, ClC-Kb, and barttin are also expressed in the inner ear, where they play an important role in the generation of endocochlear potential. Type 5 transient antenatal Bartter syndrome has a similar presentation to other antenatal forms but affects mainly male subjects and is characterized by a spontaneous resolution often in the first year of life. The classical Bartter syndrome has a milder phenotype with a later onset of signs and symptoms (polyuria, failure to thrive and nephrocalcinosis) beginning in infancy through to adolescence and

corresponds to Bartter syndrome type 3. In this last group, a profound hypochloraemia is often present, probably associated with the additional presence of the ClC-Kb channel in intercalated cells in the collecting duct, where it promotes chloride reabsorption.

Gitelman syndrome

Gitelman syndrome, the most frequent form of this group of diseases, is also the milder one. Most of the patients are diagnosed as adolescents or adults. In about 50% of patients, the fortuitous discovery of hypokalaemia allows the diagnosis. The remaining patients present with fatigue, tetany, paraesthesiae, cramps, muscle weakness, and salt craving, and less frequently with cardiac arrhythmia or failure to thrive. In addition to hypokalaemia and metabolic alkalosis, most patients present with hypomagnesaemia and hypocalciuria. Symptoms are secondary to hypokalaemia and hypomagnesaemia but there is no correlation between electrolyte imbalance and symptoms severity. By analogy with thiazide-induced hypocalciuria and hypomagnesaemia, the suggested mechanisms of these abnormalities are, respectively, an increase of proximal calcium reabsorption, and apical TRPM6 magnesium channel inhibition.

Table 6.9 summarizes the clinical characteristics of Bartter syndrome and Gitelman syndrome, and their correlation with the genetic classification.

Investigations

Diagnosis is based on the clinical presentation and biological abnormalities. Bartter syndrome and Gitelman syndrome share the presence of similar hypokalaemia levels (2.6 ± 0.69 and 2.7 ± 0.44 mmol/L in Bartter syndrome and Gitelman syndrome, respectively) of renal origin (urinary potassium over 20 mmol/L) and metabolic alkalosis (bicarbonate: 31 ± 7 and 30 ± 3 mmol/L (189 ± 43 and 183 ± 18 mg/dL) in Bartter syndrome and Gitelman syndrome, respectively). In contrast, plasma renin activity and plasma aldosterone concentration

Table 6.9 Main clinical and biological characteristics and their correlation with genetic types

Parameter	Antenatal Bartter syndrome				Classical Bartter syndrome	Gitelman syndrome
	Type 1	Type 2	Type 4	Type 3	Type 3	
Age of presentation	In utero	In utero	In utero	In utero	Infants, toddlers, preschoolers, and school children	Adolescent, adult, children (less frequent)
Polyhydramnios/prematurity	Yes	Yes	Yes	Yes	—	—
Failure to thrive	Yes	Yes	Yes	Yes	Often	Rare
Deafness	No	No	Yes	No	No	No
Polyuria	Yes	Yes	Yes	Yes	Yes	No
Tetany crisis	—	—	—	—	Occasional	Common
Magnesaemia	Normal	Normal	Normal	Normal	Normal or low	Low (sometimes normal)
Transitory hyperkalaemia	No	Yes	No	No	No	No
Hypochloraemic alkalosis	Yes	Yes	Yes (severe)	Yes (very severe)	Yes (very severe)	Yes
Calciuria	High	High	Normal or high	Yes (very severe)	Yes (very severe)	Low (sometimes normal)
Nephrocalcinosis	Yes	Yes	Yes	Sometimes	Sometimes	—
Urinary prostaglandins	High	High	High	High	Normal or high	Normal

are more prominent in patients with Bartter syndrome, particularly in the antenatal form (renin and aldosterone can be, respectively, 20–30 and 2–8 times above normal values for age in Bartter syndrome, and 2–8 and 1–2 times in Gitelman syndrome). A constant hypercalciuria (urinary calcium/creatinine ratio over 2 in the first year and over 0.7 after 5 years) is observed in patients with type 1 and 2 Bartter syndrome; patients with type 3 and 4 could have normo- or hypercalciuria. In contrast, most patients with Gitelman syndrome have hypocalciuria (urinary calcium-to-creatinine ratio lower than 0.1 mmol/mmol). Hypomagnesaemia (lower than 0.65 mmol/L (1.6 mg/dL)) is present in most of patients with Gitelman syndrome and in some patients with type 3 Bartter syndrome. In patients with Gitelman syndrome and a severe failure to thrive, a deficit of growth hormone can be associated.

Management
Bartter syndrome treatment is supportive: water and electrolyte supplementation are particularly high in the antenatal form, and patients may need enteral nutrition to meet the high fluid and sodium requirements (150–500 mL/kg per day, and 10–45 mmol/kg per day, respectively). Potassium chloride supplementation (1–3 mmol/kg per day) is also often necessary. Indometacin therapy is initiated after 2 months, at a dose ranging from 1 to 3 mg/kg per day. This drug allows a decrease of supplementation and dramatically improves growth. However, signs of intolerance or toxicity should be sought.

Gitelman syndrome treatment is based on magnesium and potassium supplementation. Magnesium deficit is often important and aggravates the hypokalaemia; some patients need only magnesium supplementation (magnesium chloride: 4–5 mg/kg per day). Nevertheless, potassium-chloride (1–3 mmol/kg per day) supplementation is often necessary. These supplements should be divided in four doses to avoid diarrhoea, and adjusted according to the serum levels of potassium and magnesium. Some patients may require anti-aldosterone drugs (i.e. amiloride).

Both Bartter syndrome and Gitelman syndrome patients are encouraged to have a high-sodium and high-potassium diet and to increase supplementation doses during periods of additional losses (warmer environmental conditions or intercurrent diseases associating vomiting or diarrhoea).

Complications and prognosis
End-stage renal failure may occur in patients with type 3 and 4 Bartter syndrome. Patients with antenatal Bartter syndrome can have neurological disabilities and cognitive dysfunction linked to prematurity. Early screening of deafness is important for a normal speech and general development.

The long-term prognosis of Gitelman syndrome is, in general, excellent. Some adult Gitelman syndrome patients present with chondrocalcinosis (calcium

pyrophosphate dehydrate crystals deposition in joint cartilage), which is related to chronic hypomagnesaemia. Joint pain and pseudogout attacks can be managed with NSAIDs. A screen for additional risk factors of cardiac arrhythmia is recommended.

Further reading
Birkenhager R, Otto E, Schurmann MJ, et al. Mutation of BSND causes Bartter syndrome with sensorineural deafness and kidney failure. *Nat Genet* 2001; 29: 310–4.

Bockenhauer D, Feather S, Stanescu HC, et al. Epilepsy, ataxia, sensorineural deafness, tubulopathy, and KCNJ10 mutations. *N Engl J Med* 2009; 360: 1960–70.

Brochard K, Boyer O, Blanchard A, et al. Phenotype-genotype correlation in antenatal and neonatal variants of Bartter syndrome. *Nephrol Dial Transplant* 2009; 24: 1455–64.

Jeck N, Konrad M, Peters M, et al. Mutations in the chloride channel gene, CLCNKB, leading to a mixed Bartter-Gitelman phenotype. *Pediatr Res* 2000; 48: 754–8.

Laghmani K, Beck BB, Yang SS, et al. Polyhydramnios, Transient Antenatal Bartter's Syndrome, and MAGED2 Mutations. *N Engl J Med* 2016; 374:1853–63.

Legrand A, Treard C, Roncelin I, et al. Prevalence of Novel MAGED2 Mutations in Antenatal Bartter Syndrome. *Clin J Am Soc Nephrol* 2018; 13:242–250.

Peters M, Jeck N, Reinalter S, et al. Clinical presentation of genetically defined patients with hypokalemic salt-losing tubulopathies. *Am J Med* 2002; 112: 183–90.

Proesmans W. Bartter syndrome and its neonatal variant. *Eur J Pediatr* 1997; 156: 669–79.

Rickheit G, Maier H, Strenzke N, et al. Endocochlear potential depends on Cl- channels: Mechanism underlying deafness in Bartter syndrome IV. *EMBO J* 2008; 27: 2907–17.

Rodriguez-Soriano J. Bartter and related syndromes: The puzzle is almost solved. *Pediatr Nephrol* 1998; 12: 315–27.

Schlingmann KP, Konrad M, Jeck N, et al. Salt wasting and deafness resulting from mutations in two chloride channels. *N Engl J Med* 2004; 350: 1314–9.

Scholl UI, Choi M, Liu T, et al. Seizures, sensorineural deafness, ataxia, mental retardation, and electrolyte imbalance (SeSAME syndrome) caused by mutations in KCNJ10. *Proc Natl Acad Sci USA* 2009; 106: 5842–7.

Simon DB, Bindra RS, Mansfield TA, et al. Mutations in the chloride channel gene, CLCNKB, cause Bartter's syndrome type III. *Nature Genet* 1997; 17: 171–8.

Simon DB, Karet F, Hamdan J, et al. Bartter's syndrome, hypokalemic alkalosis with hypercalciuria, is caused by mutations in the Na-K-2Cl cotransporter NKCC2. *Nature Genet* 1996; 13: 183–8.

Simon DB, Karet F, Rodriguez-Soriano J, et al. Genetic heterogeneity of Bartter's syndrome revealed by mutations un the K+ channel, ROMK. *Nature Genet* 1996; 14: 152–6.

Simon DB, Nelson-Williams C, Bia MJ, et al. Gitelman's variant of Bartter's syndrome, inherited hypokalaemic alkalosis, is caused by mutations in the thiazide-sensitive Na-Cl cotransporter. *Nat Genet* 1996; 12: 24–30.

Vargas-Poussou R, Dahan K, Kahila D, et al. Spectrum of mutations in Gitelman syndrome. *J Am Soc Nephrol* 2011; 22: 693–703.

Vargas-Poussou R, Feldmann D, Vollmer M, et al. Novel molecular variants of the Na-K-2Cl cotransporter gene are responsible for antenatal Bartter syndrome. *Am J Hum Genet* 1998; 62: 1332–40.

6.8 Cushing's syndrome and autonomous cortisol secretion

Introduction

Cushing's syndrome is a symptom complex that comprises signs and symptoms caused by chronic exposure to excessive amounts of glucocorticoids. It is important to recognize and treat Cushing's syndrome because it is associated with an increased standard mortality rate up to fivefold that of the general population. Remission improves or reverses the features of the syndrome, normalizing the standard mortality rate.

Epidemiology

The annual incidence of endogenous Cushing's syndrome is two to three cases per million. It is more common in women than in men, and occurs during the reproductive ages.

Pathophysiology

Exogeneous glucocorticoids cause most cases of Cushing's syndrome. Other physiologic forms of hypercortisolism may be difficult to distinguish from endogenous Cushing's syndrome. These so-called pseudo-Cushing states include psychiatric disorders, alcohol withdrawal, glucocorticoid resistance, and late pregnancy.

The causes of Cushing's syndrome can be divided into adrenocorticotrophic-hormone-independent (15%) and adrenocorticotrophic-hormone-dependent (85%) forms. In adrenocorticotrophic-hormone-independent forms, pituitary corticotrope production of adrenocorticotrophic hormone is suppressed, and any normal adrenal tissue becomes atrophic as a result. The adrenal glands produce cortisol independently, most often from a unilateral adenoma (60%) or cancer (40%). Rare bilateral disorders include primary pigmented nodular adrenal disease (PPNAD; with or without Carney complex features), macronodular adrenal hyperplasia, or McCune–Albright syndrome. Whilst McCune–Albright syndrome is almost always only seen in infancy, macronodular adrenal hyperplasia occurs mostly in older adults, and PPNAD is found in children and young adults.

Adrenocorticotrophic-hormone-dependent causes of Cushing's syndrome are characterized by inappropriate adrenocorticotrophic hormone secretion, either from a corticotrope tumour (called 'Cushing's disease'; about 80%) or from a non-pituitary tumour (called ectopic adrenocorticotrophic hormone secretion or syndrome; about 20%). Ectopic adrenocorticotrophic hormone secretion is most common from pulmonary carcinoids, but also occurs with other foregut carcinoids, phaeochromocytoma, medullary thyroid cancer, and other tumours. Very rarely, a tumour may produce CRH in excess, resulting in corticotrope stimulation and excess adrenocorticotrophic hormone secretion.

The precise defect(s) causing these disorders is largely unknown. Germ-line mutations of the regulatory sub-unit R1A of protein kinase A (encoded by *PRKAR1A*) were found in some patients with PPNAD, whilst germ-line mutations of phosphodiesterase 11A (encoded by *PDE11A*) and phosphodiesterase 8B (encoded by *PDE8B*) occur in patients with PPNAD or macronodular adrenal hyperplasia. McCune–Albright syndrome is due to a post-zygotic activating mutation in *GNAS1* gene and leads to tissue mosaicism.

Clinical features

The number and severity of characteristic features (obesity, proximal muscle weakness, plethora, moon facies, wide purple striae, psychiatric disturbances, and impaired memory; see Box 6.3) reflect the duration and amount of exposure. Patients with a less florid presentation may only have features that are common in the general population, such as depression, hypertension, and overweight.

Cushing's syndrome tends to progress, so that additional features appear over time. A thorough history is essential, with attention to the duration and tempo of the progression of signs and symptoms. Psychiatric and cognitive features should be sought. Comparison of the current facies or body habitus with old photographs may help establish progression.

The term 'subclinical Cushing's syndrome' describes patients with cortisol excess insufficient to cause overt clinical features. These patients generally have common disorders (weight gain, glucose intolerance, hypertension) that may be exacerbated by mild hypercortisolism. An astute clinician may initiate screening; more often, an adrenal incidentaloma provokes consideration of the diagnosis.

Investigation

Biochemical screening for Cushing's syndrome

Before testing is done, exclude exogenous exposure by asking about oral, rectal, inhaled, injected, or topical glucocorticoid administration. Megestrol acetate has glucocorticoid activity. Over-the-counter items such as 'tonics', herbs. and skin-bleaching creams may contain glucocorticoids.

Recent Endocrine Society guidelines recommend screening in individuals most likely to have the syndrome, including those with progressive symptoms, those with unusual features for their age (e.g. fracture in a 20-year-old), children with decreasing height and increasing weight percentiles, and patients with an adrenal incidentaloma.

The guidelines suggest performing two of three screening tests chosen based on availability, patient circumstance, and preference: measurement of 24-hour

---

Box 6.3 Signs and symptoms of Cushing's syndrome

Occurring in >80% of patients: obesity, weight gain, hypertension, plethora, round face, thin skin
Occurring in 40%–80% of patients: striae, oedema, echymoses, menstrual changes, psychiatric disturbances, osteoporosis, glucose intolerance, hirsutism
Occurring in 0%–20% of patients: recurrent infections, abdominal pain, renal calculi

UFC or LNSC, or a 1 or 2 mg DST. Each has advantages and disadvantages and can be performed in outpatients.

UFC
Urine cortisol represents the free fraction of cortisol in blood that is excreted; results above the upper reference range are compatible with a diagnosis of Cushing's syndrome. Falsely normal results occur in renal failure; cyclic Cushing's syndrome during a quiescent interval; a cortisol-producing adrenal incidentaloma; and when the 24-hour collection is incomplete. Falsely abnormal results occur if patients over-collect the sample, if the urine volume is more than 5 L, and in pseudo-Cushing states. At least two measurements should be obtained.

LNSC
LNSC measures the free fraction of cortisol in blood that is secreted into saliva. The normal sleep-entrained nocturnal nadir is lost in Cushing's syndrome, so a late-night value is abnormal. The sample is collected by passive drooling into a container or by sucking on a pledget just before bedtime (usually 23:00 h to midnight). Values above the reference range, which varies by assay, are consistent with Cushing's syndrome. Falsely abnormal results occur in individuals with erratic times of sleep onset, in those with excitement or stress at the time of collection, and with smoking. Abnormal values have been reported with increasing age, hypertension, and diabetes; the influence of co-morbidities on the normal range has not been fully evaluated. At least two measurements should be obtained.

DST
The potent glucocorticoid dexamethasone increases negative feedback so that adrenocorticotrophic hormone and cortisol levels decrease. Because Cushing's syndrome patients are resistant to negative feedback they do not suppress normally. A two-day 2 mg DST (also known as the low-dose DST) is used most often in the UK. This test involves taking dexamethasone, 500 µg, orally every 6 hours for eight doses and then measuring serum cortisol 2 or 6 hours after the last dose, using a test-specific cortisol suppression criterion (<39 or 50 nmol/L (1.4 or 1.8 µg/dL)). The 1 mg test involves measurement of cortisol between 08:00 and 09:00 h after giving dexamethasone 1 mg between 23:00 h and midnight; normal suppression is <50 nmol/L (1.8 mg/dL).

False responses to dexamethasone occur in healthy individuals who metabolize the agent quickly, or in patients with Cushing's disease who metabolize the agent slowly. Liver disease and drugs that induce or inhibit CYP3A4 (which metabolizes dexamethasone) alter its clearance. If available, measurement of a dexamethasone level when the cortisol is drawn can assess clearance. Oestrogen-induced increases in CBG (and thus total cortisol) can cause falsely abnormal responses. Patients with an adrenal incidentaloma but not Cushing's syndrome may have abnormal DST results without other biochemical abnormalities.

Other tests
In general, tests used for the differential diagnosis of Cushing's syndrome (e.g. pituitary MRI, plasma adrenocorticotrophic hormone) should not be used to make the diagnosis of Cushing's syndrome. An adrenal incidentaloma is an exception; in this setting, a suppressed adrenocorticotrophic-hormone or DHEAS level supports the diagnosis of subclinical or overt Cushing's syndrome.

Two other tests may be helpful. In an inpatient, measurement of cortisol at midnight is helpful if it is quite low; studies set different criteria for interpretation depending on whether the sample is drawn as a straight stick during sleep (<50 nmol/L (1.8 µg/dL)) or if it is drawn via an indwelling line when awake (<207 nmol/L (7.5 µg/dL)).

The dexamethasone-suppressed CRH test involves measurement of a cortisol level 2 hours after the last dexamethasone dose in the 2 mg two-day test, followed by administration of CRH (1 µg/kg, intravenous) with measurement of cortisol 15 minutes later. Cortisol values >38 nmol/L (1.4 µg/dL) initially were thought to show high discrimination for Cushing's syndrome. Subsequent studies showed high sensitivity (up to 98%), but less specificity (about 70%). Falsely abnormal results correlated with the number of administered medications in one study, but dexamethasone levels were not measured.

Interpretation of test results
For all tests, a normal result excludes Cushing's syndrome with high certainty. However, abnormal results do not predict Cushing's syndrome with similar accuracy. If two tests are normal, Cushing's syndrome is quite unlikely unless it is cyclic. If this is suspected, repeated testing should be performed over time. Two abnormal tests results are consistent with Cushing's syndrome. However, patients with pseudo-Cushing states may have mildly abnormal salivary and urine cortisol values; in this setting, a normal response to dexamethasone is against the diagnosis of Cushing's syndrome. Mixed results should prompt additional testing.

Investigation of the cause of Cushing's syndrome
Once the diagnosis of Cushing's syndrome is established, its cause must be determined. The first step is measurment of random plasma adrenocorticotrophic hormone when the patient is actively hypercortisolemic; suppressed values (<2 pmol/L (10 ng/L)) indicate adrenocorticotrophic-hormone-independent causes. Conversely, values more than 20 ng/L (4 pmol/L) indicate adrenocorticotrophic-hormone-dependent disease. Indeterminate values include all causes; in this case, a CRH test may help determine the cause.

Investigation of adrenocorticotrophic-hormone-independent Cushing's syndrome
Imaging studies identify unilateral or bilateral disease. On high-resolution CT scans, Hounsfield units are higher in cancer (>20 HU) and lower in adenoma (<10 HU) and contrast washout is low (<60%) and high, respectively. Bright MRI T2-weighted images suggest cancer.

The size of the mass(es) and evaluation of the contra-lateral gland are helpful. Most adenomas are less than 5 cm; the risk of cancer increases with size. Other features of malignancy include irregular borders and heterogeneity. The adrenal glands in macronodular adrenal hyperplasia are bilaterally enlarged (often >5 cm), with nodularity and/or hyperplasia. In McCune–Albright syndrome, glands may show bilateral (or less commonly, unilateral) nodularity and/or hyperplasia. The nodules in PPNAD are generally small (< 1 cm); the surrounding tissue may be atrophic, leading to a 'beads-on-a-string' appearance. Exogenous Cushing's syndrome should be suspected if both glands are atrophic.

Features of Carney complex (multiple lentigenes, blue nevi, large-cell calcifying Sertoli cell tumours, melanotic schwannoma, thyroid masses, acromegaly, and skin or cardiac myxomas) and a family history should be evaluated in PPNAD patients. If Carney complex is suspected, echocardiography and/or MRI should be performed, as cardiac myxomas are associated with heart failure, systemic embolization, and obstruction of cardiac blood flow, which may be fatal. Infants with McCune–Albright syndrome should be examined for characteristic skin lesions and fibrous dysplasia. Patients with adrenal cancer require staging for metastases and measurement of adrenal androgens and estrogens as tumour markers. No additional endocrine tests are needed in other patients.

Investigation of adrenocorticotrophic-hormone-dependent Cushing's syndrome

A pituitary MRI is the initial test in this evaluation. This is done to identify a pituitary macroadenoma or abnormal anatomy, given the high pretest probability of Cushing's disease (about 85%). Spin-echo T1-weighted sequences and another sensitive sequence (e.g. dynamic imaging or spoiled gradient echo) should be obtained, with and without administration of gadolinium contrast, in axial and sagittal views. It is very important to obtain dedicated pituitary sequences, not just a brain MRI. The smaller field of view and thinner sections enhance the ability to detect a tumour.

A pituitary tumour appears as a hypointense mass—often seen best on post-gadolinium images. However, a tumour is seen in only about 50% of patients with Cushing's disease. A further complication is the finding of small masses (6 mm or less) in healthy subjects and patients with ectopic secretion of adrenocorticotrophic hormone. Thus, only larger masses can be confidently considered to represent Cushing's disease.

Biochemical tests should identify Cushing's disease in more than 85% of patients (i.e. better than the pretest probability). Serum potassium and plasma adrenocorticotrophic hormone do not discriminate between Cushing's disease and ectopic adrenocorticotrophic hormone syndrome very well. Measurement of tumour marker (e.g. calcitonin, 5-hydroxyindoleacetic acid, serotonin, and catecholamines) may help to identify a neuroendocrine tumour.

Currently recommended dynamic tests include inferior petrosal sinus sampling and CRH stimulation. The DST (either 2 mg two-day or high dose, 8 mg) is still used, especially if inferior petrosal sinus sampling is not available, but its diagnostic accuracy is suboptimal. All tests should be done during a period of hypercortisolism so that normal corticotropes are suppressed. Thus, testing in cyclic Cushing's syndrome patients should be timed to occur in an active phase.

In experienced hands, inferior petrosal sinus sampling has 95% or better diagnostic accuracy and is the best test for the differential diagnosis of adrenocorticotrophic-hormone-dependent Cushing's syndrome. Each petrosal sinus is catheterized separately via a femoral approach, and blood for measurement of adrenocorticotrophic hormone is obtained simultaneously from each sinus and a peripheral vein (or inferior vena cava) at two time points just before and at 3 and 5 minutes (and possibly 10 minutes) after the administration of ovine or human CRH (1 μg/kg or 100 μg intravenous). Because adrenocorticotrophic hormone in Cushing's disease derives from the pituitary gland,

there is a gradient between one or both petrosal sinuses and the peripheral values. A maximal central-to-peripheral ratio of more than 2 before or 3 after administration of CRH at any time point indicates Cushing's disease; lower values indicate ectopic secretion of adrenocorticotrophic hormone. Comparison of the right and left values does not reliably predict the tumour location. The test can be falsely negative (i.e. give an inappropriate diagnosis of ectopic production of adrenocorticotrophic hormone) with abnormal venous anatomy (atrophic vessels or arborization). Recent studies suggest that prolactin measurement can evaluate successful catheterization and provide the correct diagnosis when the results suggest ectopic secretion of adrenocorticotrophic hormone.

Technical aspects are critical: each sinus must be correctly catheterized, the anatomy must be evaluated, and catheter placement must be confirmed. Complications include transient ear discomfort and, rarely, transient or permanent neurologic sequelae. Heparin may be given to prevent thrombosis.

The CRH stimulation test relies on the ability of corticotrope adenomas to release adrenocorticotrophic hormone in response to human or ovine CRH (1 μg/kg or 100 μg intravenous), whilst ectopic tumours do not. The test has about 90% sensitivity and specificity if ovine CRH is used. In a large series using human CRH, the best criterion for identifying Cushing's disease was an increase in cortisol of at least 14% from a mean basal (−15 and 0 minutes) to a mean of values taken at 15 and 30 minutes, giving a sensitivity of 85% and a specificity of 100%. The best adrenocorticotrophic hormone response was a maximal increase of at least 105%, giving 70% sensitivity and 100% specificity.

The DST has less ability to discriminate among adrenocorticotrophic-hormone-dependent causes. The test is based on the premise that patients with Cushing's disease (but not those with ectopic secretion of adrenocorticotrophic hormone) retain some response to negative feedback. Using a single 8 mg dose at 23:00 h, an initial criterion for suppression required a 50% or more reduction of the subsequent morning cortisol from that of the day before. However, an incorrect diagnosis would be assigned in up to 30% of patients with ectopic secretion of adrenocorticotrophic hormone, and 20% of those with Cushing's disease using this criterion. A greater than 30% suppression of mean serum cortisol at 24 and 48 hours during the 2-day low-dose DST had a sensitivity 65%, and specificity of 94% in one study, but this result has not been validated further.

Localization of the ectopic adrenocorticotrophic-hormone-producing tumour

Because these tumours occur most often in the chest, an initial chest CT scan with 1 mm slice thickness is cost-effective. An MRI is complementary and will identify these tumours as bright on T2 sequences. Scans with octreotide or its analogues are good adjunctive tests. Subsequent studies of the neck, the abdomen, and the pelvis may reveal a mass. However, many of these tumours remain occult for years.

Treatment

Surgical resection of the tumour

Identification and resection of the specific tumoural cause is the optimal treatment for all causes of Cushing's syndrome. If successful, cortisol levels fall to undetectable, and the patient requires glucocorticoid replacement. Those undergoing bilateral adrenalectomy require lifelong glucocorticoid and mineralocorticoid replacement. All other patients resume normal HPA function, generally over 6–18 months.

If surgical treatment is not possible or is not successful, other treatment is needed. Patients with adrenal cancer should be considered for mitotane and/or chemotherapy, ideally as part of adrenal cancer consortium studies. They may also require other steroidogenesis inhibitors in addition to mitotane (see 'Medical therapy'). The diagnosis should be reconsidered in patients in whom no tumour is found at trans-sphenoidal exploration. If tumour is found but the patient is not cured, repeat trans-sphenoidal surgery should be considered. However, if dural invasion was suspected (grossly or on pathology), additional surgery is not likely to be curative, and radiation therapy is indicated.

Medical therapy

Patients with failed trans-sphenoidal surgery, those in whom the surgery is too risky, and those with metastatic or occult ectopic adrenocorticotrophic-hormone-producing tumours require medical therapy. The available steroidogenesis inhibitors include ketoconazole, metyrapone, mitotane, and etomidate. The latter is an intravenous agent that is helpful in patients unable to take oral medications when adrenalectomy is not an option. Other agents are considered in 'Other medical therapy'. The first-line agent in the UK is usually metyrapone, and ketoconazole in the US. Overtreatment with any of these agents can lead to adrenal crisis.

The goal of medical treatment (except for mifepristone) is to normalize UFC values to achieve eucortisolism. Monitoring to acheive a morning serum cortisol value of 165–300 nmol/L (6–11 μg/dL) is a less cumbersome endpoint that is generally associated with normal or slightly increased UFC. Patients with cyclic Cushing's syndrome or those with marked variability in UFC may require a 'block-and-replace' strategy in which cortisol production is suppressed completely at all times, and glucocorticoid is replaced at physiologic doses.

Metyrapone inhibits 11-beta-hydroxylase activity. It is started at 0.75 to 1.50 g/day in 3–4 divided doses. Generally, 2.00 g/day is effective, although higher doses (up to 6.00 g/day) may be needed in ectopic-adrenocorticotrophic-hormone syndrome. The side effects are hirsutism and acne (due to increased adrenal androgens), gastrointestinal upset, and dizziness. Hypokalaemia, oedema, and hypertension due to increased mineralocorticoids are infrequent.

Ketoconazole inhibits multiple steps in steroidogenesis, especially side-chain cleavage. Treatment is usually started at 200 mg twice daily, with optimal doses between 400 and 1200 mg/day in four divided doses. Hepatotoxicity is the principal side effect. Reversible elevation of hepatic enzymes occurs in up to 15% of patients; the agent can be continued if levels remain below two to three times the upper normal range. Serious idiosyncratic hepatic injury occurs in approximately 1 of 15,000 patients, and can be fatal. Other adverse reactions include skin rashes and gastrointestinal upset (<15%). Ketoconazole is useful in women with hirsutism, which may be worsened with metyrapone. However, gynaecomastia and reduced libido in men may be unacceptable and require alternative agents.

Mitotane inhibits steroidogenesis and is cytolytic at higher doses. It has been used in combination with radiotherapy and other steroidogenesis inhibitors at daily doses of 0.5–4.0 g. Adverse reactions include gastrointestinal and neurologic toxicity, which may be avoided by beginning at a dose of 0.5 to 1.0 g/day and increasing gradually, by 0.5 to 1.0 g every 1 to 4 weeks. Doses are taken once daily with food. Other adverse effects include gynaecomastia, skin rash, elevated liver enzymes, and abnormal platelet function. Mitotane is teratogenic and has a long half-life so it is not recommended for women desiring fertility within 2–5 years.

Other medical therapy

The dopamine agonist cabergoline normalizes UFC in about 20% of patients with Cushing's disease; the somatostatin analogue pasireotide has similar efficacy but a 73% rate of hyperglycemic events. Patients with lower UFC are most likely to normalize UFC with these agents. The glucocorticoid antagonist mifepristone can improve glucocse tolerance; because UFC does not decrease, clinical features must be used to adjust the dose.

Radiotherapy and radiosurgery

These are used to treat Cushing's disease. Conventional pituitary radiotherapy is given at a total dose of 4500–5000 cGy (rad) in 25 fractional doses over 35 days, using a three-field technique based on stereotactic conformal field planning. When used in the setting of failed trans-sphenoidal sugery, it achieves remission rates up to 83%, beginning 9 months after treatment; most patients are in remission by 2 years.

In stereotactic radiosurgery, concentrated beams of radiation are aimed at a precisely mapped lesion and deliver very high doses to the tumour and relatively low doses to normal surrounding tissue, usually in a single session. The procedure comprises a number of techniques: using narrow beams from multiple gamma cobalt sources (gamma knife), using heavy charged particles (proton or helium beams), or using a single beam from a linear accelerator that is arced around the target (X-knife, SMART, linac). The technique may be used to deliver radiation to the entire pituitary gland when a specific target is not known. Hypopituitarism is a common side effect of both types of radiotherapy.

Bilateral adrenalectomy
for adrenocorticotrophic-hormone-dependent causes

Bilateral adrenalectomy gives rapid resolution of fulminant hypercortisolism and is potentially life-saving. It may be chosen over radiation therapy by young patients desiring fertility and who have concerns about radiation-induced loss of reproductive function and hypopituitarism. Its disadvantages include perioperative morbidity and mortality and the lifelong requirement for glucocorticoid and mineralocorticoid replacement. Surveillance for an occult tumor must continue (usually annually) in patients with occult ectopic secretion of adrenocorticotrophic hormone.

Prognosis

The prognosis for adrenal cancer is almost uniformly poor. For other forms of Cushing's syndrome, mortality is much reduced after successful therapy, although it may still not return to normal, especially in patients requiring several modes of treatment. In addition, varying co-morbidities may not necessarily resolve and require individualized treatment.

Subclinical Cushing's syndrome (Autonomous cortisol secretion)

In 5%–10% of patients with adrenal adenomas, there is evidence of significant autonomous cortisol secretion sufficient to be associated with hypertension, glucose intolerance, reduced bone density, hyperlipidaemia, and increased mortality. However, there are currently no controlled trials on the efficacy and advisability of surgical resection. Treatment of co-morbidities is indicated.

Further reading

Chiodini I. Clinical review: Diagnosis and treatment of subclinical hypercortisolism. *J Clin Endocrinol Metab* 2011; 96: 1223–36.

Debono M, Bradburn M, Bull M, et al. Cortisol as a marker for increased mortality in patients with incidental adrenocortical adenomas. *J Clin Endocrinol Metab* 2014; 99: 4462–70.

Estrada J, Boronat M, Mielgo M, et al. The long-term outcome of pituitary irradiation after unsuccessful transsphenoidal surgery in Cushing's disease. *N Engl J Med* 1997; 336: 172–7.

Findling JW and Raff H. Cushing's syndrome: Important issues in diagnosis and management. *J Clin Endocrinol Metab* 2006; 91: 3746–53.

Nieman LK, Biller BM, Findling JW, et al. The diagnosis of Cushing's syndrome: An Endocrine Society clinical practice guideline. *J Clin Endocrinol Metab* 2008; 93: 1526–40.

Nieman LK, Biller BM, Findling JW, et al. Treatment of Cushing's syndrome: An Endocrine Scoiety Clinical practice guideline. *J Clin Endocrinol Metab* 2015; 100: 2807–31.

Steffensen C, Bak AM, Rubeck KZ, et al. Epidemiology of Cushing's syndrome. *Neuroendocrinology* 2010; 92 (Suppl. 1): 1–5.

Tritos NA, Biller BM, and Swearingen B. Management of Cushing disease. *Nat Rev Endocrinol* 2011; 7: 279–89.

Valassi E, Swearingen B, Lee H, et al. Concomitant medication use can confound interpretation of the combined dexamethasone-corticotropin releasing hormone test in Cushing's syndrome. *J Clin Endocrinol Metab* 2009; 94: 4851–9.

Zemskova MS, Gundabolu B, Sinaii N, et al. Utility of various functional and anatomic imaging modalities for detection of ectopic adrenocorticotropin-secreting tumors. *J Clin Endocrinol Metab* 2010; 95: 1207–19.

6.9 Adrenal incidentalomas

Definition
The term 'adrenal incidentaloma' applies to any adrenal mass of 1 cm or more that is discovered serendipitously in the workup of clinical conditions unrelated to adrenal diseases. Adrenal incidentaloma is increasingly recognized in current practice as a byproduct of technological medicine. In the context of ageing Western societies with a widespread access to advanced radiological tests, adrenal incidentaloma should be considered a public health challenge.

Pathophysiology and epidemiology
The pathophysiology of adrenal incidentaloma remains uncertain, although it may be speculated that it is a hallmark of the ageing process of the adrenal glands. In both autopsy and clinical series, the frequency of adrenal incidentaloma peaks in the fifth to the seventh decade of age, when it approximates 7%–10% whilst being <1% in the third decade and extremely rare in childhood and adolescence. Frequency does not vary according to gender in autopsy series; in clinical series, a slight excess of adrenal incidentaloma in women is due to a referral bias. Using contemporary high-resolution scanning technology, the rate of discovery of adrenal incidentalomas is 4%, or more, in subjects of middle age. adrenal incidentalomas are bilateral in about 10% of cases.

Adrenal incidentaloma is a heterogeneous condition including a variety of diseases listed in Table 6.10. The distribution of the different adrenal incidentaloma types is affected by referral patterns and inclusion criteria. Adrenocortical cancer and phaeochromocytoma are over-represented in surgical series whilst metastases of extra-adrenal tumours are frequent seen in oncology patients. Conversely, metastases are rare in patients without a history of malignancy.

Clinical features
By definition, patients with adrenal incidentalomas should not present specific features of a definite endocrine syndrome (Cushing's, primary aldosteronism, catecholamine excess). Therefore, clinical presentation is non-specific, including a variety of signs and symptoms. The purest definition of adrenal incidentaloma excludes the overtly secreting adrenal tumours that are discovered by chance because the clinical picture was initially missed. However, adrenal incidentalomas may be functional and produce a slight hormone excess that is insufficient to cause a full-blown phenotype. Patients with silent phaeochromocytomas are normotensive or have stable, low-grade hypertension, whilst patients with subclinical Cushing's may show a metabolic syndrome without the typical cushingoid features.

Investigations
The diagnostic approach to an adrenal incidentaloma is aimed at recognizing the tumours that may harm the patients and can be effectively treated once recognized. Adrenocortical cancer is on top of the list, due to its biological aggressiveness heralded by poor 5-year survival; complete surgical resection is the only hope to improve prognosis. Phaeochromocytoma has also the potential to significantly affect patients' health if it remains undiagnosed, and surgery is the treatment of choice. The adrenal glands are sites of metastatic spread of many malignancies that are usually known when the adrenal incidentaloma is detected; rarely, an adrenal incidentaloma is the presenting feature of an occult extra-adrenal cancer.

An optimal radiological assessment is the key to differentiating between benign tumours and tumours associated with an increased mortality (malignancies or phaeochromocytomas). Unenhanced CT is most useful, allowing one to identify different imaging phenotypes (Box 6.4), although overlap between categories does exist. MRI does not offer any significant advantage

Table 6.10 Causes of adrenal incidentaloma in surgical and clinical series; data are presented as the average and range of the frequencies reported in the relevant studies

Causes of adrenal incidentaloma	Surgical series (%)	Clinical series (%)
Adrenal adenoma	55 (49–69)	75 (33–96)
Phaeochromocytoma	10.0 (1.0–15.0)	7.0 (1.5–14.0)
Adrenal carcinoma	11.0 (1.2–12.0)	8.0 (1.2–11.0)
Metastasis	7.0 (0.0–21.0)	5.0 (0.0–18.0)
Myelolypoma	8.0 (7.0–15.0)	2.0 (0.0–5.0)
Cyst	5.0 (4.0–22.0)	2.0 (0.0–8.0)
Ganglioneuroma	4.0 (0.0–8.0)	1.0 (0.0–4.0)

Box 6.4 CT imaging phenotype of the most frequent types of adrenal incidentaloma

Adrenal adenoma
Small size; usually ≤4.0 cm
   Regular shape with well-defined margins
   Homogeneous and hypodense content (attenuation value ≤10 HU on unenhanced CT scan and ≤30 HU on enhanced CT scan)

Adrenocortical carcinoma
Large size; usually >4.0 cm
   Intratumoural necrosis and haemorrhage
   Irregular shape with ill-defined margins
   Possible involvement of adjacent tissues or organs, or distant metastases
   inhomogeneous and hyperdense content (above the thresholds of adenoma)

Phaeochromocytoma
Any size; usually >3.0 cm
   Well-defined margins
   Intratumoural cystic areas and haemorrhage
   Increased vascularity
   Inhomogeneous and hyperdense content (above the thresholds of adenoma)

Metastasis
Any size; usually >3.0 cm
   Often multiple, bilateral lesions
   Irregular shape with ill-defined margins
   Inhomogeneous and hyperdense content (above the thresholds of adenoma)

and, in clinical practice, unenhanced CT should be considered the primary diagnostic test (see Figure 6.25). The CT that detects an adrenal incidentaloma is ordered for other reasons and is usually obtained with early scanning after intravenous contrast; thus, it is advised to repeat the CT in basal conditions to obtain an accurate assessment of mass density, which is the most reliable parameter for separating adrenal adenomas from non-adenomas, with the latter category including the potentially dangerous tumours. A density of ≤10 HU on unenhanced CT indicates a benign lipid-rich adenoma whilst lesions with a density >10 HU are considered indeterminate and in need of further characterization: 30% of adrenal adenomas are lipid poor and may fall in this category. The assessment of contrast washout on delayed enhanced scans is accurate in refining the diagnosis, or a functional MRI (in- and out-of-phase) may be helpful. However, FDG PET or PET–CT is increasingly used in patients with equivocal tumours at CT. Although FDG PET may miss small adrenal malignancies, although uptake is possible in some adrenal adenomas and phaeochromocytomas, it is of particular help in avoiding unnecessary surgery due to its excellent negative predictive value. Fine-needle aspiration biopsy has a limited role in patients with presumed adrenal metastases or rare adrenal tumours (e.g. lymphoma) and is not indicated to pursue the diagnosis of adrenocortical cancer because of poor differentiation from adenoma, and safety issues.

Hormonal assessment should complement radiologic workup in any adrenal incidentaloma except when CT characteristics are typical for myelolipoma or an adrenal cyst (Figure 6.25). Since phaeochromocytomas may frequently present with non-specific imaging findings, it is mandatory to perform an appropriate biochemical screening in every adrenal incidentaloma that is not categorized as a typical adenoma. Screening is usually done with measurement of 24-hour plasma or urinary fractionated metanephrines and is most needed whenever

fine-needle aspiration biopsy or surgical removal of the mass is deemed necessary. Patients with a presumed adrenocortical cancer should undergo hormonal assessment (including possibly urinary steroid profile) to detect steroid secretion, whereas hypoadrenalism has to be excluded in patients with bilateral adrenal metastases. It is advised to rule out subclinical Cushing's syndrome in most patients with a presumed adrenal adenoma, whilst primary aldosteronism should be considered when hypertension and/or unexplained hypokalaemia are present.

Subclinical Cushing's syndrome is a common disorder that may be observed in 5%–25% of adrenal incidentaloma, depending on variable diagnostic criteria, characterized by an adrenal adenoma secreting cortisol independently of pituitary feedback. A minimal-to-slight cortisol excess may ensue and contribute to metabolic syndrome, increased the risk of cardiovascular events and bone fractures. However, it remains to be definitively demonstrated whether subclinical Cushing's syndrome predisposes to the classical complications of overt cortisol excess. Subclinical Cushing's syndrome is defined by three criteria: first, incidental discovery of an adrenal adenoma without any previous suspect of adrenal disease; second, lack of a clear Cushingoid phenotype; third, documentation of autonomous (adrenocorticotrophic-hormone-independent) cortisol secretion. The best strategy to diagnose subclinical Cushing's syndrome remains controversial, and many algorithms including different tests have been proposed. However, the value of an extensive assessment of the HPA axis has been questioned, due to the lack of a clear demonstration that subclinical Cushing's syndrome may have a negative impact on patients' health. A simple approach based on the 1 mg DST, with further testing guided by clinical judgement, is presented in Figure 6.26.

Management

Surgery is the appropriate treatment for adrenal incidentaloma with a presumptive diagnosis of either

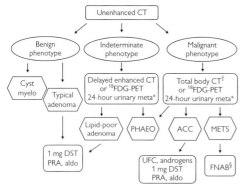

Fig 6.25 Diagnostic approach to adrenal incidentaloma, based on the results of unenhanced CT; ACC, adrenocortical cancer; aldo, aldosterone; DST, dexamethasone suppression test; [18]FDG, ^{18}F-fluorodeoxyglucose; FNAB, fine-needle aspiration biopsy; meta, metanephrines; METS, metastases; myelo, myelolypoma; PHAEO, phaeochromocytoma; PRA, plasma renin activity; UFC, urinary free cortisol.

* Plasma metanephrines are an alternative.
† Total body CT is performed for staging purposes.
§ FNAB is used in selected cases only.

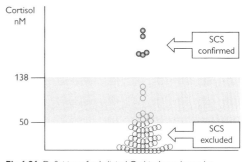

Fig 6.26 Definition of subclinical Cushing's syndrome by using different cut-off levels of cortisol after a 1 mg overnight dexamethasone suppression test. Cortisol levels <50 nmol/L (1.81 µg/dL) exclude the condition, whilst levels >138 nmol/L (5 µg/dL) are confirmatory. Cortisol levels between these are indeterminate. In the presence of clinical features suggestive of hypercortisolism, additional endocrine tests are needed to prove the condition; SCS, subclinical Cushing's syndrome.
Reproduced with permission from Terzolo A, Reimondo PG, Subclinical Cushing's syndrome: definition and management, *Clinical Endocrinology*, Volume 76, pp. 12–18, Copyright © 2011 John Wiley and Sons Ltd.

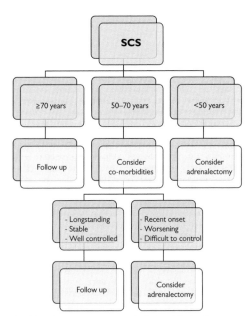

Fig 6.27 Management strategy of subclinical Cushing's syndrome; SCS, subclinical Cushing's syndrome.
Reproduced with permission from Terzolo A, Reimondo PG, Subclinical Cushing's syndrome: definition and management, *Clinical Endocrinology*, Volume 76, pp. 12–18, Copyright © 2011 John Wiley and Sons Ltd.

adrenocortical cancer or phaeochromocytoma. Both tumours are potentially lethal, and the patient's outcome can be improved by timely adrenalectomy, thus justifying a low threshold for recommending surgery in doubtful cases. Treatment of metastases of extra-adrenal tumours depends on different clinical circumstances. Surgery is also usually recommended in the event of an inconclusive diagnosis, particularly when an adrenal incidentaloma shows unsafe attenuation values or is larger than 4 cm.

The management of typical adrenal adenomas depends on whether they are functioning or not. Surgery should be considered in those cases of primary aldosteronism that represent a potentially curable form of hypertension. Treatment of subclinical Cushing's syndrome remains a dilemma, since there is currently insufficient evidence of increased morbidity associated with the condition that may reversed by adrenalectomy. Thus, data are insufficient to indicate whether surgery is superior to a conservative management for patients with subclinical

Cushing's syndrome. In case of adrenalectomy, patients should receive post-operative glucocorticoid coverage to prevent an adrenal crisis. A pragmatic strategy for managing subclinical Cushing's syndrome is presented in Figure 6.27.

The large majority of adrenal adenomas remain untreated, and the limited evidence on their natural history precludes any firm recommendation for follow-up. The value of periodic hormonal screening is uncertain and it is more important to conduct a clinical surveillance programme to detect the development of hormone excess. However, the risk of progression from subclinical to overt Cushing's syndrome is minimal. It is common practice to repeat the CT after 3–6 months from diagnosis, to recognize a rapidly growing mass. Patients with tumours less than 2 cm do not need further imaging but, for larger tumours, the need of imaging follow-up should be judged individually, taking into consideration the characteristics of the patient and the mass, and taking into account the very limited risk that a benign adrenal incidentaloma will undergo malignant transformation during follow-up.

Further reading

Aron DC. The adrenal incidentaloma: Disease of modern technology and public health problem. *Rev Endocr Metab Disord* 2001; 2: 335–42.

Barzon L, Sonino N, Fallo F, et al. Prevalence and natural history of adrenal incidentalomas. *Eur J Endocrinol* 2003; 149: 273–85.

Cawood TJ, Hunt PJ, O'Shea D, et al. Recommended evaluation of adrenal incidentalomas is costly, has high false positive rates and confers a risk of fatal cancer that is similar to the risk of the adrenal lesion becoming malignant; time for a rethink? *Eur J Endocrinol* 2009; 161: 513–27.

Grumbach MM, Biller BMK, Braunstein GD, et al. Management of the clinically inapparent adrenal mass ('incidentaloma'). *Ann Intern Med* 2003; 138: 424–9.

Kloos RT, Gross MD, Francis IR, et al. Incidentally discovered adrenal masses. *End Rev* 1995; 16: 460–84.

Mansmann G, Lau J, Balk E, et al. The clinically inapparent adrenal mass: Update in diagnosis and management. *End Rev* 2004; 25: 309–40.

Martin Fassnacht, Wiebke Arlt, Irina Bancos, Henning Dralle, John Newell-Price, Anju Sahdev, Antoine Tabarin, Massimo Terzolo, Stylianos Tsagarakis and Olaf M Dekkers, Management of adrenal incidentalomas: European Society of Endocrinology clinical practice guideline in collaboration with the European Network for the Study of Adrenal Tumors. *Eur J Endocrinol* 2016; 175: G1–34.

Terzolo M, Pia A, and Reimondo G. Subclinical Cushing's syndrome: Definition and management. *Clin Endocrinol (Oxf)* 2012; 76: 12–18.

Terzolo M, Stigliano A, Chiodini I, et al. AME position statement on adrenal incidentaloma. *Eur J Endocrinol* 2011; 164: 851–70.

Young WF. The incidentally discovered adrenal mass. *N Engl J Med* 2007; 356: 601–10.

6.10 Adrenal carcinoma

Epidemiology

Adrenocortical carcinoma is a rare and highly aggressive malignancy with an annual incidence of 0.7–2.0 cases per million population. It can occur at any age, with a peak incidence between 40 and 50 years, and women are more often affected (55%–60%). The molecular pathogenesis is still only incompletely understood.

Clinical presentation

Most patients present with steroid hormone excess, for example Cushing syndrome or virilization, or abdominal mass effects, but a growing proportion of patients with adrenocortical carcinoma (currently >15%) is initially diagnosed incidentally (see Box 6.5).

Diagnostic workup

For diagnostic workup, comprehensive hormonal assessment is required, because in most adrenocortical carcinomas evidence for autonomous steroid secretion can be found. For the preoperative laboratory workup, we currently follow the recommendation of the European Network for the Study of Adrenal Tumours (www.ensat.org/ACC.htm). It comprises assessment of basal cortisol, adrenocorticotrophic hormone, dehydroepiandrostenedione sulphate, 17-hydroxyprogesterone, androstenedione, testosterone, and estradiol, as well as a DST and a UFC. The aldosterone-to-renin ratio is measured in patients with hypertension or hypokalaemia. This panel may prove the adrenocortical origin of the lesion, suggest malignancy, and document autonomous glucocorticoid excess which, if missed, regularly entails post-operative adrenal failure.

Together with a careful endocrine workup, modern cross-sectional imaging is able to correctly diagnose an adrenal mass as adrenocortical carcinoma prior to surgery in the majority of cases. Size is an obvious criterion for differentiating an adrenal mass, since the median size of adrenocortical carcinomas is 11 cm, whereas most adenomas are <5 cm. Currently, no single imaging method can characterize with certainty a localized adrenal mass as an adrenocortical carcinoma, but a threshold of ≤10 HU in unenhanced CT or a relative washout >50% 10 min after contrast media can be used to diagnose a benign adrenal lesions. State-of-the-art MRI including chemical shift is probably equally accurate as CT. In the difficult case, additional functional imaging (FDG or metomidate PET) is often helpful. With very few exceptions, there is no role for a fine-needle biopsy of an adrenal tumour.

All patients with suspected adrenocortical carcinoma require a chest CT scan prior to surgery, since the lung is the most frequent localization of metastases (see Box 6.6).

Treatment

We recommend a multidisciplinary approach with advice and possibly referral to a major centre specializing in these tumours. As many patients as possible should be treated within clinical trials, to improve our knowledge and treatment options in this rare disease.

Surgery (see also Section 6.14) is the single most important intervention in the treatment of non-metastatic adrenocortical carcinoma. Whilst preoperative evidence of locally advanced disease undoubtedly requires open adrenalectomy, some groups have postulated that tumours with a diameter of <106 cm may be safely treated by laparoscopic adrenalectomy. However, open adrenalectomy should still be regarded as standard treatment for adrenocortical carcinoma. New data suggest that locoregional lymph node dissection improves therapeutic outcome.

As the recurrence rate even after complete resection is high, adjuvant treatment should be considered in all patients. We currently try to stratify patients according to their perceived risk of recurrence. In most patients, we recommend an adjuvant mitotane treatment (see also Box 6.7) for at least 2 years. In patients with very high risk (e.g. R1 resection or high proliferative Ki67 index >30%), we suggest additional radiotherapy of the tumour bed or cytotoxic drugs, whereas in low-risk patients (R0 resection and Ki67 ≤10%) the evidence for an adjuvant treatment is lower, and an individualized decision is needed.

In case of recurrence, we suggest the following approach: surgery should be performed in patients who have had a disease-free interval of more than 12 months and in whom a complete resection is feasible. However, we advocate against surgery if the time between surgery

---

Box 6.6 Localization of metastases in patients with metastatic disease

Lung: 80%
Liver: 60%
Skeleton: 25%
Brain: 5%–10%
Other locations: 10%–15%

Box 6.7 Mitotane treatment

- Start with 1.5 g/day and increase daily dose within 4–6 days to 6 g/day. For patients in poor clinical condition or with concomitant cytotoxic drugs, a lower dosage (e.g. 3 g/day) is recommended.
- Measure mitotane blood level every 3–4 weeks and adapt dosage according tolerability and blood level (target 14–20 mg/L).
- All patients require concomitant high-dose glucocorticoid replacement (e.g. 20–20–10 mg hydrocortisone/day).
- Mitotane influences by strong induction of CYP3A4 the metabolism of many drugs (e.g. antihypertensives, antibiotics, steroids).

Box 6.5 Clinical presentation of adrenal carcinoma

Cushing's syndrome: 30%
Hirsutism/virilization: 30%
Abdominal symptoms: 25%
Feminization: 5%–10%
Incidentaloma 15%–20%

and recurrence is less than 6 months. These patients are likely to benefit more from aggressive medical treatment. In all other patients, individualized treatment concepts (e.g. combination of medical therapy and ablative procedures) are applied.

Treatment for metastatic adrenocortical carcinoma is challenging, because the median overall survival is only about 12–15 months; however, there is significant heterogeneity. Only the combination chemotherapy of etoposide, doxorubicin, cisplatin, and mitotane has been validated in a randomized controlled trial. In selected patients with presumably less aggressive disease (e.g. slowly progressing tumour growth, only two involved organs, long disease-free interval after initial surgery), we use mitotane monotherapy as first-line treatment and add etoposide, doxorubicin, and cisplatin only in case of progression.

Unfortunately, up to now, none of the investigated 'targeted therapies' showed promising results in adrenocortical carcinoma.

As mitotane is currently the cornerstone of medical treatment for adrenocortical carcinoma it is necessary to understand its use and possible adverse effects (see also Box 6.7). Mitotane is given orally and specifically targets cells derived from the adrenal cortex. Since the bioavailability of the drug is quite variable, a certain drug level is required to be efficient, and toxicity depends on the blood level, it is recommend to monitor the plasma level, aiming at a concentration of 14–20 mg/L. Mitotane comes with significant toxicity, and patients should be followed closely. Dizziness, vertigo, and other CNS disturbances are common, and virtually all patients suffer some kind of gastrointestinal symptoms requiring active management with antiemetics and loperamide, as individually indicated. Furthermore, all patients develop adrenal insufficiency, which has to be replaced with high doses of hydrocortisone. Recent data indicate that mitotane is one of the strongest inducers of cytochrome p450 3A4 (CYP3A4) and this has a major impact on the care of adrenocortical carcinoma patients, because mitotane lowers the blood levels of many drugs frequently co-administered with mitotane (including but not limited to steroids, antihypertensives, and antibiotics).

The prognosis of adrenocortical carcinoma, with a median overall survival of 3.5 years, is still poor. However, international cooperation in the fight against this dreadful disease has undoubtedly set the stage for progress in the coming years.

Further reading

Berruti A, Baudin E, Gelderblom H, et al. Adrenal cancer: ESMO Clinical Practice Guidelines for diagnosis, treatment and follow-up. *Ann Oncol* 2012; 23 (Suppl. 7): vii 131–8.

Fassnacht M, Arlt W, Bancos I, et al. Management of adrenal incidentalomas: European Society of Endocrinology Clinical Practice Guideline in collaboration with the European Network for the Study of Adrenal Tumors. *Eur J Endocrinol* 2016; 175(2): G1–G34.

Fassnacht M, Libé R, Kroiss M, et al. Adrenocortical carcinoma: A clinician's update. *Nat Rev Endocrinol* 2011; 7: 323–35.

Fassnacht M, Terzolo M, Allolio B, et al. 2012 Combination chemotherapy in advanced adrenocortical carcinoma. *N Engl J Med* 366: 2189–97.

Terzolo M, Angeli A, Fassnacht M, et al. 2007 Adjuvant mitotane treatment for adrenocortical carcinoma. *N Engl J Med* 356: 2372–80.

6.11 Addison's disease

Definition
Addison's disease (also known as primary adrenal insufficiency) is caused by destruction of the adrenal cortex and is characterized by impaired adrenocortical function resulting in decreased production of glucocorticoids, mineralocorticoids, and androgens.

Pathophysiology
The pathophysiology of Addison's disease is as follows:
- autoimmune (commonest cause in developed world); isolated or as part of autoimmune polyendocrine syndrome type 1 or 2 (see Chapter 5, Section 5.9); may be associated with the following:
  - autoimmune polyendocrine syndrome type 1 (rare; due to mutations in the autoimmune regulator gene *AIRE*, causing hypoparathyroidism)
  - chronic mucocutaneous candidiasis
  - autoimmune polyendocrine syndrome type 2 (mainly primary hypothyroidism, atrophic gastritis, B_{12} deficiency, and type 1 diabetes mellitus)
  - vitiligo (common)
- malignancy (metastatic (lung, breast, kidney) lymphoma); although the adrenal glands are common sites for metastases as visualized on axial imaging, adrenal insufficiency is unusual
- infiltration (amyloid, sarcoidosis)
- infection (TB (commonest cause worldwide)), histoplasmosis, AIDS (CMV, *Mycobacterium intracellulare*, cryptococcus)
- vascular haemorrhage (meningococcaemia, anticoagulants, trauma)
- infarction (e.g. anti-phospholipid syndrome and thrombosis)
- adrenoleukodystrophy (X linked)
- bilateral adrenalectomy/drugs (steroid-synthesis inhibitors)

Epidemiology
The prevalence of Addison's disease is 93–140 per million, with an incidence of 4.7–6.2 per million in Caucasian populations. Women are affected more often than men. Autoimmune Addison's disease has a peak incidence in the third to the fifth decade, but may occur at any age.

Clinical features
Chronic presentation
The onset of Addison's disease is usually gradual and insidious, and may go undetected until an illness or stress precipitates an adrenal crisis. As symptoms are non-specific in chronic Addison's disease, a significant number of patients have the following signs or symptoms for a year before diagnosis:
- weight loss
- fatigue
- loss of energy
- abdominal pain
- anorexia
- weakness

- pigmentation due to high adrenocorticotrophic hormone levels, in sun-exposed areas and areas of pressure (elbows, knees), palm creases, and buccal mucosa

Mineralocorticoid deficiency, with resultant electrolyte abnormalities and postural hypotension (may also occur with cortisol deficiency), and androgen deficiency with loss of axillary and pubic hair and loss of libido are also features.

Acute presentation
Patients with acute adrenal insufficiency usually present acutely unwell, with the following:
- hypotension
- collapse
- vomiting
- abdominal pain
- fever
- history or signs of a condition precipitating the event

Typically, these patients do not respond fully to fluid resuscitation unless glucocorticoids are given. If the condition is not treated it may result in confusion, coma, and death, and is a medical emergency.

Investigation
Investigation is a two-step process:
1. Determine if Addison's disease is present.
2. Determine the cause.

Treatment must not be delayed in the acute setting or once a diagnosis has been made.

Step 1: Is adrenal insufficiency present?
A thorough history and examination for symptoms and signs directly related to adrenal insufficiency is mandatory. Further, history taking should also be directed to identifying a possible cause for adrenal insufficiency, such as a history of autoimmune conditions or malignancy, a family history of endocrine disorders, use of drugs affecting cortisol production or the use of long-term steroids (causing secondary adrenal insufficiency). The management of these patients is discussed in Section 6.12. Social history should be directed towards identification of risk factors, including risks for sexually transmitted disorders. Signs of autoimmune disorders, such as vitiligo, or signs of underlying malignancy may also be useful in suggesting the diagnosis. Oral oestrogens will increase CBG levels and falsely elevate serum cortisol.

Biochemical investigation of chronic presentation
In practice, if there is a good clinical suspicion of Addison's disease, it is safer and more time efficient to perform all basal tests at the basal sampling point of a Synacthen® test, which should be performed at the same time of the initial clinic visit—investigation should not be delayed.

Basal testing results
- Hyponatraemia, hyperkalaemia, and elevated urea may be present.
- Basal morning cortisol may be in the normal range; a level >500–550 nmol/L (18–20 µg/dL)) excludes the diagnosis.
- Elevated morning plasma adrenocorticotrophic hormone compared to level of cortisol is suggestive of Addison's disease.

- A full blood count (normochromic, normocytic anaemia, eosinophilia in Addison's disease) should be performed.
- Serum calcium may be elevated in Addison's disease.
- TFTs should be performed (cortisol deficiency may result in elevated TSH that resolves on treating adrenal insufficiency).
- The DHEAS level may be low.

Short Synacthen® (adrenocorticotrophic hormone 1–24) test
- Blood samples for serum cortisol, plasma adrenocorticotrophic hormone, and renin are taken. Elevated plasma adrenocorticotrophic hormone and renin are found in Addison's disease.
- Next, 250 μg of Synacthen® is administered intramuscularly or intravenously.
- Serum cortisol is sampled at 30 (and in some centres) 60 minutes.
- Serum cortisol >500–550 nmol/L (18–20 μg/dL) at 30 or 60 minutes indicates an adequate response.

Biochemical investigation of acute presentation
In the acutely unwell patient, when there is a high index of suspicion for adrenal insufficiency, samples for serum cortisol and plasma adrenocorticotrophic hormone should be taken, together with serum for electrolytes, glucose, calcium, and haematology, and treatment with fluids and glucocorticoids initiated immediately and before the result is available.
- Serum cortisol <250 nmol/L (9 μg/dL) and increased adrenocorticotrophic hormone is diagnostic of Addison's disease.
- Serum cortisol <400 nmol/L (14 μg/dL) and increased adrenocorticotrophic hormone is strongly suggestive of Addison's disease.
- Confirmatory testing can be performed once the patient is medically stabilized.

Step 2: Investigation of the cause
Since autoimmune adrenalitis is the commonest cause of Addison's disease in developing countries, initial testing of autoantibodies to 21-hydroxylase should be performed. In time, autoantibodies may become negative, emphasizing the need for testing early after diagnosis, and the fact that a lack of antibodies does not exclude autoimmunity.
A suggested schema for investigation is as follows:
1. Test autoantibodies to 21-hydroxylase.
2. If negative, CT of the adrenal glands is needed.
3. If normal, CT adrenal in males; analysis of very long chain fatty acids (for X-linked adrenoleukodystrophy) is indicated.
4. In younger patients with positive 21-hydroxylase autoantibodies and other clinical manifestations suggesting autoimmune polyendocrine syndrome type 1,

preferably, genetic testing for *AIRE* mutations, or an assay for anti-interferon omega or anti-interleukin-22 antibodies, is indicated to establish a diagnosis.

Management
Emergency: Known or suspected diagnosis
- Acute adrenal insufficiency is a medical emergency.
- After a blood sample is taken for serum cortisol, and if possible plasma adrenocorticotrophic hormone for later analysis, large volumes of 0.9% saline are needed—several litres over 24 hours.
- Hydrocortisone 100 mg given as an intravenous bolus, followed by 100 mg intramuscularly 6-hourly. On recovery, double replacement oral doses are given until the patient is well.
- Glucose supplementation may be necessary if hypoglycaemia develops. The precipitant should be identified and treated.

Maintenance
See Section 6.12.

Prognosis
Patients with Addison's disease, although on full replacement therapy, have a mortality rate twofold greater than that of the background population. Most deaths are from cardiovascular, malignant, endocrine, respiratory, or infectious causes. It is possible that a major contributor to cardiovascular mortality is relative overdosing with hydrocortisone.

Patient support groups
The Addison's Disease Self-Help Group (http:www.addisons.org.uk) may be useful.

Future developments
Use of high-dose Synacthen® to rescue adrenocortical cells in the stem-cell niche, and immunosuppressive therapies, are currently being evaluated in early clinical trials in patients with new-onset autoimmune Addison's disease, with reversal of adrenal failure in isolated cases. Despite the small numbers tested, this is a highly promising approach.

Further reading
Arlt W and Allolio B. Adrenal insufficiency. *Lancet* 2003; 361: 1881–93.

Gan EH, MacArthur K, Mitchell AL, et al. Residual adrenal function in autoimmune Addison's disease: Improvement after tetracosactide (ACTH1–24) treatment. *J Clin Endocrinol Metab* 2014; 99: 111–18.

Husebye ES, Allolio B, Arlt W, et al. Consensus statement on the diagnosis, treatment and follow-up of patients with primary adrenal insufficiency. *J Intern Med* 2014; 275: 104–15.

White K and Arlt W. Adrenal crisis in treated Addison's disease: A predictable but under-managed event. *Eur J Endocrinol* 2010; 162: 115–20.

6.12 Glucocorticoid replacement

Definition
Lifelong glucocorticoid replacement therapy is mandatory for anyone with Addison's disease (primary adrenal insufficiency) or secondary adrenal insufficiency. Maintenance doses aim to be as physiological as possible

Maintenance glucocorticoid replacement
Physiology
- Cortisol is secreted in a circadian fashion, with levels starting to rise at around 3:00–4:00 h and a peak at 8:00 h in people on normal day–night patterns of activity, with levels then falling over the day thereafter.
- In addition, there are pulsatile peaks and troughs (ultradian secretion).
- The average daily secretion is between 5 and 10 mg/m^2 body surface area per 24 hours.
- The oral equivalent dose for replacement therapy is 15–25 mg of hydrocortisone per day.

Limitations of glucocorticoid replacement
- Current oral glucocorticoid therapy is unable to mimic the daily secretory pattern of cortisol.
- Typically, patients with adrenal insufficiency awake with very low or undetectable levels of serum cortisol at exactly the time point when this should be at a maximum.
- No oral replacement preparation can reproduce the ultradian pattern of cortisol secretion.

Oral preparations
Hydrocortisone
- Oral hydrocortisone is the treatment of choice.
- Doses are usually given twice or thrice daily (e.g. 10 mg on waking, 5 mg at midday, and 5 mg at 18:00 h).
- Weight-adjusted dosing regimens provide optimum replacement.
- Dual-release hydrocortisone, providing a more prolonged release of hydrocortisone and a more physiological level of cortisol, is available and also under development. Whether it has any major advantages remains unclear at present.

Cortisone acetate
- Oral cortisone acetate is used in several countries
- Daily doses of 25–30 mg are usual
- The need for activation by hepatic 11-beta-hydroxysteroid dehydrogenase causes a slight delay in the onset of action.
- There is no definitive method of monitoring treatment, and clinical assessment may be as effective as repeated day serum cortisol levels.

Prednisolone
- Prednisolone is used in few select patients.
- It is possible to monitor circulating levels of prednisolone but assays are not widely available.
- The usual dosage is 3–5 mg on waking, and 1–2 mg at 14:00–15:00 h.

Monitoring of therapy
Clinical assessment is vital in determining whether dosages are appropriate. Assessment needs to take account of the time of day of symptoms and the patient's usual daily routine.

Clinical signs and symptoms of over-replacement
Clinical signs and symptoms of over-replacement include:
- weight gain
- facial plethora
- insomnia
- peripheral oedema

Clinical signs and symptoms of under-replacement
Clinical signs and symptoms of under-replacement include:
- lethargy
- tiredness
- nausea
- poor appetite
- increasing pigmentation (in primary adrenal insufficiency)

Biochemical monitoring
- Detailed biochemical 'day curves' are unnecessary in the majority.
- If malabsorption is suspected or if patients are on medication or foods that are either inducers or inhibitors of CYP3A4 (the key metabolizing enzyme of hydrocortisone) and so may result in lower or higher levels of circulating cortisol, sampling of serum cortisol when the patient is on hydrocortisone may be needed.
- If biochemical monitoring is performed when the patient is on hydrocortisone, a 2-hour post-dose serum cortisol sample with dose adjustment, combined with taking into account the value together with the clinical features, is sufficient in most circumstances.

Specific situations requiring dose adjustment
Patients on glucocorticoid replacement therapy are unable to respond appropriately to physical stress and have an absolute requirement for increased glucocorticoid at times of physical stress, infection, or surgery.

Surgical and other procedures
Surgical and other procedures that require dose adjustment are as follows (for more information see Addison's Disease Self-Help Group, http://www.Addisons.org.uk; see also Section 6.11):
- major surgery with a long recovery time:
  - 100 mg hydrocortisone intramuscularly just before anaesthesia
  - continue 100 mg hydrocortisone intramuscularly every 6 hours until the patient is able to eat and drink
  - then double the oral dose for 48 hours
  - then taper to the normal dose
- major surgery with rapid recovery:
  - 100 mg hydrocortisone intramuscularly just before anaesthesia
  - continue 100 mg hydrocortisone intramuscularly every 6 hours for 24–48 hours
  - then double the oral dose for 24–48 hours
  - then taper to the normal dose

- labour and vaginal birth:
  - 100 mg hydrocortisone intramuscularly just at the onset of labour
  - double the oral dose for 24–48 hours after delivery
  - then taper to the normal dose
- minor surgery and major dental surgery:
  - 100 mg hydrocortisone intramuscularly just before anaesthesia
  - double the oral dose for 24 hours
  - then return to the normal dose
- invasive bowel procedures requiring laxatives:
  - hospital admission overnight with 100 mg hydrocortisone intramuscularly and fluid
  - repeat dose before the start of the procedure
  - double the oral dose for 24 hours
  - then return to the normal dose
- other invasive procedures
  - 100 mg hydrocortisone intramuscularly just before the start of the procedure
  - double the oral dose for 24 hours
  - then return to the normal dose
- dental procedure:
  - extra morning dose 1 hour prior to surgery
  - double the oral dose for 24 hours
  - then return to the normal dose
- minor procedure:
  - usually not required
  - extra dose (e.g. 20 mg hydrocortisone) if symptoms are present

Pregnancy

Since there is an increase in CBG at the end of the third trimester, hydrocortisone doses may need increasing according to symptoms by 2.5–10.0 mg daily.

Physical activity

An extra dose of hydrocortisone, 5 mg, is recommended prior to prolonged physical activity, and repeated doses may be needed for ultra-endurance events.

Mineralocorticoid therapy

- Most patients with Addison's disease need 0.05–0.20 mg per day fludrocortisone.
- Monitoring is performed clinically and by monitoring plasma renin activity and electrolytes, with the aim of achieving a value at the upper end or just above the normal range for plasma renin. A suppressed plasma renin activity indicates overtreatment.
- The dose may need to be increased towards the end of pregnancy.

Androgen replacement

DHEA replacement in patients with Addison's disease may have beneficial effects on well-being, but is not recommended as routine medication.

Patients on pharmacological therapy

Patients on long-term prednisolone may need to be weaned off therapy. One approach is to transfer patients to a physiological hydrocortisone dosing when down to a daily dose of prednisolone, 3–5 mg; the hydrocortisone can be tapered and a Synacthen® test performed to assess whether there is long-term axis suppression.

Patient education

- Patient education is vital. All patients on glucocorticoid replacement therapy should be advised to carry an 'Emergency Steroid card' and preferably an emergency bracelet of necklace such as 'MedicAlert'.
- Patients need to understand that they need to double the dose of glucocorticoids during febrile illness and physical stress.
- It is recommended that patients and partners are taught to self-inject/inject soluble parenteral hydrocortisone, 100 mg intramuscularly, for emergency situations and that they carry the vial at all times. It is recommended, where possible, to have patient details on emergency service databases, indicating the absolute need for hydrocortisone in emergencies, and that patients have letters which indicate this need and which can be handed to emergency service staff.

Emergency situations

See Section 6.11. Once the emergency has passed, the dose of hydrocortisone is tapered to normal replacement doses and fludrocortisone restarted. When the patient is on high-dose parenteral hydrocortisone, fludrocortisone is not needed.

Future developments

- A long-acting hydrocortisone preparation is available in Europe but its exact role remains to be established.
- A delayed and sustained modified release hydrocortisone to be taken at bedtime with levels building up over the night and peaking in the morning is under development.
- Variable doses of hydrocortisone delivered by metered pumps via the subcutaneous infusion route may be appropriate in some patients.

Patient support groups

The following patient support groups may be helpful:

- The Addison's Disease Self-Help Group (http://www.addisons.org.uk)
- The Pituitary Foundation (http://www.pituitary.org)

Further reading

Arlt W and Allolio B. Adrenal insufficiency. *Lancet* 2003; 361: 1881–93.

Debono M, Ghobadi C, Rostami-Hodjegan A, et al. Modified-release hydrocortisone to provide circadian cortisol profiles. *J Clin Endocrinol Metab* 2009; 94: 1548–54.

Debono M, Ross RJ, and Newell-Price J. Inadequacies of glucocorticoid replacement and improvements by physiological circadian therapy. *Eur J Endocrinol* 2009; 160: 719–29.

Husebye ES, Allolio B, Arlt W, et al. Consensus statement on the diagnosis, treatment and follow-up of patients with primary adrenal insufficiency. *J Intern Med* 2014; 275: 104–15.

Johannsson G, Nilsson AG, Bergthorsdottir R, et al. Improved cortisol exposure-time profile and outcome in patients with adrenal insufficiency: A prospective randomized trial of a novel hydrocortisone dual-release formulation. *J Clin Endocrinol Metab* 2012; 97: 473–8.

6.13 Autoimmune polyglandular syndrome

Introduction

Where several of the following autoimmune diseases listed cluster together in a patient, this is known as autoimmune polyglandular syndrome (also known as autoimmune polyendocrine syndrome):

- diabetes type 1
- autoimmune thyroid disease (Graves' disease, Hashimoto's/hypothyroidism)
- coeliac disease
- Addison's disease
- vitiligo
- alopecia
- premature ovarian or testicular failure
- atrophic gastritis with B$_{12}$ deficiency
- hypoparathyroidism with hypocalcaemia

A patient with one of these has an increased risk, relative to the general population, of acquiring one or more of the others. The predisposition is genetic, and the pathogenesis is mainly autoimmune. The main characteristics are shown in Table 6.11.

Autoimmune polyendocrine syndrome type 2

Autoimmune polyendocrine syndrome type 2 is the most common form of the disease, shows a female preponderance, and typically develops in midlife. Some differentiate between autoimmune polyendocrine syndrome types 2, 3, and 4. We see no advantage in this subclassification, and include in autoimmune polyendocrine syndrome type 2 those with two or more of the manifestations listed in 'Introduction'. The prevalence is probably 5–10:10.000.

Clinical course

Each disease has a course and treatment similar to that seen in those with only one disease, and we therefore refer to other texts on this point. Each manifestation is mostly permanent, but a few may remit. Chronic autoimmune thyroiditis with high levels of anti-thyroid peroxidase antibodies (Hashimoto's disease) shows several clinical phenotypes which overlap. One phenotype is with a goitre and no hypothyroidism; another is hypothyroidism with no goitre (common). The thyroid failure develops gradually. A third phenotype with changing thyroid function from hyper- to hypothyroidism (frequently seen post partum; also called silent or painless, or cyclic thyroiditis) has a more unpredictable course.

Treatment challenges occur when two or more diseases are present: examples include diabetes and coeliac disease: a gluten-free diet increases hyperglycaemia, whilst malabsorption may give rise to hypoglycaemia. With Addison's disease and diabetes, there is a high proneness to hypoglycaemia, because the adrenal response is absent.

In Addison's and hypoparathyroidism, there is an increasing risk of hypocalcaemia when increasing the dose of glucocorticoid.

Hyperthyroidism may make the diabetes brittle, and hypoglycaemia unawareness may become a major problem because the symptoms are similar to that of hyperthyroidism. With hyperthyroidism and Addison's, one needs to treat the Addisonian condition first to avoid an adrenal crisis; the hypothyroidism may remit when the glucocorticoid is replaced.

Immunology

See also Chapter 1, Section 1.5. The normal tolerance to self-antigens is impaired: most patients have antibodies against tissue-specific antigens (Table 6.12), many of those being key enzymes. The antibodies often appear years before the disease is diagnosed, and they may also be present in many of the patient's relatives who do not develop any clinical manifestations; thus, the antibodies themselves are probably mostly not pathogenic, but rather just a marker of the trait. To proceed to a clinical manifestation, it seems necessary to have a cell-mediated attack by autoreactive helper T lymphocytes, cytotoxic T lymphocytes, macrophages, and cytokines, and complement-mediated attack may play a role. The innate immune system is also altered, impairing self-tolerance.

The antibodies may disappear, both in those who never develop autoimmune polyendocrine syndrome, and in the late stage of organ destruction, when the tissue-specific antigenic stimulus thereby is reduced or absent.

One exception to the non-pathogenic antibodies is the stimulatory antibodies to the TSH receptor causing Graves' disease. This is also an exception in that the disease often remits, and in that the antigen presents itself on the cell surface, whereas most autoimmune polyendocrine syndrome antigens are intracellular key enzymes of the affected organ or interleukins. Therefore, Graves' disease may not be a typical example of the prevailing disease mechanism in autoimmune polyendocrine syndrome type 2.

Genetics

The disposition to get autoimmune polyendocrine syndrome type 2 is inherited. The genetics are similar to that of patients who have only one of the diseases. It seems, therefore, reasonable to infer that all are part of one spectrum of different risks.

Relatives of the index patient have an increased risk of having one or more of the diseases, but it may not be the same as is present in the primary patient. Patients with diabetes and Addison's may have close relatives with coeliac disease, but there is no clear Mendelian inheritance pattern. Monozygotic twins have a much higher risk of concordance than dizygotic twins or first-degree relatives. The explanation is polygenic inheritance.

The strongest risk is determined by polymorphisms in HLA genes. *HLA DR3* seems to be the main culprit, conferring increased risk for nearly all diseases of the syndrome. But other HLA genes also contribute, and so do other genes both in the HLA region on Chromosome 6 and on other chromosomes. There are also protective genetic variants (e.g. *HLA DQ6*, against diabetes). Because the *HLA DR* and *HLA DQ* gene products present antigens to the T lymphocytes, this makes a plausible causal link between the genetics and immunology of autoimmune polyendocrine syndrome type 2.

Examples of other genes with predisposing alleles are *CTLA4* (important for T-lymphocyte interactions), *PTPN22* (which encodes protein tyrosine phosphatase non-receptor type 22, a lymphocyte-specific phosphatase), and the TSH-receptor gene. Most of the genes associated with autoimmune polyendocrine syndrome type 2 have important functions in the activation or suppression of immune cells. Accordingly, the patients show

Table 6.11 Characteristics of autoimmune polygandular syndrome type 2 and type 1

Typical manifestations	APS 2	APS 1
Diabetes type 1	+	+
Graves', Hashimoto's, hypothyroidism	+	+
Coeliac disease	+	+
Addison's disease	+	+++
Vitiligo and alopecia	+	+
Ovarian or testicular failure	+	+
Atrophic gastritis with B12 deficiency	+	+
Hypoparathyroidism		+++
Mucocutane candidiasis		+++
Criteria for diagnosis	Two or more manifestations	Two or three of the following: • Addison´s disease • Hypoparathyroidism • Mucocutaneous candidiasis
Typical age at onset	Midlife	Childhood or adolescence
Genetics	Polygenic; mainly HLA	Mutations in AIRE; recessive
Consider APS if	One typical disease plus signs of any of the others Close relatives with typical manifestations	One of the four following: • Addison´s disease • Hypoparathyroidism • Mucocutaneous candidiasis • Sibling with APS 1
Further investigations	Clinical workup Antibodies to relevant antigens listed in Table 6.12	Anti-interferon omega Test for AIRE mutations
Prevalence	Common	Rare

Table 6.12 The main antigens in autoimmune polyglandular syndromes

Diabetes type 1	GAD, IA-2/ICA512, insulin, ZNT8
Graves' disease	TSH receptor
Hashimoto's, hypothyroidism	TPO
Coeliac disease	Transglutaminase
Addison's disease	21-hydroxylase
Vitiligo and alopecia	Tyrosine hydroxylase, SOX 10
Ovarian or testicular failure	Cholesterol side-chain cleavage enzyme
Atrophic gastritis with B12 deficiency	Parietal cells, intrinsic factor
Hypoparathyroidism	NALP-5
For the diagnosis of APS 1	Interferon omega

Abbreviations: APS, autoimmune polyendocrine syndrome; GAD, glutamic acid decarboxylase; IA-2, insulinoma antigen 2; ICA512, islet cell antigen 512, which is part of the IA-2 molecule; ZNT8, islet zinc transporter isoform 8; TSH, thyroid stimulating hormone; TPO, thyroid peroxidase; SOX 10, a transcription factor; NALP-5, NACHT leucin-rich-repeat protein 5.

Note: Antibodies to these antigens indicate autoimmunity, and are of diagnostic help. Antibodies to several other antigens, mainly to intracellular enzymes and interleukins, have also been reported recently.

defective response of the regulatory suppressor T and B cells, and impaired activation-induced cell death of autoreactive T cells.

Many of the predisposing alleles are common in the normal healthy population, so the disease penetrance is low. There are most likely a number of other genes, not found yet, with predisposing alleles. Epigenetics, microchimerism, and skewed X-chromosome inactivation may contribute.

The very complex immunogenetic interplay and its uncertainties are dealt with in detail in the review by Mitchell and Pearce (2012).

Exogenous factors

Exogenous factors probably contribute, although stochastic events on a purely genetic background may be operating. Virus, pollutants, drugs, nutrition, gut microbes, the intrauterine milieu, and other factors have been proposed to precipitate the attack on specific tissues, but none has been proven.

Preclinical phase

In the preclinical phase, the decline in function develops slowly. There is often a gradual reduction in insulin secretory capacity years before diabetes is diagnosed, and similarly for cortisol before overt Addison's disease ensues. In this preclinical phase, tissue-specific antibodies are often detectable.

When to consider
Be alert to slight indications of any of the other diseases on the list in patients with one of the disorders. Relatives with one or more of the diseases should raise one's suspicion. Tissue-specific antibodies indicate a risk that tissue destruction may be going on or may develop later. Antibodies to more than one antigen, and high titers, are both associated with increased risk.

Refrain from too-active screening
In trying to detect and treat all incipient or subclinical manifestations, we may do more harm than good. For example, we could screen all patients with diabetes type 1 for anti-transglutaminase antibodies, biopsy all positives, and treat all with the slightest coeliac gut changes; however, many of these may have remained asymptomatic without treatment. They already have the burden of their diabetes, and superimposing a gluten-free diet is an additional strain. Their prognosis if untreated is unknown, and probably much better than for those who have symptomatic coeliac disease. Subclinical autoimmune thyroid disease should often be left untreated, and similarly with the others on the list.

Prophylaxis
Various general immunosuppressive treatments slow disease progression, both in the preclinical and in the clinical phase of many of these diseases, both in man and in animal models. Nevertheless, to date, the side effects of such therapy have been considered to be worse than the beneficial effects. However, if restricted and specific suppression of the various tissue-specific immune attacks could be improved from the present experimental state, this may become promising. If so, family history, genotyping, antibodies, and functional testing could help in selecting candidates for early treatment.

Autoimmune polyendocrine syndrome type 1

Autoimmune polyendocrine syndrome type 1 is a rare, monogenic, autosomal recessive disease, and much more severe than autoimmune polyendocrine syndrome type 2. Its prevalence is probably between 1:10,000 and 1:100,000. The diseases develop much earlier in life than in autoimmune polyendocrine syndrome type 2, and are more numerous in each patient. One should consider the diagnosis if there is hypoparathyroidism, Addison's disease, or mucocutaneous candidiasis, or if a sibling has autoimmune polyendocrine syndrome type 1. Antibodies to interferon omega seem to have a high diagnostic specificity and sensitivity.

There is a defect in *AIRE* in both alleles, impairing the presentation of self-antigens to the lymphocytes in the fetal and neonatal thymus, and this, in turn, allows autoreactive T lymphocytes to escape inactivation and therefore launch autoimmune attacks. Antibodies to interleukins 17A, 17F, and 22 probably impair their defence against candida infection.

Because multiple diseases are often present, treatment is challenging. One should be especially aware of the requirement for active treatment of the candidiasis, which is very disabling and may lead to mucocutaneous carcinomas. If Howell–Jolly bodies are discovered on a blood smear, check with ultrasound for asplenia; if asplenia is present, vaccination against pneumococcus, meningococcus, and haemophilus influenza needs to be administered.

The increased frequency of autoimmune polyendocrine syndrome type in patients with Down syndrome may be caused by the triplication of *AIRE*, which is located on Chromosome 21. A recent finding is that dominant-negative mutations in *AIRE* can cause a milder and less penetrant clinical presentation with a later debut than the classical autoimmune polyendocrine syndrome type 1. Some of the patients previously diagnosed as autoimmune polyendocrine syndrome type 2 may harbour this type of mutation.

Immunodeficiencies

Some primary immune deficiency disorders are associated with development of autoimmune diseases: for example, the rare immunodysregulation polyendocrinopathy enteropathy X-linked syndrome (IPEX) leads to severe autoimmune phenomena including enteropathy, chronic dermatitis, and polyendocrinopathy. Neonatal diabetes type 1 and/or thyroiditis are hallmarks of IPEX, which shows a defect in the regulatory T-cells. Omenn syndrome, another severe combined immunodeficiency, exhibit peripheral expansion of autoreactive T cells, and the patients develop autoimmunity early. In DiGeorge syndrome (22q11.2 deletion syndrome), the thymus is hypoplastic, and autoimmune diseases affecting endocrine tissues are frequent. In addition, these patients are prone to hypoparathyroidism, since the parathyroid glands are hypoplastic. IgA deficiency is associated with both systemic and organ-specific autoimmunity, such as diabetes type 1 and coeliac disease.

Anti-cancer immunostimulatory drugs

Antibodies to key regulatory molecules on T cells are increasingly used to treat cancer patients. These antibodies augment the T-cell attacks on cancer cells, but may also induce autoimmunity. Dermatitis, colitis, thyroid disease, and hypophysitis seem frequent, but also broader polyendocrine attacks can occur. The frequency is uncertain, but may possibly be around 20% of treated cancer patients. Thyroid function tends to fluctuate. Hypophysitis with adrenocorticotrophic hormone deficiency or Addison's disease requires steroid substitution. Other autoimmune manifestations may need high-dose glucocorticoid treatment.

Other autoimmune associations

More and more manifestations are reported in the autoimmune polyendocrine syndromes. These are either less frequent or less established than the main manifestations:

• rheumatoid arthritis
• lupus erythematosus
• Sjögren's syndrome
• anti-phospholipid syndrome
• haemolytic anaemia and trombopenia
• asplenia
• unspecified anaemia
• diarrhoea and malabsorption
• autoimmune hypophysitis
• hepatitis
• nephritis
• bronchiolitis
• habitual abortion and preterm birth
• atrioventricular block

- Parkinson-like encephalopathy
- myasthenia gravis
- stiff man's syndrome
- multiple sclerosis

There seems to be a broad tendency to attacks on tissue-specific antigens, enzymes, and interleukins.

References and further reading

Cutolo M. Autoimmune polyendocrine syndromes. *Autoimmune Rev* 2014; 13: 85–9.

Husebye ES, Perheentupa J, Rautemaa R, et al. Clinical manifestations and management of patients with autoimmune polyendocrine syndrome type 1. *J Intern Med* 2009; 265: 514–29.

Lima K, Abrahamsen TG, Wolff AB, et al. Hypoparathyroidism and autoimmunity in the 22q11.2 deletion syndrome. *Eur J Endocrinol* 2011; 165: 345–52.

Michels AW and Eisenbarth GS. Autoimmune polyendocrine syndrome type 1 (APS-1) as a model for understanding autoimmune polyendocrine syndrome type 2 (APS-2). *J Intern Med* 2009; 265: 530–40.

Mitchell AL and Pearce SHS. Autoimmune Addison disease: pathophysiology and genetic complexity. *Nat Rev Endocrinol* 2012; 8: 306–16.

6.14 Phaeochromocytoma

Definition
Phaeochromocytomas are rare neuroendocrine tumours derived from chromaffin cells in the adrenal medulla. Similar tumours arising outside the adrenal glands from sympathetic or parasympathetic paraganglia are called paragangliomas. Unless otherwise specified in this section, the term phaeochromocytomas will refer to both phaeochromocytomas and paragangliomas.

Epidemiology
Phaeochromocytomas occur at a rate of about 1 per 2500–6500 in Western countries, although about 50% are not discovered until autopsy, suggesting a higher prevalence. Phaeochromocytomas are diagnosed in patients of any sex, race, or age, although most phaeochromocytomas are diagnosed between the ages of 30 and 50.

Diagnosis of phaeochromocytoma
Symptoms
The symptoms of phaeochromocytoma are non-specific and can therefore be mistaken for other diseases. However, phaeochromocytoma should always be considered in patients presenting with headaches, palpitations, and sweating. Additional symptoms are numerous, and can include hypertension, tachycardia, and anxiety, among others (see Table 6.13).

Biochemistry
Previously, phaeochromocytomas were diagnosed based on elevated catecholamine levels. However, not all phaeochromocytomas secrete catecholamines, but almost all metabolize them. Whilst the release of catecholamines can be episodic, their metabolites, metanephrines, are released continuously and independently of catecholamine release. Therefore, measurements of metanephrine and normetanephrine are considered the most specific diagnostic markers for phaeochromocytoma. These can be measured in plasma or urine; plasma is preferable, although there are no current studies to support its superiority.

In addition to metanephrine and normetanephrine, methoxytyramine, the O-methylated metabolite of dopamine, has been introduced as a novel biomarker for phaeochromocytoma. Methoxytyramine is useful for:

- diagnosing tumours that secrete primarily dopamine
- head and neck paragangliomas
- metastatic lesions
- diagnosing SDHB- and SDHD-related phaeochromocytomas; approximately 70% of patients with SDHB- or SDHD-related phaeochromocytoma have elevated methoxytyramine levels

Almost unequivocal diagnosis of phaeochromocytoma is based on elevations of metanephrines greater than three to four times the upper reference limit. However, many patients have elevated results that do not meet this threshold. In these patients, it is important to rule out the interference of medications and food that could cause false-positive results (see Section 6.2). If medication and food interferences have been ruled out, patients may need to undergo a clonidine suppression test. Note that this test cannot be used for epinephrine (adrenaline) or metanephrine-secreting phaeochromocytomas. Baseline levels should be checked before the administration of a small dose of clonidine. Metanephrines and catecholamines should be drawn before and 3 hours after administration of clonidine. Suppression is defined by a decrease in plasma normetanephrine to within normal limits or by at least 40%. Patients who fail to suppress should be evaluated further for the presence of phaeochromocytoma. With the use of plasma normetanephrine, this test has a sensitivity of 97% and a specificity of 100%. The previously used glucagon stimulation test for diagnosis in patients with equivocal biochemical results is not recommended, due to its low sensitivity (less than 50%) and the potential for hypertensive crisis.

Table 6.13 Signs and symptoms associated with phaeochromocytoma

Signs		Symptoms	
Hypertension	++++	Headaches	++++
Sustained hypertension	++	Palpitations	++++
Paroxysmal hypertension	++	Anxiety/nervousness	+++
Postural hypotension	+	Tremulousness	++
Tachycardia or reflex bradycardia	+++	Weakness, fatigue	++
Excessive sweating	++++	Nausea/vomiting	+
Pallor	++	Pain in chest/abdomen	+
Flushing	+	Dizziness or faintness	+
Weight loss	+	Paresthesias	+
Fasting hyperglycemia	++	Constipation (rarely diarrhea)	+
Decreased gastrointestinal motility	+	Visual disturbances	+
Increased respiratory rate	+		

Reproduced from Pacak K, Preoperative management of the pheochromocytoma patient, *Journal of Clinical Endocrinology & Metabolism*, 2007, Volume 92, Issue 11, pp. 4069–4079, by permission of Oxford University Press; Data from Eisenhofer, G., Rivers, G., Rosas, A.L. et al., 30, *Drug-Safety*, Adverse Drug Reactions in Patients with Phaeochromocytoma, 2007.

Table 6.14 Sensitivity and specificity of imaging modalities for phaeochromocytoma

Imaging modality	Primary (non-metastatic)		Head/neck PGL (%)	Metastatic (%)	SDHB metastatic (%)	Non-SDHB metastatic (%)	Bone metastases (%)
	Sensitivity (%)	Specificity (%)					
FDG PET	77–88	90	67–76	74–82	83–100	49–67.3	76–93
FDOPA PET	67–93	100	92–100	45	20	75–93	—
FDA PET	78–88	90	40–46	76	79–82	76–78	79–100
^{68}Ga-DOTATATE PET	73–100	86–100	100	92–100	98	97–100	100
MIBG	67–87	82–100	31–33	50–93	44–57	59–66	61–76
Octreoscan	28.5	75	64	68–89	59–81	—	—
CT/MRI	95–100	40–90	42–80	74	78	71–82	65–96

Abbreviations: FDA, ^{18}F-fluorodopamine; FDG, ^{18}F-fluorodeoxyglucose; FDOPA, ^{18}F-fluorodopa; MIBG, metaiodobenzylguanidine; PGL, paraganglioma.

Imaging

After confirmation of the biochemical diagnosis of phaeochromocytoma, patients should undergo anatomic imaging to localize the tumour, either by CT or by MRI. CT is the preferred technique, but MRI can be useful for:

- pregnant women
- children
- patients in whom radiation exposure should be limited
- the evaluation of extra-adrenal tumours, particularly cardiac paragangliomas and head and neck paragangliomas

Anatomic imaging should proceed in the following order:

1. Adrenals.
2. Abdomen and pelvis.
3. Chest and neck.

If no tumour can be identified after comprehensive anatomic imaging, it may be necessary to proceed to specific functional imaging.

In addition to aiding in the localization of phaeochromocytoma, functional imaging can be valuable in characterizing phaeochromocytoma. The sensitivity and specificity of various functional imaging modalities are listed in Table 6.14. Clinical recommendations for imaging are summarized in Table 6.15.

There are several PET radiotracers that have been studied in phaeochromocytoma patients. For the diagnosis of non-metastatic, non-SDHB-related phaeochromocytomas, FDA PET appears to be the best imaging modality in general. FDA is an analogue of dopamine, which is transported into cells via the norepinephrine transporter system. FDA PET can also be used for the detection of metastatic disease, although it is less sensitive than FDG PET. FDA PET is not recommended for the detection of head and neck paragangliomas, due to low sensitivity.

For the detection of head and neck paragangliomas, ^{18}F-fluorodopa (FDOPA) is an excellent radiotracer, with a sensitivity of 95%–100%. FDOPA is a catecholamine precursor, which enters the cells through the amino-acid transporter. This imaging modality can also be used for non-metastatic phaeochromocytomas, although it is less sensitive than FDA PET. FDOPA PET is not recommended for the detection of metastatic lesions.

The use of ^{68}Ga-labelled somatostatin analogues is an emerging PET imaging technique that has shown promising preliminary results. These analogues are preferable to ^{18}F-based technologies because they do not require a cyclotron for their production and so are more easily acquired. However, the spatial resolution may not be as good as ^{18}F-PET technologies, although high tumour-to-background uptake ratios partially overcome this limitation. Studies suggest that ^{68}Ga-DOTATATE PET may be especially useful in detecting metastatic phaeochromocytoma, including SDHB-related metastatic disease and head and neck paraganglioma.

To localize metastatic or SDHB-related phaeochromocytomas, FDG PET is recommended as the preferred functional modality. FDG measures glucose uptake by tumour cells. It can also be used to detect non-metastatic phaeochromocytoma or head and neck paragangliomas, although its sensitivity for these lesions is inferior to those of FDA and FDOPA, respectively.

In the future, new PET tracers to measure cellular processes such as proliferation, hypoxia, and angiogenesis may become valuable in further characterizing tumours non-invasively and monitoring responses to treatment.

Non-PET functional imaging includes octreoscan, and $^{123/131}$I-MIBG single-photon-emission CT (SPECT).

Table 6.15 Clinical recommendations for functional imaging modalities

Type of PHEO/PGL	Suggested functional imaging modality
Non-metastatic PHEO/PGL except some hereditary tumors (MEN2, VHL, NF1) for which data is missing	FDA PET
SDHB-related PHEO/PGL (including metastatic)	FDG PET, 68Ga-DOTATATE PET
Head/neck PGL	FDOPA PET, 68Ga-DOTATATE PET
Adrenal tumours <5 cm with elevated EPI/MN	No functional imaging recommended except for some hereditary EPI-secreting tumors to rule out multiplicity

Abbreviations: EPI, epinephrine; FDA, ^{18}F-fluorodopamine; FDG, ^{18}F-fluorodeoxyglucose; FDOPA, ^{18}F-fluorodopa; MIBG, metaiodobenzylguanidine; MN, metanephrine; PGL, paraganglioma; PHEO, phaeochromocytoma.

Octreoscan has low sensitivity and specificity for non-meta-static phaeochromocytomas and should not be used as a diagnostic imaging modality for these tumours. They can be valuable in evaluating metastatic phaeochromocytomas, particularly when considering treatment with radio-actively labelled somatostatin analogues. However, ^{68}Ga-DOTATATE PET also can be used for this purpose, with greater sensitivity and specificity. Therefore, octreoscan is only rarely used, primarily when ^{68}Ga-DOTATATE PET is not available.

MIBG is structurally similar to norepinephrine and enters phaeochromocytoma cells through the norepin-ephrine transporter. ^{123}I-MIBG is preferred over ^{131}I-MIBG for imaging. Whilst MIBG scintigraphy can be comparable to other functional imaging modalities for primary tumours, its sensitivity for metastatic lesions is low; therefore, MIBG scintigraphy should only be used in metastatic cases to evaluate eligibility for ^{131}I-MIBG therapy. In addition, false-negative ^{123}I-MIBG results occur more frequently with SDHB mutations and higher rates of metastases, so genetic testing and close follow-up is recommended in patients with known lesions which are not positive on MIBG scintigraphy.

Genetics of phaeochromocytoma

See also Sections 13.3 and 13.8. Phaeochromocytomas can occur sporadically or as a result of underlying germ-line genetic mutations. The known susceptibility genes for phaeochromocytoma can be divided into two groups:
- major susceptibility genes
- minor susceptibility genes

Major susceptibility genes
- VHL, which is linked to Von Hippel–Lindau disease, en-codes a protein involved in the regulation and degrad-ation of hypoxia-inducible factor (HIF) alpha.
- RET, which is mutated in multiple endocrine neoplasia type 2, encodes Ret, a tyrosine kinase that plays a role in cell proliferation and apoptosis regulation.
- NF1 mutations, which lead to neurofibromatosis type 1, affect a protein inhibitor of the ras and mTOR path-ways involved in cell growth.
- SDHB, which is associated with familial paraganglioma syndrome type 4, encodes SDHB, one of the four sub-units of succinate dehydrogenase, which is also known as mitochondrial complex 2. Succinate dehydrogenase plays a role in both the electron transport chain and the Krebs cycle, giving it a critical role in cellular metabolism.
- SDHD, associated with paraganglioma syndrome type 1, encodes SDHD, another of the four subunits of suc-cinate dehydrogenase.

Minor susceptibility genes
- SDHA encodes the succinate dehydrogenase subunit SDHA.
- SDHC, which is linked to paraganglioma syndrome type 3, encodes the succinate dehydrogenase subunit SDHC.
- SDHAF2, which is linked to paraganglioma syndrome type 2, encodes a protein involved in the flavination of the succinate dehydrogenase subunit SDHA.
- Mutations in FH (which encodes fumarate hydratase) and MDH2 (which encodes malate dehydrogenase) af-fect proteins involved in the Krebs cycle.
- HIF2A encodes HIF-2 alpha, which is a transcription factor that can induce a pseudohypoxic state, leading to tumour development.

- PHD1 and PHD2 encode prolyl hydroxylase domain proteins 1 and 2, which are involved in the regulation of HIF-2 alpha.
- MAX encodes the transcription factor max, which is a member of the myc–max–mdx1 pathway, which plays a role in multiple cellular processes, including prolifer-ation, differentiation, and apoptosis.
- TMEM127 encodes transmembrane protein 127, which appears to be linked to the mTOR signalling pathway, although its function is not well known.
- Mutations in KIF1B, which encodes a protein involved in apoptosis induction, have been reported in patients with phaeochromocytoma and neuroblastoma.

The clinical characteristics associated with these muta-tions are outlined in Table 6.16. Genetic testing is critical for patients with phaeochromocytoma, as this can help guide treatment and imaging strategies and can lead to screening and earlier diagnosis in carrier family members. Recent studies have determined an algorithm for genetic testing based on biochemical profile and clinical char-acteristics; this can minimize the costs of testing whilst accurately diagnosing patients with underlying genetic mutations (see Figure 6.28). Next-generation sequencing techniques and the development of gene panels may eventually permit the affordable simultaneous evaluation of all susceptibility genes.

Immunohistochemistry, in conjunction with biochemical phenotype, can play a role in the diagnosis of SDHx mutations if genetic testing has not been performed before the removal of the phaeochromocytoma. Immunostaining for the suc-cinate dehydrogenase subunit SDHB can distinguish SDHA-, SDHB-, SDHC-, and SDHD-related phaeochromocytomas from VHL-related phaeochromocytomas, which also have a noradrenergic phenotype. Patients with negative immunostaining for SDHB should undergo genetic testing for SDHx mutations. Further immunostaining for the suc-cinate dehydrogenase subunit SDHA can help distinguish SDHA-related tumours from other SDHx-related tumours, since the rarity of SDHA mutations can make finding a centre for genetic testing difficult.

Somatic mutations
In addition to frequent germ-line mutations that predis-pose individuals to phaeochromocytoma development, particular somatic mutations play an important role in the genetic landscape of these tumours.
- Tumours from individuals without identified germ-line genetic mutations may harbour somatic muta-tions in known susceptibility genes such as RET, NF1, or VHL.
- Recurrent driver genes, including HRAS, HIF2A, and CSDE1, have been identified via exome sequencing of phaeochromocytoma tumours.
- Somatic mutations in ATRX have been observed in tumours from some individuals with germ-line SDHB mutations.
- MAML3 fusion proteins have been found as the pri-mary driver in a subset of phaeochromocytoma tu-mour samples.
- Hypermethylation of 52 loci has been associated with metastatic phaeochromocytoma development inde-pendently of underlying genetic mutations.
- Somatic mutations in HIF2A occurring shortly after fer-tilization can lead to Pacak–Zhuang syndrome, which consists of polycythaemia, somatostatinoma, and mul-tiple phaeochromocytomas.

Table 6.16 Clinical characteristics of genetic mutations associated with phaeochromocytoma/paraganglioma

Gene	Syndrome	PHEO/PGL penetrance (%)	De novo mutations (%)	Mean age	Biochemical phenotype	Common PHEO/PGL sites	Bilateral PHEO	Malignancy	Other associated clinical characteristics/tumours
VHL	VHL	10–20	20	30	Noradrenergic	Adrenal PHEOs (rarely, sympathetic or head and neck PGLs)	50%	<5%	Haemangioblastomas Renal cell carcinoma Islet cell tumours of the pancreas
RET	MEN2	50	5 (MEN2A) 50 (MEN2B)	30–40	Adrenergic	Adrenal PHEOs	50–80%	<5%	Medullary thyroid carcinomas (95% MEN2A, 100% MEN2B) MEN2A: hyperparathyroidism (15%–30%) MEN2B: marphanoid habitus, mucosal ganglioneuromas
NF1	NF1	<6	50	42	Adrenergic	Adrenal PHEOs (rarely, sympathetic PGLs)	16%	9%–12%	Café-au-lait spots Neurofibromas Freckles Benign iris hamartomas Optic-nerve gliomas Sphenoid bone dysplasia/pseudoarthritis
SDHB	PGL4	42–50	Further study needed	30	Noradrenergic and/or dopaminergic (Rarely biochemically silent)	Sympathetic PGLs (rarely, adrenal PHEOs and head and neck PGLs)	Rare	31%–71%	Renal cell carcinomas Gastrointestinal stromal tumours Breast carcinomas Papillary thyroid carcinomas
SDHD	PGL1	90 (Paternal transmission)*	Further study needed	35	Noradrenergic, dopaminergic, or silent	Head and neck PGLs, commonly multiple (rarely, extra-adrenal abdominal PGLs or adrenal PHEOs)	Rare	<5%	Carney-Stratakis syndrome Gastrointestinal stromal tumour
SDHC	PGL3	Further study needed	Further study needed	40–50	Noradrenergic, dopaminergic, or silent	Head and neck PGLs, sometimes multiple (rarely, sympathetic PGLs or adrenal PHEOs)	Further study needed	Rare	Carney-Stratakis syndrome Gastrointestinal stromal tumour
SDHA	—	39	Further study needed	40	Adrenergic and noradrenergic	Head and neck PGLs Adrenal PHEOs	Rare	0%–14%	Homozygous patients: Leigh syndrome
SDHAF2	PGL2	100 (Paternal transmission)	Further study needed	30–40	Further study needed	Head and neck PGLs, often multiple (rarely, adrenal PHEOs)	No known cases	No known cases	—

(continued)

Table 6.16 Continued

Gene	Syndrome	PHEO/PGL penetrance (%)	De novo mutations (%)	Mean age	Biochemical phenotype	Common PHEO/PGL sites	Bilateral PHEO	Malignancy	Other associated clinical characteristics/tumours
MAX	—	73 (Paternal transmission)	Further study needed	32	Adrenergic and noradrenergic	Adrenal PHEOs	67%–73%	7%–25%	—
TMEM127	—	41	Further study needed	43	Adrenergic and noradrenergic	Adrenal PHEOs Head and neck PGLs	33%–50%	0%–10%	Possibly linked to breast carcinoma Possibly linked to papillary thyroid carcinoma
HIF2A	Somatic mutations: Pacak–Zhuang	Further study needed	Further study needed	—	Noradrenergic	Multiple extra-adrenal PGLs	Rare	29%	Polycythemia Somatic mutations early in development linked with Pacak–Zhuang syndrome (recurrent PGL, polycythemia, and somatostatinoma)
FH	—	Further study needed	Further study needed	40	Noradrenergic	Adrenal PHEOs Multiple extra-adrenal PGLs	Rare	3/8 cases	Leiomyoma Renal cell carcinoma
KIF1B	—	Further study needed	Further study needed	—	Noradrenergic	Adrenal PHEOs	2/3 cases	No known cases	One case also had a history of neuroblastoma, ganglioneuroma, and leiomyosarcoma
MDH2**	—	Further study needed	Further study needed	—	Noradrenergic	Further study needed	Further study needed	Further study needed	—
PHD2**	—	Further study needed	Further study needed	—	Noradrenergic	Further study needed	Further study needed	Further study needed	Polycythaemia
PHD1**	—	Further study needed	Further study needed	—	Noradrenergic	Further study needed	Further study needed	Further study needed	—

Abbreviations: MEN2, multiple endocrine neoplasia type 2; MEN2A, multiple endocrine neoplasia type 2a; MEN2B, multiple endocrine neoplasia type 2b; NF1, neurofibromatosis type 1; PGL, paraganglioma; PGL1, paraganglioma syndrome type 1; PGL2, paraganglioma syndrome type 2; PGL3, paraganglioma syndrome type 3; PGL4, paraganglioma syndrome type 4; PHEO, phaeochromocytoma; VHL, Von Hippel–Lindau disease.

*Rare cases of maternal transmission have been reported.

**Germ-line mutations in these genes have only been identified in one or two cases with PHEO/PGL, so clinical information is limited.

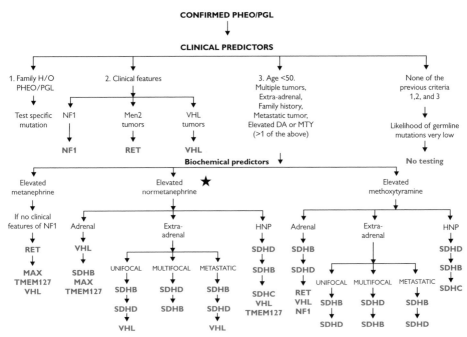

Fig 6.28 Algorithm for genetic testing; DA, dopamine: H/O, history of; HNP: head and neck paragangliomas; MEN2, multiple endocrine neoplasia type 2; MTY: methoxytyramine; NF1, neurofibromatosis type 1; PHEO, phaeochromocytoma; PGL, paraganglioma.

Note: If both normetanephrine and methoxytyramine are elevated, then follow the algorithm for methoxytyramine. If both normetanephrine and methoxytyramine are elevated, then follow the algorithm for metanephrine. SDHAF2 and SDHA gene mutations are not listed since their biochemical phenotypes are not known. If age >50, adrenal tumour, benign, no family history, consider TMEM27 testing.

* In a patient with elevated normetanephrine in whom clinical features and investigations do not clearly indicate the gene to be tested, perform immunohistochemistry for SDHB and SDHA before proceeding with testing.

Reprinted by permission from Macmillan Publishers Ltd: *Journal of Human Hypertension*, Karasek D, Shah U, Frysak Z et al., An update on the genetics of pheochromocytoma, Volume 27, Issue 3, copyright (2013).

Management of phaeochromocytoma

Surgery

Surgical resection is the preferred treatment method for phaeochromocytomas, if feasible. Patients with secreting tumours must be blocked with appropriate antihypertensive medications for at least 2 weeks prior to surgery, to significantly reduce the risk of perioperative complications. Blockade should be initiated with an alpha-adrenoceptor antagonist, followed by the addition of a beta-adrenoceptor blocker, if needed. Beta blockade should only start after at least 2 days of alpha blockade, as unopposed beta-adrenoceptor blockade can lead to beta-adrenoceptor-mediated vasodilatation and hypertensive crisis. The blockade should be titrated to achieve a blood pressure of no more than 130/80 mm Hg and a heart rate of 60–70 bpm, although this target varies depending on the centre. After surgery, patients should be followed up annually with plasma or urinary metanephrines and imaging for non-secretory tumours indefinitely to monitor development of new tumours or metastases. Follow-up should be lifelong for patients with genetic mutations, large tumours, or a young age at presentation.

Alpha-adrenoceptor blocking agents

- The most commonly used and preferred alpha-adrenoceptor blocking agent is phenoxybenzamine. The initial dose is typically 10 mg twice a day, which is then adjusted until normotension or mild hypotension is achieved. Because of the long half-life of phenoxybenzamine, a dose should not be given on the morning of surgery.
- Other alpha blockers include prazosin, terazosin, and doxazosin. Doses of these drugs can usually be adjusted more rapidly than phenoxybenzamine to achieve blood pressure control. Because of their shorter half-lives, these drugs should also be administered on the morning of surgery.
- With the use of any alpha-adrenoceptor blocking agent, post-operative hypotension can occur.

Beta-adrenoceptor blocking agents

- Beta-adrenoceptor blocking agents should be used in patients with tachyarrhythmia resulting from catecholamine excess or alpha blockade.
- Cardioselective beta-1-adrenoceptor blockers are preferable, including atenolol and metoprolol.

- The non-selective beta blocker propranol can also be used.

Combined alpha- and beta-adrenoceptor blockers, such as labetalol, are not recommended for preoperative blockade.

Calcium channel blockers
Calcium channel blockers can be of value in preoperative blockade in the following circumstances:

- when adequate blood pressure control cannot be achieved with alpha- and beta-adrenoceptor antagonists
- when side effects of alpha- and beta-blocking agents are severe enough to warrant replacement
- to avoid severe hypotension resulting from adrenoceptor blockade in patients with mild episodic hypertension

Amlodipine, nicardipene, nifedipine, and verapamil can all be given as part of preoperative blockade.

Drugs that inhibit catecholamine synthesis

- Drugs that inhibit catecholamine synthesis can be valuable in decreasing perioperative complications.
- They can be given in conjunction with adrenoceptor blocking agents for patients with biochemically active tumours.
- Metyrosine is used in some centres as a standard part of preoperative blockade. Because metyrosine also crosses the blood–brain barrier and inhibits catecholamine synthesis, side effects can include sedation, depression, anxiety, and galactorrhoea.
- Patients who are normotensive can still become hypertensive during surgery, so low doses of alpha-adrenoceptor antagonists or calcium channel blockers should be given preoperatively.

Radiofrequency ablation
Radiofrequency ablation can be a successful management strategy for metastatic lesions to the liver or bone, with complete tumour necrosis achieved in many patients. Patients should be appropriately blocked with alpha- and beta-adrenoceptor antagonists for 7–21 days before treatment to reduce the potential for intraprocedural complications. Studies on this treatment for metastatic phaeochromocytomas have shown complete ablation of bone and liver metastases, but studies with larger patient populations and longer follow-up are necessary to determine the long-term efficacy of this treatment modality. However, in patients with rapidly growing metastatic lesions or severe symptoms, radiofrequency ablation can be valuable in prolonging survival and reducing tumour burden.

Radiotherapy
Treatment with ^{131}I-MIBG is often a valuable therapeutic approach for patients with metastatic phaeochromocytoma and positive ^{123}I-MIBG scintigraphy. In preparation for treatment, the following steps should be taken:

- certain drugs, such as labetalol, tricyclic antidepressants, reserpine, and cocaine, are known to inhibit MIBG uptake and should be discontinued before treatment
- patients should be on appropriate blockade with antihypertensives to avoid complications resulting from catecholamine release
- patients must take a potassium iodine solution to block accumulation of iodine in the thyroid, from 24–48 hours before treatment to 10–15 days after treatment

The dosing and timing of ^{131}I-MIBG therapy varies greatly among different institutions. Lower doses of approximately 100–200 mCi appear to be well tolerated by patients, and repeated treatments can be done on shorter intervals. Depending on the disease progression and growth rate, intervals between treatments typically range from 3–6 months, and treatments have been repeated up to 11 times in some reports. Higher-dose treatments have also been performed, with as much as 1160 mCi given in one dose. The side effects, particularly on the bone marrow, are more significant with high-dose treatment, so repeat doses are infrequently given. Some centres offering high-dose ^{131}I-MIBG therapy also give stem cell transplants after treatment. The clinical advantages of low-dose versus high-dose therapy are still being evaluated, but studies of both strategies have shown positive responses in disease progression and symptom reduction.

Radiolabelled somatostatin analogues have also been evaluated in the treatment of phaeochromocytoma, due to the presence of somatostatin receptors in many phaeochromocytoma tumours. Three somatostatin analogues, DOTATATE, DOTATOC, and DOTANOC, have been used in neuroendocrine tumours, labelled with radioactive indium (^{111}In), yttrium (^{90}Y), or lutetium (^{177}Lu). Studies with small phaeochromocytoma-patient sample sizes have shown therapeutic benefit in some patients, with partial responses or stable disease and symptom relief reported. Further study is needed to determine the efficacy and benefit of varying doses and treatment schedules for somatostatin analogues. Bone marrow toxicity can also result from treatment with radiolabelled somatostatin analogues.

Chemotherapy
Chemotherapy can be a valuable treatment strategy for metastatic phaeochromocytoma. The combination of cyclophosphamide, vincristine, and dacarbazine (CVD) has shown the most success, leading to reported partial responses and symptom relief. As with other therapeutic options, CVD can induce catecholamine release, and therefore patients should be blocked with appropriate antihypertensive medications. Once CVD is initiated, it should be continued indefinitely until there is clear evidence of disease progression or until the patient can no longer tolerate treatment. This treatment modality appears to be particularly effective for *SDHB*-related metastatic phaeochromocytoma.

Alternative chemotherapeutic agents have also been evaluated on a limited basis in neuroendocrine tumours, including phaeochromocytomas. Temozolomide has been used in neuroendocrine tumours, both alone and in combination with thalidomide, and could be of use in metastatic phaeochromocytoma, although further study is needed to determine the utility of this chemotherapeutic agent.

Targeted therapy
Recent research on new treatment options for metastatic phaeochromocytoma has focused on targeted therapies that would directly target specific features of phaeochromocytoma cells. One target of interest is VEGF, which is involved in angiogenesis. Sunitinib, a tyrosine kinase inhibitor, has shown success in treating metastatic renal cell carcinoma and has recently been studied in cases of metastatic phaeochromocytoma. There are conflicting reports regarding the success of sunitinib,

but it appears to have limited success in *SDHB* patients. However, sunitinib may still be of value in non-*SDHB*-related metastatic phaeochromocytoma. Clinical trials with sunitinib and similar tyrosine kinase inhibitors are ongoing to determine their utility in treating metastatic phaeochromocytoma.

Inhibitors of mTOR have also been studied, since the mTOR pathway is activated in hypoxic cells. Everolimus, a therapy targeted to mTORC1, did not inhibit disease progression in metastatic phaeochromocytoma patients. This may be attributed to a lack of inhibition of both forms of HIF alpha and/or the existence of a secondary pathway that can compensate in the absence of mTORC1. Therefore, therapy with drugs targeting both mTORC1 and mTORC2 has been proposed as a potential option. Combined therapies with mTOR inhibitors and ERK inhibitors have also been proposed to target alternative pathways that the cell may use to circumvent mTORC1 inhibition.

Immunotherapy has also been considered in treatment of metastatic phaeochromocytoma. It has been suggested that the pseudohypoxic tumour environment may decrease recognition of the tumour by the immune system. Clinical trials of pembrolizumab, an antibody against lymphocytic programmed cell death protein 1 receptors, have been initiated in patients with metastatic phaeochromocytoma, but no results are yet available.

Future therapy

Future therapy will most likely focus on the development or application of existing drugs to target proteins and pathways overexpressed in metastatic phaeochromocytoma. Potential targets include:

- the Ret protein and other tyrosine kinases
- heat-shock proteins, which are involved in protein folding and assembly
- apoptotic mechanisms
- HIF-2 alpha, using specific HIF-2 alpha inhibitors that are currently being tested in other forms of cancer

Repurposing existing approved drugs for metastatic phaeochromocytoma could also represent an important strategy for the introduction of novel therapies. For example, radium dichloride 223 (Xofigo) is an alpha emitter approved for prostate cancer bone metastases and could prove valuable for phaeochromocytoma patients with metastatic bone disease.

Prognosis

The prognosis of patients diagnosed with phaeochromocytoma depends on the number, size, and location of the tumour(s), and the patient's underlying genetic disorder. Patients with small benign adrenal lesions have low rates of recurrence and high survival rates, with almost all still alive 5 years after resection. Patients with larger tumours, multiple tumours, or tumours caused by a germ-line genetic mutations (particularly in *SDHB*) have higher rates of recurrence and metastasis. Once a phaeochromocytoma metastasizes, the 5-year survival rate is generally below 50%. Current recommendations suggest lifelong follow-up for all patients.

Patient support groups/useful websites

- The Pheo/Para Alliance was founded to support research efforts for phaeochromocytoma/paraganglioma and spread awareness of the disease to physicians and patients. Their website (http://www.

pheo-para-alliance.org/) is a resource for patients and physicians to learn more about phaeochromocytoma/paraganglioma.
- The Pheo Para Troopers is an organization dedicated to supporting patients with phaeochromocytoma/paraganglioma. Their website (http://pheoparatroopers.org/) provides valuable information to patients diagnosed with phaeochromocytoma/paraganglioma.

Further reading

Adjalle R, Plouin PF, Pacak K, et al. Treatment of malignant pheochromocytoma. *Horm Metab Res* 2009; 41: 687–96.

Archier A, Varoquaux A, Garrigue P, et al. Prospective comparison of 68Ga-DOTATATE and 18F-FDOPA PET/CT in patients with various pheochromocytomas and paragangliomas with emphasis on sporadic cases. *Eur J Nucl Med Mol Imaging* 2016; 43: 1248–57.

Bausch B, Schiavi F, Ni Y, et al. Clinical characterization of the pheochromocytoma and paraganglioma susceptibility genes SDHA, TMEM127, MAX, and SDHAF2 for gene-informed prevention. *JAMA Oncol* 2017; 3: 1204–12.

Carrasquillo JA, Pandit-Taskar N, and Chen CC. Radionuclide therapy of adrenal tumours. *J Surg Oncol* 2012; 106: 634–42.

Castinetti F, Kroiss A, Kumar R, et al. 15 years of paraganglioma: Imaging and imaging-based treatment of pheochromocytoma and paraganglioma. *Endocr Relat Cancer* 2015; 22: T135–45.

de Cubas AA, Korpershoek E, Inglada-Perez L, et al. DNA methylation profiling in pheochromocytoma and paraganglioma reveals diagnostic and prognostic markers. *Clin Cancer Res* 2015; 21: 3020–30.

Eisenhofer G, Goldstein DS, Walther MM, et al. Biochemical diagnosis of pheochromocytoma: How to distinguish true-from false-positive test results. *J Clin Endocrinol Metab* 2003; 88: 2656–66.

Eisenhofer G, Lenders JW, Siegert G, et al. Plasma methoxytyramine: A novel biomarker of metastatic pheochromocytoma and paraganglioma in relation to established risk factors of tumour size, location and SDHB mutation status. *Eur J Cancer* 2012; 48: 1739–49.

Eisenhofer G, Lenders JW, Timmers H, et al. Measurements of plasma methoxytyramine, normetanephrine, and metanephrine as discriminators of different hereditary forms of pheochromocytoma. *Clin Chem* 2011; 57: 411–20.

Fishbein L, Leshchiner I, Walter V, et al. Comprehensive molecular characterization of pheochromocytoma and paraganglioma. *Cancer Cell* 2017; 31: 181–93.

Gupta G and Pacak K. Precision medicine: An update on genotype-biochemical phenotype relationships in pheochromocytoma/paraganglioma patients. *Endocr Pract* 2017; 23: 690–704.

Havekes B, King K, Lai EW, et al. New imaging approaches to pheochromocytomas and paragangliomas. *Clin Endocrinol (Oxf)* 2010; 72: 137–45.

Ilias I, Chen CC, Carrasquillo JA, et al. Comparison of 6–18F-fluorodopamine PET with 123I-metaiodobenzylguanidine and 111in-pentetreotide scintigraphy in localization of nonmetastatic and metastatic pheochromocytoma. *J Nucl Med* 2008; 49: 1613–19.

Imani F, Agopian VG, Auerbach MS, et al. 18F-FDOPA PET and PET/CT accurately localize pheochromocytomas. *J Nucl Med* 2009; 50: 513–19.

Janssen I, Blanchet EM, Adams K, et al. Superiority of [68Ga]-DOTATATE PET/CT to other functional imaging modalities in the localization of SDHB-associated metastatic pheochromocytoma and paraganglioma. *Clin Cancer Res* 2015; 21: 3888–95.

Janssen I, Chen CC, Millo CM, et al. PET/CT comparing 68Ga-DOTATATE and other radiopharmaceuticals and in comparison with CT/MRI for the localization of sporadic metastatic pheochromocytoma and paraganglioma. *Eur J Nucl Med Mol Imaging* 2016; 43: 1784–91.

Janssen I, Chen CC, Zhuang Z, et al. Functional imaging signature of patients presenting with polycythemia/paraganglioma syndromes. *J Nucl Med* 2017; 58: 1236–42.

Janssen I, Taieb D, Patronas NJ, et al. [68Ga]-DOTATATE PET/CT in the localization of head and neck paragangliomas compared to other functional imaging modalities and CT/MRI. *J Nucl Med* 2016; 57: 186–91.

Karasek D, Shah U, Frysak Z, et al. An update on the genetics of pheochromocytoma. *J Hum Hypertens* 2013; 27: 141–7.

King KS, Chen CC, Alexopoulos DK, et al. Functional imaging of SDHx-related head and neck paragangliomas: comparison of 18F-fluorodihydroxyphenylalanine, 18F-fluorodopamine, 18F-fluoro-2-deoxy-D-glucose PET, 123I-metaiodobenzylguanidine scintigraphy, and 111In-pentetreotide scintigraphy. *J Clin Endocrinol Metab* 2011; 96: 2779–85.

Lenders JWM, Duh QY, Eisenhofer G, et al. Pheochromocytoma and paraganglioma: An Endocrine Society Clinical Practice Guideline. *J Clin Endocrinol Metab* 2014; 99: 1915–42.

Naswa N, Sharma P, Nazar AH, et al. Prospective evaluation of 68Ga-DOTA-NOC PET-CT in phaeochromocytoma and paraganglioma: preliminary results from a single centre study. *Eur Radiol* 2012; 22: 710–19.

Pacak K. Preoperative management of the pheochromocytoma patient. *J Clin Endocrinol Metab* 2007; 92: 4069–79.

Pacak K, Jochmanova I, Prodanov T, et al. New syndrome of paraganglioma and somatostatinoma associated with polycythemia. *J Clin Oncol* 2013; 31: 1690–8.

Plouin PF, Amar L, Dekkers OM, et al. European Society of Endocrinology clinical practice guidelines for long-term follow-up of patients operated on for a phaeochromocytoma or a paraganglioma. *Eur J Endocrinol* 2016; 174: G1–G10.

Pillai S, Gopalan V, Smith RA, et al. Updates on the genetics and the clinical impacts on phaeochromocytoma and paraganglioma in the new era. *Crit Rev Oncol Hematol* 2016; 100: 190–208.

Roman-Gonzalez A, Jimenez C. Malignant pheochromocytoma-paraganglioma: Pathogenesis, TNM staging, and current clinical trials. *Curr Opin Endocrinol Diabetes Obes* 2017; 24: 174–83.

Tan TH, Hussein Z, Saad FF, et al. Diagnostic performance of (68)Ga-DOTATATE PET/CT, (18)F-FDG PET/CT and (131)I-MIBG scintigraphy in mapping metastatic pheochromocytoma and paraganglioma. *Nucl Med Mol Imaging* 2015; 143–51.

Timmers HJ, Carrasquillo JA, Whatley M, et al. Usefulness of standardized uptake values for distinguishing adrenal glands with pheochromocytoma from normal adrenal glands by use of 6–18F-fluorodopamine PET. *J Nucl Med* 2007; 48: 1940–4.

Timmers HJ, Chen CC, Carrasquillo JA, et al. Staging and functional characterization of pheochromocytoma and paraganglioma by 18F-fluorodeoxyglucose (18F-FDG) positron emission tomography. *J Natl Cancer Inst* 2012; 104: 700–8.

Timmers HJ, Chen CC, Carrasquillo JA, et al. Comparison of 18F-fluoro-L-DOPA, 18F-fluorodeoxyglucose, and 18F-fluorodopamine PET and 123I-MIBG scintigraphy in the localization of pheochromocytoma and paraganglioma. *J Clin Endocrinol Metab* 2009; 94: 4757–67.

Timmers HJ, Eisenhofer G, Carrasquillo JA, et al. Use of 6-[18F]-fluorodopamine positron emission tomography (PET) as first-line investigation for the diagnosis and localization of non-metastatic and metastatic phaeochromocytoma (PHEO). *Clin Endocrinol (Oxf)* 2009; 71: 11–17.

Timmers HJ, Kozupa A, Chen CC, et al. Superiority of fluorodeoxyglucose positron emission tomography to other functional imaging techniques in the evaluation of metastatic SDHB-associated pheochromocytoma and paraganglioma. *J Clin Oncol* 2007; 25: 2262–9.

Venkatesan AM, Locklin J, Lai EW, et al. Radiofrequency ablation of metastatic pheochromocytoma. *J Vasc Interv Radiol* 2009; 20: 1483–90.

Wiseman GA, Pacak K, O'Dorisio MS, et al. Usefulness of 123I-MIBG scintigraphy in the evaluation of patients with known or suspected primary or metastatic pheochromocytoma or paraganglioma: Results from a prospective multicenter trial. *J Nucl Med* 2009; 50: 1448–54.

Zelinka T, Timmers HJ, Kozupa A, et al. Role of positron emission tomography and bone scintigraphy in the evaluation of bone involvement in metastatic pheochromocytoma and paraganglioma: Specific implications for succinate dehydrogenase enzyme subunit B gene mutations. *Endocr Relat Cancer* 2008; 15: 311–23.

Zhuang Z, Yang C, Lorenzo F, et al. Somatic HIF2A gain-of-function mutations in paraganglioma with polycythemia. *N Engl J Med* 2012; 367: 922–30.

6.15 Adrenal surgery

Introduction
The name of the early twentieth-century Boston neurosurgeon Harvey Cushing is associated with the eponymous syndrome characterized by clinical signs resulting from excessive chronic exposure to glucocorticoid excess.

Medical treatment of Cushing's syndrome
Medical treatment aims to optimize the patients preoperatively and to provide long-term support postoperatively (see also Section 6.8).

Metyrapone and ketoconazole can be used preoperatively to decrease cortisol synthesis but their efficacy is limited and poor compliance is common. Occasionally, etomidate can be used for the same purpose [1].

Cortisol replacement after unilateral or bilateral adrenalectomy is vital. Patients with solitary adrenal tumours have the contralateral adrenal gland atrophied and it may take 6 months (or more) for a return to normal function. Patients should be informed about the possibility of an Addisonian crisis triggered by any illness that could impair their ability to continue oral medication (e.g. severe diarrhoea/vomiting episodes). They should wear a bracelet and carry a card with details of their condition.

In a group of 170 patients undergoing retroperitoneoscopic adrenalectomy for manifest Cushing's syndrome (n = 99) or subclinical Cushing's syndrome (n = 71), postoperative oral steroids supplementation was administered in 136 patients (all with manifest disease, and 37 with subclinical Cushing's syndrome) for a mean duration of therapy of 12.3 months and 10.3 months, respectively [2].

Mineralocorticoid replacement (fludrocortisone 0.1 mg) is necessary only after bilateral adrenalectomy.

Surgical treatment of Cushing's syndrome
- Surgical resection of a pituitary adenoma could be curative for Cushing's syndrome. Because many adrenocorticotrophic-hormone-secreting pituitary adenomas are small in size (<1 cm), the success of the operation is dependent on the experience of the neurosurgeon (see Section 6.8).
- Adrenal adenomas are removed via laparoscopic adrenalectomy. The transperitoneal approach is widely used but the retroperitoneal approach is increasing in popularity in recent years.
- Adrenocortical cancers raise more challenges. Most patients present with large tumours (>10 cm); hence, ensuring a complete resection implies multi-organ resection of the tumour in continuity with the perinephric fat, the kidney, the tail of the pancreas, and the spleen. Such patients should be treated where a multidisciplinary approach can be offered and where there is previous (surgical) experience with the condition.

In a historical synopsis of surgery over a 10-year period at the Mayo Clinic (1996–2005), 298 patients underwent 322 operative procedures for Cushing's syndrome. One-quarter of the patients had adrenocorticotrophic-hormone-independent Cushing's syndrome (n = 67; 22%) and the majority had adrenocorticotrophic-hormone-dependent Cushing's syndrome (n = 231; 78%), either pituitary-dependent Cushing's syndrome (n = 196; 66%) or ectopic adrenocorticotrophic-hormone syndrome (n = 35; 12%). Cure rates were 80% for first-time pituitary operations, and 55% for reoperations. Five-year survival rates (all causes) were 90%, 51%, and 23% for adrenocortical adenomas, ectopic adrenocorticotrophic-hormone syndrome, and adrenocortical carcinomas, respectively [3].

In a retrospective study of 50 patients after adrenalectomy for adrenocorticotrophic-hormone-independent hypercortisolism, after a mean follow-up of 134 months, 100% of patients were biochemically cured, and a clinical recovery was observed in most cases: obesity in 60% and hypertension in 58%. In addition, bone mass density significantly improved (+20%). The long-term mortality rate did not differ from that of the normal population. Subjectively, a full recovery was confirmed by 95.6% of the patients, who reported the subjective feeling of physical recovery (95.6%) and regained working ability (93.3%). Despite biochemical and clinical cure, no subjective improvement of the psychological conditions was observed in a quarter of cases [4].

Treatment of subclinical Cushing's syndrome
Currently, it is considered that 4% of subjects older than 60 years of age harbour adrenal incidentalomas (see Sections 6.8 and 6.9), of which a fifth could be associated with subclinical Cushing's syndrome. Some consider that subclinical Cushing's syndrome is associated with insulin resistance, hypertension, obesity, dyslipidemia, impaired glucose tolerance, and diabetes mellitus as frequently as is overt Cushing's syndrome; hence, a case for treating such patients could be made. There are, however, no Level 1 data to confirm this hypothesis.

In a small study of 16 patients with subclinical Cushing's syndrome, the prevalence of hypertension, impaired glucose tolerance, diabetes mellitus, and dyslipidemia and obesity was 56%, 50%, 50%, and 19%, respectively. Eight cases underwent unilateral adrenalectomy (operated group) and the remaining eight cases were a conservative-treatment group (non-operated group). The number of cardiovascular risk factors decreased significantly in the operated group, but not in the non-operated group [5]. Overall, a small number of retrospective analysis of cohorts of patients who had subclinical Cushing's syndrome and were observed or operated on suggest that adrenalectomy decreases accumulated cardiovascular risk factors in subclinical Cushing's syndrome; hence, this hypothesis should be tested in a formal randomized trial. Such a project could only be organized on a multicentre basis and would need prolonged follow-up; hence, the challenge is considerable.

Laparoscopic adrenalectomy for Cushing's syndrome
Patients with Cushing's syndrome due to unilateral adrenal adenoma are generally operated on without the need for pharmacological control of the raised cortisol. In the presence of severe clinical signs (more likely in patients with adrenocortical cancer), the cortisol synthesis inhibitor metyrapone can be used preoperatively. For all patients, it is crucial to correct hypokalaemia before the planned operation.

For laparoscopic adrenalectomy, most surgeons use a transperitoneal approach with four ports situated under the costal margin. Conversion to open adrenalectomy is seldom necessary; it should be done either when the macroscopic appearance of the tumour suggests malignancy or if uncontrolled bleeding is encountered during control of the adrenal vein. In the British Association of Endocrine and Thyroid Surgeons national audit, which recorded just under 1400 adrenalectomies, conversion to open adrenalectomy was commoner for malignant cases (25.3%; 22/87) than for benign (6.5%; 52/796). In the same report, median post-operative stay was 4 days for Cushing's syndrome, which is longer than that for Conn adenomas (2 days), equal to that for phaeochromocytomas (4 days), and shorter than that for adrenocortical cancer (7 days), with significantly longer admission after open operation (7 days vs 3 days) [6].

In recent years, retroperitoneoscopic adenalectomy has been increasing in popularity because of its alleged better post-operative pain control and possibly shorter in-hospital stay. The experience with this technique in the UK remains limited.

Perioperative care for patients with Cushing's syndrome
An adrenal adenoma causes profound suppression of the normal contralateral adrenal cortex as a result of the inhibition of adrenocorticotrophic-hormone secretion. This inhibition persists after removal of the tumour, and patients require hydrocortisone replacement for up to 12 months post-operatively. Intravenous hydrocortisone 100 mg four times per day should be started intraoperatively and be used until oral intake is restarted. Oral hydrocortisone should then be started at a high dose (20–20–10 mg) and tapered slowly towards the physiological dose (10–5–5 mg) within the following few weeks/months.

In view of the increased risk of post-operative infections, prophylactic antibiotics should be used, and urinary catheters and intravenous lines regularly monitored.

These patients are at increased risk of venous thromboembolism; hence, thromboembolic deterrent stocking should be used throughout the admission, flowtron pumps should be used intraoperatively, and subcutaneous heparin (Fragmin/Daltaprin/Clexane) should be used daily.

Radical adrenalectomy for adrenocortical cancer

See also Section 6.10. Despite increased use of cross-sectional imaging, adrenocortical cancer continue to be diagnosed at a late stage in the development of these tumours, and the majority of patients have locally advanced disease (Stages 2–3) or metastatic disease (Stage 4). Surgery plays a major role in the management of these patients. For those with localized disease (Stages 1–2), a radical operation could prevent the risk of local recurrence. For those with more advanced disease (Stage 3), a radical operation should still be able to achieve good local control. For patients with metastatic disease, the operation is beneficial, as removal of the large adrenal mass reduces the amount of cortisol secretion, limits the morbidity related to severely abnormal biochemical changes, and allows time for systemic chemotherapy to be effective. The decision on which patients are or are not candidates for a surgical intervention should be made in a multidisciplinary setting with contribution from an experienced surgical team. In view of the poor prognosis of these tumours, it is unreasonable for the patient to be

managed by surgeons with no previous experience with this condition.

In many patients, radical extensive local resection of the tumour requires resection of the surrounding viscera. In our own centre, a total of 46 patients with adrenocortical cancer were operated on in the last decade; of these, 21 patients had adrenalectomy only whilst, for the others, the operation involved simultaneous nephrectomy ($n = 23$), splenectomy ($n = 10$), distal pancreatectomy ($n = 11$), or limited liver resection ($n = 2$). Particular attention is given to CT scans to assess the possibility of direct invasion in the inferior vena cava. Such locally advanced tumours need particular care, and their management should be centralized in hospitals where collaboration with the cardiovascular surgeons and/or liver surgeons ensures a safe multidisciplinary approach. Based on a personal experience of five such cases in Oxford, a survey of members of the European Society of Endocrine Surgeons identified a total of 38 patients operated on for adrenocortical cancer with inferior vena cava invasion; there was a 14% 30-days in-hospital mortality rate (related to uncontrolled intraoperative bleeding) but 13 patients of the patients were alive at 2–58 months (median 16 months) with known metastatic disease ($n = 7$) or with no signs of distant disease ($n = 6$) [7].

In view of the complexity of the operative approach and the need for support from different surgical specialities, the operative care of patients with adrenocortical cancer should be centralized in nominated regional centres. This aim is yet to be achieved, as the rarity of these tumours makes referrals unlikely, and the majority of patients are being operated on in hospitals with minimal previous experience in adrenal surgery (Hospital Episode Statistics data, personal communication). It is the responsibility of the medical profession and of the funding bodies to reorganize the care pathway for such patients in coming years. More immediate support and information for patients and their relatives are increasingly being offered by patient support groups (http://www.amend.org.uk/guide-to-the-disorders/acc.html).

Adrenalectomy for phaeochromocytoma

Once a diagnosis has been made, pharmacological treatment should be commenced to control symptoms and prevent cardiovascular complications (see also Section 6.14). Classically, this is achieved with the alpha blocker phenoxybenzamine, together with propranolol. Some advocate the use of the selective alpha-1 blocker doxazosin as a single drug, as it lacks the side effects associated with the alpha-2 effects of phenoxybenzamine (nasal stuffiness, postural hypotension, somnolence).

Doses of medication that adequately control blood pressure and symptoms without excessive side effects may provide insufficient protection from the cardiovascular changes that occur during surgical manipulation. In the authors' unit, the practice is to admit patients a few days before surgery, to measure lying/standing pulse and blood pressure regularly, and titrate up the dose of medication towards the following endpoints:

- controlled systolic blood pressure, preferably ≤ 120 mm Hg
- significant postural drop in blood pressure
- controlled heart rate, preferably ≤ 80 bpm
- no significant increase in heart rate on standing

Patients are likely to suffer side effects from the doses required to achieve these goals; indeed, some use their presence as further reassurance that the patient is adequately blocked.

Surgical manipulation of the tumour, whether open or laparoscopic, is associated with release of catecholamine and surges of blood pressure. Antihypertensives should be given to treat (and, ideally, pre-empt) these surges. A pre-eminent concern is preventing the cardiac and cerebrovascular complications that may result from extremes of blood pressure. It is usually possible to identify the moment the surgeon ligates the main adrenal vein, as the blood pressure becomes almost immediately less labile.

Post-operative management for phaeochomocytomas

After successful excision of a phaeochomocytoma, cardiovascular stability is usual. Somewhat surprisingly, the presence of high-dose alpha and beta blockade rarely leads to post-operative hypotension. In such cases, a period of post-operative vasopressor support may be required. Post-operative hypertension is rarer still, and may suggest undetected bilateral or extra-adrenal disease. Hypoglycaemia may occasionally occur in diabetics, as a result of the withdrawal of the anti-insulin effects of catecholamines. An hour or two of invasive blood pressure monitoring in recovery is appropriate, after which patients can be discharged to a general ward. Although, in our experience, post-operative management in the intensive care unit or high-dependency unit is rarely required, some centres use it routinely. Phenxoybenzamine (or doxazosin) can be stopped immediately post-operatively.

Propranolol is usually weaned off over a period of days, to prevent rebound tachycardia.

References and further reading

1. Preda V, Chen J, Karavitaki N, et al. The use of etomidate in the treatment of Cushing's syndrome. *Eur J Endocrinol* 2012; 167: 137–43.
2. Alesina PF, Hommeltenberg S, Meier B, et al. Posterior retroperitoneoscopic adrenalectomy for clinical and subclinical Cushing's syndrome. *World J Surg* 2010; 34: 1391–7.
3. Porterfield JR, Thompson GB, Young WF Jr, et al. Surgery for Cushing's syndrome: An historical review and recent ten-year experience. *World J Surg* 2008; 32: 659–77.
4. Iacobone M, Mantero F, Basso SM, et al. Results and long-term follow-up after unilateral adrenalectomy for ACTH-independent hypercortisolism in a series of fifty patients. *J Endocrinol Invest* 2005; 28: 327–32.
5. Akaza I, Yoshimoto T, Iwashima F, et al. Clinical outcome of subclinical Cushing's syndrome after surgical and conservative treatment. *Hypertens Res* 2011; 34: 1111–15.
6. Chadwick D, Kinsman R, and Walton, P. *The British Association of Endocrine and Thyroid Surgeons Fourth National Audit Report*, 2012. Dendrite Clinical Systems Ltd. Available at http://www.baets.org.uk/wp-content/uploads/2013/05/4th-National-Audit.pdf (accessed 27 Dec 2017).
7. Mihai R, Iacobone M, Makay O, et al. Outcome of operation in patients with adrenocortical cancer invading the inferior vena cava: A European Society of Endocrine Surgeons (ESES) survey. *Langenbecks Arch Surg* 2012; 397: 225–31.
8. Iacobone M, Citton M, Scarpa M, et al. Systematic review of surgical treatment of subclinical Cushing's syndrome. *Br J Surg* 2015; 102: 318–30.
9. Mihai R. Diagnosis, treatment and outcome of adrenocortical cancer. *Br J Surg* 2015; 102: 291–306.

Chapter 7

Female hormone metabolism

Chapter contents

7.1 Anatomy and physiology

Introduction

Human ovaries are cyclically active endocrine organs responsible for the periodic process of egg maturation and ovulation and for the production of the main steroid hormones estradiol and progesterone. Both functions are tightly meshed with feedback mechanisms to the hypothalamus and pituitary glands in the hypothalamo-pituitary–ovarian axis. Other endocrine organs such as the thyroid and the adrenal glands are equally important for normal reproductive functions. This well-orchestrated process normally results in regular ovulation and leads to cyclic changes in the endometrium and the predictable monthly menses in adult females.

Anatomy

The adult human ovaries are oval bodies averaging 14 g each and lie over the ovarian fossae at the posterolateral pelvic wall and are attached to the posterior leaflet of the broad ligaments by the mesovarium. The ovary consists of three major distinct portions:

1. The outer cortex, which contains two regions: the outermost region is a single layer of cuboidal epithelium, referred to as the surface germinal epithelium, and the inner region contains the follicles embedded in stromal tissue derived from mesenchymal cells which have the ability to respond to LH or hCG.
2. The central medulla consists of stroma, which is derived mainly from mesonephric cells.
3. The rete ovarii (the hilum) in the area of attachment of the ovary to the mesovarium. It contains nerves, blood vessels, and the hilar cells, which can potentially become active in steroidogenesis.

Follicles

The follicle represents the basic structural and functional complex in the ovary with respect to oocyte maturation and steroidogenesis. The primordial follicles start to form at 18–20 gestational weeks. Each primordial follicle contains an oocyte arrested at the prophase stage of the first meiotic division, enveloped by a single layer of pregranulosa cells surrounded by a basement membrane. They are embedded in the loose connective tissue of the ovarian cortex. Only a minority of primordial follicles are recruited during a woman's reproductive lifetime; most undergo the process of atresia. The recruitment of primordial follicles into growing follicles induces changes in granulosa cell growth and maturation, as well as follicular structural and functional changes. They typically grow and develop through primary, preantral, and antral follicle stages. The early stages of follicular growth are FSH independent and are probably controlled by local intra-ovarian factors such as anti-Müllerian hormone. Full maturity, as expressed by ovulation, typically occurs in the reproductive age only, as the dominant ovulating follicle is selected during the early days of the same cycle. At 16–20 gestational weeks, there are 6–7 million germ cells. At birth, the number of oocytes is nearly 1 million. At the onset of puberty, the oocyte number is reduced to about 500,000 and, throughout the reproductive life, only 300–500 oocytes will be selected to ovulate. The vast majority of eggs are lost in a process of atresia or apoptosis (programmed cell death).

Follicular growth and egg maturation

The early stages of follicular growth occur over a time period of several preceding cycles, about 85 days prior to achieving pre-ovulatory status. Reaching this stage, either the follicles are recruited by an FSH-dependent process at about the transition time between the preceding cycle's luteal phase and the early days of the current cycle's follicular phase, or they become arrested and undergo atresia. Typically, a cohort of FSH-dependent 2–6 mm antral follicles is recruited by the late luteal phase due to the FSH rise of the preceding cycle. The average time for the development of the selected dominant follicle to the ovulation stage is 10–14 days.

Reproductive physiology

Normal reproductive function with cyclic menses requires the pulsatile secretion of GnRH from the hypothalamus. This pulsatile rhythmic release must be within a critical range of frequency and amplitude for normal control to occur. GnRH has a positive effect on the anterior pituitary, resulting in increased gonadotrophin synthesis, storage, and pulsatile secretion. Lower GnRH pulse frequencies favour FSH secretion, and higher frequencies favour LH secretion. The variation in GnRH pulse frequencies is modulated by the ovarian steroid feedback. Estradiol increases GnRH pulse frequency, whereas elevated progesterone levels decrease it. Estradiol and progesterone levels are important in determining gonadotrophin regulation.

Oestrogen levels

Low estradiol levels enhance FSH and LH synthesis and storage and have negative effects on FSH secretion, with little effect on LH secretion. However, it is the high estradiol levels that induce the LH surge at mid-cycle.

Progesterone levels

Low levels enhance the LH response to GnRH and are responsible for the FSH surge at mid-cycle. The increased level of progesterone in the luteal phase inhibits gonadotrophin secretion by inhibiting hypothalamic GnRH pulses and inhibiting the pituitary response to GnRH. It is the raised progesterone levels at the end of the luteal phase that decrease GnRH pulsatile frequency, leading to preferential FSH secretion in the late luteal phase and the start of the next ovarian cycle with follicular cohort recruitment.

GnRH pulsatility is also modulated by neurotransmitters such as dopamine, noradrenaline, endorphins, kisspeptins, and others. The half-life of GnRH is short (2–4 minutes), as it is degraded rapidly by peptidases in the hypothalamus and the pituitary gland.

Gonadotrophs are the target cells of GnRH at the level of the anterior pituitary gland and are responsible for the synthesis, storage, activation, and secretion of LH and FSH. Each gonadotrophin is a heterodimer and is made of two peptide subunits termed alpha and beta, respectively. The alpha subunits are structurally identical but the beta subunits are unique and confer the specific activity. During the late luteal phase, FSH levels start to rise, reaching a peak around Day 3 of menstruation in the next cycle. This causes FSH-dependent antral follicular recruitment and growth; granulosa cell proliferation and differentiation;

aromatase action; oestrogen production; and inhibin B secretion. The last two hormones exert negative feedback at the hypothalamus and the pituitary. FSH induces LH receptors within the dominant follicle. Estradiol levels derived from the dominant follicle increase steadily and exert suppressive feedback on FSH release, leading to a lack of support for and consequent atresia of the non-dominant follicles. The mid-follicular rise in estradiol leads to a switch from negative to positive feedback on LH release, resulting in the mid-cycle surge. This surge lasts 36–48 hours and is responsible for the resumption of oocyte meiotic maturation, triggering of ovulation, luteinization of granulosa cells, and synthesis of progesterone and prostaglandins within the follicle.

Two-cell, two-gonadotrophin theory for ovarian steroidogenesis

Estradiol and progesterone are the main steroid hormones secreted by the ovaries. Ovarian steroidogenesis in the follicles takes place through two mechanisms:

1. LH action on theca cells, mediated largely by cAMP, StAR, and SF-1, leading to androgen synthesis, predominantly androstenedione, which then diffuses to the granulosa cells.
2. FSH action on granulosa cells through cAMP, LRH-1 and/or SF-1 binding activity, and promotion of aromatase expression in granulosa cells and subsequent estradiol formation by aromatization of androstenedione and other androgens.

Estradiol is the most important oestrogen; its main functions are endometrial development and triggering of the mid-cycle LH surge leading to follicular rupture and ovulation. In addition, the suppression of FSH secretion by negative estradiol feedback is key to preventing multifollicular development in the mid-follicular phase, once a single dominant follicle has been recruited.

Estradiol levels rise rapidly after menstruation to reach a peak in the late follicular phase, which induces the mid-cycle LH surge. During the luteal phase, estradiol is produced by the corpus luteum; in the absence of an endogenous rise in hCG from an implanting embryo, the corpus luteum involutes, leading to a sharp decline in estradiol (and progesterone) levels and consequent menstruation.

The granulosa lutein cells have high levels of LH receptors and produce progesterone, the main luteal phase hormone. Progesterone stimulates secretory changes in the endometrium, and these are critical for achieving an environment receptive for embryo implantation. Progesterone levels rise following ovulation and decline with the demise of the corpus luteum before menstruation. Peak progesterone levels are reached in the mid-luteal phase, and a blood sample (taken 7 days before the estimated day of the following menstrual bleed) is commonly used to confirm ovulation.

Extra-ovarian steroidogenesis

Estradiol production can take place in peripheral tissues, such as subcutaneous fat and skin fibroblasts. Peripheral tissue aromatase is responsible for the aromatization of androstenedione, resulting in the production of the weaker oestrogen, oestrone. Oestrone is further metabolized and converted to the more biologically active estradiol in target tissues such as the breast and endometrium. This extra-ovarian production is potentially clinically important in obese women because of the increased mass of fat tissue.

Peptide hormones produced by the ovary

The ovaries produce a number of peptides that can act in an autocrine, paracrine, or endocrine manner. These peptides include numerous cytokines, growth factors, and other regulatory proteins such as inhibin, activin, and follistatin that are produced by granulosa cells under the control of FSH and LH and take part in the hypothalamo-pituitary–ovarian feedback loops. For further reading, see the suggested references.

Further reading

Reed LP. *Williams Textbook of Endocrinology* (10th edition), 2003. Saunders.

Speroff L, Glass RH, Kase NG, et al. *Clinical Gynecologic Endocrinology and Infertility* (6th edition), 1999. Lippincott Williams & Williams.

Strauss JF and Barbieri RL. *Yen and Jaffe's Reproductive Endocrinology* (6th edition), 2009. Saunders.

Wass JAH and Stewart PM. *Oxford Textbook of Endocrinology and Diabetes* (2nd edition), 2011. Oxford University Press.

7.2 Investigation

Introduction

Female reproductive hormone dysfunction is often manifested by disruption of the regular cyclic menses, oligo/anovulation, infertility, or a presentation of clinical hyperandrogenism. History taking and physical examination are still the mainstay of any diagnostic workup. Based on clinical presenting symptoms and the physical signs obtained, further investigative workup including biochemical, hormonal, and genetic tests and imaging studies can then be used to make a diagnosis.

History

A detailed history should be taken with the aim of understanding the main presenting complaints, including guided questions to assess the possible underlying hormonal disruptions. Thorough knowledge of the physiological effects of the different female hormones is critical for establishing the correct diagnosis. Possible involvement of the hypothalamic-pituitary—ovarian axis as well as non- hypothalamic-pituitary—ovarian-axis glands (e.g. the adrenal glands or the thyroid) should be thoroughly evaluated by organ-targeted questions.

The history should include careful evaluation of the menses, their regularity, their frequency, the duration and quantity of bleeding, the age of menarche, and the relationship to puberty. Other areas include past medical and surgical history; intercurrent systemic illnesses or use of medications; primary versus secondary amenorrhea; galactorrhoea and/or visual disturbances; clinical presentation of hyperandrogenism (i.e. hirsutism, acne or signs of virilization); gradual versus sudden onset of hirsutism; evaluation of reproductive and obstetric histories; weight, weight changes, eating disorders, and related complaints; physical activity; hot flushes; fertility history; and previous contraception. Family history may prove important.

Physical examination

The physical examination should aim to elicit evidence of abnormality in the primary endocrine organ (e.g. the thyroid gland) and/or the target organ (e.g. the skin). The BMI should be calculated for patients; the severity of hirsutism and acne, if indicated, should be assessed; and signs of virilization (i.e. clitoromegaly, voice deepening, or hair loss) should be looked for. Physical examination of the breasts and Tanner staging should be undertaken, if indicated. Careful gynaecological examination with attention to any vulvo-vaginal, cervical, uterine, or adnexal lesions or pathologies should be undertaken.

Based on careful history taking and physical examination, a tentative differential diagnosis is offered. The final diagnosis is most often established or confirmed with completion of the laboratory workup, including biochemical and/or genetic tests. The different tests that are routinely used in the evaluation of female hormonal metabolism dysfunction are discussed in this section. A structured detailed approach and specific algorithms for the different pertinent diagnoses will be dealt with separately in the relevant sections.

Biochemical

Determining an early follicular-phase (Day 2–5) hormonal profile is the initial step in a female endocrine workup. The test can be taken on a random day in a woman with absent or very irregular menses. If the patient is already on hormonal treatment (i.e. the combined oral contraceptive pill), then blood tests should be taken on the seventh off-pill day. These tests will commonly include tests for FSH, LH, total and free testosterone, prolactin, TSH, and FT4. Based on the clinical presentation and the results of the initial workup, further tests are arranged as necessary. The differential diagnosis and the stepwise diagnostic workup will be dealt with in more detail in the relevant sections (Section 7.4 for PCOS; Chapter 3, Section 3.5 for prolactinoma/galactorrhoea; Sections 7.4–7.6 for hirsutism/hyperandrogenism; and Section 7.7 for ovarian failure).

The FSH and LH levels are mainly used to differentiate between primary and secondary ovarian dysfunction. Abnormal tests should be repeated after at least 1 month to confirm the results. Table 7.1 shows a classification of oligo/amenorrhoea, common causes, and hormonal profiles.

Tests measuring total and free testosterone are the initial tests in hyperandrogenism states. Further tests may be then sent if abnormal results are achieved, as follows.

DHEAS and androstenedione are usually tested if the serum testosterone is greater than 5 nmol/L (144.21 ng/dL), in the presence of a rapidly progressive hyperandrogenic state or in cases of virilization. Androstenedione is elevated in both ovarian and adrenal aetiologies. DHEAS is a useful hyperandrogenic adrenal marker. In cases of adrenal tumours, it is in excess of >20 µmol/L (7.4 µg/ml).

17-Hydroxyprogesterone (taken at 8:00 h) is measured to screen for late-onset congenital adrenal hyperplasia (see Section 7.5). It is indicated when testosterone levels are greater than 5 nmol/L or in cases of virilization. The blood sample should be taken in the follicular phase of the menstrual cycle, to avoid false-positive results that may occur in the luteal phase, since it is also secreted by the corpus luteum.

17-Hydroxyprogesterone is measured 60 minutes after intravenous adrenocorticotrophic hormone, and cortisol (8:00 h) measured after 1 mg dexamethasone at midnight if the 17-hydroxyprogesterone (8:00 h) screening test is abnormal. Typically, an exaggerated rise in 17-hydroxyprogesterone is seen in non-classic congenital adrenal hyperplasia. Most patients have levels of >45 nmol/L (1487 ng/dL). Levels <30 nmol/L (991 ng/dL) post-adrenocorticotrophic hormone rule out the diagnosis. Levels 30–45 nmol/L suggest heterozygosity or non-classic congenital adrenal hyperplasia. Abnormal levels should be confirmed by genotyping.

Depending on the clinical context and degree of suspicion of Cushing's syndrome, blood tests for free cortisol or an overnight DST are used.

Prolactin is measured to exclude hyperprolactinemia as a cause of galactorrhoea, or ovulatory dysfunction leading to oligo/amenorrhoea or infertility. Assays for macroprolactin should be used in patients with hyperprolactinaemia and regular ovulatory cycles.

TSH and FT4 are the screening tests for thyroid dysfunction, especially if either hypothyroidism or hyperthyroidism is clinically suspected.

In the progesterone challenge test, progesterone withdrawal bleeding is induced using 10 mg oral

Table 7.1 Follicle-stimulating hormone and luteinizing hormone profiles in common causes of WHO groups of oligo/amenorrhea

WHO group	Pathology definition	Common causes	FSH, LH profile
1	Hypothalamic-pituitary failure (Hypogonadotrophic hypogonadism)	Kallmann's syndrome	Very low FSH and LH
		Functional hypothalamic amenorrhea	
		Weight loss	
		Eating disorders	
		Exercise	
		Stress related	
		Brain tumours	
		Hypophysectomy	
		Cranial irradiation	
2	Hypothalamic-pituitary dysfunction	PCOS	Normal or low FSH
		Adult type CAH	Normal or high LH
		Cushing's syndrome	
3	Ovarian failure	Premature ovarian failure	High FSH and LH
		Idiopathic/familial gonadal dysgenesis	
		Autoimmune disorder	
		Surgery/irradiation	
		Chemotherapy	
		Mumps oophoritis	
		Resistant ovary	
4	Hyperprolactinaemia	Pituitary adenoma	Normal FSH and LH
5	Outflow tract defect	Imperforate hymen	Normal FSH and LH
		Tranverse vaginal septum	
		Asherman's syndrome	
		Müllerian agenesis (Mayer–Rokitansky–Kuster–Hauser syndrome)	
		Cervical stenosis	
		Testicular feminization	
		(Androgen insensitivity)	

Abbreviations: CAH, congenital adrenal hyperplasia; FSH, follicle-stimulating hormone; LH, luteinizing hormone; PCOS, polycystic ovary syndrome.

Data from *International Classification of Diseases* (ICD), version 10. Copyright (1992) World Health Organization.

medroxyprogesterone acetate twice daily for 7 days. If a bleed ensues after progesterone administration is stopped, then there is evidence of adequate oestrogen priming of the endometrium and a normal outflow tract.

Dyslipidaemia and impaired glucose tolerance screening may be used in patients with PCOS, as they are at higher risk of cardiometabolic syndrome, with a predisposition towards hypertriglyceridaemia, hyper-cholesterolaemia, low HDL cholesterol, and impaired glucose tolerance. Screening blood tests for blood lipids and fasting glucose are indicated in patients with PCOS, especially if they have other metabolic risk factors. If the fasting glucose is abnormal, the glucose challenge test should follow.

Genetic investigation

Karyotype

The main indication for chromosomal analysis is premature ovarian insufficiency (see Section 7.7). Women who present with hypergonadotrophic hypogonadism and are below the age of 40 should be karyotyped. Turner syndrome and other X-chromosomal abnormalities are responsible for the majority of cases of premature ovarian insufficiency.

Fragile X syndrome

See also Section 7.7. Testing for *FRAXA* is indicated in premature ovarian insufficiency in the UK. *FMR1* should ideally be tested for in all cases of premature ovarian insufficiency, as the pre-mutation (50–200 CCG repeats in *FMR1*) may lead to a mild phenotype but infertility or premature ovarian insufficiency. Several other genes are potentially implicated in premature ovarian insufficiency, with variable degrees of evidence.

7.3 Imaging of functional ovarian tumours

Functional ovarian tumours

Functional ovarian tumours are rare, accounting for less than 3% of all ovarian tumours and 40% of solid ovarian tumours. Unlike epithelial neoplasms, which usually present at advanced stages, functioning tumours usually present as small Stage 1 lesions and therefore have a better prognosis.

Any ovarian tumour can have hormonal activity from its stromal cells, including epithelial tumours and metastases. The tumours usually produce sex hormones, either female or male, but occasionally tumours producing renin, aldosterone, adrenocorticotrophic hormone, and corticosteroids have been described. However, the majority are non-epithelial primary ovarian tumours classified by cell origin (germ cell or sex cord–stromal origin) or as feminizing or masculinizing tumours (Table 7.2).

Sex cord–stromal tumours arise from structural cells that hold the ovary together and produce female or male hormones. They can occur at any age, but are most common in the third to fifth decades. These tumours are the most common type of hormonally active ovarian tumour, usually slow growing, causing pain and discomfort at presentation, and secreting hormones like oestrogen or testosterone. The most common tumour is the granulosa cell tumour, accounting for 80% of all stromal tumours.

Germ cell tumours arise from ovarian reproductive cells and may be germinomatous (e.g. dysgerminoma), non-germinomatous (e.g. teratomas, yolk cell tumours, choriocarcinomas), or mixed. Germ cell tumours account for 30% of ovarian tumours and are more common in younger women under the age of 21. In children and women under 21 years, 60% of ovarian tumours are of germ cell origin, and up to one-third are malignant. Germ cell cancers usually grow rapidly. They can become very large and cause significant pain and abdominal distension. They can produce various hormones, including alpha-fetoprotein and hCG. In spite of their aggressive nature, germ cell cancers are highly curable. Treatment involves surgery and chemotherapy.

Other than tumours, polycystic ovaries, ovarian oedema, and torsion have been known to produce virilizing syndromes through unexplained mechanisms.

Imaging appearances

The role of imaging in patients presenting with signs and symptoms of a functioning ovarian tumour is to localize the tumour and assist in planning surgery. The first-line imaging investigation is transvaginal ultrasound or, in the paediatric group, trans-abdominal ultrasound. This allows localization of the tumour and limited characterization when combined with Doppler ultrasound. The endometrial thickness, uterine size, ascites, and pelvic nodal disease can also be assessed by ultrasound.

For further characterization or when ultrasound does not detect a lesion, MRI is recommended. CT may be used in women unable to undergo MRI and in staging malignant lesions; in addition, larger ovarian masses may be detected incidentally. Ovarian venous sampling is limited to instances where an androgen-secreting tumour is highly likely but imaging is negative.

Although there is a great deal of overlap in the imaging appearances of epithelial, stromal, and germ cell tumours, certain radiologic findings predominate for each type of tumour. Sex cord–stromal tumours vary from small solid to large multicystic masses. Granulosa cell tumours are usually large multicystic masses with solid components. Fibrothecomas, sclerosing stromal tumours, and Sertoli–Leydig cell tumours are usually solid masses. Fibromas and Brenner tumours have very low signal intensity on T2-weighted MRI images. Ovarian teratomas demonstrate areas of fat on CT and MRI. Malignant germ cell tumours manifest as a large, complex abdominal masses with both solid and cystic components. Associated ascites and peritoneal disease confirms a malignant nature of the mass.

We describe key features of the more common functional tumours which may be helpful in developing a differential diagnosis for these tumours.

Sex cord–stromal tumours

The key imaging suggestive feature of sex cord–stromal tumours is the presence of low T2-signal-intensity solid areas. As the fibrous component increases, the T2 signal intensity decreases.

Ovarian masses with fibrous components include fibroma, fibrothecoma, cystadenofibroma, Sertoli–Leydig cell tumours, and Brenner tumours.

Table 7.2 Summary of the functional ovarian tumours

		Sex cord–stromal	**Germ cell**	**others**
Feminizing (oestrogen secreting)	Premenopausal	Granulosa cell (juvenile)	Dysgerminoma Teratomas	Mucinous cystadenoma
		Sclerosing stromal cell		
		Lutenized thecoma		
	Postmenopausal	Granulosa cell (adult)		
		Thecoma		
		Fibroma		
		Brenner tumours (transitional cell tumours)		
Masculinizing (androgen secreting)	Premenopausal	Sertoli–Leydig cell	Teratomas	Ovarian metastases (esp. gastric and colorectal)
		Sclerosing stromal cell		
		Lutenized thecoma		Carcinoids
	Postmenopausal	Steroid cell		
		Brenner tumours (transitional cell tumours)		

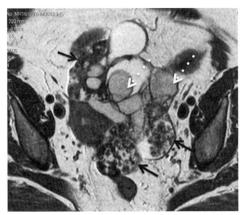

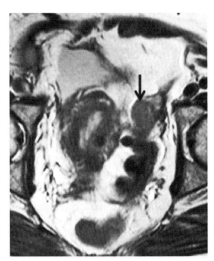

Fig 7.1 Large granulosa cell tumour. Axial T2-weighted MRI demonstrating a large multicystic mass with solid, low-T2-signal-intensity nodules (arrows). Several of the cystic locules have intermittent signal intensity consistent with haemorrhage (dashed arrow). The mass was present in a woman presenting with postmenopausal bleeding. The presence of low-T2-signal-intensity nodules and the symptoms are suggestive of a sex-cord stromal tumour. The predominantly cystic nature and haemorrhage supports a granuloma cell tumour, confirmed on histology.

Fig 7.2 Small granulosa cell tumour. Axial T2-weighted MRI showing a small, solid, intermittent-T2-signal-intensity mass (arrowed) in the left ovary. Very small tumours have non-specific appearances, and diagnosis rests on elevated oestrogens. Very small tumours may not be demonstrated on MRI or transvaginal ultrasound, and localization requires ovarian venous catheterization.

Granulosa cell tumours

Granulosa cell tumours are the most common functional ovarian stromal tumours. The juvenile form of granulosa cell tumour affects prepubertal children resulting in precocious puberty. Adult forms account for 95% of granulosa cell tumours, secrete oestrogens, and occur in peri- and postmenopausal women causing endometrial hyperplasia and endometrial cancer (3%–25%) manifesting as postmenopausal bleeding (Fink et al., 2001).

Most tumours are solid–cystic masses with haemorrhage. Smaller tumours are mainly solid with increasing cystic components in larger lesions (see Figures 7.1 and 7.2). The imaging appearances may be indistinguishable from epithelial cancers. Adult granulosa cell tumours have a malignant potential and late recurrence.

Sertoli–Leydig cell tumours

These are the commonest virilizing ovarian tumours, containing an admixture of Sertoli, Leydig, and fibroblast cells. They are commonly unilateral and occur in young patients; 75% are in women below 30 years. Virilization occurs in 30%. The majority of the tumours are small, solid with intermediate to low T2 signal intensity and intratumoral cysts on MRI (Outwater et al., 2000; also see Figure 7.3). Rarely, in patients presenting with virilization, the tumour may be too small to detect on transvaginal ultrasound and MRI, making ovarian venous catherization or exploratory laparotomy necessary.

Thecomas

Thecomas occur mainly in older women, with 80% occurring in postmenopausal women; 20% have associated endometrial cancer on a background of endometrial hyperplasia due to the excess oestrogens produced by the tumour. They may also be associated with Meigs syndrome and ascites. Most are an admixture of fibrous and thecoma components and hence usually termed fibrothecomas. These are characteristically homogeneously solid, vary in size, and rarely have cystic changes within larger tumours. On ultrasound, they are a homogeneous hypoechoic mass with posterior acoustic shadowing. The tumours demonstrate homogeneous intermediate T1 and low T2 signal intensity on MRI. The degree of contrast enhancement which varies on amount of fibrous (low enhancement) and thecoma components (avid enhancement) (see Figures 7.4 and 7.5). CT shows a homogeneous solid tumour with delayed enhancement and dense calcification. Luteinizing thecomas represent

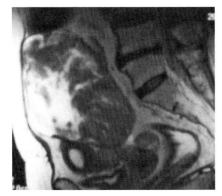

Fig 7.3 Sertoli–Leydig cell tumour. Sagittal T2-weighted MRI demonstrating a large pelvic mass in a 20-year-old woman presenting with irregular menstrual bleeding. The mass is predominantly solid with large areas of cystic change. The endometrium is thickened, and hyperplastic secondary to the elevated hormones.

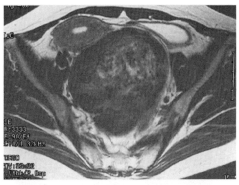

Fig 7.4 Ovarian fibrothecoma. Axial T2-weighted MRI showing a large solid mass with a whorled, low T2 signal intensity. The mass has the characteristic appearance of a fibrothecoma. The signal intensity is lower in tumours with high fibrous content, whilst thecomas have a more intermediate signal intensity.

(a)

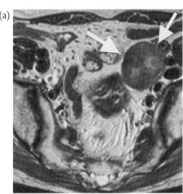

(b)

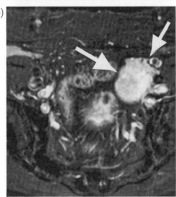

Fig 7.5 (a) Axial T2-weighted MRI demonstrating a left ovarian solid mass consistent with a fibrothecoma (arrowed). (b) Axial T1 fat-saturated MRI following administration of intravenous gadolinium. The mass (arrowed) demonstrates the significant post-contrast enhancement more frequently seen in thecomas, whilst fibromatous components demonstrate no or little contrast enhancement.

a subgroup of tumours which occur in younger women and may be feminizing (50%), virilizing (40%), or non-functional (10%) lesions.

Sclerosing stromal tumours

Sclerosing stromal tumours are seen mainly in young women below 30 years and hence present mainly as menstrual irregularities or, rarely, with virilization. These benign predominantly cystic tumours have increased amounts of collagen and hence demonstrate solid, low-T2-signal-intensity nodules on a background of high T2 signal intensity and with a lobulated contour. Following dynamic contrast enhancement, centripetal avid enhancement has been described due to tumour hypervascularity (Ihara et al., 1999).

Brenner tumours

The presence of solid areas with very low T2 signal intensity on T2-weighted MRI corresponds to dense fibrous stroma, a key feature of Brenner tumours. The tumour may be a multilocular cystic mass with a solid components or a small, mostly solid mass with low T2 signal intensity (see Figure 7.6). On CT and MRI, the solid components are mildly or moderately enhancing. Extensive amorphous calcification is often present within the solid component (see Figure 7.6). Brenner tumours are associated with other ovarian tumours in 30% of cases (Moon et al., 2000).

Germ cell tumours

Of all the germ cell tumours, only mature teratomas are benign, and they are the most common lesion in this group. Malignant germ cell tumours account for 5% of all ovarian malignancy and are generally large and non-specific with a complex but predominantly solid imaging appearance. Elevated tumour markers are key in the diagnosis.

Teratomas

Mature teratomas (dermoids) are composed of mature tissue from two or more embryonic germ cell layers. Mature cystic teratomas are unilocular with sebaceous material lined by squamous epithelium. There is usually a raised solid tissue projecting into the cyst known as Rokitansky nodule. Most of the hair, bone, or teeth

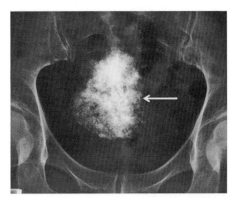

Fig 7.6 Ovarian Brenner tumour. A histologically confirmed right ovarian Brenner tumour (arrowed) with dense amorphous calcification mimicking fibroid calcification, seen on an abdominal X-ray.

(a)

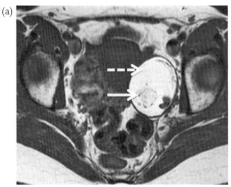

(b)

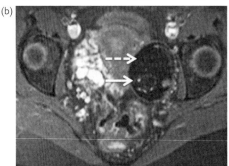

(a)

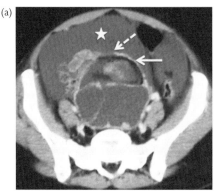

(b)

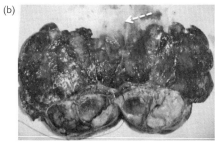

Fig 7.8 (a, b) Large cystic mass with calcification and fat (arrow) in keeping with a teratoma. The mass has an irregular anterior capsule with a defect (dashed arrow). A large amount of ascites is present in the abdomen and pelvis (star). Ascites is more frequently present in malignant tumours. At surgery, a large defect was present in the anterior capsule of the tumour, which was confirmed as a malignant immature teratoma.

Fig 7.7 (a) Axial T1-weighted MRI showing a left ovarian dermoid cyst. On the T1-weighted image, there is a large amount of high-signal-intensity (dashed arrow) fat within the cyst. A solid nodule is seen within the cyst, in keeping with a Rokintansky nodule (arrow). This solid nodule is an admixture of multiple tissue including collage, fat, osseous tissue, and endocrine tissues. (b) Axial T1-weighted MRI with fat saturation. On this sequence, the loss of signal in areas of high T1 signal confirms the fatty nature of the cyst (dashed arrow).

typically arise from the Rokitansky nodule. Hair follicles, skin glands, muscle, and other tissues lie within the wall.

On all imaging modalities, dermoids demonstrate a broad spectrum of findings, ranging from purely cystic, to a mixed mass with all the components of the three germ cell layers, to a mass composed predominantly of fat.

On ultrasound, dermoids vary from a cystic lesion with a densely echogenic Rokitansky nodule, to a diffusely or partially echogenic mass. On CT, fat attenuation within a cyst, with or without calcification in the wall, is diagnostic for mature cystic teratoma (see Figure 7.7). On MRI, the adipose component of dermoid cysts has very high signal intensity on T1-weighted images similar to that of pelvic fat. This high T1 signal is suppressed on fat-saturated sequences, pathognomonic for dermoids.

Immature teratomas

Immature teratomas represent less than 1% of all teratomas and contain immature tissue from all three germ cell layers. Immature teratomas are large, complex masses, have prominent solid components, and may demonstrate internal necrosis or haemorrhage with a poorly defined capsule. Mature tissue elements similar

to those seen in mature cystic teratoma are invariably present. Small foci of fat are also seen in immature teratomas. These tumours grow rapidly and frequently demonstrate perforation of the capsule (see Figure 7.8; Outwater et al., 2001).

Dysgerminomas

Dysgerminomas are rare and occur predominantly in young women. Five per cent of dysgerminomas contain syncytiotrophoblastic giant cells which cause elevation of serum hCG levels. Characteristic imaging findings include multilobulated solid mass and calcification may be present in a speckled pattern (see Figures 7.9 and 10). Anechoic, low-signal-intensity, or low-attenuation areas on ultrasound, MRI, and CT, respectively, represents necrosis and haemorrhage.

Key imaging features

- Functional ovarian tumours associated with endometrial hyperplasia or carcinoma are oestrogen-secreting tumours.
- A predominantly solid ovarian tumour with a very low signal intensity on T2-weighted MRI include fibroma, Brenner tumour, and fibrothecoma.
- Solid–cystic tumours with low-signal-intensity solid areas with highly enhancing solid areas are likely to be sex cord–stromal tumours (e.g. sclerosing stromal, Sertoli–Leydig cell tumours, or cystadenofibromas).

(a)

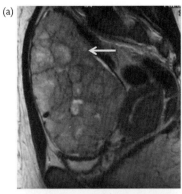

(b)

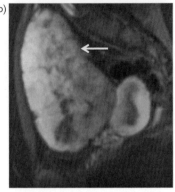

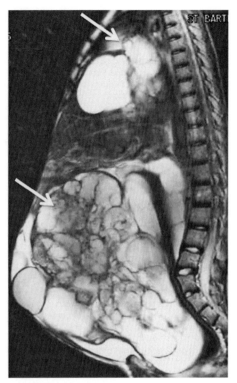

Fig 7.9 (a) Sagittal T2-weighted MRI showing a mass (arrowed). (b) Sagittal T1-weighted MRI with fat saturation and contrast enhancement, from a 17-year-old woman presenting with abdominal distension. The MRI appearances are characteristic, with a solid, lobulated, intermediate-T2-signal-intensity mass with smooth homogenous enhancement (arrowed). Dysgerminomas usually have no or only minimal cystic change, and this appearance in a young woman is highly suggestive of a dysgerminoma. Lymphoma and metastases may have similar appearances, but the latter are rare in this age group.

Fig 7.10 Malignant mixed germ cell tumour. Sagittal T2-weighted MRI of the chest, abdomen, and pelvis in a 6-year-old girl. The image demonstrates a very large heterogeneous pelvic mass and a mediastinal metastasis (arrows). The MRI appearances are of a malignant mixed solid–cystic mass filling the whole abdomen and pelvis, typical of malignant germ cell tumours at presentation.

- The presence of fat in an ovarian lesion is highly specific for a teratoma. Mature teratomas (dermoids) are predominantly cystic with dense calcifications and Rokitansky nodules, whereas immature teratomas are predominantly solid with small foci of lipid material, irregular capsules, and scattered calcification.
- Malignant germ cell tumours (e.g. dysgerminoma and endodermal sinus tumours) are large, lobulated, predominantly solid masses that are more common in younger women (second and third decades of life). Serum tumour markers are useful in making the diagnosis of malignant germ cell tumour.

References and further reading

Athey PA and Malone RS. Sonography of ovarian fibromas/thecomas. *J Ultrasound Med* 1987; 6: 431–6.

Fink D, Kubik-Huch RA, and Wildermuth S. Juvenile granulosa cell tumor. *Abdom Imaging* 2001; 26: 550–2.

Hill WE and Clark JF. Functional ovarian tumors: A ten year study at Freedmen's Hospital. *J Natl Med Assoc* 1964; 56: 66–70.

Ihara N, Togashi K, Todo G, et al. Sclerosing stromal tumor of the ovary: MRI. *J Comput Assist Tomogr* 1999; 23: 555–7.

Kim SH and Kang SB. Ovarian dysgerminoma: Color Doppler ultrasonographic findings and comparison with CT and MR imaging findings. *J Ultrasound Med* 1995; 14: 843–8.

Moon WJ, Koh BH, Kim SK, et al. Brenner tumor of the ovary: CT and MR findings. *J Comput Assist Tomogr* 2000; 24: 72–6.

Outwater EK, Marchetto B, and Wagner BJ. Virilizing tumors of the ovary: Imaging features. *Ultrasound Obstet Gynecol* 2000; 15: 365–71.

Outwater EK, Siegelman ES, and Hunt JL. Ovarian teratomas: Tumor types and imaging characteristics. *RadioGraphics* 2001; 21: 475–90.

Troiano RN, Lazzarini KM, Scoutt LM, et al. Fibroma and fibrothecoma of the ovary: CT and MR imaging findings. *Radiology* 1997; 204: 795–8.

7.4 Polycystic ovary syndrome

Definition

PCOS (for polycystic ovary syndrome) is a highly prevalent heterogeneous endocrine disorder in women of reproductive age. The main features of PCOS are clinical or biochemical androgen excess, oligo- or anovulation, polycystic ovaries, dysregulation of the hypothalamo-pituitary–ovarian axis, and metabolic derangements. Currently, three different definitions of PCOS exist:

- the 1990 National Institute of Child Health and Human Development (NICHD) criteria for PCOS include hyperandrogenism and/or hyperandrogenaemia, oligo/anovulation, and the exclusion of similar disorders (Cushing's syndrome, androgen-producing tumours, non-classic adrenal hyperplasia, hypothyroidism, hyperprolactinaemia, and acromegaly)
- the 2003 Rotterdam criteria recommend there be at least two of the following three features for a diagnosis of PCOS: clinical and/or biochemical hyperandrogenism, oligo/anovulation, and polycystic ovaries on ultrasound, excluding other endocrinopathies
- the 2006 Androgen Excess and Polycystic Ovary Syndrome Society (AES–PCOS) criteria include obligatory clinical and/or biochemical hyperandrogenism, with either oligo/anovulation and/or polycystic ovaries on ultrasound, excluding related disorders

Including polycystic ovaries morphology on ultrasound as a criterion made the PCOS definition even more confusing, as 20%–30% of normally ovulating women with normal androgen levels have such ovarian morphology, as well as do 40%–50% of adolescent girls.

As the Rotterdam criteria are widely used, it is important to stress that, by implying different combinations of these criteria, four different phenotypes of PCOS emerge, ranging from the most severe to the milder forms:

- Type A: hyperandrogenism, chronic anovulation, and polycystic ovaries
- Type B: hyperandrogenism and chronic anovulation
- Type C: hyperandrogenism and polycystic ovaries
- Type D: chronic anovulation and polycystic ovaries

The Rotterdam criteria do not grade the importance of individual criteria, whilst NICHD and AES–PCOS emphasize the hyperandrogenism as the main, sine qua non feature of the syndrome, being closely related with insulin resistance and consequent hyperinsulinaemia, thus raising the awareness of metabolic dysfunction in PCOS. Despite these several definitions, PCOS is still a diagnosis of exclusion of other hyperandrogenic disorders (e.g. see the NICHD criteria above); these include:

- Cushing's syndrome
- acromegaly
- congenital adrenal hyperplasia
- androgen-secreting tumours
- severe insulin resistance
- hyperthecosis (post-menopausal hyperandrogenism)
- drugs (e.g. phenytoin)

Pathophysiology

PCOS is a cluster of symptoms which cannot be ascribed to a common aetiologic factor. The increase in ovarian androgen production by the increased activity of theca cells is a fundamental characteristic of PCOS. The aetiology of PCOS is not well understood, but there is increasing evidence that it may have developmental origins. This theory suggests that, due to genetic and/or epigenetic factors, the human fetal ovary produces excess androgens and thus influences the hypothalamus, the pancreas, and itself to develop the endocrine and metabolic phenotype of PCOS at puberty and later in life. In animal studies, androgenization of the foetus in sheep and non-human primates, as well as excess androgen production in congenital adrenal hyperplasia, produces an adult PCOS phenotype. Excess androgens cannot come from the mother, as her androgens are tightly bound to SHBG and would be aromatized by the placenta before they could reach the foetus. It seems that the fetal ovary in PCOS is genetically predisposed to secrete higher-than-normal levels of androgens by itself. Familial studies have demonstrated the heritability of PCOS. The concordance of symptoms of PCOS is much greater in identical than in non-identical twin pairs (estimated genetic influence 79%, environment 21%). The mode of inheritance is unclear but, given the clinical and biochemical heterogeneity of the syndrome, it is more likely to be polygenic or oligogenic. Attempts to identify causative loci using a candidate gene approach have been largely disappointing, although genomic familial linkage studies have identified two regions linked to PCOS, one of which is close to the follistatin gene. Another, the dinucleotide repeat microsatellite marker D19S884, maps to Intron 55 of the fibrillin 3 gene. Both fibrillin 3 and follistatin regulate the activity of members of the transforming growth factor (TGF) beta superfamily. TGF beta stimulates fibroblast function (production and deposition of collagen). In the PCOS ovary, all stromal compartments are grossly increased in volume. The specialized stromal theca interna layer around antral follicles has an elevated capacity for producing androgens. Fibrillin 3 is present in the stromal compartments of fetal ovaries and is highly expressed at a critical stage early in developing fetal ovaries when stroma is expanding and follicles are forming. This could be the genetic data linking fibrillin 3 with the physiological mechanism, in line with animal models and clinical observations, of fetal development predisposing to PCOS phenotype in adult life. Recently, genome-wide association studies identified PCOS candidate loci, including *DENND1A*, which encodes a protein associated with clathrin-coated pits where cell-surface receptors reside. An alternatively spliced form of *DENND1A* (DENND1A.V2) was found to be increased in PCOS theca cells and could represent the source of the excess androgens. Exosomal DENND1A.V2 RNA was significantly elevated in urine from PCOS women compared to normal cycling women. Forced expression of DENND1A.V2 in normal theca cells increased the expression of genes encoding steroidogenic enzymes, leading to augmented androgen biosynthesis, whereas silencing of DENND1A.V2 in PCOS theca cells caused them to revert to a normal phenotype.

Adult PCOS ovaries have increased numbers of primordial follicles in the ovarian cortex that develop during fetal life due to the trophic effect of androgens, and an increase in the proportion of preantral follicles that have initiated growth. The abundance of these is the first abnormality of folliculogenesis in PCOS. The second abnormality is follicular arrest—the inability to select and stimulate the dominant follicle from the excessive follicular cohort, due to inefficient FSH. FSH is low or low normal in PCOS. In addition, there is a local self-inhibitory effect of the small follicles on FSH action by exaggerated secretion of anti-Müllerian hormone, one of many members of the TGF beta superfamily involved in ovarian (patho)physiology. Serum anti-Müllerian hormone levels correlate with the number of small preantral and antral follicles and there is also an increased production of anti-Müllerian hormone per follicle. Anti-Müllerian hormone is suspected to inhibit the FSH-dependent aromatase activity and conversion of androgens to estradiol, thus causing follicular arrest. Anti-Müllerian hormone serum levels are a good marker of menstrual irregularity and hyperandrogenism in PCOS.

Increased androgen synthesis is intrinsic to the polycystic ovaries, although there are additional factors like LH and insulin, stimulating theca-interstitial cells to overproduce testosterone and androstenedione. Excess androgen during fetal life or later at puberty may reduce the sensitivity of the GnRH pulse generator to steroid feedback at the hypothalamic level, resulting in an increased pulse frequency of GnRH and thus causing accelerated LH pulses with increased amplitude.

The majority of women with PCOS are insulin resistant, with compensatory hyperinsulinaemia. Insulin acts as a co-gonadotrophin stimulating steroidogenic enzymes in the ovary and inhibits hepatic SHBG production, resulting in an increase in free androgens. The presence of obesity worsens insulin resistance, the degree of hyperinsulinaemia, the severity of ovulatory and menstrual dysfunction, and pregnancy outcome in PCOS, and is associated with an increasing prevalence of metabolic syndrome, glucose intolerance, cardiovascular risk factors, and sleep apnoea. PCOS is associated with a greater propensity for obesity and weight gain, which, in turn, aggravates the features of PCOS.

Epidemiology

PCOS is the most common endocrine disorder in women of reproductive age. The actual prevalence of PCOS depends on the criteria used. The prevalence based on the strict NICHD criteria is 6%–10%; with the implementation of the Rotterdam criteria, the prevalence increases to 15%–20%, whilst, by the AES–PCOS criteria, PCOS prevalence is 10%–15%. The prevalence is remarkably similar across different populations and different geographic areas. It is increased in subgroups of women with obesity, type 1, type 2, or gestational diabetes mellitus, oligo/anovulatory infertility, premature adrenarche, and a positive family history for PCOS among first-degree relatives. Women with PCOS have insulin resistance that is independent and additive with that of obesity. Insulin resistance occurs in approximately 60%–80% of women with PCOS and in 95% of obese women with PCOS. The prevalence of obesity among women with PCOS is 50%–60%.

Clinical features

PCOS is a syndrome, reflecting multiple potential etiologies and variable clinical presentations. The key features of PCOS are hyperandrogenism, menstrual dysfunction, polycystic ovaries on pelvic ultrasonography, infertility, obesity, and insulin resistance.

Hyperandrogenism

Hyperandrogenism is the first defining characteristic of PCOS. This is manifested clinically by hirsutism, acne, and/or male pattern balding.

Hirsutism is the most common clinical manifestation of hyperandrogenism, affecting 60%–70% of women with PCOS. It is defined as excessive terminal (thick, pigmented) facial and body hair growth in a male-type pattern and is caused by androgen excess. In clinical practice, excessive hair growth is generally evaluated using the Ferriman–Galwey scoring system, which grades terminal hair growth from 0–4 on nine anatomical sites with sexual hair (on the upper lip, the chin, the chest, the upper abdomen, the lower abdomen, the back, the thighs, and the upper arms). Scores above 7 are confirmative of hirsutism (see Figure 7.11). The system is highly subjective and therefore useful only when applied by the same physician.

Other manifestations of hyperandrogenism are acne persisting after adolescence, and male pattern baldness.

Hyperandrogenaemia

Hyperandrogenaemia constitutes one of the cardinal features of PCOS, as 60%–90% of patients have elevated circulating androgen levels. The adrenal cortex can contribute to the excess androgens derived from the ovary. Ovaries and adrenals secrete testosterone and androstenedione, whilst dehydroepiandrosterone is almost exclusively secreted by the adrenals. Serum SHBG concentrations are decreased by androgens and insulin in PCOS. Thus, among women with PCOS, the proportion of women with elevated serum free testosterone concentrations is higher than that with elevated serum total testosterone concentrations. Androgen levels in some women with PCOS may be normal when assayed in a single blood specimen.

Menstrual dysfunction

Menstrual dysfunction in PCOS is characterized by oligo- or amenorrhoea and, therefore, by oligo-anovulation. Some women may have a normal menarche followed by irregular cycles. Others may have regular cycles at first and subsequently develop menstrual irregularity in association with weight gain.

Anovulatory infertility

Due to oligo/anovulation, women with PCOS have fertility problems. Many eventually undergo ovulation induction therapies. Women with PCOS may have other reasons for infertility as well, since they have a reduced rate of conception relative to the rate of ovulation after therapy with clomiphene citrate, and an increased rate of early pregnancy loss.

Endometrial cancer

Chronic anovulation leads to deficient progesterone secretion, and the chronic unopposed oestrogen exposure may increase the risk of endometrial carcinoma. In PCOS, excess oestrogens are produced by peripheral aromatization of androgens. Additional risk factors for endometrial cancer are hyperinsulinaemia, hyperandrogenaemia, and obesity.

Polycystic ovarian morphology

The key ovarian findings in PCOS include multiple small preantral and antral follicles in a peripheral location, with an increased volume of stroma. With high-frequency transvaginal ultrasonography, the histological findings

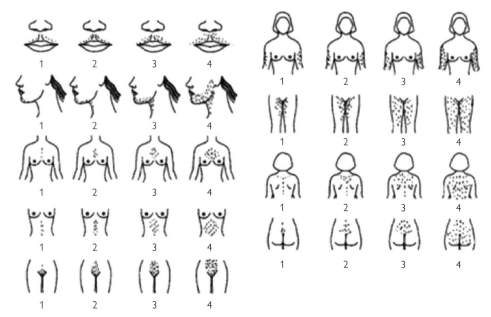

Fig 7.11 Modified Ferriman–Gallwey score for semi-quantitative assessment of hirsutism: nine regions are evaluated for their degree of hair growth, from 0–4.

Reproduced from Yildiz BO, Bolour S, Visually scoring hirsutism, *Human Reproduction Update*, Volume 16, Issue 1, pp. 51–64. doi: 10.1093/humupd/dmp024. Copyright (2010) by permission of Oxford University Press on behalf of Human Reproduction Update.

can be corroborated non-invasively. The Rotterdam ultrasound criteria for polycystic ovaries include the presence of 12 or more follicles in each ovary, with the follicles measuring 2–9 mm in diameter, and/or increased ovarian volume (>10 mL; calculated using the formula 0.5 × length × width × thickness). Both situations are suggestive of polycystic morphology, even if they are detected in only one ovary. The finding is not specific for PCOS, as 20%–30% of normally ovulating women without hyperandrogenism have such ovarian morphology, as do even more adolescent girls in whom it may be a transient feature.

Mood disorders
Women with PCOS may be more likely to have depression and anxiety, when compared to women of similar BMI without PCOS. The prevalence of depression might be as high as 60%. Both depression and anxiety are major risk factors for cardiovascular disease. They also appear to have impaired quality of life, and are at risk for eating disorders (binge eating in 23%). Therefore, AES–PCOS suggests screening all women with PCOS for mood disorders.

Metabolic derangements
Insulin resistance
At least half of PCOS women are obese with predominant central fat accumulation. Even more are hyperinsulinaemic and insulin resistant, independent of obesity. Insulin resistance is most prevalent and severe in classical PCOS phenotypes A and B, with hyperandrogenism and chronic anovulation. Insulin resistance is intrinsic to the disorder and additive with that of obesity. In vivo insulin action is profoundly decreased in skeletal muscle, secondary to signalling defects, but hepatic insulin resistance is present only in obese women with PCOS. There is a post-receptor defect in insulin signalling: increased serine/threonine instead of tyrosine phosphorylation of the insulin receptor substrates impairs the metabolic phosphatidylinositol 3 kinase-dependent pathway and glucose uptake, leaving the non-metabolic mitogen-activated protein kinase pathway unaffected. Insulin resistance plays a central pathogenetic role in the development of metabolic derangements of the syndrome, such as impaired glucose tolerance, type 2 diabetes, atherogenic dyslipidaemia, chronic inflammation, fatty liver disease, and others. In severe cases of insulin resistance, acanthosis nigricans occurs on the neck and in the axillae and elbows.

Impaired glucose tolerance and type 2 diabetes
Impaired glucose tolerance and type 2 diabetes are highly prevalent among PCOS adolescents, and up to 40% of women with classic PCOS develop impaired glucose tolerance or type 2 diabetes by the fourth decade of life, with age and weight gain worsening the glycaemic control. Women with a first-degree relative with type 2 diabetes are particularly at risk. A meta-analysis of 35 studies found that PCOS is associated with a 2.5-fold increased prevalence of impaired glucose tolerance and a fourfold increased prevalence of type 2 diabetes.

Metabolic syndrome
The prevalence of the metabolic syndrome in women with PCOS appears to be two- to threefold higher than that of age-matched women in the general

population. Metabolic syndrome in PCOS is an inflammatory, atherothrombotic, insulin-resistant state that promotes atherogenesis.

Dyslipidaemia
Women with PCOS show higher prevalence of atherogenic dyslipidaemia, with low HDL, high triglyceride levels, and small dense LDL particles, as is consistent with their insulin resistance. A form of dyslipidaemia with high LDL cholesterol is less frequent, less obesity correlated, and more related to hyperandrogenism.

Non-alcoholic fatty liver disease
The prevalence of non-alcoholic fatty liver disease and non-alcoholic steatohepatitis is also increased in women with PCOS, due to insulin resistance, dyslipidaemia, and central adiposity. Patients may have mild or moderate elevations in aspartate aminotransferase (AST) and alanine aminotransferase (ALT), although normal aminotransferase levels do not exclude non-alcoholic fatty liver disease. When elevated, the AST-to-ALT ratio is <1. Non-alcoholic fatty liver disease is under-diagnosed in women with PCOS but is threatening, as it can progress to cirrhosis.

Obstructive sleep apnoea
Adult (but not adolescent) PCOS patients were reported to have at least fivefold higher risk for obstructive sleep apnoea as similarly obese women without PCOS. Obstructive sleep apnoea is an independent risk factor for cardiovascular disease. It is associated with activated pathways that lead to insulin resistance (or aggravate it), to hypertension, and to increased levels of a group of pro-inflammatory and prothrombotic factors that are involved in the atherogenic process. Therefore, obstructive sleep apnoea may be an under-recognized yet significant risk factor for cardiometabolic derangements in PCOS.

Cardiovascular disease
PCOS patients are often obese, hypertensive, dyslipidaemic, and insulin resistant; they have obstructive sleep apnoea, mood disorders, and higher aldosterone levels, in comparison to normal healthy controls. Many studies exploring subclinical atherosclerosis in PCOS by measuring flow-mediated dilatation, intima media thickness of carotid arteries, arterial stiffness, and coronary artery calcification, as well as circulating cardiovascular risk markers, point towards an increased cardiovascular risk and early atherogenesis. Studies like the Nurses' Health Study, the Women's Ischemia Syndrome Evaluation study, the Rancho Bernardo Study, and others have shown increased incidence of cardiovascular events in women with PCOS after menopause, whilst, in few other studies, the incidence of cardiovascular disease and cardiovascular death was the same as in background population. Undoubtedly, all surrogate markers of cardiovascular risk are higher in PCOS (adjusted for age and BMI), but the association of these with cardiovascular events and especially with cardiovascular death remains unclear. The early subclinical atherosclerosis evident already in young women with PCOS is largely reversible with lifestyle changes and insulin sensitizers.

Investigations

PCOS is a syndrome and a diagnosis of exclusion of other endocrinopathies, such as:

- Cushing's syndrome (via an overnight 1 mg DST; cortisol <50 nmol/L (1.8 µg/dL); see Chapter 6, Section 6.8)

- virilizing adrenal or ovarian tumour (history of rapid onset of symptoms, signs of virilization (increased muscle mass, deepening of the voice, clitoromegaly); assessment of testosterone, DHEAS, and LH; see Section 7.6)
- non-classical congenital adrenal hyperplasia (by assessment of basal 17-hydroxyprogesterone; basal <6 nmol/L (198 ng/dL); see Section 7.5)
- acromegaly (clinical judgement and assessment of IGF-1)
- hyperprolactinaemia (assessment of prolactin)
- hypothyroidism (TSH, FT4)
- premature ovarian failure (FSH),
- drug-related condition (history)

The occurrence of a gradual development of signs of hyperandrogenism starting usually at puberty, accompanied by slow deterioration of menstrual cycle, especially with weight gain, are highly suggestive of PCOS, as is a family history of hyperandrogenism, oligomenorrhoea, and type 2 diabetes.

Ovarian ultrasound evaluation is not obligatory if two out of three diagnostic criteria for PCOS have been confirmed, namely hyperandrogenism and oligo/anovulation.

Measurement of free testosterone or total testosterone and SHBG to calculate the free androgen index (= total testosterone × 100/SHBG) is recommended. Androstenedione should also be assessed, as it seems to be a more sensitive indicator of PCOS-related androgen excess than serum total testosterone. Gonadotrophins should be assessed only in cases of oligo/amenorrhoea. As 40% of hirsute patients with 'regular' episodes of vaginal bleeding are actually oligo/anovulatory, the mid-luteal serum progesterone level should be measured on Day 22–24 of the menstrual cycle. Values greater than 10 nmol/L (5 ng/L) confirm ovulation.

Lately, assessment of anti-Müllerian hormone has emerged as a valuable surrogate marker of hyperandrogenism and menstrual irregularity in patients with PCOS.

A meticulous, in-depth medical history accompanied by a detailed clinical examination can reduce the need for an expensive laboratory workup. BMI and waist circumference should be measured, with the latter pointing to an increased cardiometabolic risk if >80 cm. Other parameters of metabolic syndrome should be looked for. Patients need to be screened for impaired glucose tolerance with an oral glucose tolerance test, with measurement of fasting and 2-hour glucose levels, and for dyslipidaemia. It is suggested that rescreening with an oral glucose tolerance test be conducted every 3–5 years, or more frequently if clinical factors such as central adiposity, substantial weight gain, and/or symptoms of diabetes develop. Patients with impaired glucose tolerance should be screened annually for the development of type 2 diabetes. No tests of insulin resistance are necessary to make the diagnosis of PCOS in a clinical setting, nor are they needed to select treatment. Blood pressure should be measured once yearly.

Management

Treatment of PCOS must be tailored to the specific needs of each patient; goals of therapy are ameliorating hyperandrogenic symptoms, inducing ovulation, regulating the menstrual cycle, and preventing cardiometabolic complications.

Lifestyle intervention

Lifestyle modification is the mainstay of PCOS treatment. Weight loss with healthy diet and regular exercise improves clinical signs and symptoms and substantially reduces cardiometabolic risk in PCOS women. Modest weight loss may result in restoration of normal ovulatory cycles. Regular physical activity without substantial weight loss is beneficial in improving cardiopulmonary capacity and insulin sensitivity by directly affecting muscle metabolism. It has been shown that even modest, short-term weight loss of less than 10% decreases abdominal fat and improves insulin sensitivity, hyperglycaemia, hyperandrogenism, depression, ovulation, conception, and quality of life. Up to 60% of PCOS women had improvement in either their menstrual cycle or ovulation after lifestyle changes and subsequent weight loss. Overweight/obese PCOS women should initially attempt 5%–10% weight loss to reduce obesity-related cardiovascular-disease risk factors, with long-term goals of achieving and maintaining a reduced weight of 10%–20 % and a waist circumference of less than 80–88 cm. Actually, lifestyle intervention produces long-term positive results only in the minority of highly motivated patients. The majority of PCOS patients lack compliance and willpower; therefore, in many patients, medical intervention can be used as a therapeutic tool in addition to lifestyle changes.

Medical therapy

There are several treatments for each of the symptoms of PCOS. Lately, the awareness of complex cardiometabolic risk influences the choice of treatment.

Treatment of hyperandrogenism

Hirsutism can be treated by suppressing levels of circulating androgens with combined oral contraceptives. Oestrogens increase SHBG production in the liver and suppress LH secretion. Oral contraceptive preparations contain 30–35 µg of ethinylestradiol combined with a progestin with minimal androgenicity, such as norethindrone, norgestimate, desogestrel, or drospirenone. The latter has a weak anti-androgenic and anti-mineralocorticoid activity. When compared with insulin sensitizers and insulin-lowering agents, oral contraceptives are more effective in improving the menstrual pattern and reducing serum androgen levels. Although some studies report unfavourable metabolic effects, such as a worsening of insulin resistance, in individuals using certain oral contraceptives, meta-analyses do not support these findings. Differences may depend on the specific progestin used. Additionally, obesity prone women with PCOS often gain substantial weight when put on oral contraceptives, worsening the metabolic risk. In addition to the usual risks of oral-contraceptive therapy, including the risk of thromboembolic complications (deep vein thrombosis, pulmonary embolism, myocardial infarction, and stroke) and breast cancer, it has been suggested that patients with PCOS may also experience a modest, albeit measurable, worsening of their insulin resistance, but this finding has not been confirmed in all studies. Thus, the actual effect of oral contraceptives on insulin action in PCOS remains to be determined. One potential strategy to offset worsening insulin resistance is to combine oral contraceptives with the insulin sensitizer metformin.

Recently, an oral-contraceptive preparation used for treating acne (35 µg ethinylestradiol and 2 mg cyproterone acetate) has been withdrawn from the French market due to four thromboembolic deaths and 125 other serious life-threatening adverse events in the last 25 years. The European Medicines Agency has issued a special warning and proposed to strictly limit the use of the drug for the treatment of acne in patients without any risk for thromboembolic events.

If the cosmetic response to oral contraceptives is suboptimal, peripheral androgen blockade can be achieved by adding androgen receptor blockers like spironolactone, 50–200 mg daily. A significant reduction in hair growth may not occur for up to 6 months, the approximate half-life of a hair follicle. After 6 months, if the patient feels that the response has been suboptimal, options to consider include a change in dose or drug, or the addition of a second agent. Pharmacological therapy is usually continued during the reproductive years, with short-term interruptions every few years, as the underlying condition typically persists during this window and hirsutism recurs when treatment is discontinued. Spironolactone should be gradually down titrated before discontinuation after 2–3 years of treatment, to avoid water retention and rebound body hair growth. Other anti-androgens such as flutamide, 62.5–250.0 mg per day, cyproterone acetate, 10–100 mg per day intermittently, or finasteride, 2.5–5 mg per day, can also be used, usually in combination with oral contraceptives. During anti-androgen treatment, appropriate contraception is mandatory to avoid potential malformation of external genitalia in a male foetus.

Eflornithine hydrochloride (11.5%) is a topical drug that inhibits hair growth when used continuously. Hirsutism can also be treated by removal of hair by mechanical means such as shaving, depilation, or laser treatment.

Anovulatory uterine bleeding and endometrial protection

The chronic anovulation in PCOS is associated with an increased risk of endometrial hyperplasia, associated with thickened fragile endometrium resulting from endometrial proliferation owing to oestrogen action unopposed by progesterone. The consequence is dysfunctional uterine bleeding, which can occasionally be very severe, and possibly endometrial cancer. Oral contraceptives or intermittent progestins are used for endometrial protection in these patients. A progestin-releasing intrauterine device is an alternative option. Progestin therapy alone will not reduce the symptoms of acne or hirsutism, nor will it provide contraception.

The insulin sensitizer metformin is a potential alternative to restore menstrual cyclicity, induce ovulation, and protect the endometrium.

Sometimes an endometrial ablation or hysterectomy may be required, due to intractable uterine bleeding.

Ovulation induction

Anovulatory infertility requires ovulation induction; the first-line treatment is clomifene citrate, 50–100 mg per day. Via oestrogen-receptor antagonism at the hypothalamo-pituitary level, clomifene citrate stimulates pituitary gonadotrophin release. Clomifene citrate therapy for ovulation induction is typically started on the fifth day of a cycle, following either spontaneous or induced bleeding. The starting dose is 50 mg for 5 days. If ovulation does not occur in the first cycle of treatment, the dose is increased to 100 mg in the second and to 150 mg in the third cycle. Approximately 80% of women with PCOS ovulate in response to clomifene citrate and approximately 50% conceive.

Alternative ovulation induction agents are metformin, 2000–2550 mg per day (combined with diet and exercise), and the aromatase inhibitor letrozole, 2.5–5.0 mg per day, which inhibits oestrogen production and stimulates endogenous FSH secretion. Clomifene citrate acts rapidly and causes 10% multiparity, whereas metformin gradually reduces hyperinsulinaemia, inducing ovulatory cycles in 6 months, with low multiparity. Life birth rates are higher with clomifene.

Thiazolidinediones have shown some beneficial effects but are not recommended for the induction of ovulation, as concern has been raised about their cardiovascular safety and potential teratogenicity.

The second-line method for inducing ovulation is the administration of exogenous gonadotrophins, but women with PCOS treated with gonadotrophins are at high risk for ovarian hyperstimulation syndrome (a combination of ovarian enlargement due to multiple ovarian cysts and an acute fluid shift out of the intravascular space with abundant ascites, a restrictive type of pulmonary dysfunction due to intraabdominal or pleural fluid accumulation, and, in severe cases, pericardial effusion, hyponatraemia, hyperkalaemia, hypovolaemia, and hypovolaemic shock). It is a potentially life-threatening complication of ovulation induction.

An alternative to the ovarian wedge resection used in old times, laparoscopic ovarian drilling or laser electrocautery, might induce ovulation in some women with PCOS. However, given the other pharmacologic options for ovulation induction, surgery is rarely indicated.

Insulin resistance and prevention of type 2 diabetes
The primary method for the prevention of type 2 diabetes is lifestyle management. The addition of the insulin-sensitizing agent metformin, a biguanide that primarily inhibits hepatic gluconeogenesis and lipogenesis and also enhances peripheral glucose uptake, is indicated to reduce insulinaemia and androgen levels, increase SHBG, and improve metabolic status.

The off-label indications of metformin use in PCOS are:
- oligo/amenorrhoea
- anovulatory infertility
- treatment of type 2 diabetes and gestational diabetes
- prevention of PCOS in adolescence

Metformin has a limited effect on hirsutism and other signs of androgen excess. Side effects like nausea and abdominal discomfort are transient in most cases.

Thiazolidinediones, which bind to the peroxisome proliferator-activated receptor (PPAR) gamma to improve insulin sensitivity, are an alternative treatment for insulin resistance and its consequences in PCOS. They have beneficial effects that are similar to those of metformin, but often induce weight gain. Metformin is preferred, given its long history of safe use in PCOS and helping in weight reduction.

In morbidly obese women with PCOS, bariatric surgery is indicated for weight loss, restoring ovulatory cycles, and improving insulin resistance, hyperandrogenaemia, and even hirsutism scores.

Prevention of cardiovascular disease
The prevention of cardiovascular disease, likewise, requires lifestyle management, treatments targeting cardiovascular-disease risk factors, and the amelioration of insulin resistance, using insulin sensitizers. These have been shown to reverse early atherosclerotic changes like endothelial dysfunction and intima media thickening of the carotid artery in young PCOS women.

Obstructive sleep apnoea
Being an independent risk factor for cardiovascular disease and reducing quality of life, obstructive sleep apnoea has to be actively searched for in women with PCOS and treated with a continuous positive-airway pressure device in combination with lifestyle changes.

Postmenopausal hyperthecosis
Postmenopausal hyperthecosis is the commonest cause of hirsutism following menopause, although the differential diagnosis described in 'Investigations' should be considered. Testosterone suppression in response to depot GnRH establishes gonadotrophin dependence.

Prognosis

PCOS is not just a cosmetic or fertility disorder but represents a general health problem. It carries considerable morbidity and long-term risk, particularly for glycaemic abnormalities and type 2 diabetes, cardiovascular disease, and mood and affective disorders. Data on increased mortality for cardiovascular disease are inconsistent. The comparison with the background population is complicated by making the diagnosis of PCOS in retrospect. Nevertheless, the present epidemiological data suggest more frequent cardiometabolic derangements in classical phenotypes of PCOS, mostly mediated through increased total and abdominal adiposity, and interacting with PCOS-related hyperandrogenism.

Patients support groups/useful websites

Patient support groups/useful websites are as follows:
- http://www.managingpcos.org.au/pcos-evidence-based-guidelines
- http://www.womenshealth.gov/publications/our-publications/fact-sheet/polycystic-ovary-syndrome.cfm
- http://www.hormone.org/public/polycystic.cfm
- http://www.uptodate.com/contents/polycystic-ovary-syndrome-pcos-beyond-the-basics

Further reading

Bajuk Studen K, Jensterle Sever M, and Pfeifer M. 'Cardiovascular risk and subclinical cardiovascular disease in PCOS', in Macut D, Pfeifer M, Yildiz BO, et al., eds, *Polycystic Ovary Syndrome: Novel Insights into Causes and Therapy*, 2013. Frontiers of Hormone Research, Vol. 40. Karger, pp. 64–82.

Catteau-Jonard S and Dewailly D. 'Pathophysiology of PCOS: The role of hyperandrogenism', in Macut D, Pfeifer M, Yildiz BO, et al., eds, *Polycystic Ovary Syndrome: Novel Insights into Causes and Therapy*, 2013. Frontiers of Hormone Research, Vol. 40. Karger, pp. 22–7.

de Groot PCM, Dekkers OM, Romijn JA, et al. PCOS, coronary heart disease, stroke and the influence of obesity: A systematic review and meta-analysis. *Hum Reprod Update* 2011; 17: 495–500.

Fauser BCJM, Tarlatzis BC, Rebar RW, et al. Consensus on Women's Health Aspects of Polycystic Ovary Syndrome (PCOS): The Amsterdam ESHRE/ASRM-Sponsored 3rd PCOS Consensus Workshop Group. *Fertil Steril* 2012; 97: 28–38.

Franks S and Berga SL. A debate: Does PCOS have developmental origins? *Fertil Steril* 2012; 97: 2–6.

Goodarzi MO, Dumesic DA, Chazenbalk G, et al. Polycystic ovary syndrome: Etiology, pathogenesis and diagnosis. *Nat Rev Endocrinol* 2011; 7: 219–31.

Hatzirodos N, Bayne RA, Irving-Rodgers HF, et al. Linkage of regulators of TGF-beta activity in the fetal ovary to polycystic ovary syndrome. *FASEB J* 2011; 25: 2256–65.

Livadas S and Diamanti-Kandarakis E. 'Polycystic ovary syndrome: Definitions, phenotypes and diagnostic approach', in Macut D, Pfeifer M, Yildiz BO, et al., eds, *Polycystic Ovary Syndrome: Novel Insights into Causes and Therapy*, 2013. Frontiers of Hormone Research, Vol. 40. Karger, pp. 1–21.

McAllister JM, Modi B, Miller BA, et al. Overexpression of a DENND1A isoform produces a polycystic ovary syndrome theca phenotype. *Proc Natl Acad Sci USA* 2014; 111: E1519–27.

Moran LJ, Misso ML, Wild RA, et al. Impaired glucose tolerance, type 2 diabetes and metabolic syndrome in polycystic ovary syndrome: A systematic review and meta-analysis. *Hum Reprod Update* 2010; 16: 347–63.

O'Reilly MW, Taylor AE, Crabtree NJ, et al. Hyperandrogenemia predicts metabolic phenotype in polycystic ovary syndrome: The utility of serum androstenedione. *J Clin Endocrinol Metab* 2014; 99: 1027–36.

Wild RA, Carmina E, Diamanti-Kandarakis E, et al. Assessment of cardiovascular risk and prevention of cardiovascular disease in women with the polycystic ovary syndrome: A consensus statement by the Androgen Excess and Polycystic Ovary Syndrome (AE–PCOS) Society. *J Clin Endocrinol Metab* 2010; 95; 2038–49.

7.5 Congenital adrenal hyperplasia

Clinical symptoms

Congenital adrenal hyperplasia due to 21-hydroxylase deficiency is traditionally categorized into the classic form (salt wasting and simple virilizing) and the non-classic form. Patients with classic congenital adrenal hyperplasia suffer from glucocorticoid deficiency and adrenal androgen excess with (salt wasting) or without (simple virilizing) mineralocorticoid deficiency [1]. Patients with non-classic congenital adrenal hyperplasia typically do not experience glucocorticoid or mineralocorticoid deficiency but do, however, suffer from adrenal androgen excess. Most patients with non-classic congenital adrenal hyperplasia only present during adolescence or early adulthood, with a phenotype resembling polycystic ovary syndrome. The term 'late-onset congenital adrenal hyperplasia' should be avoided, as patients with classic congenital adrenal hyperplasia are also sometimes identified early in life. All patients with congenital adrenal hyperplasia should undergo a structured assessment of their glucocorticoid and mineralocorticoid reserves.

The clinical symptoms are defined by the hormonal deficits, and these depend on the severity of the underlying mutations.

Glucocorticoid deficiency clinically manifests with fatigue, exhaustion, loss of energy, weakness, muscle and joint aches, weight loss, loss of appetite, hypoglycaemia (children!), and fever.

Mineralocorticoid deficiency clinically manifests with salt craving, postural hypotension, dizziness, dehydration, nausea, vomiting, abdominal pain, diarrhoea, and somnolence.

Adrenal androgen excess clinically manifests as follows:
- in classic congenital adrenal hyperplasia:
  - masculinization of the external genitalia in newborn 46, XX females (46, XX disordered sex development)
  - precocious pseudopuberty, premature pubarche, genitoscrotal hyperpigmentation, and increased penile and testicular growth in 46, XY children

- early growth acceleration and advanced bone age, followed by early growth cessation resulting in short stature
- acne, hirsutism, and seborrhoea
- in non-classic congenital adrenal hyperplasia:
  - premature pubarche/adrenarche
  - acne, hirsutism, and seborrhoea
  - primary amenorrhoea, oligomenorrhoea, anovulation, and subfertility
  - only very rarely, bone age acceleration and clitoral hypertrophy

Biochemical findings

The following biochemical findings can be observed in untreated or undertreated congenital adrenal hyperplasia (see Table 7.3):
- classic congenital adrenal hyperplasia:
  - excessively increased baseline 17-hydroxyprogesterone
  - excessively increased 21-deoxycortisol (generated from 17-hydroxyprogesterone only in the absence of notable 21-hydroxylase activity)
  - increased androstenedione
  - increased testosterone
  - raised renin and low aldosterone in salt-wasting congenital adrenal hyperplasia
- non-classic congenital adrenal hyperplasia:
  - slightly to moderately increased baseline 17-hydroxyprogesterone; alternatively, it may be normal but markedly elevated after Synacthen® (a short Synacthen® test assessing the increase in 17-hydroxyprogesterone after adrenocorticotrophic-hormone stimulation differentiates between non-classic congenital adrenal hyperplasia and healthy individuals [2]; a 30-minute value <30 nmol/L (991 ng/dL) in the follicular phase excludes the diagnosis)
  - increased levels of androstenedione and testosterone

Table 7.3 Typical biochemical findings in 21-hydroxylase deficiency without therapy or with poor disease control

	SW 21-OHD	SV 21-OHD	NC 21-OHD
Sodium	Decreased	Normal	Normal
Potassium	Increased	Normal	Normal
Renin	Increased	Normal	Normal
Aldo	Decreased	Normal	Normal
17OHP	Highly increased	Highly increased	Mildly/moderately increased
Cortisol at baseline	Low or normal	Low or normal	Normal
Cortisol after ACTH	Low	Low	Normal or low
Δ4-A	Highly increased	Highly increased	Mildly/moderately increased
17HP, PT	Highly increased	Highly increased	Mildly/moderately increased
PTONE	Highly increased	Highly increased	Mildly/moderately increased
(Free) T	Increased	Increased	Normal or moderately increased

Abbreviations: 17HP, 24-hour urinary 17-hydroxypregnanolone; 17OHP, serum 17-hydroxyprogesterone; 21-OHD, 21-hydroxylase deficiency; Δ4-A, serum androstenedione; ACTH, adrenocorticotrophic hormone; Aldo, plasma aldosterone; NC, non-classical; PT, 24-hour urinary pregnanetriol; PTONE, 24-hour urinary pregnanetriolone; SV, simple virilizing; SW, salt wasting; T, serum testosterone.

Table 7.4 Recommended gluco- and mineralocorticoid substitution in classic congenital adrenal hyperplasia

Steroid	Recommended daily dose in children	Dosing frequency	Recommended daily dose in adults (mg)	Dosing frequency
HC	10–15 mg/m^2	2^c–3^{b,c}	15–25	3
Pred	—	2	5.0–7.5	2
Predlone	—	2	4–6	2
Dex^a	—	1	0.25–0.50	1
FC	0.05–0.20 mg	1^c–2^b	0.05–0.30	1
SCS	1–2 g/day in infancy	Divided into several feedings	—	—

Abbreviations: HC, hydrocortisone; Pred, prednisone; Predlone, prednisolone; Dex, dexamethasone; FC, fludrocortisone, SCS sodium chloride supplements.

^{a} Avoid if possible or limit to short time (e.g. for fertility treatment).

^{b} In growing patients.

^{c} In fully grown patients.

Adapted from Speiser PW, Azziz R, Baskin LS et al., Congenital Adrenal Hyperplasia Due to Steroid 21-Hydroxylase Deficiency: An Endocrine Society Clinical Practice Guideline, *Journal of Clinical Endocrinology & Metabolism* 2010; Volume 95, pp. 4133–4160. This article is published under the terms of the Creative Commons Attribution-Non Commercial-No Derivatives License (CC-BY-NC-ND; http://creativecommons.org/licenses/by-nc-nd/4.0/).

Ideally, urinary steroid hormone profiling (via gas chromatography–mass spectrometry) should be performed, which comprehensively detects the characteristic steroid fingerprint of the disease (increased excretion of the urinary metabolites of 17-hydroxyprogesterone, 17-hydroxypregnanolone, and pregnanetriol, and the urinary metabolite of 21-deoxycortisol, pregnanetriolone) [3, 4].

Molecular genetics

The 21-hydroxylase gene *CYP21A2* is located in HLA region 3 at Chromosomal position 6p21.3. About 65%–75% of congenital adrenal hyperplasia patients are compound heterozygotes. Only approximately 1% of cases of 21-hydroxylase deficiency are due to de novo mutations. The genetics follows an autosomal recessive trait, and the allele harbouring the less severe mutation drives the phenotype, specifically by defining the severity of glucocorticoid and mineralocorticoid deficiency. Severe mutations result in combined glucocorticoid and mineralocorticoid deficiency whilst very mild mutations result in adrenal androgen excess only, with normal glucocorticoid and mineralocorticoid reserves.

The clinical and biochemical diagnosis should be confirmed by molecular genetics, in order to be able to predict the clinical disease expression and provide data for genetic counselling [5]. Partners of affected patients should be tested prior to planned pregnancy, to ascertain carrier status, which has a prevalence of 1:50 in the normal population.

Follow-up

Children

In children and adolescents, the following parameters need to be carefully looked at each follow-up visit: height, weight, BMI, growth and growth velocity, signs of virilization, hirsutism, striae, tiredness, hyperpigmentation, blood pressure, pubertal stage (pubic hair, breast, testes), and bone age (see Table 7.4). Follow-up visits should take place at least every 3 months during infancy and every 4–6 months thereafter [6]. In addition to clinical monitoring, biochemical monitoring of blood, urine, and/or saliva is performed.

At the age of 16–24 years, medical issues change from a focus on growth and development to preservation of fertility and long-term prevention of co-morbidities, in particular adverse metabolic complications [7]. At this stage, patients should be transferred to an adult endocrinologist. An ideal setting for this transition is a transition clinic, where the patient is seen by both the paediatric and the adult endocrinologist to ensure optimal transfer of information about the patient's history and introduce the adult endocrinologist to the patient (and parents) [8]. A smooth process of transition will help to reduce the number of cases lost to follow-up and, thus, reduce complications in this vulnerable period.

Adults

After a successful transition, adult patients require specialist review every 6–12 months, although more frequent reviews may be necessary (see Tables 7.4 and 7.5). Biochemical monitoring should include 17-hydroxyprogesterone (normal levels indicate overtreatment with glucocorticoids) and androstenedione and testosterone (increased levels indicate glucocorticoid undertreatment), with blood drawn after intake of the normal morning glucocorticoid dose.

Plasma renin should be regularly monitored in patients on fludrocortisone replacement, aiming at levels in the upper normal range. Mineralocorticoid reserves should be reassessed in young adults, ideally at the transition stage, as dose requirements differ between childhood and adulthood.

Clinical assessment should include weight, BMI, and symptoms and signs of androgen excess (virilization, hirsutism) or glucocorticoid excess (striae, high blood pressure, glucose tolerance). In addition, glucocorticoid deficiency (fatigue, hyperpigmentation) should be checked, as well as sitting and standing blood pressure, to rule out postural hypotension.

In women, the regularity of the menstrual cycle should be documented and, if fertility treatment is required, additional parameters may require testing. In men, testicular ultrasound should be performed in order to rule out testicular adrenal rest tissue (TART) or, if present, to follow-up on it [9–11]. This should be offered to all male patients at the time of transition. In patients with evidence of TART, a sperm count and motility assessment (and, where appropriate, sperm banking) should be offered.

At each clinic visit, patients and parents/partners should be educated with regard to the risk of adrenal crises and to prevention strategies (Sick day rule 1: double the dose of glucocorticoids in intercurrent

Table 7.5 Follow-up in adult congenital adrenal hyperplasia patients

To do	Interval
History; ask about the following:	At least annually
• ability to cope with daily life	
• fatigue	
• regular menstrual cycle	
• adrenal crisis since last review	
• doubling of hydrocortisone for illness since last review	
• steroid emergency card	
• knowledge of sick day rules	
• steroid emergency injection kit	
Clinical examination:	Once yearly
• BMI	
• blood pressure (sitting and standing)	
• acne	
• hirsutism	
• striae	
• hyperpigmentation	
Biochemistry (blood):	Once yearly
• sodium	
• potassium	
• plasma renin	
• 17OHP	
• androstenedione	
• testosterone	
• (SHBG in women)	
• LH	
Genetic assessment and counselling	Once at transition and when fertility is planned
Gynaecological assessment	Once at transition and then as required
Testicular ultrasound (check for presence of testicular adrenal rest tumours)	Once at transition, thereafter according to findings
Fasting lipid profile	Once at transition, thereafter if clinically justified
HOMA-IR	Once at transition, thereafter if clinically justified
BMD	Once at transition, thereafter if clinically justified

Abbreviations: 17OHP, 17-hydroxyprogesterone; BMD, bone mineral density; HOMA-IR, homeostatic model assessment for insulin resistance; LH, luteinizing hormone; SHBG, sex hormone-binding globulin.

Note: The transition to adult endocrinology care takes place between the ages of 16 and 24.

Table 7.6 Recommended intravenous glucocorticoid dosing during critical illness or surgery

Age	Steroid	Bolus (single dose) at admission or induction of anaesthesia	Maintenance dose[†]
≤3 years	HC	25 mg IV	25–30 mg IV/24 hours [‡]
>3 years and <12 years	HC	50 mg IV	50–60 mg IV/24 hours
12–16 years	HC	100 mg IV	100 mg IV/24 hours
Adults >16 years	HC	100 mg IV	100–200 mg IV/IM qds

Abbreviations: HC, hydrocortisone; IM, intramuscular; IV, intravenous; qds, four times daily.

[†] Continue until transfer from the intensive therapy unit to normal ward and back on oral medication; thereafter, taper according to clinical performance.

[‡] Continuous intravenous infusion preferred; if not possible, split into 6-hourly doses by intravenous/intramuscular injection.

Data from: *Journal of Clinical Endocrinology & Metabolism*, Volume 87, Consensus statement on 21-hydroxylase deficiency from the Lawson Wilkins Pediatric Endocrine Society and the European Society for Paediatric Endocrinology, 2002, pp. 4048–53; *European Journal of Endocrinology*, Volume 167, Reisch N, Willige M, Kohn D et al., Frequency and causes of adrenal crises over lifetime in patients with 21-hydroxylase deficiency, 2012, pp. 35–42.

illness with fever, bed rest, antibiotics; Sick day rule 2: inject hydrocortisone and seek medical treatment in case of persistent vomiting, acute trauma, or serious illness; see Table 7.6) [12]. All patients need to have a steroid emergency card and should be offered a steroid emergency self-injection kit and training to use it.

The clinical care of congenital adrenal hyperplasia patients is an interdisciplinary effort. Therefore, the patient should also be introduced to a gynaecologist, a urologist, a geneticist, and a psychologist, as appropriate [13, 14]. All women should be offered a gynaecological review at transition (or at the first adult appointment, if no transition took place), particularly those women who previously underwent genital corrective surgery.

References and further reading

1. Speiser PW, Azziz R, Baskin LS, et al. Congenital adrenal hyperplasia due to steroid 21-hydroxylase deficiency: An Endocrine Society clinical practice guideline. *J Clin Endocrinol Metab* 2010; 95: 4133–60.
2. New MI, Lorenzen F, Lerner AJ, et al. Genotyping steroid 21-hydroxylase deficiency: Hormonal reference data. *J Clin Endocrinol Metab* 1983; 57: 320–6.
3. Krone N, Hughes BA, Lavery GG, et al. Gas chromatography/mass spectrometry (GC/MS) remains a pre-eminent discovery tool in clinical steroid investigations even in the era of fast liquid chromatography tandem mass spectrometry (LC/MS/MS). *J Steroid Biochem Mol Biol* 2010 121:496–504.
4. Kamrath C, Hartmann MF, and Wudy SA. Androgen synthesis in patients with congenital adrenal hyperplasia due to 21-hydroxylase deficiency. *Horm Metab Res* 2013; 45:86–91.
5. Krone N and Arlt W. Genetics of congenital adrenal hyperplasia. *Best Pract Res Clin Endocrinol Metab* 2009; 23: 181–92.

6. Joint LWPES/ESPE CAH Working Group. Consensus statement on 21-hydroxylase deficiency from the Lawson Wilkins Pediatric Endocrine Society and the European Society for Paediatric Endocrinology. *J Clin Endocrinol Metab* 2002; 87: 4048–53.

7. Auchus RJ and Arlt W. Approach to the patient: The adult with congenital adrenal hyperplasia. *J Clin Endocrinol Metab* 2013; 98: 2645–55.

8. Kruse B, Riepe FG, Krone N, et al. Congenital adrenal hyperplasia: How to improve the transition from adolescence to adult life. *Exp Clin Endocrinol Diabetes* 2004; 112: 343–55.

9. Reisch N, Flade L, Scherr M, et al. High prevalence of reduced fecundity in men with congenital adrenal hyperplasia. *J Clin Endocrinol Metab* 2009; 94: 1665–70.

10. Reisch N, Rottenkolber M, Greifenstein A, et al. Testicular adrenal rest tumors develop independently of long-term disease control: A longitudinal analysis of 50 adult men with congenital adrenal hyperplasia due to classic 21-hydroxylase deficiency. *J Clin Endocrinol Metab* 2013; 98: E1820–6.

11. Reisch N, Scherr M, Flade L, et al. Total adrenal volume but not testicular adrenal rest tumor volume is associated with hormonal control in patients with 21-hydroxylase deficiency. *J Clin Endocrinol Metab* 2010; 95: 2065–72.

12. Reisch N, Willige M, Kohn D, et al. Frequency and causes of adrenal crises over lifetime in patients with 21-hydroxylase deficiency. *Eur J Endocrinol* 2012; 167: 35–42.

13. Reisch N, Arlt W, and Krone N 2011 Health problems in congenital adrenal hyperplasia due to 21-hydroxylase deficiency. *Horm Res Paediatr* 76: 73–85.

14. Arlt W, Willis DS, Wild SH, et al. Health status of adults with congenital adrenal hyperplasia: A cohort study of 203 patients. *J Clin Endocrinol Metab* 2010; 95: 5110–21.

15. Kim CJ, Lin L, Huang N, et al. Severe combined adrenal and gonadal deficiency caused by novel mutations in the cholesterol side chain cleavage enzyme, P450scc. *J Clin Endocrinol Metab* 2008; 93: 696–702.

16. Miller WL and Strauss JF, 3rd. Molecular pathology and mechanism of action of the steroidogenic acute regulatory protein, StAR. *J Steroid Biochem Mol Biol* 1999; 69: 131–41.

17. Simard J, Ricketts ML, Gingras S, et al. Molecular biology of the 3beta-hydroxysteroid dehydrogenase/delta5-delta4 isomerase gene family. *Endocr Rev* 2005 26: 525–82.

18. Nimkarn S and New MI. Steroid 11beta- hydroxylase deficiency congenital adrenal hyperplasia. *Trends Endocrinol Metab* 2008; 19: 96–9.

19. Yanase T, Simpson ER, and Waterman MR. 17 Alpha-hydroxylase/17,20-lyase deficiency: From clinical investigation to molecular definition. *Endocr Rev* 1991; 12: 91–108.

20. Krone N, Reisch N, Idkowiak J, et al. Genotype–phenotype analysis in congenital adrenal hyperplasia due to P450 oxidoreductase deficiency. *J Clin Endocrinol Metab* 2012; 97: E257–67.

7.6 Androgen-secreting tumours

Physiologic androgen production in females

In women, androgens are derived from the ovary, from the adrenals, and through peripheral conversion of prohormones. Testosterone and dihydrotestosterone are considered true androgens which bind to the androgen receptor to exert their androgenic action, whilst androstenedione, DHEA, and DHEA-S are prohormones with weak or no androgenic potency. These prohormones are converted to androgens that bind to androgen receptors. About 25% of testosterone is produced by the ovaries, 25% is produced by the adrenal glands, and 50% is produced from the peripheral conversion of androstenedione (from the ovaries and the adrenal glands) in fat or skin. In hair follicles, testosterone is converted to dihydrotestosterone by 5-alpha reductase; in adipose tissues, it is converted to estradiol via aromatase. Physiologic prohormone and androgen production in women is illustrated in Figure 7.12.

Aetiology and subtypes

See Section 7.3 for imaging appearances. Increased prohormone conversion in peripheral tissues or androgen secretion leads to hirsutism and virilization in women. Virilization consists of hirsutism, acne, and signs of masculinization, such as deepening of the voice, increased muscle mass, temporal balding, clitoromegaly, and, at times, increased libido. In premenopausal women, hirsutism, acne, and oligomenorrhoea are usually due to PCOS, ovarian hyperthecosis, congenital adrenal hyperplasia, familial hirsutism, exogenous androgenic medications, or decreased SHBG levels. Virilization results from severe hyperandrogenism and may be due to an androgen-secreting tumour. Most commonly, androgen-secreting tumours originate in the ovaries. Whilst adrenal tumours that exclusively secrete androgens are rare, it is important to remember that adrenocortical adenomas and carcinomas can present with clinical and biochemical manifestations of Cushing's syndrome along with virilization. Table 7.7 outlines the types of androgen-secreting tumours.

Gonadal tumours

Ovarian tumours can be subdivided into non-functional and functional neoplasms. Both types may secrete excess androgen and lead to a clinical presentation of hyperandrogenism. Non-functional tumours, such as benign epithelial cystadenomas, cystoadenocarcinomas, Brenner tumours, or Krukenberg tumours, can result in prohormone and androgen production from normal stroma. Rarely, androgen production may be severe and lead to virilization. Functional ovarian tumours, shown in Table 7.7, are more commonly associated with clinical features of hyperandrogenism.

Ovarian sex cord–stromal tumours

Ovarian sex cord–stromal tumours represent 1.2% of all ovarian neoplasms. This is a heterogeneous group of benign or malignant tumours which are characterized histologically as granulosa cell tumours, Sertoli–Leydig cell tumours, and gynandroblastomas.

Granulosa stromal cell neoplasms include granulosa cell tumours, granulosa–theca cell tumours, thecomas, and fibromas. Compared to other ovarian sex cord–stromal tumours, fibromas are usually not hormonally active. Although the sex cord–stromal tumours are generally considered to have low-grade malignant potential, granulosa cell ovarian tumours are more often malignant than thecomas or fibromas.

Granulosa cell tumours are usually large and unilateral and can be subdivided into two categories: juvenile and adult. Juvenile tumours typically develop before puberty and have a higher proliferative rate and a lower risk of recurrence than the adult types. Adult granulosa tumours more commonly present in middle age and in older, non-Caucasian, obese women with a family history of breast and/or ovarian cancer (most patients' age range: 31–70). Patients present with an abdominal mass, ascites, increased abdominal distension, and abdominal pain. Granulosa tumours are often hormonally active and can produce oestrogen or testosterone, so symptoms related to hyperoestrogenism (breast tenderness, endometrial hyperplasia, abnormal uterine bleeding) or, occasionally, hyperandrogenism (hirsutism and virilization) are common at diagnosis. An inhibin level is a useful serum marker for granulosa cell tumours. Studies suggest that an

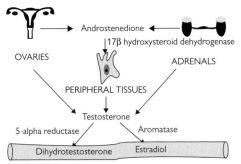

Fig 7.12 Testosterone production in women.

Table 7.7 Types of androgen-secreting tumours

Ovarian tumours	Adrenal tumours
Granulosa and granulosa–theca cell tumour[†]	Adenoma[†]
Thecoma[‡]	Carcinoma[†]
Fibrothecoma[‡]	Bilateral macronodular adrenal hyperplasia[†]
Sertoli—Leydig cell tumour[§]	
Gynandroblastoma[†]	
Hilus cell tumour[§]	
Luteoma of pregnancy[§]	
Theca–lutein cyst[§]	
Adrenal rest tumour of the ovary[§]	

[†] Both pre- and postmenopausal.

[‡] Postmenopausal.

[§] Premenopausal.

increased inhibin B level has 89%–100% sensitivity and up to 100% specificity. Elevated inhibin B levels in a woman presenting with an ovarian mass, amenorrhea, infertility, and signs of hyperoestrogenism or hyperandrogenism is suggestive of a granulosa cell tumour. Anti-Müllerian hormone has also been reported as a marker for granulosa cell tumours, with high specificity (close to 95%) but a lower sensitivity of 76%–91%.

Thecomas are usually benign ovarian stromal tumours containing theca cells. These tumours present as a unilateral mass in postmenopausal women with symptoms of hyperoestrogenism or hyperandrogenism, but without ascites. In approximately 20% of patients with oestrogen-secreting thecomas, endometrial hyperplasia and/or carcinoma are also detected. Fibrothecomas share features with fibromas, thecomas, and hormonally active tumours. The clinical presentation of fibrothecomas is similar to that of thecomas.

Sertoli–Leydig cell tumours can present as pure Sertoli cell tumours, pure Leydig cell tumours, or tumours with a mixed population. These rare tumours represent only 0.5% of ovarian tumours and are more common in young women aged 20–40. Hilus cell tumour is the terminology primarily reserved for a pure Leydig cell neoplasm located at the hilus of the ovary. Unlike the case with granulosa cell tumours, the hallmark of Sertoli–Leydig tumours is androgen production, with presentation of severe virilization in approximately 30% of patients. Whilst pure Sertoli tumours usually secrete more oestrogen, pure Leydig cell tumours secrete only androgens. Clinically, patients present with increased abdominal pain and distension, severe virilization, and a unilateral large ovarian mass. The diagnosis in premenopausal women presenting with a unilateral ovarian mass, severe virilization, and testosterone levels >7 nmol/L (200 ng/dL) is highly suggestive of a Sertoli–Leydig cell tumour.

Gynandroblastomas contain both granulosa and Sertoli–Leydig cell populations. They are very rare neoplasms, with only 23 cases reported in literature, and are usually small in size, presenting with symptoms of either hyperoestrogenism or hyperandrogenism.

Pregnancy-related hyperandrogenism

Normal testosterone levels during pregnancy are up to threefold that of non-pregnant controls, due to an increased production of SHBG. The free testosterone level, however, is not altered; thus, new onset hirsutism and virilization are pathologic. The two most common causes of pregnancy-related hyperandrogenism are luteomas and theca–lutein cysts of the ovary.

Luteomas present as either unilateral or bilateral (up to 50%) hyperplasic masses of lutein cells which usually spontaneously regress in the post-partum period. Approximately 35% of women with a luteoma have significant hirsutism and virilization, suggesting that the frequency of these tumours might be under-reported, as most of them have subclinical presentation with minimal or no androgen excess. Patients with clinically evident luteomas have increased serum testosterone, dihydrotestosterone, androstenedione, and urinary 17-ketosteroid levels, compared to normal pregnant controls. In patients with luteomas and evidence of virilization, up to 80% of female infants are virilized whereas, in non-virilized mothers, infants are normal. Previous studies have reported that the placenta normally protects the foetus from maternal androgens through metabolism or aromatization but, when maternal testosterone levels reach 28 nmol/L (800 ng/dL) or higher, the placental aromatization mechanism is saturated, and the risk of virilization of the female foetus is increased.

Theca–lutein ovarian cysts can be quite large and present with adnexal pressure or pain and elevated chorionic gonadotrophin hormone production. Most often, these cysts are associated with multiple gestations, molar pregnancies, and trophoblastic disease. Approximately 30% of pregnant women with theca–lutein cysts demonstrate hirsutism and/or virilization. Unlike the case with luteomas, however, female infants of mothers with theca–lutein cysts are not virilized, despite maternal hyperandrogenism and elevated cord blood levels of testosterone.

Adrenal rest tumours

The hormone-producing cells of the gonads and adrenals are both derived from the same embryologic structure, the genital ridge. Precursor adrenal cells remain with the mesonephros, whilst gonadal cells migrate caudally. It has been suggested that, in the case of adrenal rest cells, some of the adrenal cells either get misdirected caudally or remain as undifferentiated stem cells within gonads. The most common clinical example of adrenal rest cells within the gonads has been described in young patients with uncontrolled congenital adrenal hyperplasia. Adrenal rest tumours have also been described. These are pleomorphic tumours found in premenopausal women, and microscopically resemble Leydig cell tumours. Women with adrenal rest tumours often present with a clinical picture of hyperandrogenism together with cushingoid features. In addition to having increases in testosterone and androstenedione, patients often have elevated serum cortisol and urinary 17-ketosteroids. Adrenal rest tumours larger than 8 cm have increased number of mitosis and ~20% malignant potential.

Adrenal tumours

Although the major adrenal androgen prohormones DHEA and DHEAS have weak androgenic potency, these precursors convert into more potent testosterone and dihydrotestosterone, which in turn can cause adrenal-related hirsutism and virilization. Congenital adrenal hyperplasia with 21-hydroxylase deficiency shunts the steroidogenic pathway towards androgen production, resulting in hirsutism and virilization of the female offspring. Androgen-secreting tumours of the adrenal glands, on the other hand, are uncommon.

Adrenal adenoma

Pure androgen-secreting tumours are rare and can be malignant, accounting for 2.4%–5.3% of the bulk adrenalectomies performed. The malignant tumours are usually larger at presentation and have up to 2.5-fold higher testosterone levels compared to benign tumours. The primary prohormones secreted by these tumours are DHEA, DHEA-S, and androstenedione, which are converted into testosterone, resulting in masculinization. There have been only 14 reports of pure testosterone secreting adrenal tumours, although they may be under-reported. In children, androgen-secreting tumours produce a clinical picture similar to that of congenital adrenal hyperplasia, with accelerated muscle and growth development, and precocious puberty, whereas in adults the degree of hirsutism and virilization depends on the potent androgen levels. Cushing's syndrome due to benign cortisol-secreting adenomas can also produce androgens, but the androgen serum levels are usually too low to produce clinically apparent virilization.

Adrenal carcinoma

Although rare, adrenal carcinomas more commonly secrete pro-androgens than adrenal adenomas, with most patients having very high serum DHEA, DHEAS, and urinary 17-ketosteroids which do not suppress in response to dexamethasone. Virilization is particularly prominent in children, in whom this is the hallmark presentation of adrenocortical carcinoma. Most of these tumours are larger than 4 cm, and often capsular invasion with micrometastases is present, even in patients with smaller tumours.

Bilateral macronodular adrenal hyperplasia

Whilst most of the patients with bilateral macronodular adrenal hyperplasia present with overt Cushing's syndrome, a small subset of these patients have cortisol and androgen co-secretion, causing virilization in women. Very rarely, exclusively androgens are secreted with bilateral macronodular adrenal hyperplasia.

Diagnostic investigations

In a patient presenting with signs and symptoms of hyperandrogenism, hirsutism, and virilization, a detailed history and a physical examination including direct laboratory and radiological testing should be carried out. It is important to keep in mind that ovarian/adrenal androgen-secreting tumours are rare, and non-tumorous causes of hyperandrogenism such as PCOS, obesity-induced hyperandrogenism, hyperthecosis, congenital adrenal hyperplasia, and familial idiopathic hirsutism need to be excluded first. When taking a history, it is essential to inquire about the timing of menarche, the regularity of menses, any evidence of hirsutism or virilization, and the timing of their onset and progression. It is also important to ask about the patient's weight history and family history of hirsutism, infertility, and diabetes mellitus, as well as medication history, with an emphasis on medication that can increase or alter androgen levels and action. In women with a history of regular menses and presenting with a sudden onset of severe hirsutism and virilization, an ovarian or adrenal androgen-secreting tumour should be suspected.

Testosterone levels >5 nmol/L (200 ng/dL) or DHEAS greater than 2171 nmol/L (800 ng/mL) suggests that imaging for ovarian or adrenal neoplasm, retrospectively, is indicated. Some studies have suggested that these thresholds are variable, and that even lower testosterone values in presence of rapid onset virilization might warrant investigation for ovarian androgen-secreting tumour. The literature also suggests that a failure of testosterone, androstenedione, and DHEA to suppress in response to the 2- to 5-day low DST might indicate an ovarian source, although this has not been validated through well-designed studies.

When an androgen-secreting tumour of the ovary is suspected, imaging with pelvic ultrasound is indicated. Ovarian tumours are usually small, and asymmetry between ovaries might represent the only evidence of a tumour by an ultrasound. Axial CT or MRI of the adrenal is indicated in patients with high DHEAS or with symptoms suggestive of Cushing's syndrome. Although androgen-secreting tumours are far more common in the ovaries than in the adrenals, it is important to exclude adrenal tumours.

Ovarian and adrenal vein sampling has been used in an attempt to determine the source of hyperandrogenism, with variable success. The procedure is expert dependent and technically difficult since there is no clear marker to ensure proper placement of the catheter into the ovarian vein. The literature suggests that it is often difficult to distinguish between hyperthecosis and tumours; thus, the procedure is very rarely used.

Management

When managing hyperandrogenism in women, the treatment options are dependent on the underlying aetiology. PCOS, obesity, and congenital adrenal hyperplasia are usually treated medically, whilst ovarian and adrenal tumours are managed surgically.

The approach to ovarian androgen-secreting tumours is based on intraoperative findings, the patient's age, and fertility issues. Malignant ovarian tumours secreting androgens are treated and staged as primary ovarian cancer, with the exception that these tumours rarely have lymph-node metastasis, so pelvic lymphadenectomy is not usually performed. The tumour stage is the most important predictor of prognosis and usually guides the treatment of these tumours. If a young patient, desiring fertility, presents with a unilateral ovarian androgen-secreting tumour, with either benign or indeterminate frozen sections, preservation of the contralateral ovary is reasonable.

In patients presenting with hormone-secreting adrenal tumours, surgery is the treatment of choice. In cases of unilateral hormone-secreting adrenal adenomas, one-gland adrenalectomy is performed. Adrenocortical carcinoma, however, presents as an aggressive malignant tumour. Surgery is the first-line therapy but is usually not curative, as micrometastases are often present, even in early stages. In the case of persistent or recurrent disease, mitotane in combination with other cytotoxic agents is usually used. Mitotane is an adrenolytic, and most patients require glucocorticoid as well as mineralocorticoid replacement. In patients with advanced or metastatic disease, palliative radiation therapy has also been used.

In summary, severe and sudden onset of hirsutism and virilization in the setting of a three- to fourfold elevation of testosterone or DHEAS warrants an investigation for androgen-secreting tumours. Although rare, ovarian sex cord–stromal tumours, particularly Sertoli–Leydig tumours, are the most common tumours that cause excess testosterone. In virilized patients presenting with elevation of DHEAS and normal testosterone, an adrenal androgen-secreting tumour must be excluded. After a careful history and physical and biochemical diagnosis confirmation, targeted (either ovarian or adrenal) imaging is indicated. The surgical approach is the first-line therapy for androgen-secreting tumours, regardless of their aetiology.

Further reading

Chivukula M, Hunt J, Carter G, et al. Recurrent gynandroblastoma of ovary: A case report: A molecular and immunohistochemical analysis. *Int J Gynecol Pathol* 2007; 26: 30–3.

Cordera F, Grant C, van Heerden J, et al. Androgen-secreting adrenal tumors. *Surgery* 2003; 134: 874–80; discussion 880.

Freeman DA. Steroid hormone-producing tumors of the adrenal, ovary, and testes. *Endocrinol Metab Clin North Am* 1991; 20: 751–66.

Geerts I, Vergote I, Neven P, et al. The role of inhibins B and antimüllerian hormone for diagnosis and follow-up of granulosa cell tumors. *Int J Gynecol Cancer* 2009; 19: 847–55.

Lobo RA. Ovarian hyperandrogenism and androgen-producing tumors. *Endocrinol Metab Clin North Am* 1991; 20: 773–805.

Molta L, Schwartz U. Gonadal and adrenal androgen secretion in hirsute females. *Clin Endocrinol Metab* 1986; 15: 229–45.

7.7 Primary ovarian failure and premature ovarian insufficiency

Definition
Primary ovarian insufficiency is defined as the presentation of hypergonadotrophic amenorrhea before the age of 40. Diagnosis is based on obtaining serum FSH measurements that are >20 mU/L on two occasions.

Pathophysiology and immunogenetics
At birth, each ovary contains about 1 million germ cells, which decline in number through apoptosis at a rate of between 20 and 150 germs cells per day until menopause. Any process that accelerates apoptosis will result in early ovarian insufficiency. Germ cell production ceases before birth.

Causes of ovarian failure can be classified into four groups:
- genetic anomalies:
  - Turner syndrome (see Section 7.8) and variants
  - other X chromosome defects
  - Swyer syndrome (46, XY disorder of sex development)
  - fragile X syndrome (pre-mutation in *FMR1*)
  - over 20 single-gene associations
- autoimmune:
  - isolated or part of polyendocrinopathy (e.g. with hypothyroidism, Addison's disease, or type 1 diabetes mellitus)
- iatrogenic:
  - treatment for childhood cancer
  - pelvic surgery
- idiopathic:
  - most cases

Epidemiology
The average age of the onset of menopause is 50 years, with 1% of women menstruating after the age of 60, and 1% entering menopause before the age of 40. The age of onset of natural menopause is closely inherited and is also affected by environmental factors such as smoking. Menopause before the age of 40 is most commonly taken to be the definition of primary ovarian insufficiency. Estimates of the prevalence of primary ovarian insufficiency range between 0.3% and 1.0%, and this condition accounts for approximately 25% of women presenting with amenorrhoea.

Clinical features
History key points
Key points to note when taking the history are:
- a family history of primary ovarian insufficiency, consanguinity, and fragile X syndrome
- early feeding problems and otitis media (common in Turner syndrome)
- deafness (in Turner syndrome and Perrault syndrome; autosomal inheritance: sensorineural deafness and gonadal dysgenesis)
- previous surgery, radiotherapy, or chemotherapy
- a history of other autoimmune diseases, especially hypothyroidism (in up to 10% of cases)

Examination key points
Key points to note when performing the examination are:

- short stature (Turner syndrome and Perrault syndrome)
- features that are characteristic of fragile X syndrome, and any learning difficulties
- tall stature (Swyer syndrome)
- ptosis, blepharophimosis, and epicanthus inversus (blepharophimosis, ptosis, and epicanthus inversus syndrome; BPES)
- vaginal examination is not informative and is unnecessarily distressing

Investigations
The following investigations should be performed:
- repeat LH, FSH, estradiol, and TFTs, as results may vary
- serum anti-Müllerian hormone (is of no value if FSH is already raised (see Figure 7.13))
- karyotype, especially in early onset primary amenorrhoea (mandatory) and when there is a positive family history
- *FMR1* genetic analysis, if indicated

Note that pelvic ultrasound shows relatively normal appearances in 50% and fails to identify ovaries in <30%. These variable appearances make it useful for general information only; it is not of diagnostic value.

Ovarian biopsy offers no useful diagnostic or prognostic information and is not recommended.

Management
The main stay of medical management is oestrogen replacement, for which the main treatment goal is quality of life, together with secondary aims such as maintaining bone density. Oestrogen replacement can be based on the use of a combined oral contraceptive, especially in those who require contraception (conception is possible in 5% of women with primary ovarian insufficiency). Oral or transdermal estradiol are options, often offering improved quality of life. The transdermal oestrogen patch or gel is indicated for those with thrombotic risk and those in older age groups. Oestrogen replacement should continue until the age of 50. Progestogens are required for all women with a uterus.

Ovum donation is the only realistic fertility option. Even though 5% of women with primary ovarian insufficiency can conceive, there is no treatment to make this more likely and no reliable predictive factor. Oocyte cryopreservation is available for women at risk of ovarian failure, such those with a recent diagnosis of cancer.

Psychological support should be provided; this is a devastating diagnosis, and referral should be made to a unit experienced in the long-term psychological and fertility issues so that accurate information can be provided at an early stage. Advice on sexual function is required along with oestrogen use.

Monitoring should include an assessment of quality of life, including sexual function, bone density, and autoimmune screening every 5 years.

Complications/risks of treatment
Oral oestrogen confers a 2–4 fold increase in the risk of thrombosis. In young women, the absolute risk of

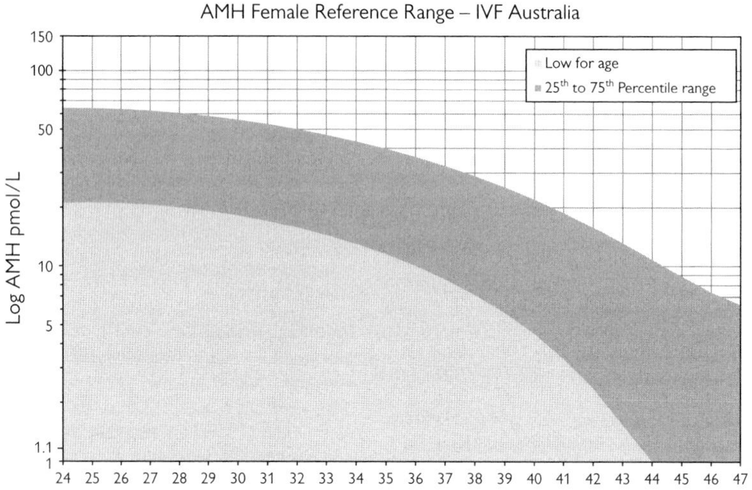

Fig 7.13 Beckmann GenII AMH assay.
Courtesy of IVF-Australia. Laboratories need to generate local normal ranges for AMH assay.

thrombosis is low but this becomes an important issue in older groups where transdermal oestrogen is favoured.

Women with primary ovarian insufficiency have a tendency to have low self-esteem and reduced sexual satisfaction, which can be improved with psychological input and optimization of sex-steroid replacement.

Prognosis

Women with menopause before the age of 45 have an excess risk of osteoporosis and cardiovascular disease but a reduced risk of breast cancer. These risks are thought to return to normal with oestrogen replacement. Most of the risks of oestrogen replacement have been defined in women over 50 and do not apply to young women with primary ovarian insufficiency.

Patient support groups/useful websites

The following patient support groups/websites may be useful:

- The Daisy Network (http://www.daisynetwork.org.uk/>): a registered charity for women who have experienced premature menopause
- The International Premature Ovarian Failure Association (http://www.ipofa.org/): a non-profit, international organization whose mission is to provide community support and information to women with premature ovarian failure
- The Human Fertilisation and Embryology Authority (http://www.hfea.gov.uk/): an independent regulator overseeing the use of gametes and embryos in fertility treatment and research in the UK; a useful resource for information on ovum donation

Future developments

The most important gap in our knowledge is that, in the majority of women, the aetiology of primary ovarian insufficiency is unknown. Research into mechanisms of apoptosis may lead to an improved understanding of the factors that determine the life span of the ovary.

In vitro maturation of oocytes is an advancing field that does not yet apply to primary ovarian insufficiency, as the success of this technique relies on being able to obtain relatively mature follicles of about 10 mm, which are rarely found in primary ovarian insufficiency. Future research may succeed in maturing primordial follicles to successful fertilization. Similarly, oocyte cryopreservation is only possible if ovarian function is normal. Once FSH is raised, then too few oocytes are obtained to make this worthwhile.

Further reading

Chlebowski RT and Anderson GL. Changing concepts: Menopausal hormone therapy and breast cancer. *J Natl Cancer Inst* 2012; 104: 517–27.

De Vos M, Devroey P, and Fauser BC. Primary ovarian insufficiency. *Lancet* 2010; 376: 911–21.

Graziottin A. Menopause and sexuality: Key issues in premature menopause and beyond. *Ann N Y Acad Sci* 2010; 1205: 254–61.

Lobo RA. Hormone-replacement therapy: current thinking. *Nat Rev Endocrinol*. 2017; 13(4): 220–31.

Oktem O, Kim SS, Selek U, Schatmann G, and Urman B. Ovarian and uterine functions in female survivors of childhood cancers. *Oncologist* 2018; 23(2): 214–24.

Rocca WA, Grossardt BR, Miller VM, et al. Premature menopause or early menopause and risk of ischemic stroke. *Menopause* 2012; 19: 272–7.

Rossetti R, Ferrari I, Bonomi M, and Persani L. Genetics of primary ovarian insufficiency. *Clin Genet* 2017; 91(2): 183–98.

Simon JA. What's new in hormone replacement therapy: Focus on transdermal estradiol and micronized progesterone. *Climacteric* 2012; 15 (Suppl. 1) :3–10.

Wallace WH. Oncofertility and preservation of reproductive capacity in children and young adults. *Cancer* 2011; 117 (Suppl. 10): 2301–10.

7.8 Turner syndrome

Definition

Turner syndrome is a relatively common genetic disorder affecting 1/2500 live-born females. It is characterized by loss or structural anomalies of an X chromosome. Clinical features vary among patients, and multiple organ systems can be affected. Thus, Turner syndrome patients commonly require a multidisciplinary approach. Endocrinologists are more commonly involved in the management of short stature, delayed puberty, infertility, and osteoporosis.

Genetics

Turner syndrome is caused by complete or partial loss of the X chromosome, or complex rearrangements affecting the X chromosome. Structural abnormalities can include deletions of the short or long arms of the X chromosome, duplications, or ring chromosomes. Some women are mosaic and carry one or more additional cell lines. Approximately 45% of patients with Turner syndrome have a 45, X karyotype and tend to have more clinical features than those who are mosaic with a normal cell line (e.g. 45, X/46, XX. Table 7.8). About 10% of Turner syndrome patients have mosaicism involving a cell line containing Y chromosome material. This condition is associated with an increased risk of gonadoblastoma.

Clinical features

Short stature is the most common abnormality in Turner syndrome. Growth failure begins prenatally, with poor growth often evident within the first 3 years of age. Adult height is about 20 cm below than that of the general female population. *Other skeletal* abnormalities and phenotypic features are short fourth metacarpals, cubitus valgus, Madelung deformity of the forearm and wrist, a broad chest with widely spaced nipples, a short neck with a webbed appearance, a low hairline at the back of the neck, and low-set ears (Table 7.9).

Ovarian failure is one of the most common features of Turner syndrome, and Turner syndrome is one of the most common causes of premature ovarian failure (see Section 7.7). Spontaneous puberty occurs in about 15% of girls with 45, X and in 30% of girls with a second cell line with more than one X chromosome. Only a small percentage will have spontaneous menarche, and only about 5% of women with Turner syndrome maintain normal menstrual cycles by 20 years of age.

Cardiovascular health issues include congenital abnormalities (more commonly bicuspid aortic valve, aortic coarctation, and elongation of the transverse aortic arch) and an aortic dilatation that can led to aortic dissection. Complications of congenital cardiovascular disease and systemic hypertension are the leading cause of morbidity and premature mortality in Turner syndrome. Aortic dissection is significantly increased (40 per 100,000/year) and occurs at a younger age (29–35 years) compare to that of the female population (75 years).

Renal anomalies include collecting system malformations, and horseshoe, duplicated, or absent kidneys. The majority of patients with these anomalies do not have secondary morbidity.

Metabolic syndrome and diabetes mellitus are more common in Turner syndrome. An increased frequency of central obesity, insulin resistance, type 2 diabetes, and dyslipidemia has been reported in young and adult women with Turner syndrome. An increased risk of hypertension at a younger age has also been reported, even after excluding Turner syndrome patients with cardiac or renal defects. Given these adverse cardiometabolic profiles, in addition to congenital and renal malformation, Turner syndrome patients are at increased risk of cardiovascular diseases.

Abnormal liver enzymes occur with a higher frequency in young and adult women with Turner syndrome, occasionally with progression to cirrhosis. The cause and

Table 7.8 Turner syndrome karyotypes (frequencies, %) and suggested correlation with phenotypes

Karyotypes	%	Phenotypes
45, X	45–50	Most severe phenotype
		Highest incidence of cardiovascular and renal malformations
45, X mosaicism:		Clinical phenotype often milder:
• 45, X/46, XX		• less severe phenotype
• 45, X/46, XX/47, XXX	45–50	• increased mean height
• 45, X/47, XXX		• spontaneous puberty and menses
		• higher probability of spontaneous pregnancy
		Phenotype similar to that for 45, X/46, XX, with a higher probability of fertility
46, Xi(Xq)	—	Higher risk of autoimmune disorders
Ring X chromosome	5–10	Sometimes associated with variable intellectual disability
45, X/46, XY or 45, X/46, X, idic(Y)	5–10	Increased risk of gonadoblastoma
Xq deletion	—	Variable phenotype
		Higher risk of ovarian insufficiency with no other TS features

Abbreviations: TS, Turner syndrome.

Table 7.9 Major clinical features in Turner syndrome and reported frequencies

Clinical feature	Reported frequency (%)
Short stature	95–100
Ovarian failure	90–95
Micrognatia	60
Low posterior hairline	40
Neck webbing	25
Cubitus valgus	50
Short fourth metacarpal	35
Madelung deformity	5
High, arched palate	35
Cardiac malformations:	50
• elongated transverse aortic arch	50
• bicuspid aortic valve	20
• coarctation of the aorta	10
Autoimmune thyroiditis	50
Celiac disease	6
Recurrent otitis media	50
Renal abnormalities	24–42
Multiple nevi	25
Scoliosis	11
Ptosis	10–30

clinical significance is unclear. Obesity is one of the common causes thought to contribute to this finding. Oestrogen therapy appears to be associated with improvement of the liver function tests.

Autoimmune disorders, most importantly, Hashimoto's thyroiditis (50%) and celiac disease (6%), are more frequent in the Turner syndrome population.

Hearing abnormalities in Turner syndrome include a high risk for recurrent otitis media with associated conductive hearing problems, and progressive sensorineural hearing loss which tends to worsen with age.

Eye problems are common among patients with Turner syndrome and include a wide range of diseases, such as strabismus, ptosis, epicanthal folds, glaucoma, and early cataract.

Concerning *psychological and educational issues*, the majority of patients with Turner syndrome have normal intelligence, although women with a small ring X chromosome have an increased risk of mental retardation. There are increased risks for selective neuropsychological impairments including visual–spatial organization deficits, difficulty with social cognition and problem-solving (e.g. mathematics), and motor deficits. Overall, behavioural function is normal in Turner syndrome; however, there may be an increased risk for social isolation, immaturity, anxiety, and reduced self-esteem.

Diagnosis

The diagnosis of Turner syndrome is often delayed, particularly for individuals with minimal stigmata. Prompt diagnosis is important to permit effective treatment of short stature and management of co-morbidities. More commonly, Turner syndrome is diagnosed during evaluation for short stature, often with primary amenorrhea in girls aged 10–16 years. Clinicians need to be alert to the clinical features associated with Turner syndrome, especially short stature, delayed puberty, primary amenorrhea, or premature ovarian failure. Nevertheless, physicians need to stay aware of the possibility of Turner syndrome diagnosis throughout the entire adult life. The diagnosis is confirmed by karyotype analysis.

Management

Management of short stature

Therapy with recombinant human growth hormone, starting in early childhood (around 4–6 years of age), is recommended to maximize adult height. Turner syndrome girls can achieve adult height within the normal range with optimum growth-hormone treatment. Patients with Turner syndrome require higher doses of growth hormone, compared with patients with growth-hormone deficiency.

Management of primary hypogonadism

Almost all girls with Turner syndrome need exogenous oestrogen. The timing and dosing of oestrogen therapy should be selected to reflect normal puberty. Beginning treatment with low-dose estradiol around 11–12 years of age permits a normal timing and pace of puberty without compromising adult height. The dose should be increased gradually during the following 2–3 years to a young-adult dose. Transdermal oestrogen preparations are preferred. To allow for normal breast and uterine development, it seems advisable to delay the addition of progestin for at least 2 years after starting oestrogen or until breakthrough bleeding occurs. Oestrogen–progestin therapy should be continued until the average age of menopause.

If *Y chromosome material* is detected, patients should undergo prophylactic removal of the gonads. Hysterectomy is not recommended, to preserve the possibility of pregnancy using donor oocytes.

Initial evaluation and monitoring

At the time of diagnosis, all patients with Turner syndrome should have a comprehensive *cardiovascular* evaluation, ideally by a cardiologist with Turner syndrome expertise, including transthoracic echocardiography and ECG. Cardiac magnetic resonance (CMR) is recommended as soon as feasible. Girls found to have coarctation of the aorta should undergo surgical correction. Repeat imaging should be done every 5–10 years, and more often if aortic dilatation or other cardiovascular risk factors are detected. *Blood pressure* should be monitored regularly. If hypertension develops, it should be treated vigorously.

Patients should undergo *renal* ultrasonography at the time of diagnosis. If structural abnormalities are identified, patients should be monitored clinically for urinary tract infection.

Monitoring of *thyroid function* (TSH and FT4) is recommended annually, and *celiac* screening with tissue transglutaminase IgA, combined with total IgA, should begin in childhood and should be repeated every 2–5 years.

An *ophthalmologic* examination is recommended at the time of diagnosis, and regular monitoring of *hearing* is recommended throughout life.

Neuropsychological and educational testing is recommended before enrollment in preschool. Any identified issues should be addressed by specific implementation of educational strategies.

Adult monitoring

Few women with Turner syndrome go on to receive optimal care and surveillance as adults.

Women with Turner syndrome should be seen *annually* for physical examination and *biochemical testing* for glucose intolerance, dyslipidaemia, liver abnormalities, and thyroid function. Many of the problems of adult life in women with Turner syndrome are compounded by obesity. *Lifestyle education* must be included in a programme of prevention of hypertension, diabetes, hepatic steatosis, and osteoporosis.

To minimize the risk for aortic dissection, close *blood pressure and cardiovascular* monitoring are required in patients with a dilated ascending aorta. Because body size is a major determinant of normal aortic dimensions, it is appropriate in Turner syndrome population to evaluate it in relation to body surface area. The ascending aorta is the most affected and informative site, and an aortic size index (the ratio of the diameter of the ascending aorta to the body surface area) >2.0 cm/m^2 should be considered to indicate mild aortic dilatation. Approaches to managing woman with aortic dilatation include exercise restriction and aggressive blood pressure control; when the index is ≥ 2.3 cm/m^2, a beta blocker and/or an angiotensin-receptor blocker should be started. Elective operations should be considered when the index is ≥ 2.5 cm/m^2. Any symptoms consistent with aortic dissection need urgent evaluation, and all Turner syndrome patients should be educated accordingly.

Women with Turner syndrome have an increased risk for *osteoporosis* and fractures. DXA should be used to monitor bone health after the start of oestrogen replacement therapy, with follow-up depending on the initial result. Additional evaluation of bone mineral density is recommended when considering discontinuation of oestrogen therapy. Management of low bone mineral density is the same as for the general female population.

Most women with Turner syndrome are infertile due to primary ovarian failure. However, 4.8%–7.6% experience spontaneous *pregnancy*. IVF with donor oocytes can be used to achieve pregnancy. Thus, all young women with Turner syndrome should receive counselling on the timing of pregnancy, because of the risk of premature ovarian failure, and the possibility of assisted reproductive technologies, along with the elevated risk of miscarriage and the possibility of chromosomal abnormalities in the offspring.

Specific risks of pregnancy for Turner syndrome include higher rates of spontaneous abortion, fetal anomaly, and maternal morbidity and mortality. It is reported that the risk of pregnancy-associated death and aortic dissection in women with Turner syndrome undergoing IVF pregnancy is approximately 2%. It is likely that pregnancy-associated hemodynamic and hormonal factors promote deterioration in the compromised cardiovascular system of women with Turner syndrome. Therefore, before pregnancy can be contemplated, a complete medical evaluation, with particular attention to the cardiovascular system, is mandatory. Echocardiography and CMR need to be performed before any pregnancy consideration. All pregnancies should be followed by a multidisciplinary team, including high-risk pregnancy specialists, endocrinologists, and cardiologists, at a tertiary care centre.

Ongoing *psychological* assessment and support should be considered at each visit. Premature ovarian failure and infertility are reported as being the hardest part about Turner syndrome. Problems are responsive to targeted clinic psychology support.

Patient support groups/useful websites

The following patient support groups/websites may be useful:

- The Turner Syndrome Society of UK (http:// www. tss.org.uk/)
- The Premature Ovarian Failure Support Group (www. daisynetwork.org.uk)

Further reading

Bondy C. Pregnancy and cardiovascular risk for women with Turner syndrome. *Womens Health (Lond)* 2014; 10: 469–76.

Bondy CA. Turner Syndrome Study Group. Care of girls and women with Turner syndrome: A guideline of the Turner Syndrome Study Group. *J Clin Endocrinol Metab* 2007; 92: 10–25.

Gravholt CH, Andersen NH, Conway GS, et al. On behalf of the International Turner Syndrome Consensus Group. Clinical practice guidelines for the care of girls and women with Turner Syndrome: Proceedings from the 2016 Cincinnati International Turner Syndrome Meeting. *Euro J Endocrinol* 177: G1–70.

Hewitt JK, Jayasinghe Y, Amor DJ, et al. Fertility in Turner syndrome. *Clin Endocrinol (Oxf)* 2013; 79: 606–14.

Lee MC and Conway GS. Turner's syndrome: Challenges of late diagnosis. *Lancet Diabetes Endocrinol* 2014; 2: 333–8.

Mortensen KH, Andersen NH, and Gravholt CH. Cardiovascular phenotype in Turner syndrome: Integrating cardiology, genetics, and endocrinology. *Endocr Rev* 2012; 33: 677–714.

Pinsker JE. Clinical review: Turner syndrome: Updating the paradigm of clinical care. *J Clin Endocrinol Metab* 2012; 97: E994–1003.

Roulot D. Liver involvement in Turner syndrome. *Liver Int* 2013; 33: 24–30.

Trolle C, Hjerrild B, Cleemann L, et al. Sex hormone replacement in Turner syndrome. *Endocrine* 2012; 41: 200–19.

7.9 Approach to the assessment of disorders of menstrual function

Introduction

Menopause is a universal phenomenon among women who live long enough to experience it. The mean age of menopause in Western societies has remained relatively constant at about 51 years of age over many years, although there are signs that this may be slowly increasing. As the mean age of menarche has fallen substantially over the past 150 years, from >18 to <14, the female reproductive lifespan has increased. Girls now experience menarche earlier due to better nutrition and earlier attainment of an adequate body fat mass to activate the hypothalamo-pituitary–ovarian axis and begin the ovarian cycle.

Epidemiology and physiology

Menopause is defined as the cessation of menses, and hence occurs at the time of the last menstrual period. However, this is a point which can only be recognized in retrospect, and a working definition requires a year to pass following the last recorded menses before menopause can be said to have occurred. Even then, it is possible for a late ovulation to occur with an episode of postmenopausal bleeding. Most women will experience a change in their menstrual cycle in the years leading up to menopause, with a shortening and then, in some cases, lengthening of the cycle as ovulation becomes less frequent and the hormone changes that underlie growth and then shedding of the superficial endometrium become less coordinated. As ovarian follicle growth, ovulation, and formation of the corpus luteum occur less frequently, and the follicle produces less oestrogens, the woman may experience symptoms of oestrogen withdrawal such as hot flushes and sweats, particularly at night, and mood disturbance. These symptoms are very variable both in severity and duration.

Age at menopause is strongly familial. Women who have a family history of late menopause are likely to continue to experience monthly periods, and to remain fertile, for longer than those with family history of earlier menopause. Some families seem to be at the extreme of this distribution, with natural menopause occurring in the late thirties or early forties. This physiological variation was not a major problem in previous generations in which pregnancies occurred in the teens and twenties. However, the deferral of attempts to conceive until later life, which has become one of the demographic phenomena of our time, has resulted in an increasing incidence of infertility in this group as they run out of their ability to conceive before they reach a point in their lives at which they wish to start their family.

It has been known for many years that the length of the ovarian lifespan is largely determined by events that occur during fetal life. The primordial germ cells migrate into the developing gonad by 6–7 weeks of embryonic life and undergo a finite number of waves of mitosis, followed by the early stages of meiosis to create the resting pool of primordial follicles. The size of this pool is maximal at about 5 months of fetal life and then declines in a regulated manner over the life of the woman. The majority of the resting primordial follicles never develop to the early pre-antral stage but enter apoptosis shortly after re-entering their growth phase. Recent studies have highlighted the complexity of this regulatory process, involving an interaction between the oocyte and its adjacent cumulus cells. The physiology of follicle dormancy and later growth is fundamental to understanding of the duration of the reproductive lifespan and its regulation. It is clear that many factors, including treatments for cancer (chemotherapy and radiotherapy), cigarette smoking, and environmental toxins, are gonadotoxic and can shorten the woman's reproductive life, but little is known about methods to lengthen this period of time. Animal studies have demonstrated the importance of antioxidants in slowing the rate of follicle attrition, but it remains to be seen whether this can be extrapolated to the human.

Clinical features

There is a simple feedback loop between the ovary and hypothalamus/pituitary that maintains regular ovulation and hence menstruation during health for many years. Pituitary secretion of FSH is elevated by about 30% above baseline during the menstrual phase of the cycle. This rise is sufficient to induce follicle growth and development in a young woman. As the size of the follicle pool diminishes with age, more FSH is needed to induce this response. Hence, FSH rises with age in the early follicular phase of the cycle. As the follicle grows and becomes dominant, it secretes increasing amounts of oestrogens, particularly estradiol, into the circulation. This secretion does not vary significantly with ageing—the total amount of estradiol secreted from a large follicle will lead to a plasma estradiol of approximately 1000 pmol/L (27 ng/dL), whatever the age of the woman. However, the time taken for a follicle to develop varies significantly and determines most of the length of the cycle. Hence, older women experience more shorter or longer cycles than their younger counterparts as the lifespan of the growing follicle becomes less well regulated.

Ovulation occurs as the rise in circulating estradiol triggers the LH surge in the mid-cycle. This process also remains usually intact with reproductive ageing, although the frequency of anovular cycles, due either to poor follicle growth or an inadequate LH surge, increases with age. The length of the luteal phase is fixed at about 14 days post LH surge, and varies less with ageing than the length of the follicular phase. Menstruation frequently becomes heavier as women age, due in part to pathologies, including fibroids and endometrial polyps, and in part to less efficient myometrial contractility and regulation of menstrual bleeding by the spiral arterioles of the basalis endometrium and superficial myometrium.

Assessment

Proximity to menopause

Menopause occurs at the time of the last menstrual period. However, many women wish to know whether they are close to their menopause. This has relevance to their fertility, particularly for those who have deferred starting to try for a family, and also to those who wish to stop use of contraception. Symptoms of perimenopause, such as flushes, sweats, and heavy menses, are

---

Box 7.1 Consequences of menopause

Immediate
Sweats, flushes, mood swings
Insomnia, anxiety, memory loss
Fatigue, poor concentration
Loss of libido, vaginal dryness

Intermediate
Collagen loss, leading to:
• loss of skin turgor
• vaginal epithelial thinning and atrophy with vaginal bleeding
• urinary tract infections, dysuria, urgency, frequency
• easy bruising
• joint and muscle pain

Long term
Activation of bone resorption, leading to osteoporosis
    Reduced HDL and increased LDL and cholesterol, leading to cardiovascular disease
    Loss of cerebral perfusion and increased amyloid deposition, leading to dementia

---

non-specific and should not be attributed to menopause without adequate investigation (see Box 7.1). Assessment of proximity to menopause has been made easier in recent years by availability of assays for anti-Müllerian hormone. This is secreted into the circulation by developing small antral follicles. The size of the small antral follicle pool reflects the size of the dormant primordial follicle pool, and hence a simple measurement of anti-Müllerian hormone in serum can give an early indication of a fall in the size of the primordial follicle pool—the ovarian reserve. The level of anti-Müllerian hormone is reported in relation to the age of the woman (see Figure 7.13). Those with anti-Müllerian hormone levels lower than the mean for their age have a smaller follicle pool and lower ovarian reserve than average, whereas those with higher than average levels for their age have a larger follicle pool. Low levels for age indicate closer proximity to menopause. However, the hormone becomes undetectable in the circulation several years before cessation of menses, and is also temporarily suppressed during chemotherapy. Many pregnancies, both natural and after IVF, have been reported for women with undetectable levels of anti-Müllerian hormone, although fertility is generally low in this group. Anti-Müllerian hormone levels are not significantly altered by the stage of the menstrual cycle, so they can be measured at any time, but they are variably suppressed by use of the oral contraceptive pill. Therefore, caution should be exercised in this group. It is often helpful to measure anti-Müllerian hormone and FSH together in an early follicular phase blood sample (Days 2–3 of the period). FSH rises with LH in the mid-cycle, so a random measurement may give a falsely high reading and an erroneous diagnosis of perimenopause if the sample is collected by chance during the mid-cycle surge.

Ultrasound can also be used to assess ovarian reserve. Transvaginal ultrasound during the early follicular phase of the cycle allows the number of antral follicles (2–4 mm diameter) to be assessed, giving an antral follicle count.

This generally correlates with the concentration of anti-Müllerian hormone in serum but can be used as a second means of measuring ovarian reserve in women with an unexpectedly low level of anti-Müllerian hormone, or other paradoxical findings. Ultrasound can also be used to study uterine anatomy in order to investigate causes of irregular or heavy bleeding, such as fibroids or polyps. If other causes of menstrual irregularity are suspected, then the woman should have a full reproductive endocrine assessment including measurement of thyroid function, prolactin, androgens, and SHBG for polycystic ovary syndrome, and luteal phase progesterone, to test for ovulation.

HRT remains the mainstay for treatment of perimenopausal symptoms. Importantly, women who reach menopause before their late forties should be offered screening for bone mineral density and, if it is low, should be offered oestrogen HRT and/or bisphosphonate, along with calcium and vitamin D replacement. These women are at high risk of early onset of osteoporosis, especially if there is a family history. Oestrogen HRT in this group is true replacement and should not carry any excess risk of breast cancer above that of the majority of women who still experience regular menstrual cycles at this age. Relatively high doses of oestrogens may be necessary for symptom relief in this young group.

After a normal menopause (Box 7.2), minimum effective doses of oestrogen should be used for HRT (Box 7.3), although there is no good evidence that the risk of breast cancer is dose dependant. However, lower doses

---

Box 7.2 Assessment after menopause

General
Weight, blood pressure, fasting lipids
    Mammography every 3 years up to age 65, or older if still using HRT
    Cervical cytology

Abnormal vaginal bleeding
Single episode within 5 years of last menses
    Bimanual and speculum examination for atrophic change
    Pipelle office endometrial biopsy and transvaginal ultrasound (normal endometrial thickness 4 mm or less)
    Repeated bleeds, or greater than 5 years since last menses
    Bimanual and speculum examination
    Transvaginal ultrasound
    Hysteroscopy (local or general anaesthetic) with endometrial biopsy

Urinary symptoms
Bimanual and speculum examination for atrophy or prolapse
    Urine microbiology
    Urodynamics
    Rarely, cystoscopy

Osteoporosis risk
Dual energy X-ray absorptiometry of lumbar spine and hip
    Less useful: peripheral X-ray, ultrasound screening
    Treatment

Box 7.3 **Minimum effective doses of oestrogens**

Systemic
Micronized estradiol/estradiol valerate: 1–2 mg
Oral conjugated equine oestrogens: 0.300–0.625 mg
Transdermal estradiol: 25–50 µg
Estradiol implant: 25–50 µg
Estradiol silicone ring: 50 µg

Local vaginal oestrogen
Estriol: 0.1% or 0.01%
Vaginal tablet: 25 µg/24 hours estradiol
Silicone ring: 7.5 µg/24 hours

carry less risk of mastalgia and breakthrough vaginal bleeding.

The route of administration should be decided with the patient. Oral oestrogens are subject to extensive first pass metabolism. Transdermal patches are available with sequential oestrogen, sequential oestrogen and progesterone, and continuous oestrogen and progesterone formulations. Oral and transdermal oestrogen should be used in conjunction with a progestogen for women with a uterus, to avoid the possibility of endometrial hyperplasia and adenocarcinoma if unopposed oestrogen is given long term. Those without a uterus can safely use oestrogen alone and avoid the fluid retention and PMS-like side effects of progestogens. Progestogen can be given as a continuous low dose, provided that at least a year has passed since the last menstrual bleed, or as an intermittent regime for 12–14 days per month. The duration of exposure to progestogen can be extended, or doses increased, if there is persistent breakthrough bleeding with HRT. Progestogens can be administered orally, transdermally, vaginally, or via the Mirena® levonorgestrel-containing intrauterine system. Alternatives for women with troublesome progestogenic side effects include use of the synthetic oestrogen/gestagen analogue tibolone, and use of a drospirinone-containing combined HRT.

Risks and benefits of HRT

The Women's Health Initiative (WHI) and Million Women Study both showed an excess risk of breast cancer using oestrogen and progestogen HRT when compared with oestrogen alone. The Million Women Study showed that, after 10 years of oestrogen–progesterone HRT, there were 19 additional cases of breast cancer per 1000 women but no additional cases of endometrial cancer. In contrast, after 10 years of oestrogen-only HRT, there were 5 additional cases of breast cancer per 1000 women per year, but 10 additional cases of endometrial cancer. There was also an increase in the number of cases of irregular bleeding, with considerable extra resource implications. Hence, progestogens are still recommended, and alternative routes of administration such as vaginal gel or the intrauterine system are under investigation. Long-term data for the incidence of breast cancer with these approaches are not yet available.

The Heart Estrogen Replacement Study of secondary prevention of coronary heart disease using HRT failed to confirm earlier observations concerning reduction in risk of coronary heart disease in HRT users, and WHI failed to demonstrate benefit in a primary prevention setting.

WHI also showed a small but significant increase in risk of heart disease in combined HRT users when compared with placebo after 5 years, with an age-related increase in stroke. There was no increase in risk of coronary heart disease in the oestrogen-only arm of the WHI study. Overall, women who use HRT below age 60 appear to have a significantly lower all-causes mortality than those who do not.

The current practice is to use low-dose HRT for women who are troubled by symptoms of menopause for up to 5 years during the perimenopausal transition. Many patients will not experience severe menopausal symptoms when HRT is stopped later. Women who wish to continue HRT over age 55 must be counselled about the risks of breast cancer and screened regularly. It is prudent to avoid long-term oestrogen HRT in women with significant family history of breast cancer. As with any medication, the risks of use must be balanced against the benefits, with an individual risk assessment based on age, family history, past medical history, and concurrent disorders being made for each individual woman, and carefully annotated.

Deep vein thrombosis

There is a two- to threefold increase in risk of venous thromboembolism among HRT users when compared with non-users. The majority of these events occur in the first year of use, and problem-free long-term use of oral contraceptives in the past may identify a group of women who are less likely to experience a thromboembolic event on HRT. Risks may be lessened by use of a transdermal preparation.

A number of potential benefits of use of combined HRT have stood the test of time. These include a reduction in the risk and severity of osteoporosis, a reduction in the risk of colorectal cancer (combined HRT only), and possibly a reduction in the risk of later dementia if HRT is started in the immediate few years after menopause. This effect was not observed in the WHI memory study, in which HRT was started at older age (mean 67 years).

Testosterone

Recent years have seen an increase in pharmacological interest in treatment of low female libido using androgens. 'Hypoactive sexual desire disorder' may respond to treatment with low-dose testosterone, usually using a transdermal gel. Side effects of androgenization are rare with low-dose therapies, although response to treatment varies considerably from one patient to the next. DHEA, purchased as a food supplement, may also have weak androgenic effects and is widely used.

Non-HRT treatments

Many women resort to complementary approaches to management of perimenopausal symptoms, given the scare stories concerning risks of HRT that continue to appear in the popular press. Results vary from patient to patient. Preparations of black cohosh have become the most widely used in recent years, while other women use acupuncture and homeopathy with apparent benefit. Some of these alternative medications may contain significant levels of pesticides or compounds that may cross react with anti-epileptic or other medications. Phytoestrogens, compounds that contain natural oestrogens, which contain the isoflavones genistein and daidzein derived from soy, chickpeas, and red clover, may work via the oestrogen receptor and be no more dangerous or safe than conventional oestrogen HRT. Other commonly used remedies include evening primrose oil, Ginkgo biloba, and St John's wort extract. The latter compound induces hepatic cytochrome P450 enzymes and interacts with a large number of medications, including warfarin.

The benefit of exercise and healthy lifestyle in the reduction of the risk of osteoporosis are more clearly researched. Exercise regimes should be low impact, sustained, and regular. Reduction in alcohol intake and cessation of smoking are also prudent.

Specific treatments for perimenopausal flushes and sweats have moved in recent times, away from alpha-2 agonists such as clonidine and beta blockers towards SSRIs, particularly venlafaxine. Potential benefits should be weighed against the well-known side effects of this class of compounds. Gabapentin has also been shown to be effective in small studies.

An increasing number of pharmacological interventions for the prevention or treatment of osteoporosis (see Chapter 12, Section 12.6) has become available in recent years. These include bisphosphonates, selective oestrogen modulators, strontium ranelate, and parathormone. These have been reviewed by NICE (see http://www.nice.org.uk) for fracture prevention.

Patient support groups/useful websites

The following patient support groups/websites may be useful:

- The British Menopause Society (http://www.thebms.org.uk/)
- National Osteoporosis Society (http://www.nos.org.uk/)

The following websites have information about dietary supplements:

- http://health.nih.gov
- http://www.mhra.gov.uk/Howweregulate/Medicines/Herbalmedicinesregulation/RegisteredTraditionalHerbalMedicines/LIstofproductsgrantedaTraditionalHerbalRegistrationTHR/

Further reading

Beral V, Bull D, Reeves G et al. Endometrial cancer and hormone-replacement therapy in the Million Women Study. *Lancet* 2005; 365: 1543–51.

Dólleman M, Faddy MJ, van Disseldorp J, et al. The relationship between anti-Mullerian hormone in women receiving fertility assessments and age at menopause in subfertile women: Evidence from large population studies. *J Clin Endocrinol Metab* 2013; 98: 1946–53.

Freeman EW, Sammel MD, Lin H, et al. Anti-mullerian hormone as a predictor of time to menopause in late reproductive age women. *J Clin Endocrinol Metab* 2012; 97: 1673–80.

Hulley S, Grady D, Bush T, et al. Randomized trial of estrogen plus progestin for secondary prevention of coronary heart disease in postmenopausal women. *JAMA* 1998; 280: 605–13.

Landgren BM, Collins A, Csemiczky G, et al. Menopause transition: Annual changes in serum hormonal patterns over the menstrual cycle in women during a nine-year period prior to menopause. *J Clin Endocrinol Metab* 2004; 89: 2763–9.

Ledger WL. Clinical utility of measurement of anti-mullerian hormone in reproductive endocrinology. *J Clin Endocrinol Metab* 2010; 95: 5144–54.

Million Women Study Collaborators. Breast cancer and hormone-replacement therapy in the Million Women Study. *Lancet* 2003; 362: 419–27.

Morris EP and Rymer J. Menopausal symptoms, search date December 2006. *Clin Evid (Online)* 2007; 2007.

NICE. The clinical effectiveness and cost effectiveness of technologies for the secondary prevention of osteoporotic fractures in postmenopausal women: Technology appraisal guidance [TA87], 2005. Available at https://www.nice.org.uk/guidance/ta87 (accessed 1 Jan 2017).

NICE. Menopause: diagnosis and management. NG23. Available at http://www.niceguidance[ng23].

Panay N and Fenton A. A global consensus statement on menopause hormone therapy: Aims, aspirations and action points. *Climacteric* 2013; 16: 201–2.

Rossouw JE, Anderson GL, Prentice RL, et al. Risks and benefits of estrogen plus progestin in healthy postmenopausal women: Principal results from the Women's Health Initiative randomized controlled trial. *JAMA* 2002; 288: 321–33.

Stuenkel CA, Davis SR, Gompel A, et al. Treatment of symptoms of the menopause: An Endocrine Society clinical practice guideline. *J Clin Endocrinol Metab* 2015; 100: 3975–4011.

Thacker HL. Assessing risks and benefits of nonhormonal treatments for vasomotor symptoms in perimenopausal and postmenopausal women. *J Womens Health (Larchmt)* 2011; 20: 1007–16.

Shumaker SA, Reboussin BA, Espeland MA, et al. The Women's Health Initiative Memory Study (WHIMS): A trial of the effect of estrogen therapy in preventing and slowing the progression of dementia. *Control Clin Trials*. 1998; 19: 604–21.

Chapter 8

Male hormone metabolism

Chapter contents

8.1 Anatomy and physiology

Introduction
The testis has two major functions: first, to synthesize and secrete testosterone and, second, to produce mature sperm.

Anatomy
The testicular parenchyma is surrounded by a fibrous capsule known as the tunica albuginea. The testes consist mainly of seminiferous tubules, which account for 85%–90% of the testicular volume. The gametes (spermatozoa) are produced by the Sertoli cells, which are situated within the walls of the seminiferous tubules. Sertoli cells are attached to the basement membrane and extend with maturity into the lumen of the seminiferous tubule. The Sertoli cells form a blood testicular barrier which is impermeable to large molecules.

The testicular parenchyma is divided into 200–300 lobules by septa made of connective tissue. The lobules each contain two or three convoluted seminiferous tubules which are individually approximately 50 cm in length. The newly formed sperm flow through the tubules, which eventually merge to form the rete testis in the hilum. The spermatozoa then pass into the epididymis via efferent ducts from the mediastinum of the hilum. The epididymis is divided into the head (caput), the body (corpus), and the tail (cauda). In the epididymis, the sperm mature, acquiring the potential for fertilization and forward motility. The sperm are then stored in the cauda, where they remain immotile, prior to ejaculation. During ejaculation, the vas deferens via peristalsis transports the sperm through the tract, where seminal fluid is increased by secretions from the prostate, the seminiferous vesicles, and other accessory glands. The sperm acquire motility and further mature during the transit through the genital tract.

Full maturation of the sperm occurs in the female reproductive tract through a process known as capacitation.

Leydig cells, which synthesize and secrete testosterone, are situated between the seminiferous tubules.

Physiology
Hypothalamo-pituitary–testicular axis
Testosterone is mainly (95%) synthesized and secreted but not stored by the Leydig cells of the testis. The remaining testosterone is produced by the zona reticularis of the adrenal cortex. The testis produces and releases approximately 5–7 mg of testosterone per day into the circulation. Testosterone is synthesized from cholesterol via the biochemical pathway shown in Figure 8.1.

Testosterone synthesis and secretion is dependent on the pulsatile release of GnRH from the hypothalamus; this, in turn, stimulates pulses of LH and FSH from the gonadotrophs of the anterior pituitary (see Figure 8.2). Kisspeptin is a neuropeptide released by hypothalamic neurons in the arcuate and antero-ventral periventricular nuclei which initiate and control pusatile GnRH secretion. LH stimulates testosterone synthesis and secretion by a direct action on the LH receptor, increasing intracellular cAMP. FSH has a negligible effect on testosterone production. Although hCG is not normally produced in males, it can stimulate the LH receptor. This is clinically important in men who develop hCG-secreting testicular tumours and is used pharmacologically to stimulate testosterone production and release in

puberty and in adult secondary hypogonadism. In the latter condition, hCG can stimulate spermatogenesis in post-pubertal onset of secondary hypogonadism. Prepubertal onset invariably requires adjunctive therapy with FSH. Testosterone then exerts a negative feedback on both the hypothalamus and the pituitary. Prolactin inhibits GnRH release from the hypothalamus. This is clinically important, as hyperprolactinaemia leads to hypogonadotrophic hypogonadism by suppression of the hypothalamo-pituitary–testicular axis. Chronic glucocorticoid administration inhibits LH-induced cAMP-mediated testosterone release. Chronic opioid therapy also suppresses testosterone production by an inhibitory action at all three levels of the hypothalamo-pituitary-testicular axis, with the central effect being dominant.

FSH stimulates the release of inhibin from Sertoli cells. Inhibin, which exists in two forms (A and B), negatively feeds back at the level of the pituitary, suppressing FSH synthesis and secretion. Inhibin does not affect GnRH release. Activin produced in the testes and pituitary stimulates FSH synthesis and secretion.

Serum testosterone has a circadian rhythm, with highest levels in the early morning (06:00–08:00 h)

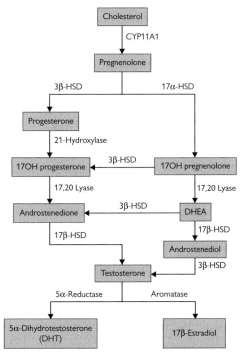

Fig 8.1 Pathway of testosterone synthesis and metabolism. Note that testosterone is also broken down to form inactive metabolites; DHEA, dehydroepiandrosterone; HSD, hydroxysteroid dehydrogenase.
Reproduced from Jones H, *Testosterone Deficiency in Men, Second edition*, Fig. 2.2, p. 12. Copyright © 2012 with permission from Oxford University Press.

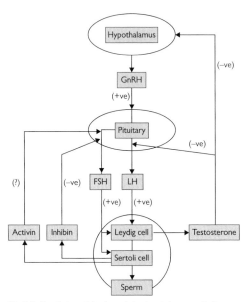

Fig 8.2 Regulation of the hypothalamic–pituitary–testicular axis; −ve; +ve; FSH, follicle-stimulating hormone; GnRH, gonadotrophin-releasing hormone; LH, luteinizing hormone. Reproduced from Jones H, *Testosterone Deficiency in Men, Second edition*, Fig. 2.3, p. 13. Copyright © 2012 with permission from Oxford University Press.

and lowest levels in the early evening (18:00–20:00 h). The biological function of this circadian rhythm is not understood. Fit and healthy men maintain this circadian rhythm at least up to their seventh decade. Circulating testosterone is comprised of three major components: free testosterone (2%–3%), albumen-bound testosterone (20%–50%), and SHBG-bound testosterone (50%–80%). The relative proportions of each of these fractions varies between individuals. Free testosterone has a half-life of 10 minutes, so it has to be rapidly replenished from the albumen-bound testosterone. Testosterone is tightly bound to SHBG and is therefore considered to be mainly biologically inactive, although there is some evidence that SHBG-binding sites are present on cell membranes. Free testosterone and albumen-bound testosterone are considered to be biologically active or bioavailable testosterone. Levels of free and bioavailable testosterone have been shown to correlate more closely with known biological actions of testosterone (e.g. bone turnover, muscle strength, erectile function, and cardiac ischaemia) than levels of total testosterone do.

Testosterone is metabolized either to 17-beta-estradiol (by the action of aromatase) or to dihydrotestosterone (by 5-alpha-reductase), both of which are active metabolites. It is important to recognize that the metabolism of testosterone is tissue specific; for example, in the prostate, it is preferentially converted to dihydrotestosterone whereas, in adipose tissue, it is preferentially converted to estradiol. Testosterone is also converted to inactive substances which are excreted by the kidneys and liver. Approximately 2% of natural testosterone is excreted in the urine.

Androgen receptor

The gene for the androgen receptor is situated on the long arm of the X chromosome. The majority of the biological actions of testosterone and dihydrotestosterone are mediated through the androgen receptor. The androgen receptor is a nuclear receptor which is a member of a large superfamily of master regulators of nuclear transcription factors; this family also includes the retinoid X receptor, PPAR alpha, PPAR gamma, and the liver X receptor. Testosterone binds to the androgen receptor in the cytosol and is then transported to the nucleus, where the complex acts as a transcription factor, binding to specific target genes. Coactivators enhance the binding of testosterone. Androgen binding to the androgen receptor can rapidly affect signal transduction pathways within the cytoplasm.

In the transactivation domain of the androgen receptor (Exon 1), there is a clinically relevant CAG repeat polymorphism which encodes for a variable-length polyglutamine stretch. The number of CAG repeats varies between 9 and 35 in the population. The lower the number of repeats, the greater is the sensitivity of the androgen receptor. Men with a more sensitive androgen receptor are more likely to have higher sperm concentrations, increased bone mineral density, and lower HDL cholesterol and are at greater risk of benign prostatic hypertrophy and prostate carcinoma. Men with a less sensitive androgen receptor have a higher BMI, a higher waist circumference, greater body fat content, and higher leptin and insulin levels. Having a less sensitive androgen receptor is associated with higher testosterone and LH levels, as a homeostatic adjustment for androgenic bioactivity. Importantly, the CAG repeat number predicts the severity of the phenotypic features in Klinefelter's syndrome (the greater the number of repeats, the worse is the phenotype; see also Sections 8.2 and 8.3). Expansion of the CAG repeat number to greater than 35 increases the risk of Kennedy's syndrome. This is a rare disorder presenting in the fifth decade with motor neuron loss in the spinal cord and the brainstem, leading to progressive neuromuscular weakness, hypogonadism, and diabetes.

Androgen-receptor-independent actions

Testosterone has been shown to have rapid direct effects on ion channels in vascular smooth muscle cells, macrophages, and T cells. For example, testosterone is an L-channel calcium blocker (which binds at the nifedipine binding site) in vascular smooth muscle cells and may account in part for testosterone-induced arterial vasodilatation.

Age

In the average population, mean levels of testosterone fall by 1%–2% annually. Healthy, active men are less likely to demonstrate significant falls but those with obesity and/or one or more co-morbidities have greater reductions in testosterone. Assessment of androgen status using total testosterone is confounded by increasing SHBG with free testosterone declining more significantly (see Figure 8.3).

Obesity

Obesity is associated with a higher prevalence of low testosterone levels, with increased percentage body fat also being a clinical feature of hypogonadism. This can be explained by the hypogonadal–obesity–adipocytokine hypothesis (see Figure 8.4). Adipose tissue, in particular central fat, secretes pro-inflammatory adipocytokines

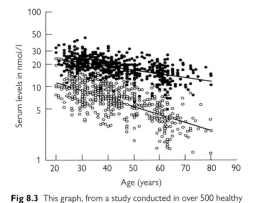

Fig 8.3 This graph, from a study conducted in over 500 healthy men, demonstrates the relation of advancing age to lower testosterone levels. The observation is markedly stronger in bioavailable testosterone, as sex hormone-binding globulins increase with advancing age.
Reproduced from Leifke E, Gorenol V, Wichers C et al., Age-related changes of serum sex hormones, insulin-like growth factor-1 and sex hormone-binding globulin levels in men: cross-sectional data from a healthy male cohort, *Clinical Endocrinology*, Volume 53, pp. 689–695, Copyright (2000) with permission from John Wiley and Sons.

(TNF alpha, interleukin 6), which inhibit the hypothalamo-pituitary release of LH and can cause hypothalamic leptin resistance in human obesity, and leptin, which suppresses testosterone secretion via a direct inhibitory action on the testes. Furthermore, increased aromatase activity in fat converts testosterone to 17-beta-estradiol. A 'tipping point' is reached when homeostatic mechanisms fail to maintain normal testosterone levels. Significant weight loss (>10%) can increase total testosterone levels by 2–4 nmol/L (58–115 ng/L), whereas bariatric surgery can raise testosterone by up to 10 nmol/L (288 ng/dL).

Type 2 Diabetes
Testosterone deficiency is common in men with type 2 diabetes (up to 42% and other clinical states of insulin resistance e.g. obesity and metabolic syndrome. Insulin resistance is the central biochemical defect in type 2 diabetes. Testosterone replacement improves insulin sensitivity hence reducing insulin resistance. There is in vitro evidence that testosterone improves pathways of glucose utilisation.

Biological functions
Metabolic and vascular health
Normal tissue androgenization has a fundamental role in inducing insulin sensitivity and controlling carbohydrate utilization. In addition, testosterone has beneficial

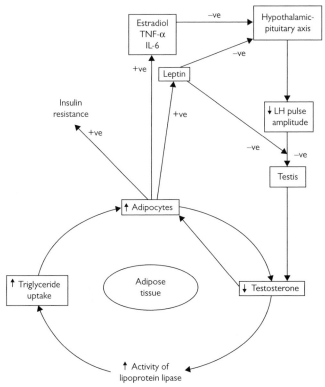

Fig 8.4 The hypogonadal–obesity–adipocytokine cycle hypothesis; −ve, negative; +ve, positive; IL-6, interleukin 6; LH, luteinizing hormone; TNF-α, tumour necrosis factor alpha.
Reproduced from Jones H, *Testosterone Deficiency in Men, Second edition*, Fig. 11.3, p. 103. Copyright © 2012 with permission from Oxford University Press.

effects on lipid, cholesterol, and protein metabolism. Testosterone stimulates erythropoiesis by primarily inducing differentiation of erythroid progenitor cells and promoting erythropoietin release. Anaemia can be a feature of hypogonadism. Testosterone is an arterial vasodilator. Testosterone deficiency is associated with hypertension, cardiovascular disease, and chronic cardiac failure. Testosterone deficiency is associated with a prolonged QT interval and an increased association with atrial fibrillation. The QT length can be shortened by testosterone therapy and evidence has shown that this may occur by direct stimulation of opening of ultrarapid potassium channels. Testosterone also activated carotid sinus baroreceptors.

Sexual health

Testosterone is important for a normal libido, with the loss or reduction of libido being the most common symptom related to hypogonadism. Erectile function is dependent on a normal androgen milieu. Animal studies have demonstrated that testosterone is essential for the maintenance of the normal morphology and function of vascular smooth muscle cells, penile blood flow of the corpus cavernosum, nerve function, elasticity of the tunica albuginea, and effacement of the engorged cavernosal vessels against the tunica on erection to prevent venous leak (low testosterone leads to fat cells being formed between these tissues). Testosterone deficiency is associated with venous leak due to this deposition of fat. Reduced vascular reactivity, neuronal function and increased stiffness of the tunica albuginea. In humans, there is a higher rate of phosphodiesterase 5 (PDE5) inhibitor therapy failure rate in untreated men with hypogonadism. Testosterone treatment convert over half of men with sildenafil failure to responders. In addition, it is clinically relevant that erectile dysfunction is a marker of ill health and may be the first symptom of cardiovascular disease.

Testosterone promotes prostate growth to achieve normal prostate size and function.

Bone and muscle health

Testosterone stimulates the accretion of bone mass in puberty, with peak bone mass being reached between 20 and 22 years of age. Testosterone and its conversion to 17-beta-estradiol is important for the maintenance of bone density in the adult. Testosterone also plays an essential role in epiphyseal closure. Prepubertal onset of hypogonadism is associated with lower peak bone mass and, in some instances, excessive height. In men, oestrogens are the major hormones involved in normal bone biology. Aromatase deficiency or malfunction or lack of estradiol receptors is associated with osteoporosis.

Testosterone is involved in the development and maintenance of muscle mass, strength, and power. Testosterone promotes the differentiation of multipotent mesenchymal cells to form myocytes and enable protein synthesis within the cells. In particular, testosterone stimulates hypertrophy of both type 1 and type 2 muscle fibres.

Neurological health

Normal testosterone is essential for the development and function of the brain in early life (fetal, neonatal, and pubertal), as well as maintenance of normal function in adult life. In particular, testosterone is involved in sexual behaviour and cognitive function such as, for example, visuospatial ability, verbal memory, mathematical ability, mental acuity, and concentration. Testosterone is also important for mood.

8.2 Investigation

Genetic

Chromosomal analysis
Chromosomal analysis should be performed in men with primary hypogonadism without an identified aetiology.

Klinefelter's syndrome
The commonest cause of primary hypogonadism is Klinefelter's syndrome (see also Section 8.3), which has a prevalence of 1 in 500 male births. Men with Klinefelter's syndrome have more than one X chromosome. The commonest chromosomal complement is 47, XXY, which occurs in 90% of cases (see Figure 8.5). There are also variant forms which include mosaic types, for example, 47, XXY/46, XY; also, 48, XXY and 49, XXXY may occur. Diagnosis is therefore made by karyotyping from a blood sample (taken in EDTA). The diagnosis can also be made via the detection of Barr bodies from a mouth mucosal swab sample. The Barr body represents the extra X chromosome.

Only 75% of men with Klinefelter's syndrome are diagnosed in life and many of those who are diagnosed are >20 years old. The reason why some men are not diagnosed is that symptoms may be mild. Men with Klinefelter's syndrome have an increased risk of type 2 diabetes and hospitalization due to respiratory infections and have an increased mortality compared to a healthy male population.

XX male syndrome, variant of Klinefelter's syndrome, occurs in 1 in 20,000 male births. In 75% of those affected, part of the Y chromosome has translocated to one end of an X chromosome; as the translocated region contains *SRY*, which is involved in the development of the testis, these cases are termed 'SRY positive'. SRY-positive men are more virilized than SRY-negative men.

The latter have a greater incidence of undescended testes and hypospadias.

XYY syndrome
Men with XXY syndrome have a normal phenotype and usually no evidence of hypogonadism but may have delayed puberty. However, some may require testosterone substitution.

Noonan's syndrome
In Noonan's syndrome, men have clinical features similar to those seen in Turner's syndrome (e.g. webbed neck, short stature, low-set ears) and small testes size or cryptorchidism. They have a normal chromosome complement.

Mixed gonadal dysgenesis: 45, X0/46, XY
Men with mixed gonadal dysgenesis mainly have a female phenotype but some have a male phenotype. The gonads are located in the abdomen.

Gene analysis
Androgen receptor defects and mutations
Androgen insensitivity syndrome, also known as testicular feminization, is where cells have partial or complete inability of cells to respond to androgens. The karyotype in this syndrome is XY. Androgen receptor gene sequencing may identify a mutation but the absence of such a mutation does not exclude the condition, especially in the partial form of the disease.

Androgen receptor defects which result in androgen insensitivity syndrome occur as a result of inherited or spontaneous mutations. Inherited androgen insensitivity syndrome is caused by an X-chromosome recessive transmission. A large number of different mutations have been identified and amount to an excess of 250.

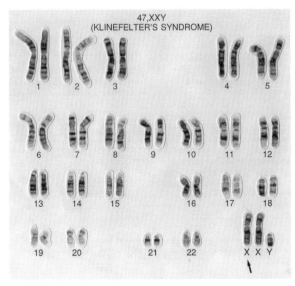

Fig 8.5 Klinefelter's syndrome XXY karyotype.
Klinefelter's syndrome karyotype 47,XXY' by Wessex Reg. Genetics Centre. https://wellcomecollection.org/works/sdyubqf2?query=xxy+chromosomes+klinefelter%27s+syndrome. Creative Commons Attribution (CC BY 4.0) terms and conditions https://creativecommons.org/licenses/by/4.0.

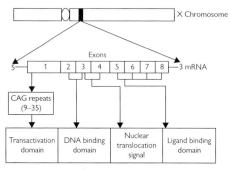

Fig 8.6 The androgen receptor gene on the X chromosome in Section Xq11–12, which encodes eight exons. The androgen receptor has four main functional domains, which comprise (1) the transactivation domain, which, in the inactive state, binds chaperone proteins, which optimize ligand affinity, and in the active state, binds co-activator proteins, which enhance ligand binding; (2) a DNA-binding domain with two zinc fingers; (3) a nuclear translocation signal, to transport the active receptor from the cytosol to the nucleus; and (4) a ligand-binding domain. Reproduced from Jones H, *Testosterone Deficiency in Men, Second edition*, Fig. 2.4, p. 15. Copyright © 2012 with permission from Oxford University Press.

The CAG-repeat polymorphism occurs in Exon 1 of the androgen receptor (see Figure 8.6). In men with symptoms of hypogonadism with elevated LH and low to mid-normal total testosterone, a long number of CAG repeats indicating a less sensitive androgen receptor may explain the clinical presentation.

Kennedy's syndrome may be confirmed in the presence of >38 CAG repeats (see Section 8.1, 'Androgen receptor', p. 240).

Defects of testosterone synthesis
Conditions involving defects of testosterone synthesis are autosomal recessive and are rare. Gene mutations can affect the following enzymes:
- 17-alpha-hydroxylase
- 3-beta-hydroxysteroid dehydrogenase

Kallmann's syndrome and isolated hypogonadotrophic hypogonadism
See also Section 8.4. These syndromes can occur sporadically as well as be inherited.

Kallmann's syndrome (100% associated with anosmia) is caused by an X-linked recessive *KAL1* mutation.

In the case of isolated hypogonadotrophic hypogonadism, most common mutations are either autosomal dominant with variable penetrance (*FGFR1*), or autosomal recessive (*GNRHR* and *KISS1*). Other gene mutations have been identified but are less common.

Biochemical

Total testosterone
Total testosterone is a good predictor of hypogonadism but an assessment of free and/or bioavailable testosterone is required in borderline cases.

Testosterone should be measured between 06:00 h and 11:00 h, when production is highest. Reference ranges are based on morning levels. Testosterone production can be as much as 25%–40% lower in the afternoon and

evening; therefore, blood taken at this time can lead to misdiagnosis. The timing of assessment should be used in older as well as younger men, as the circadian rhythm can persist into later life.

A diagnosis of hypogonadism can only be made based on at least two testosterone values taken 1 week apart, as levels can be affected by viral and other infections and inflammation. If the testosterone results are borderline, further measurements (up to five) may be needed to support a diagnosis.

It is not appropriate to measure testosterone in the presence of acute systemic illness, as inflammatory cytokines inhibit the hypothalamo-pituitary–testicular axis, resulting in significant suppression of testosterone.

Testosterone is currently measured in the majority of laboratories by fully automated, multichannel immunoassay analysers. As testosterone assays differ between assay kits and between hospital laboratories, there is no definitive normal range. It is advised that a healthy normal range should be used for each assay (based on a morning testosterone before 1100 h), which should be used for all age groups. In the male range for testosterone, the Endocrine Society (US) concluded that most assays available had adequate sensitivity and were reasonable for use for clinical diagnosis. There is, however, an increasing use of mass spectroscopy, which provides a more sensitive and specific assessment of testosterone levels. It is important that individual laboratories develop their own reference range based on a normal local population sample. The majority of assays give ranges of the order of ~8–35 nmol/L (~231–1009 ng/dL).

SHBG
Total testosterone is affected by changes in SHBG levels. SHBG should therefore be measured when total testosterone is in the low borderline range (6–12 nmol/L (173–346 ng/dL)), in conditions known to affect SHBG and in cases with classical symptoms with or without elevated gonadotrophins, as the SHBG levels could be very high in these. SHBG levels increases with age and decrease with obesity and states of insulin resistance (e.g. metabolic syndrome and type 2 diabetes; other factors are listed in Table 8.1). SHBG levels can thus be used to calculate free and bioavailable testosterone.

Free and bioavailable testosterone
In routine clinical practice, free and/or bioavailable testosterone is calculated using published equations derived

Table 8.1 Parameters which affect sex hormone-binding globulin levels

Low SHBG	Raised SHBG
Obesity	Age
Insulin resistance	Smoking
Type 2 diabetes	Oestrogens
Metabolic syndrome	Anticonvulsants
Glucocorticoids	HIV
Atorvastatin	Acromegaly
Hypothyroidism	Thyrotoxicosis
Anabolic steroids	Liver cirrhosis
Low albumin states (nephrotic syndrome)	

Abbreviations: SHBG, sex hormone-binding globulin.

from regression analysis. These require values for measured testosterone and SHBG, with or without albumen. The most commonly used and accessible equations are those formulated by Vermeulen (http://www.issam.ch/freetesto.htm). The calculated values will depend on the assay measurements of total testosterone and SHBG. Ideally, a normal range for the calculated free testosterone should be produced for individual laboratories. However, when calculating free testosterone based on the Vermeulen formula, it is generally accepted that a level <225 pmol/L (6 ng/dL) provides supportive evidence for a diagnosis of hypogonadism.

Free testosterone can be assayed using equilibrium dialysis and bioavailable testosterone ammonium sulphate precipitation assays. However, these are time-consuming, not routinely available, and usually but not always confined to research laboratories.

Analogue assays for free testosterone are available but are affected by SHBG levels and inaccurate.

The free androgen index [100 × (total testosterone/SHBG)] was derived from female testosterone levels, not male. It has been shown to be a poor predictor of bioavailable testosterone and hypogonadism in men and should only be used in women.

LH and FSH

LH and FSH should be measured in all subjects investigated for hypogonadism. LH and FSH levels above the normal range are consistent with primary hypogonadism. In secondary hypogonadism, LH levels are low or in the low normal range. These levels are inappropriate for a low testosterone states. Undetectable LH and FSH indicate that there is profound hypogonadism and that a classical cause of pituitary failure such as pituitary adenoma is likely.

Prolactin

Prolactin should be measured in all subjects with LH and FSH levels below or in the low-normal range. Hyperprolactinaemia suppresses the hypothalamo-pituitary production of LH and FSH. Elevated prolactin should be confirmed with cannulated prolactin measurement to exclude the effect of stress at time of the venepuncture.

17-Beta-estradiol

17-Beta-estradiol should be measured in the presence of gynaecomastia. Osteoporosis in a younger male may be caused by either aromatase deficiency or estradiol receptor resistance. Causes of elevated 17-beta-estradiol include obesity, adrenal adenomas, adrenal carcinomas, testicular tumours, (Leydig and Sertoli cell), chorionic carcinomas, hepatomas, androgen resistance, cirrhosis, thyrotoxicosis, oestrogen receptor defects, hCG, anti-androgens, and anti-oestrogen therapy. On testosterone gel therapy if the testosterone level is elevated this could be due to skin contamination of the gel over the venepuncture site. If this is the case then estradiol levels will be low. Also estradiol levels are elevated in association with high testosterone then this confirms the testosterone dose is too high. If the estradiol is low or normal with a high testosterone this should be repeated as there may be variable testosterone absorption.

Anterior pituitary hormones

In the presence of hypogonadotrophic hypogonadism, patients should be assessed for evidence of other pituitary hormone deficiencies (e.g. levels of FT4, TSH, prolactin, cortisol and IGF-1, as well as a short Synacthen® test for secondary adrenocortical insufficiency).

Ferritin

Haemochromatosis is a cause of primary and secondary hypogonadism. Serum ferritin should be measured in these conditions. If the ferritin level is elevated, blood should be sent for haemochromatosis gene analysis.

Diabetes and cardiovascular disease

There is a high prevalence of hypogonadism and erectile dysfunction in type 2 diabetes (up to 70%) and cardiovascular disease. Fasting blood glucose, glycated haemoglobin, and a fasting lipid profile should be assessed.

Liver and renal function

Liver disease (including haemochromatosis) and renal failure are both associated with low testosterone.

hCG

hCG should be assayed in men with elevation of testosterone to diagnose or exclude an hCG-secreting testicular tumour.

Safety Tests

A full blood count for haematocrit and haemoglobin. PSA to screen for prostate cancer.

Box 8.1 Diagnosis of hypogonadism

In the presence of symptoms of hypogonadism:
- total testosterone <8 nmol/L (231 ng/dL) is consistent with hypogonadism
- total testosterone 8–12 nmol/L (213–346 ng/dL)[†‡] could have hypogonadism and may respond to testosterone replacement
- total testosterone >12 nmol/L (346 ng/dL) does not generally support the diagnosis, unless LH and FSH levels are elevated, or there is a previously-documented testosterone level that was significantly higher (e.g. prior to pituitary surgery, or radiotherapy)

[†] A calculated free testosterone level <220 pmol/L (6.3 ng/dL) in the presence of reduced libido, erectile dysfunction, and loss of morning erections supports the diagnosis of hypogonadism.
[‡] Those with a total testosterone level <10.4 nmol/L (300 ng/dL) are more likely to be at risk of bone loss and increased body fat deposition.
Abbreviations: FSH, follicle-stimulating hormone; LH, luteinizing hormone.
Note: Total testosterone suggested cut-off values should be adjusted for those assay ranges which significantly differ from those more commonly used.

Interpretation of testosterone results

Hypogonadism

Hypogonadism is a clinical syndrome complex which includes symptoms with or without clinical signs and biochemical evidence of testosterone deficiency.

Consensus meetings and published guidelines have agreed criteria for a diagnosis of hypogonadism (Box 8.1). The European Male Ageing Study has shown that a total testosterone <11 nmol/L (317 ng/dL) and a calculated free testosterone <220 pmol/L (6.3 ng/dL; see Box 8.1) in the presence of at least three sexual symptoms of testosterone deficiency (loss or reduced libido, lack of morning erections, erectile dysfunction) defines a diagnosis of late-onset hypogonadism.

A diagnosis of hypogonadism is supported by either elevated or low levels of LH and FSH. Increased FSH with high normal LH also supports a diagnosis of primary testicular failure. FSH levels correlate inversely with spermatogenesis, with higher levels being linked to germinal cell failure. There may be sufficient Leydig cell function to maintain testosterone production. A finding of normal LH and FSH in the presence of low or low normal testosterone is consistent with secondary or hypogonadotrophic hypogonadism, demonstrating an inability of the hypothalamo-pituitary insufficiency to maintain a normal androgen environment. LH and FSH levels below or in the low-normal range indicate a greater likelihood of a structural lesion or an infiltrative or inflammatory cause affecting the hypothalamic and pituitary tissues. The presence of a pituitary or parasellar neoplasm is more likely but not exclusively to be found when the total testosterone level is less than 5 nmol/L (144 ng/dL), in the presence or absence of other anterior pituitary hormone deficiencies. Testosterone can also be low due to excess prolactin (hyperprolactinaemia) and cortisol (Cushing's syndrome) production.

Elevated testosterone

The most common cause of an elevated testosterone level is the abuse of testosterone-containing preparations. It is important to recognize that several anabolic steroids are not detected by the measurement of serum testosterone. Anabolic steroid abuse is associated with an elevated haematocrit and suppressed gonadotrophin levels.

An elevated testosterone in the presence of raised LH and FSH occurs in the presence of androgen resistance. Further investigation with genetic analysis is indicated.

Raised testosterone with low LH and FSH can be associated with an hCG-secreting tumour of the testis or a testosterone-secreting adrenal tumour.

Semen analysis

Semen analysis is not normally part of the clinical workup of a subject with hypogonadism. The indications for semen analysis are usually infertility, and when an individual wanting to know his potential for fertility requests the test. Counselling the patient prior to the test and after the results is important. Abnormalities of semen may be found in any subject with hypogonadism; however, the semen analysis may be normal. A guide to the interpretation of semen analyses is provided in Box 8.2.

Imaging

MRI pituitary

Pituitary imaging should be considered in all patients with secondary hypogonadism. A pituitary macroadenoma or parasellar mass is more likely to be present when

---

Box 8.2 Semen analysis: Basic WHO criteria (more detailed testing may be required)

Lower reference limits for semen characteristics (between 2 and 7 days of abstinence)
Volume of ejaculate: >1.5 mL
  Sperm concentration: >15 × 10⁶ spermatozoa/mL
  Total spermatozoa count per ejaculate: >39 × 10⁶
  Total motility: >40% spermatozoa (progressive + non-progressive motility) or >32% with progressive motility
  Normal sperm morphology: >4%
  Vitality: >58% of sperm
  Leucocytes: <1 × 10⁶/mL
  Seminal neutral glucosidase: >20 mU/ejaculate
  Fructose: >13 µmol/ejaculate
  Zinc: >2.4 µmol/ejaculate

Common abnormalities
Oligospermia: <15 × 10⁶ spermatozoa/mL
  Asthenozoospermia: <32% spermatozoa with progressive motility
  Teratozoospermia: <4% spermatozoa with normal morphology Oligoasthenoteratospermia: all of the three components described above
  Azoospermia: no spermatozoa
  Absent ejaculate (aspermia)

Adapted from *WHO laboratory manual for the examination and processing of human semen*, Fifth edition, World Health Organization, Department of Reproductive Health and Research, pp. 224. © World Health Organization 2010.

---

testosterone levels are less than 5 nmol/L (144 ng/dL) or when low testosterone is associated with deficiency of other anterior pituitary hormones. MRI should also be performed in men with hyperprolactinaemia and symptoms of headache, visual disturbance, visual field defect, or any other clinical symptoms or signs suggestive of a mass effect.

The congenital condition combined pituitary hormone deficiency, which may present in adulthood as well as childhood, can be associated with sellar hypoplasia and/or an ectopic posterior bright spot.

There is, however, no clear guidance as to whether or not an MRI pituitary scan should be carried out in men with isolated hypogonadotrophic hypogonadism. When levels of LH and FSH are both below the normal range, most endocrinologists would arrange a scan. Certainly, imaging should be done in subjects with delayed puberty and low levels of gonadotrophins. There is no evidence that, in the normal range of LH and FSH, there is a cut-off level determining where imaging should or should not be performed. With no evidence, individual clinical opinion is important; however, many endocrinologists would scan patients with LH and FSH in the low normal range (e.g. LH and FSH below 4 IU/L). Structural lesions in the pituitary may be detected but are less likely to require intervention, although they can at least identify a cause for the hypogonadism (e.g. partial or complete empty sella syndrome).

CT pituitary

If a patient cannot tolerate an MRI scan under normal or general anaesthesia, due to claustrophobia or medical co-morbidities, then, if there is a high index of clinical suspicion of a mass lesion, a CT pituitary should be considered.

MRI brain
Normally, the brain is visualized at pituitary scanning. However, it is important to recognize that, in the conditions of Kallmann's syndrome and septo-optic dysplasia, abnormalities may be identified. These include hypoplasia of the visual and olfactory pathways. The corpus callosum may be absent in Kallmann's syndrome.

Ultrasound genito-urinary tract
Testes
Ultrasound would provide an accurate assessment of testicular volume and position of the testes. In the presence of lumps found on palpation, ultrasound is the investigation of choice to determine their nature. Abnormalities detected will include tumours within the testes, epididymal cysts, hydroceles, spermatoceles, and post-vasectomy changes. There is an increased prevalence of testicular tumours found in men presenting to infertility clinics. Hyperechoic changes within the testis can indicate fibrotic change after orchitis. Microlithiasis may also be present. Extra-testicular neoplasms may also be found which are usually benign adenomatoid lesions or lipomas.

Varicoceles can also be identified and show increased drainage of the veins (i.e. a flow reversal) during a Valsalva manoeuvre.

Inguinal region
Inguinal region imaging may be used for the detection of undescended testes.

Renal
Renal imaging will show absent kidneys and horseshoe kidneys, which may occur in Kallmann's syndrome.

Prostate
Ultrasound of the prostate may be required before or after initiation of testosterone replacement therapy to assess prostate size if there are symptoms of prostatic enlargement.

Cavernosography
Cavernosography is used in erectile dysfunction to demonstrate venous leakage which could be as a result of hypogonadism. Contrast medium is introduced into the corpus cavernosum at a high flow rate. This abnormality can be corrected by testosterone replacement therapy. This test should only be arranged by a urologist if required.

Bone age
Hand X-rays
Bone age is assessed by hand X-rays in delayed puberty, to determine whether or not there is a retardation of bone age compared to chronological age. The left hand is used for assessment. This may occur in constitutional delayed puberty as well as prepubertal onset of permanent types of hypogonadism, such as congenital (e.g. Kallmann's syndrome) and acquired (e.g. trauma, tumours, radiotherapy) disorders. Bone age is assessed by using Greulich and Pyle charts.

Suspected slipped capital epiphysis
Hip X-ray
Adolescent males with hypogonadism may present with pain in the hip or thigh and difficulty walking usually with a limp. X-ray of the hip demonstrates a slipped capital femoral epiphysis.

Suspected vertebral fracture or osteoporosis
Thoracic and lumbosacral spine X-ray
Plain X-rays of the spine may show evidence of osteoporosis, loss of vertebral height, fracture, and/or kyphoscoliosis.

Bone mineral density
DXA is used for the assessment of fracture risk in male hypogonadism. The presence of osteoporosis in a man with hypogonadism supports the requirement of testosterone replacement therapy. Interval DXA scanning, usually every 2 years, is used to monitor the effect of therapy on bone density. DXA can also assess the percentage body fat and lean mass, although this is not used routinely at present in the clinic.

All men with hypogonadism should have a DXA scan performed on diagnosis. If osteoporosis is present or there has been a low trauma fracture, it is recommended that interval DXA scans are performed every 1–2 years after initiation of testosterone replacement therapy, based on clinical need. Testosterone therapy increases vertebral but not femoral neck bone density. No studies have been performed to determine whether testosterone treatment reduces fracture risk. Bisphosphonates or other treatments for osteoporosis may be required.

Further reading

Achermann JC and Hughes IA. 'Disorders of sex development', in Melmed S, Polonsky KS, Reed Larsen PR, et al., Williams Textbook of Endocrinology (12th edition), 2011. Saunders, pp. 886–934.

Bhasin S, Cunningham GR, Hayes FJ, et al. Testosterone therapy in men with androgen deficiency syndromes: An Endocrine Society clinical practice guideline. *J Clin Endocrinol Metab* 2010; 95: 2536–59.

deRonde W, van der Schouw YT, and Pols HA. Calculation of bioavailable and free testosterone in men: A comparison of 5 published algorithms. *Clin Chem* 2006; 53: 1777–84.

Dohle GR, Arver S, Bettochi C, et al. EAU guidelines on male hypogonadism, 2017. Available at http://www.uroweb.org/guideline/male-hypogonadism/ (accessed 16 March 2018).

Ferreira L, Silveira G, and Latronico AC. Approach to the patient with hypogonadotrophic hypogonadism. *J Clin Endocrinol Metab* 2013; 98: 1781–88.

Jones, TH, ed. Testosterone Deficiency in Men (2nd edition), 2013. Oxford University Press.

Jones TH and Kelly DM. Randomized controlled trials - mechanistic studies of testosterone and the cardiovascular system. *Asian J Androl* 2018; 20: 120–30.

Kelly DM and Jones TH. Testosterone and obesity. *Obesity Reviews* 2015; 16: 581–606.

Lewkowitz-Shpuntoff HA, Hughes VA, Plummer L, et al. Olfactory phenotypic spectrum in idiopathic hypogonadotrophic hypogonadism: Pathophysiological and gentic implications. *J Clin Endocrinol Metab* 2012; 97 :E136–44.

Rosner W, Auchus RJ, Azziz R, et al. Position statement: Utility, limitations, pitfalls in measuring testosterone: An Endocrine Society position statement. *J Clin Endocrinol Metab* 2007; 92: 405–13.

Wang C, Nieschlag E, Swerdloff R, et al. Investigation, treatment and monitoring of late-onset hypogonadism. *Eur J Endocrinol* 2008; 159: 507–14.

8.3 Primary hypogonadism

Introduction

In the normal testes, testosterone secretion is governed by the interstitial (Leydig) cells; production of male gametes (spermatogenesis) is governed by the germ cells/seminiferous tubules. Testicular Sertoli cells support and nourish the germ cells and secrete inhibin B. Primary hypogonadism refers the clinical syndrome of testosterone deficiency *and/or* lack of spermatogenesis due to congenital or acquired pathologies that directly damage the testes. The resultant fall in testosterone and inhibin B levels lead to a loss of negative feedback at the hypothalamus/pituitary, and cause supraphysiologic elevation in serum concentrations of LH and FSH (hypergonadotrophic hypogonadism).

Pathophysiology

Primary hypogonadism is more common than organic secondary hypogonadism. Although most testicular diseases damage all testicular cellular components, primary hypogonadism can have variable testicular defects, with spermatogenic failure being affected preferentially over testosterone deficiency. Primary hypogonadism can be either congenital or acquired, but is typically of progressive, post-pubertal onset, even when congenital.

Congenital causes
Klinefelter's syndrome
Klinefelter's syndrome (see Box 8.3) is a genetic disorder representing the most common cause of primary hypogonadism, affecting ~1 in 500–600 live male births. Klinefelter's syndrome results from X chromosomal aneuploidy leading to a classic non-mosaic 47, XXY karyotype in ~90% of cases. The supernumerary X chromosome can be derived equally from a paternal or a maternal meiotic defect. In contrast to the case in other chromosomal aneuploidies, the role of parental age on the likelihood of Klinefelter's syndrome is unclear. The remaining cases have mosaic variants (47, XXY/XY and other rare combinations), double/triple aneuploidies (48, XXXY; XXYY; 49, XXXXY), or structurally abnormal extra X

chromosomes. The number of additional X chromosomes correlates well with disease severity. In some cases, mosaicism may exist only in the testicular tissue.

Testicular histopathology in the classic adult Klinefelter's patient displays total seminiferous tubular atrophy/hyalinization with Leydig cell aplasia and absent germ cells. However, variable patterns can be observed with occasional foci of active spermatogenesis. The precise timing of the onset of germ cell failure/seminiferous tubular atrophy is unclear but accelerated failure is recognized at the time of puberty. Leydig cell failure can be less severe, but Leydig cell function is abnormal, with an increase in oestrogen secretion resulting in gynaecomastia.

The phenotypic spectrum is wide, with classic textbook descriptions reflecting the most severe end of the spectrum. Population-based studies suggest that up to 50% of Klinefelter's males go undetected during their lifetime, although increasing numbers are now presenting, with incidentally found azoospermia during infertility workup.

Other chromosomal abnormalities
XX males (~1 in 20,000 male births) are characterized by a combination of male external genitalia, gonadal differentiation into testes, and a XX karyotype. Nearly 75% of XX males are SRY positive, with Y-chromosome material translocated onto one of the X chromosomes, and clinically resemble those with Klinefelter's syndrome. The remaining patients are SRY negative and so are less virilized and display ambiguous genitalia. In contrast, XYY males are typically normal, although delayed puberty and testosterone therapy may be required in some subjects. Other rare structural chromosomal abnormalities may be present in some men with oligospermia.

Cryptorchidism
Cryptorchidism can be unilateral (commonly, on the right side) or bilateral and is common in preterm infants. Cryptorchid testes are usually palpable in the neck of the scrotum or groin. Congenital cryptorchidism is usually idiopathic, but can be associated with other developmental disorders, chromosomal abnormalities,

---

Box 8.3 Klinefelter's syndrome

Most common cause of primary hypogonadism
   90%: non-mosaic 47, XXY karyotype
   10%: mosaic forms (e.g. 47, XXY/XY); double/triple aneuploidies; structurally abnormal X chromosomes
   (Multiple tissues may need to be sampled if mosaicism is suspected and lymphocyte karyotype is normal; rarely, mosaicism may be limited to the testes)

Clinical features
Absent or delayed puberty (pubertal onset may be normal but may fail to progress)
   Absent/reduced body and sexual hair
   Eunuchoid habitus
   Gynaecomastia (in ~50%)
   Small testes (firm in consistency; usually <2 mL in volume)
   Azoospermia
   Testosterone levels usually frankly hypogonadal but may be normal in some men for many years
   Learning and social skills may be impaired in childhood
   Other disease associations: venous ulcerations, varicose veins, type 2 diabetes, and thyroid disorders
   Increase in overall mortality in adult men with relative increase in incidence of some cancers (mediastinal germ cell tumours, breast cancer, non-Hodgkin's lymphoma, lung cancer)

or congenital disorders of the reproductive endocrine axis (particularly if bilateral). Cryptorchid testes may be associated with spermatogenic defects and infertility in adults, particularly if orchidopexy is delayed, but testosterone secretion is usually unaffected in the absence of an underlying hormonal defect. High malpositioned testes are at increased risk of malignancy.

Anorchia
Anorchia can be unilateral or bilateral (vanishing testes syndrome). Bilateral anorchia must be distinguished from bilateral cryptorchidism by measuring serum anti-Müllerian hormone (undetectable in anorchia) or the more traditional hCG stimulation test (testosterone response is absent in anorchia).

Leydig cell hypoplasia
Males with partially inactivating recessive mutations of the LH receptor present with mild androgen deficiency due to Leydig cell hypoplasia (nota bene: complete inactivating mutations necessarily result in full external feminization).

Myotonic dystrophy
Testicular failure may be present in males with myotonic dystrophy, which is a complex, autosomal-dominant, multisystemic disorder characterized by myotonia, progressive skeletal muscle weakness, premature cataract, diabetes, and muscle wasting.

Acquired causes
Orchitis
Viral orchitis caused by mumps (or, rarely, echovirus (a Group B arbovirus)) may occasionally cause testicular failure if both testes are affected.

Testicular trauma and torsion
Physical trauma to the testes and testicular torsion may cause permanent damage if not treated promptly. Although anti-personnel mines were banned by the 1997 Ottawa Treaty, extensive deployment of IEDs has been a major feature of several ongoing conflicts. IEDs cause focused blast trauma to lower limbs and testes, which are typically unprotected by military-grade body armour.

Radiation damage
Testicular germinal epithelium is extremely sensitive to damage from radiation, as encountered in the treatment of leukaemia and lymphoma. Radiation doses of 15 cGy cause transient loss of spermatogonia, with increasing doses leading to permanent damage to germ cells, and more so with fractionated radiation exposure. Leydig cells are relatively resistant, but permanent damage may occur with doses of 2000–3000 cGy, as would be received in the treatment of acute lymphoblastic leukaemia.

Drugs
Drugs impair testicular function by several mechanisms: inhibition of testosterone synthesis (ketoconazole), antagonism of androgen action (spironolactone), and inhibition of spermatogenesis (chemotherapy). Alcohol intake, especially over long period of time, may impair testicular function through the inhibition of testosterone biosynthesis.

Antineoplastic drugs are particularly gonadotoxic, and the type, dose, and duration determine the degree of damage. Alkylating agents (cyclophosphamide, busulfan) are particularly toxic to germ cells. Almost all men with Hodgkin's lymphoma treated with the MOPP (for meclorethamine, vincristine, procarbazine, and prednisolone) regimen become azoospermic. However, Leydig cells are relatively resistant to antineoplastic agents, and testicular steroidogenesis is often unaffected.

Polyglandular autoimmune insufficiency
See also Chapter 6, Section 6.13. Polyglandular autoimmune insufficiency can result in sperm antibodies and testicular failure.

Systemic diseases
Systemic disease can sometimes cause primary testicular dysfunction, in addition to central inhibition of hypothalamo-pituitary function. This has been described in chronic liver and renal failure, chronic anaemia (sickle cell disease), granulomatous disorders, congestive cardiac failure, and chronic pulmonary disease.

Late-onset hypogonadism
The European Male Ageing Study demonstrated that most of the 'age-related' decline in serum testosterone levels relates to functional secondary hypogonadism caused by obesity and/or chronic disease burden, but the study did identify a small subgroup of men with age-related primary hypogonadism and elevated gonadotrophins, reflecting that, like other organs and body systems, the testes may also accumulate defects at tissue and cellular level with advancing age.

Clinical features
Primary and secondary hypogonadism share similar clinical features, but the precise clinical presentation depends on both the aetiology (e.g. muscle weakness, cataracts, baldness in myotonic dystrophy) and timing of the hypogonadism. Congenital causes of primary hypogonadism (e.g. Klinefelter's syndrome) may present in childhood (although, unlike congenital secondary hypogonadism, only rarely with failure of pubertal initiation), whilst acquired causes usually present in adult life. Neonatal or late in utero testosterone deficiency results in microphallus and/or cryptorchidism (early in utero onset deficiency of testosterone action necessarily results in feminization of external phenotype). Characteristic features of absent or arrested puberty include absent secondary sexual characteristics (e.g. absent/reduced sexual hair, failure of deepening of voice); small testes; absent spermatogenesis; gynaecomastia (~50% of boys with Klinefelter's syndrome); absent pubertal growth spurt; eunuchoidal habitus (long bones fail to fuse, resulting in >5 cm difference in arm span over height, and >5 cm difference in lower body segment over upper body segment); and delayed bone age. Libido is poor, and erections are typically absent but may be present, especially to visual erotic stimuli.

Symptoms and signs of post-pubertal hypogonadism include sexual features (which are more specific) and systemic physical and psychological features (which are often non-specific). Threshold levels of serum total testosterone that lead to post-pubertal symptoms of hypogonadism may vary from individual to individual and also vary for different symptoms. Sexual features include a decrease in facial and body hair; reduced libido; a lack of spontaneous erections; erectile dysfunction; poor ejaculate volume; and/or impaired spermatogenesis. Physical and psychological features include gynaecomastia, decreased muscle mass/strength, hot flushes/sweats, decreased bone density, fatigue, depressed mood, decreased vitality/sense of well-being, impaired concentration/cognition, frailty, increased body fat/BMI, and anaemia. Clinical features specific to Klinefelter's syndrome are shown in Box 8.3

Treatment

Irrespective of the aetiology, once primary hypogonadism is diagnosed, treatment goals are twofold: restoring testosterone levels to physiological levels, and treatment of infertility (spermatogenesis). The latter often poses a considerable clinical challenge, depending on the degree of testicular damage. As the primary defect is in the testes, gonadotrophin/pulsatile GnRH therapy is ineffective in patients with primary hypogonadism. Testosterone replacement therapy is the treatment of choice in these patients. Testosterone replacement therapy is used to initiate puberty in males with pre-pubertal onset of hypogonadism and to protect against the long-term sequelae of testosterone deficiency in males with post-pubertal hypogonadism. The benefits of testosterone replacement therapy in patients with post-pubertal hypogonadism is most pronounced in those with unambiguous frank hypogonadism at initial presentation (serum total testosterone levels <3.5 nmol/L (101 ng/dL)). The testosterone trials have shown that testosterone replacement in 'age-related' hypogonadism may improve sexual function, bone density and anaemia but does not improve vitality or cognition. The most common options for testosterone replacement therapy are described in Table 8.2.

Table 8.2 Testosterone replacement therapy formulations

Intramuscular injections	Usual dose/range	Advantages	Disadvantages
Short-acting esters			
Testosterone propionate, cypionate, enantate, or mixture of esters (Sustanon®)	200 mg/2 weeks	Effective and relatively inexpensive	Peak/trough testosterone level fluctuations
			Gynaecomastia
			Lipid microembolism
Long-acting ester			
Testosterone undecanoate (Nebido®; Aveed® in USA)	1 g[†], followed by 1 g[†] at 6 weeks, followed by 1 g[†] every 10–14 weeks	Stable testosterone levels with no peak/trough fluctuation	Lipid microembolism
Transdermal preparations			
Skin patch:		Stable testosterone levels	Skin irritation
• Androderm®	5–10 mg/day		Redness
			Itching
Transdermal gels:		Stable testosterone levels	Erythema
Testogel®	5–10 mg/day		Raised haematocrit
Testim®	5–10 mg/day		Gynaecomastia
Androgel®	5–10 mg/day		Inadvertent
Androgel® 1.62%	20.25–81 mg/day		Transfer to partners or to children
Fortesta® 2%	10–70 mg/day		
Tostran® 2%	40–60 mg/day		
Axiron® 2% solution	30–120 mg/day		
Oral testosterone			
Testosterone undecanoate	120–160 mg/day	Ease of use	Weak efficacy
			Drug interactions
			Gynaecomastia
Nasal testosterone gel			
Natesto®	33 mg/day	Ease of use	Nasal irritation
		Reduced risk of inadvertent transfer	Long-term safety data not available
Testosterone implants			
Testopel®	100–600 mg/every 4–5 months	Stable testosterone levels	Bleeding
			Extrusion
			Infection

[†] Use 750 mg for Aveed®.

and after testosterone replacement therapy is shown in Box 8.4

Box 8.4 Monitoring testosterone replacement

Clinical workup before testosterone therapy initiation

Absolute contraindications: breast or prostate cancer
  Relative contraindications: severe heart failure, untreated sleep apnoea, raised haematocrit levels
  Men >40 years: prostate evaluation

Clinical monitoring after initiation

At 3, 6, and 12 months: serum total testosterone
  Haematocrit
  Digital prostate exam, PSA (if over 40 years)

Induction of puberty is described in the section on secondary hypogonadism (Section 8.4), because failure to initiate male puberty in primary hypogonadism is exceptionally rare, occurring only when anorchia has developed after in utero sexual differentiation, but before the normal age of pubertal onset.

The choice of the type of testosterone replacement therapy for an individual patient should be based on patient preference, the pharmacokinetic properties of the testosterone replacement therapy preparation, and the side-effect profile. The target serum total testosterone level for testosterone replacement therapy is the mid-normal reference range for young adults (or, for injectables, the lower end of the reference range), but haematocrit, serum LH, and bone density data will also inform therapy adjustments. Indeed, for a younger man with poor bone density, testosterone replacement might sensibly be titrated up to the limit imposed by the haematocrit. The suggested clinical workup of patients before

Treatment of infertility (see also Chapter 9, Section 9.3) due to defective/absent spermatogenesis in patients with primary hypogonadism can be challenging. For some congenital causes, no rational therapies exist. Offending drugs should be withheld whenever possible and any other contributory systemic diseases treated appropriately. Preventative treatment should be considered to preserve fertility in some instances (e.g. treatment of cryptorchidism, gonadal protection, or cryopreservation of sperm during chemo/radiotherapy). ICSI is a therapeutic option for some patients with Klinefelter's syndrome, if sperm is found either in the ejaculate (very rare) or through microtesticular sperm extraction (mTESE). Reports indicate that mTESE may be successful in ~50% of Klinefelter's patients, depending as much on post-surgical sample processing in the andrology laboratory as on patient selection and surgical expertise.

Further reading

Bhasin S and Basaria S. Diagnosis and treatment of hypogonadism in men. *Best Pract Res Clin Endocrinol Metab* 2011; 25: 251–70.

Hugh Jones, T, ed. *Testosterone Deficiency in Men* (2nd edition), 2013. Oxford University Press.

Wass, JAH, Steward PM, Amiel SA et al, eds. 'Part 9: Male hypogonadism and infertility', in Wass, JAH, Steward PM, Amiel SA et al, eds, *Oxford Textbook of Endocrinology and Diabetes* (2nd edition), 2011. Oxford University Press, pp. 1333–483.

Woods DR, Philip R, and Quinton R. Managing endocrine dysfunction following blast injury to the male external genitalia. *JRAMC* 2013; 159 :i45–8.

Wu FC, Tajar A, Beynon JM, et al. Identification of late-onset hypogonadism in middle-aged and elderly men. *N Engl J Med* 2010; 363: 123–35.

8.4 Secondary hypogonadism

Introduction

Normal functioning of the testes requires an intact hypothalamo-pituitary axis. Pulsatile secretion of GnRH by the hypothalamus stimulates the pituitary to secrete two gonadotrophins, LH and FSH, which in turn, govern testicular steroidogenesis and spermatogenetic function, respectively. Secondary hypogonadism refers to clinical conditions in which testicular failure results secondary to disorders of the hypothalamus and/or pituitary, resulting from hypogonadotropism (decreased/absent LH and FSH secretion). In contrast to primary hypogonadism, the serum biochemical profile in these patients show hypogonadotrophic hypogonadism (i.e. low testosterone levels) in the face of inappropriately normal/low LH and FSH levels.

Pathophysiology

Secondary hypogonadism is not a final diagnosis, but requires additional evaluation to identify pituitary or hypothalamic lesions/dysfunction. In contrast to primary hypogonadism, in patients with secondary hypogonadism, the testes themselves are functionally competent and can initiate and maintain steroidogenesis and spermatogenesis upon appropriate exogenous/endogenous gonadotrophin stimulation. Secondary hypogonadism can be congenital or acquired. Whilst congenital secondary hypogonadism is typically organic, acquired secondary hypogonadism can be either organic or functional.

Congenital causes of secondary hypogonadism
Idiopathic hypogonadotrophic hypogonadism
Idiopathic hypogonadotrophic hypogonadism is a rare congenital genetic disorder resulting from an isolated deficiency of hypothalamic GnRH secretion or from defective GnRH action at the pituitary (see Box 8.5). The pituitary is anatomically and functionally intact and no other organic or functional cause for the hypogonadotropism is present. The condition is rare with an incidence of ~1:50,000, with a 3:1 male predominance. Half of the patients also have congenital anosmia, and this association defines Kallmann syndrome. The pathophysiological association between idiopathic hypogonadotrophic hypogonadism and anosmia reflects the combined developmental failure of GnRH neurons and olfactory neurons, which arise and migrate together from the embryonic nasal placode. From their common origin, the GnRH neurons traverse the olfactory axons and enter the forebrain through the cribriform plate and finally coalesce in the medio-basal hypothalamus, where they mature into a neural network delivering pulsatile secretory bursts of GnRH into the hypophyseal portal circulation, eliciting synchronous LH pulses from the pituitary. Any defect in olfactory neuronal development indirectly results in GnRH deficiency.

The remaining ~50% of patients have idiopathic hypogonadotrophic hypogonadism patients with normosmia, a condition referred to as 'normosmic idiopathic hypogonadotrophic hypogonadism'; in these patients, the defect is primarily a neuroendocrine failure of GnRH secretion, without any developmental failure of GnRH migration. Although nearly two-thirds of cases of Kallmann syndrome and normosmic idiopathic hypogonadotrophic hypogonadism occur sporadically, almost all cases are thought to result from mutations in one or more genes governing the developmental and functional ontogeny of GnRH neurons. To date, 20 genes are linked to this condition, with all three traditional modes of inheritance (X linked, autosomal recessive, and autosomal dominant; see Box 8.5). Mutations in some genes may exclusively cause either Kallmann syndrome or normosmic idiopathic hypogonadotrophic hypogonadism, whilst some may cause both forms of idiopathic hypogonadotrophic hypogonadism. More recently, a digenic/oligogenic inheritance has also been documented.

Syndromic idiopathic hypogonadotrophic hypogonadism
In addition to isolated presentations, idiopathic hypogonadotrophic hypogonadism sometimes can be associated with the following syndromic presentations:
- X-linked adrenohypoplasia congenita, idiopathic hypogonadotrophic hypogonadism, and adrenal insufficiency; secondary to DAX1 mutations
- CHARGE syndrome (for coloboma, heart defects, choanal atresia, retardation of growth/development, genitourinary anomalies, and ear abnormalities; secondary to CHD7 mutations)
- childhood-onset congenital obesity with secondary hypogonadism; secondary to LEP, LEPR, and PCSK1 mutations
- obesity, mental retardation, and secondary hypogonadism: Prader–Willi syndrome (deletions in paternally imprinted 15q11.2–12 region) and Bardet–Biedl syndrome (multiple genes)
- Moebius syndrome: Kallmann syndrome with multiple cranial nerve defects (third, fourth, sixth, seventh); secondary to TUBB3 mutations
- Gordon–Holmes syndrome: normosmic idiopathic hypogonadotrophic hypogonadism with cerebellar ataxia; secondary to OTUD4 and RNF216 mutations
- Boucher–Neuhauser syndrome: normosmic idiopathic hypogonadotrophic hypogonadism with cerebellar ataxia and chorioretinal dystrophy; secondary to PNPLA6 mutations

Combined pituitary hormone deficiency
Secondary hypogonadism is sometimes seen in conjunction with multiple pituitary hormone deficiencies. These patients typically have a genetic aetiology, and the phenotype may be either restricted to the pituitary (PROP1 mutations) or associated with extra-pituitary features (mutations in LHX3, SOX2, SOX3, HESX1, FGF8, FGFR1, or PROKR2). Similarly, the clinical presentation can be either severe (neonatal panhypopituitarism) or mild, with progressive, stepwise loss of pituitary hormones during later life.

Acquired secondary hypogonadism
Hypothalamic/pituitary organic diseases
Hypothalamic/pituitary organic diseases are caused by the following:
- tumours (often benign) in the parasellar region: pituitary adenoma (with or without apoplexy), craniopharyngioma, Rathke's cleft cyst, and parasellar

---

Box 8.5 Idiopathic hypogonadotrophic hypogonadism

Rare; incidence: 1:50,000; 3:1 male predominance

Clinical features

Absent or arrested pubertal development (a rare form of adult-onset presentation of hypogonadotrophic hypogonadism has been described)

Microphallus/cryptorchidism (this may prompt evaluation in infancy)

Anosmia or hyposmia is seen in ~50% (Kallmann syndrome), whilst the remaining have normosmic idiopathic hypogonadotrophic hypogonadism

Genetic aetiology

Mutations with the following types of inheritance cause Kallmann syndrome *and/or* normosmic idiopathic hypogonadotrophic hypogonadism (the specific phenotype associated with each mutation is given in parenthesis):

- X-linked inheritance:

  KAL1: causes Kallmann syndrome (mirror movements (synkinesia); unilateral renal agenesis)

- autosomal dominant/digenic inheritance:

  FGF8: Kallmann syndrome/normosmic idiopathic hypogonadotrophic hypogonadism (dental agenesis; midline clefts/bone defects)

  FGFR1: Kallmann syndrome/normosmic idiopathic hypogonadotrophic hypogonadism (dental agenesis; midline clefts/bone defects)

  CHD7: Kallmann syndrome/normosmic idiopathic hypogonadotrophic hypogonadism (deafness)

  SOX10: Kallmann syndrome (deafness)

  SEMA3A: Kallmann syndrome

  WDR11: Kallmann syndrome/normosmic idiopathic hypogonadotrophic hypogonadism

- autosomal recessive/digenic inheritance:

  PROK2: Kallmann syndrome/normosmic idiopathic hypogonadotrophic hypogonadism

  PROKR2: Kallmann syndrome/normosmic idiopathic hypogonadotrophic hypogonadism

  TAC3: normosmic idiopathic hypogonadotrophic hypogonadism

  TACR3: normosmic idiopathic hypogonadotrophic hypogonadism

  GNRH1: normosmic idiopathic hypogonadotrophic hypogonadism

  GNRHR: normosmic idiopathic hypogonadotrophic hypogonadism

  KISS1: normosmic idiopathic hypogonadotrophic hypogonadism

  KISS1R: normosmic idiopathic hypogonadotrophic hypogonadism

  FEZF1: Kallmann syndrome

- digenic/undetermined inheritance:

  HS6ST1: Kallmann syndrome/normosmic idiopathic hypogonadotrophic hypogonadism

  NELF: Kallmann syndrome/normosmic idiopathic hypogonadotrophic hypogonadism

  IL17RD: Kallmann syndrome/normosmic idiopathic hypogonadotrophic hypogonadism

  FGF17: Kallmann syndrome/normosmic idiopathic hypogonadotrophic hypogonadism

  FLRT3: Kallmann syndrome/normosmic idiopathic hypogonadotrophic hypogonadism

  DUSP4: Kallmann syndrome/normosmic idiopathic hypogonadotrophic hypogonadism

  SEMA3E: Kallmann syndrome

---

meningioma (direct pressure effect by tumour and/or surgical/treatment)

- hyperprolactinemia secondary to pituitary lactotroph adenomas or stalk interruption from other pituitary lesions
- head injuries, particularly military blast trauma
- haemochromatosis, or transfusion-related iron overload
- infiltrative sellar disorders (neurosarcoidosis, Langerhans cell histiocytosis, Wegener's granulomatosis, lymphocytic hypophysitis)
- Sheehan's syndrome (post-partum pituitary necrosis)
- CNS infections (e.g. tuberculous meningitis)
- CNS irradiation for childhood malignancy

Functional hypothalamic/pituitary disorders

Relative to organic causes, functional hypothalamic/pituitary dysfunction is a more common cause of secondary hypogonadism.

- Acute critical illness of any kind can cause severe secondary hypogonadism.
- Chronic systemic illness (e.g. obesity, type 2 diabetes, cardiovascular disease, AIDS, chronic liver/renal failure) typically causes mild secondary hypogonadism.
- Hypoleptinaemia secondary to an eating disorder or excessive exercise can cause secondary hypogonadism (although the male reproductive axis is much less susceptible than the female; by contrast, the male axis is uniquely susceptible to the suppressive effect of obesity).

- Drugs can also cause secondary hypogonadism; for example:
  - drug-induced hyperprolactinaemia (antipsychotics)
  - secondary hypogonadism due to androgen/testosterone abuse
  - secondary hypogonadism due to exogenous GnRH-analogue therapy
  - secondary hypogonadism due to chronic glucocorticoid therapy (e.g. for Duchenne muscular dystrophy)
  - secondary hypogonadism due to chronic opiate therapy (prescriptions for opiates have undergone an exponential rise in recent years for non-cancer pain in the Western world)

Clinical features

The clinical features of secondary hypogonadism are similar to those for primary hypogonadism (see Section 8.3), and the aetiology and timing of hypogonadism define the precise clinical presentation. Congenital causes of secondary hypogonadism present typically with a prepubertal onset of symptoms but, occasionally, patients with both combined pituitary hormone deficiency and idiopathic hypogonadotrophic hypogonadism may present secondary hypogonadism in the post-pubertal period. Patients with acquired secondary hypogonadism almost always present with a post-pubertal onset of symptoms. Neonatal or in utero testosterone deficiency results in microphallus and/or cryptorchidism, which should prompt referral for paediatric endocrine evaluation and follow-up, preferably within the post-natal diagnostic window afforded by male minipuberty.

The commonest prepubertal presenting symptom of secondary hypogonadism is the failure of boys to enter or progress through puberty. Characteristic features include absent secondary sexual characteristics (e.g. absent/reduced sexual hair, failure of deepening of voice); small testes; absent spermatogenesis; absent pubertal growth spurt; eunuchoidal habitus (long bones fail to fuse, resulting in >5 cm difference in arm span over height; >5 cm difference in lower body segment over upper body segment); and delayed bone age. In contrast to the case for primary hypogonadism, gynaecomastia is less common in secondary hypogonadism. Whilst small-volume testes are characteristic of severe secondary hypogonadism, partial pubertal presentations resulting in relatively larger testicular volumes are also recognized ('fertile eunuch' syndrome). In prepubertal secondary hypogonadism, libido may be poor, but erections may occur in response to visual erotic stimuli. Symptoms and signs of post-pubertal hypogonadism are identical in primary and secondary hypogonadism.

Clinical features specific to idiopathic hypogonadotrophic hypogonadism are shown in Box 8.5. An important differential diagnosis for idiopathic hypogonadotrophic hypogonadism at puberty is constitutional delay in puberty. Whilst a clear distinction between idiopathic hypogonadotrophic hypogonadism and constitutional delay in puberty may not be always possible, in the absence of serum testosterone, check in the postnatal minipuberty window for the presence of microphallus/cryptorchidism, a family history of idiopathic hypogonadotrophic hypogonadism, and non-endocrine clinical features, as these may help distinguish between the two conditions.

Clinical features of other causes of secondary hypogonadism

Clinical evaluation may also reveal other features of syndromic idiopathic hypogonadotrophic hypogonadism presentations (e.g. adrenal insufficiency, childhood-onset obesity, Bardet–Biedl syndrome features). Similarly, in patients with combined pituitary hormone deficiency, other pituitary hormone deficiencies and specific non-endocrine features may also be evident, depending on the genetic aetiology (microphthalmia: SOX2; mental retardation: SOX3; septo-optic dysplasia: HESX1). A history of headaches and the presence of visual field abnormalities may indicate presence of sellar/parasellar masses. A detailed review of systems may reveal chronic illnesses or drugs that may underlie secondary hypogonadism.

Treatment

Treatment of congenital secondary hypogonadism

Treatment goals include the induction of secondary sexual characteristics at presentation, restoring and maintaining testosterone levels to physiological levels, and treatment of infertility (spermatogenesis). As the primary defect in these patients is at the level of the hypothalamo-pituitary axis, with otherwise functionally competent testes, in addition to testosterone replacement therapy, gonadotrophin therapy and pulsatile GnRH therapy (currently available only in research settings) are effective physiological treatment options, especially when fertility is desired. If fertility is not desired, testosterone replacement therapy is the treatment of choice in these patients. For testosterone replacement therapy options, see Table 8.1 in Section 8.2 and, for clinical workup prior to and after initiation of testosterone replacement therapy, see Box 8.4 in Section 8.3.

Induction of puberty

In adolescent males presenting with congenital secondary hypogonadism, fertility is not a personal priority at that point, and the goal is to initiate secondary sexual characteristics. Testosterone replacement therapy using intramuscular testosterone injections or transdermal testosterone preparations have been successfully used in this setting. Typically, testosterone replacement therapy is initiated at low doses (50–100 mg intramuscular testosterone enantate/cypionate or 2.5 g daily of 1% testosterone gel), and the dose can be increased gradually with monitoring of testosterone levels, linear growth, and bone age maturation. This approach mimics the physiological progression of puberty and optimizes adequate adult height. However, as exogenous testosterone therapy suppresses any residual endogenous GnRH activity, spermatogenesis (if present at baseline) is typically suppressed in these patients. In teenagers, we aim to achieve completion of puberty over at least 2 years, so as to recapitulate normal physiology and maximize opportunity for linear growth; however, a faster tempo, taking around a year to completion, is required in older men who have already achieved adequate height and are at risk of segmental disproportion. These men can also become frustrated and disenchanted when treated with 'paediatric doses' of testosterone; dosimetry for pubertal induction in older men is thus similar to that for virilizing female-to-male transsexuals. Advanced old age, learning disability, and concomitant physical or psychiatric disease should present no obstacle or contraindication to pubertal induction and testosterone replacement therapy, although the bone-density increment resulting from testosterone therapy tends to be less good in those over 70.

Once serum total testosterone levels are optimized, serum testosterone levels should be monitored annually, along with monitoring for the safety of the testosterone replacement therapy (see Box 8.4 in Section 8.3).

Fertility induction
See also Chapter 9, Section 9.3. If fertility is desired in patients with congenital secondary hypogonadism, this is usually achieved via gonadotrophin therapy. Several gonadotrophin preparations are available: hMG contains both LH (75 IU) and FSH (75 IU) per vial, but the LH activity is virtually non-significant in respect of Leydig cell stimulation. hCG has only a LH-like activity. Recombinant FSH is now available. Several treatment regimens are used, but the likelihood of success depends on the degree of pubertal development at initiation. For those with post-pubertal testicular volumes (> 4 mL), hCG therapy alone may be sufficient for spermatogenesis. For those with prepubertal testicular volumes (<4 mL), combined therapy with both hCG and FSH is required for the successful induction of fertility. A suggested initial starting dose for hCG is 1500–2500 units, given subcutaneously twice or thrice weekly, with trough testosterone and estradiol levels measured after 6–8 weeks. The hCG dose should be titrated to achieve a serum total testosterone level in the mid-normal adult range, but slightly lower levels may need to be accepted if estradiol levels risk becoming supraphysiological. Sperm counts should be monitored every 2–3 months once the testicular volume reaches 6–8 mL. If spermatogenesis fails to initiate despite a pretreatment testicular volume of >4 mL, and attainment of adequate testosterone levels within 6–8 months, FSH should be added, starting at an initial empirical dose of 75 IU every other day, but increased if necessary to 150 IU daily, in order to achieve serum FSH levels of 4–8 IU/L, until spermatogenesis ensues, which may take up to 18–24 months.

Because FSH tends to promote germ cell proliferation and LH (or hCG) promotes differentiation, there is logic and some preliminary data to support administering at least 3 months of FSH therapy to patients with congenital secondary hypogonadism *before* starting hCG (rather than vice versa); for men with bilateral cryptorchidism, an even longer pretreatment period, potentially continued until inhibin B levels have plateaued, offers theoretical promise. Historic 'hCG-first' regimes were largely determined by the respective needs of regulators and pharma in clinical trials, the former wishing to exclude men who developed sperm on hCG alone, and the latter wishing to exclude men who failed to normalize serum testosterone with hCG alone as they could potentially harbour a primary testis defect (in fact, achieving normal serum testosterone levels is much easier in men receiving both hCG and FSH simultaneously).

We reserve hCG-first regimes for men with testicular volumes >4 mL and secondary hypogonadism acquired post-puberty. We use FSH pretreatment in men with congenital secondary hypogonadism and cryptorchidism

or testicular volumes ≤4 mL, Men with congenital secondary hypogonadism and testicular volumes >4 mL can simply start taking both hCG and FSH simultaneously.

Predictors of poor response to fertility induction include a history of cryptorchidism; testicular volumes <4 mL at initiation; certain gene mutations (e.g. mutations in *KAL1*); and a low baseline inhibin B level.

Treatment of acquired secondary hypogonadism
In those with acquired causes of secondary hypogonadism, treatment should be directed to treat any underlying cause (e.g. surgery for pituitary adenoma, dopamine agonist therapy for hyperprolactinaemia). Chronic disease treatment should be optimized and any offending drugs stopped (or doses reduced or alternative drugs substituted), if possible. In those situations where such measures are not feasible, testosterone replacement therapy should definitely be used in the context of organic disease and considered in the context of functional secondary hypogonadism. For those who require fertility, hCG therapy alone is usually sufficient. For men who desire fertility but have functional secondary hypogonadism due to morbid obesity and/or use of opiate analgesics, there are data to support the effectiveness of anti-oestrogen therapy with clomifene (50–250 mg per week), or anastrozole (1.5–7.0 mg per week). Empirically, anastrozole should be chosen where an obesity-related thromboembolism risk is paramount, and clomifene when bone health is of greater concern.

Further reading
Balasubramanian R and Crowley WF Jr. Isolated GnRH deficiency: A disease model serving as a unique prism into the systems biology of the GnRH neuronal network. *Mol Cell Endocrinol* 2011; 346: 4–12.

Balasubramanian R and Quinton R. 'Secondary hypogonadism', in Hugh Jones T, ed., *Testosterone Deficiency in Men* (2nd edition), 2013. Oxford University Press, 45–56.

Bhasin S, and Basaria S. Diagnosis and treatment of hypogonadism in men. *Best Pract Res Clin Endocrinol Metab* 2011; 25: 251–70.

Boehm U, Bouloux PM, Dattani MT, et al. European consensus statement on congenital hypogonadotrophic hypogonadism: Pathogenesis, diagnosis and treatment. *Nat Rev Endocrinol* 2015; 11: 547–64.

Dwyer AA, Jayasena CN, and Quinton R. Congenital hypogonadotrophic hypogonadism: Implications of absent minipuberty. *Minerva Endocrinol* 2016; 41: 188–95.

Dwyer AA, Raivio T, and Pitteloud N. Gonadotropin replacement for induction of spermatogenesis in hypogonadal men. *Best Pract Res Endocrinol Metab* 2015; 29: 91–103

Dunkel L and Quinton R. Transition in endocrinology: Induction of puberty. *Eur J Endocrinol* 2014; 170: R229–39.

Wass, JAH, Steward PM, Amiel SA et al, eds. 'Part 9: Male hypogonadism and infertility', in Wass, JAH, Steward PM, Amiel SA et al, eds, *Oxford Textbook of Endocrinology and Diabetes* (2nd edition), 2011. Oxford University Press, pp. 1333–483.

8.5 Erectile dysfunction

Definition and epidemiology

Normal sexual function in a male is a multifaceted process, requiring an intact libido and the ability to attain and maintain a penile erection, ejaculate semen, and return the penis to the flaccid state. Erectile dysfunction is defined as the persistent or recurrent inability to attain or maintain an adequate erection until completion of sexual activity. Although erectile dysfunction is not considered a normal part of the natural ageing process, its prevalence typically ranges from 1%–10% in men younger than 40, and 20%–40% in men aged 60–70, increasing substantially to over 50% in men older than 70 years. The worldwide prevalence of erectile dysfunction is projected to rise substantially over the next 15 years in healthy ageing men, making this a significant public health concern. Erectile dysfunction is linked to several medical conditions, including diabetes mellitus, obesity, hypertension, hyperlipidaemia, and lower urinary tract symptoms. Moreover, meta-analysis data show that erectile dysfunction is strongly associated with an increased risk of cardiovascular disease, coronary heart disease, type 2 diabetes, stroke, and all-cause mortality, so the finding of erectile dysfunction constitutes an important early warning sign to prompt disease-modifying interventions such lifestyle changes, lipid-, glucose-, or blood pressure-lowering therapy, and, potentially, antiplatelet agents.

Pathophysiology

Normal penile erection results from a complex interplay of psychological, endocrine, vascular, and neurological processes. Penile tumescence depends on the increased flow of blood into the sinusoidal spaces (lacunae) of the corpora cavernosa, accompanied by complete relaxation of the corporal arteries. Subsequent compression of the trabecular smooth muscles causes passive closure of the emissary veins and accumulation of blood in the corpora. Nitric oxide, released from the endothelium and parasympathetic nerve terminals, is one of the primary neural inputs mediating the relaxation of the vascular smooth muscles. The erectile response is then mediated by a combination of central (psychogenic) and peripheral innervations of the penis. Erectile dysfunction results from psychogenic, organic, or iatrogenic disorders that cause failure of initiation of erections, and/or vasculogenic failure: reduced arterial inflow into the penis or impaired veno-occlusive mechanisms.

Psychogenic erectile dysfunction

An increased sympathetic tone resulting in increased vascular smooth muscle tone is thought to be a possible mechanism of psychogenic erectile dysfunction. Psychogenic erectile dysfunction is commonly associated with generalized anxiety disorder, performance anxiety (fear of failure of erections), relationship conflicts, sexuality disorders (disorders of sexual orientation, sexual inhibition, traumatic childhood sex abuse experiences) and fear of pregnancy or sexually transmitted diseases. Psychogenic factors frequently coexist with organic disorders and require evaluation and therapy.

Vasculogenic erectile dysfunction

Impaired arterial inflow into the penis and/or an impaired penile veno-occlusive mechanisms are frequent causes of erectile dysfunction. Atherosclerosis is the most common cause of arterial occlusion; therefore, vasculogenic erectile dysfunction is associated with classical atherosclerotic risk factors such as age, cigarette smoking, dyslipidaemia, diabetes, hypertension, and metabolic syndrome. Thromboembolic occlusion of the major abdominal vessels or the iliac or pelvic arteries may also cause vasculogenic erectile dysfunction. Veno-occlusive impairment is commonly due to fibrotic changes in the tunica albuginea (e.g. Peyronie's disease) or in the trabecular smooth muscle (diabetes, atherosclerosis).

Neurogenic erectile dysfunction

Erectile dysfunction is commonly associated with Parkinson's disease, stroke, Alzheimer's disease, and temporal lobe epilepsy. Spinal cord diseases (congenital: spina bifida, syringomyelia; acquired: trauma, multiple sclerosis) also result in erectile dysfunction. Autonomic and peripheral neuropathy (due to diabetes, vitamin B_{12} deficiency, or alcoholism) and surgical injuries to the cavernous nerves (e.g. radical prostatectomy) can also result in erectile dysfunction.

Endocrine erectile dysfunction

Erectile dysfunction is reported by men with primary or secondary hypogonadism. Although sleep-related erections are impaired in hypogonadal subjects, men with castrate levels of testosterone (e.g. Kallmann syndrome) retain erectile function to visual/tactile stimuli, suggesting that erectile function is not completely androgen dependent. Recent data suggest that testosterone may be important for nitric oxide synthase expression within the penis, in addition to putatively entraining erections with sexual imagination, but the precise role of testosterone in erectile function remains surprisingly unclear. Similarly, although hyperprolactinemia is associated with erectile dysfunction through central inhibition of the hypothalamopituitary–testicular axis, a direct effect on libido and sexual function has been postulated.

Iatrogenic erectile dysfunction

Several drugs are associated with erectile dysfunction, although a clear cause–effect relationship has not been established for most known associations. Antihypertensive medications, particularly, diuretics, beta blockers, and calcium channel blockers are frequently associated with erectile dysfunction. Alpha blockers are the least likely hypotensive agents to cause erectile dysfunction. Psychotrophic drugs, including commonly used antidepressants such as SSRIs, tricyclics, and neuroleptics, are associated with erectile dysfunction. Anti-androgens (e.g. GnRH analogues, spironolactone, cimetidine, flutamide, and finasteride) are also frequently implicated.

Erectile dysfunction associated with systemic diseases

Erectile dysfunction is commonly seen in patients with diabetes and, in a small minority, may actually be the presenting symptom of undiagnosed disease. The aetiology of erectile dysfunction in diabetes is multifactorial and includes vasculogenic, neurogenic, and psychogenic components. Similarly, other systemic diseases, including chronic renal disease, chronic pulmonary disease, and chronic liver disease, may also be associated with erectile dysfunction, and the prevalence of erectile dysfunction in these patients rises with increasing age.

Box 8.6 Common medical conditions associated with erectile dysfunction

Psychogenic erectile dysfunction
Anxiety disorders

Vasculogenic erectile dysfunction
Atherosclerosis
Dyslipidaemia
Hypertension
Thromboembolism (abdominal/iliac/pelvic vessels)
Peyronie's disease (veno-occlusion)

Neurogenic erectile dysfunction
Parkinson's disease
Alzheimer's disease
Spinal cord diseases (spina bifida; multiple sclerosis)
Vitamin B_{12} deficiency

Mixed psychogenic, vasculogenic, and neurogenic erectile dysfunction
Ageing
Diabetes
Alcoholism
Chronic renal disease
Chronic liver disease

Endocrine erectile dysfunction
Hypogonadism (primary or secondary)
Hyperprolactinaemia

Iatrogenic erectile dysfunction
Drugs (antihypertensives, psychotrophics, neuroleptics, anti-androgens)
  Surgical (nerve damage during radical prostatectomy)

The major causes of erectile dysfunction are shown in Box 8.6.

Evaluation

The diagnostic goals include establishing the diagnosis, identifying underlying causes, and assessing risk factors and any associated serious co-morbidities. A complete sexual history should be obtained to assess whether erectile dysfunction is psychogenic or organic. Some patients may not have true erectile dysfunction but may be describing other sexual symptoms such as premature ejaculation or impaired orgasm. Explicit sexual history should be obtained including sexual orientation, sexual partner(s), and sexual habits. Sexual partners should be interviewed along with the patient, if possible. Abrupt onset, preserved early morning erections, and inconsistent nature of symptoms (e.g. symptoms with one partner, not another) may indicate psychogenic causes of erectile dysfunction. Organic erectile dysfunction symptoms are typically constant and progressive in nature. Psychogenic factors often coexist with an organic cause; hence, specialist psychological assessment can be invaluable. If libido is also poor, endocrine causes for erectile dysfunction should always be sought. Standardized sexual health questionnaires exist (e.g. Sexual Health Inventory for Men, Sexuality Experience Scales Manual), but their utility in improving diagnostic categorization is unclear. A full medical and surgical (e.g. bladder, bowel, vascular, prostate) history must be obtained to exclude other

systemic diseases and identify specific risk factors that may contribute to erectile dysfunction. A detailed drug history including recreational drug use should be obtained. Since erectile dysfunction may indicate underlying cardiovascular disease, all subjects should undergo cardiac risk assessment even if they are symptomatic.

Physical examination should review genital anatomy and identify any abnormalities (hypospadias, penile size, Peyronie's disease, fibrosis, testicular atrophy). The general examination should review the BMI, blood pressure, secondary sexual characteristics, gynaecomastia, peripheral pulses, the abdomen (aortic aneurysm), and peripheral nerves, and potentially include a digital prostate exam. Signs of cardiac, hepatic, renal, or pulmonary disease should be looked for.

Laboratory investigations

Spuriously low serum testosterone levels are associated with general ill health, sleep deprivation, and afternoon or postprandial venepuncture, so the testing tests are best performed between 8:00 h and 10:00 h and fasted, avoiding periods of concomitant non-gonadal illness, or night-shift working:

- blood sugar, lipids, and glycated haemoglobin, to assess glycaemic status and vascular risk
- a complete blood count, to exclude anaemia
- serum total testosterone
- SHBG (useful in estimating the free testosterone level and, if low, in highlighting the future risk of type 2 diabetes)
- LH and FSH, to exclude primary or secondary hypogonadism
- ferritin, prolactin, and other anterior pituitary hormones if secondary hypogonadism is suspected
- baseline PSA, if testosterone replacement therapy is contemplated

Additional specialist testing is not usually not required for establishing the diagnosis of erectile dysfunction. The following tests are typically reserved for specialist and research settings:

- nocturnal penile tumescence testing
- intracavernosal injections of vasoactive drugs
- cavernography
- penile Doppler
- colour Doppler ultrasound/arteriography
- neurological testing

Treatment

The goal of therapy should be guided by patient choice and the underlying aetiology of erectile dysfunction. Patient and partner education plays a critical role in erectile dysfunction management. Lifestyle counselling should be undertaken to address associated risk factors (smoking, alcohol, diet, recreational drugs).

Erectile dysfunction and hypogonadism

If erectile dysfunction is associated with unequivocal biochemical hypogonadism, a detailed clinical evaluation should be undertaken to clarify the aetiology of the hypogonadism. Primary hypogonadism should be treated with testosterone replacement therapy. Testosterone replacement therapy (or gonadotrophins, if fertility is desired) should be used in men with organic secondary hypogonadism. Hyperprolactinemia-associated hypogonadism should be treated appropriately with dopamine agonists, or by substituting prolactin-neutral (e.g. cyclizine) or prolactin-lowering drugs (e.g. aripiprazole) for existing anti-emetic, or antipsychotic therapies.

Chronic use of non-prescription testosterone and androgenic anabolic steroids for body building, or sporting-performance enhancement is increasingly common and can result in prolonged suppression of the hypothalamo-pituitary–gonadal axis, lasting up to a year from the last injection. Prescribed testosterone therapy will merely perpetuate androgen-induced azoospermic hypogonadism and is therefore absolutely contraindicated; clinicians thus need to be firm, reassuring, and resolute in the face of patient demands that may be emotionally charged. Bringing the partner (who may be wondering why she has failed to fall pregnant) into the consultation can be very helpful in this respect. Indeed, a partner in her mid-late thirties desiring fertility is probably the only reason to consider intervening with prescribed gonadotrophin or anti-oestrogen therapy.

Erectile dysfunction in a man with borderline–low serum testosterone and normal gonadotrophins: The clinical context is key

It is not uncommon, especially in an older and/or obese male, for symptoms of erectile dysfunction to initially appear to be associated with borderline–low serum testosterone level. If a borderline level is found, serum total testosterone levels, SHBG levels, and gonadotrophin levels should be rechecked in at least two early morning, fasted samples. If borderline testosterone levels are confirmed but the SHBG level lies towards either extreme of the normal range, free testosterone levels may be calculated using the mass-action formula, or checked with equilibrium dialysis. Low testosterone/free testosterone associated with elevated gonadotrophins is diagnostic of compensated primary hypogonadism (e.g. late-onset hypogonadism, or late-presenting Klinefelter's syndrome), and testosterone replacement therapy should be initiated unless there is an unequivocal contraindication, such as erythrocytosis, or active androgen-dependent prostate cancer. However, if gonadotrophins are normal, consistent with secondary hypogonadism, management needs to be more nuanced, as outlined in 'Symptomatic medical management of erectile dysfunction'.

Organic secondary hypogonadism can typically be framed in the context of a defined disease known to impact on hypothalamo-pituitary function, such as iron overload (readily identifiable from the baseline laboratory screen), new diagnosis of pituitary disease, or a history of cranial irradiation. Under these circumstances, even a borderline serum testosterone level is likely to be clinically significant and typically mandates testosterone replacement therapy if it is not otherwise correctable. However, it should be noted that MRI rarely detects clinically significant parasellar lesions when testosterone is borderline and pituitary function is otherwise unequivocally normal.

However, if no such disease entity can be identified, potential causes of functional/reversible secondary hypogonadotrophic hypogonadism (see Section 8.4) should be sought, Functional/reversible gonadotrophin deficiency usually signposts an underlying non-gonadal illness that needs to be addressed, and the benefit and safety of testosterone replacement therapy in this context are lacking. For instance, low total testosterone/free testosterone levels associated with severe obesity are only rarely associated with either anaemia, or osteopenia, and levels usually improve with lifestyle modification alone.

However, if no organic or functional/reversible secondary cause is found (or if the functional cause is judged to be properly monitored opiate therapy for properly characterized pain), a trial of testosterone replacement therapy for at least 6 months should be offered with clinical monitoring, unless fertility is being actively sought—in which case, gonadotrophin or possibly anti-oestrogen therapy is indicated instead. If there is no improvement in erectile dysfunction or other putative hypogonadal symptoms, symptomatic management of erectile dysfunction should be considered and, unless testosterone replacement therapy has resulted in clinically significant improvement from baseline anaemia, or osteopenia, it should be discontinued.

Lessons from studies on ageing males

Data from community-based surveys and from the recruitment process into the NIH-funded 'Testosterone Trials' have emphasized just how rare it is for a fit, healthy older man to have a low testosterone level in the absence of either raised gonadotrophins or a discernible secondary cause of hypogonadism (functional or organic). In the unusual and unrepresentative group of older men with acquired partial secondary hypogonadism, testosterone replacement therapy resulted in modest improvements in sexual function (comparable to those achievable with oral PDE5 inhibitors), with little discernible impact on other domains of age-related functional decline. Indeed, when, in a different study, testosterone replacement therapy was used to treat age-related frailty, adverse events exceeded any putative benefits.

The use of testosterone replacement therapy in men with obesity/metabolic syndrome, or age-related frailty, without classical hypogonadism, is presently best confined to clinical trials, and its use in eugonadal men with erectile dysfunction is definitely not recommended. Diagnosing 'testosterone-deficiency syndrome' based on questionnaires or random blood tests is unacceptable.

Symptomatic medical management of erectile dysfunction

Oral PDE5 inhibitors form the mainstay of medical therapy for erectile dysfunction resulting from both psychogenic and organic causes. PDE5 inhibitors block the hydrolysis of cyclic GMP, thereby maintaining high levels of it and thus maintaining penile smooth muscle relaxation, resulting in rigid penile erections. Sildenafil (25, 50, and 100 mg), vardenafil (2.5, 5, 10, and 20 mg), and tadalafil (2.5, 5, 10, and 20 mg) are three widely available PDE5 inhibitors. Their onset of action ranges from 60 minutes to 120 minutes, and graduated doses of each of these drugs should be tried to identify the best one suitable for any given patient. PDE5 inhibitors should not be used in patients concomitantly taking nitrates, as life-threatening hypotension may result from their interaction. Side effects associated with PDE5 inhibitors include headaches, dyspepsia, facial flushing, nasal congestion, a visual blue-halo effect, priapism, and back pain. In patients with treatment failure with PDE5 inhibitors, adjuvant testosterone therapy may be tried in those with hypogonadism. Alternatives include switching to other PDE5 inhibitors or the other measures detailed in this section.

Prostaglandin E1 (alprostadil)

Prostaglandin E1 (alprostadil) can be used either via the intracavernosal route (1–40 μg) or via the intra-urethral route (125–1000 μg) as an alternative to PDE5 inhibitors. Various combinations of alprostadil with other vaso-active agents (e.g. phentolamine and/or papaverine) are sometimes used. Intra-urethral insertion is associated with a markedly reduced incidence of priapism in comparison to intracavernosal injection. In addition, fibrosis may result from intravenous injections.

Vacuum constriction devices
Vacuum constriction devices are a reasonable treatment alternative for select patients who cannot take PDE5 inhibitors or who have failed treatment with all PDE5 inhibitors. The devices work by drawing venous blood into the penis by applying continuous negative pressure to the penile shaft and use an elastic band at the penis base to restrict venous return and maintain tumescence. Adverse events include non-physiological feel to patients; pain; petechiae; penile numbness; and altered ejaculation.

Surgery
Rarely, invasive surgical implantation of a semi-rigid or inflatable penile prosthesis may considered for refractory erectile dysfunction, but perioperative infection and poor erectile response limit its widespread use.

Further reading

Eardley, I. 'Sexual dysfunction', in Warrell DA, Cox TM, and Firth JD, eds, *Oxford Textbook of Medicine* (5th edition), 2012. Oxford University Press, pp. 1942–7.

Hugh Jones T. What should I do with a 60 year old man with a slightly low serum total testosterone concentration and normal levels of serum gonadotrophins? *Clin Endocrinol* 2010; 72: 584–8.

Shamloul R and Ghanem H. Erectile dysfunction. *Lancet* 2013; 381: 153–65.

Snyder PJ, Bhasin S, Cunningham GR, et al. Effects of testosterone treatment in older men. *N Engl J Med* 2016; 374: 611–24.

8.6 Gynaecomastia

Definition and epidemiology

Gynaecomastia refers to palpable enlargement of the glandular tissue in men. It is fairly common and can cause both physical discomfort and psychological distress. Breast tissue development and growth is stimulated by oestrogens and progesterone and is inhibited by androgens. A relative increase in the stimulatory-to-inhibitory hormonal milieu results in either physiological or pathological gynaecomastia. Physiological gynaecomastia in normal males is observed during the neonatal period and at puberty. Most newborns display transient gynaecomastia due to maternal/placental exposure to oestrogens. Nearly 60% of pubertal boys may experience transient, sometimes tender, asymmetrical gynaecomastia secondary to relative excess of oestrogen production from the testes during the early stages of puberty. Asymptomatic palpable breast tissue may be present in nearly a third of normal adult men (nearly 55% prevalence in autopsy studies), and prevalence increases sharply with ageing, especially in those with chronic medical illness. Pathological gynaecomastia is less common and typically is due to abnormal sex steroid production or is drug induced.

Pathophysiology

Oestrogens stimulate breast tissue proliferation whilst androgens potently inhibit breast growth. Gynaecomastia results from a relative dominance of oestrogenic action over androgenic inhibition in breast tissue. Regardless of its aetiology, initially, florid ductal proliferation and hyperplasia is seen, with an increase in stromal and periductal connective tissue and increased vascularity and periductal oedema. Once gynaecomastia has been present for several months, ductal dilatation is accompanied by periductal fibrosis, stromal hyalinization, and increased sub-areolar fat.

Gynaecomastia can result from a variety of pathophysiological states. Often, in a single patient, multiple pathophysiological defects may coexist. Box 8.7 shows the major causes of gynaecomastia.

Oestrogen excess

In addition to a direct stimulatory action of oestrogen on breast tissue, elevated levels also inhibit gonadotrophin-driven testosterone synthesis and increase hepatic SHBG synthesis (thus reducing free testosterone levels). The hormonal imbalance is, thereby, further exacerbated, and worsens the gynaecomastia.

Oestrogen excess may be absolute or relative. Absolute excess of oestrogens can result from therapeutic or unintentional exposure to oestrogens. Rarely, endogenous oestrogen excess results directly from overproduction of oestrogen by testicular (Leydig or Sertoli cell) or adrenal tumours, or indirectly from overproduction of weak androgens that can be aromatized peripherally to oestrogens (testicular/extra-testicular (e.g. lung) tumours secreting hCG; feminizing adrenal neoplasms).

Relative oestrogen excess is far more common. Ageing is associated with increased adiposity and consequent increase in aromatization of androgens to oestrogens. In addition, serum testosterone levels decline with age, and SHBG levels increase with age, thus altering the oestrogen-to-androgen ratio. Relative oestrogen excess

is also seen in patients with chronic liver disease (increased aromatization, increased SHBG, inhibition of the hypothalamo-pituitary–testicular axis); hyperthyroidism (increased SHBG and increased aromatization); or an altered oestrogen-to-androgen ratio (chronic renal failure, starvation/refeeding-gynaecomastia, HIV-positive men on retroviral therapy). Familial aromatase excess syndromes can also cause gynaecomastia, but are extremely rare.

Testosterone deficiency/androgen insensitivity

Primary hypogonadism of any cause, including partial androgen insensitivity syndrome, can result in gynaecomastia through a combination of low testosterone levels and the enhancement of testicular aromatase activity by elevated LH level. Secondary hypogonadism is less commonly associated with gynaecomastia, except during treatment with hCG therapy. Hyperprolactinemia (leading to suppression of gonadotrophin production) and androgen deprivation therapy for prostate cancer can also cause gynaecomastia.

Drugs

Drug-induced gynaecomastia is common and is often multifactorial. Mechanisms include oestrogen-like activity, increased testicular production of oestrogens, impaired testosterone production, potentiation of oestrogen action, or antagonism of androgen action. Gynaecomastia is a particular problem for recreational or sporting users of non-prescription testosterone or androgenic anabolic steroids. It principally results from aromatization to oestrogen of supraphysiological serum testosterone levels, but may be compounded by episodic secondary hypogonadism during breaks in testosterone abuse, and/or by concomitant or cyclical use of hCG in an attempt to minimize testicular atrophy secondary to suppression of gonadotrophin secretion—a technique known as 'stacking'. Even when men have genuinely ceased using testosterone or androgenic anabolic steroids, supplements described as 'herbal' or 'protein based' may contain unlisted, orally active androgenic anabolic steroids. For several drugs, the precise mechanism is still unknown. A list of drugs associated with gynaecomastia is given in Box 8.7.

Idiopathic gynaecomastia

The cause of gynaecomastia may not directly evident in several cases. Dietary supplements, herbal additives, or environmental disruptors may underlie some of these cases. Virtually any drug may be associated with gynaecomastia.

Evaluation

Incidental identification of long-standing palpable breast tissue in asymptomatic men is common and often does not require further assessment. In recent-onset gynaecomastia, a detailed history should be obtained to ascertain the presence of any of the potential clinical conditions listed in Box 8.7. A thorough medication history should be obtained, including dietary supplements, recreational drugs, and non-prescription medications. A family history may indicate the possibility of pubertal gynaecomastia, androgen insensitivity syndrome, familial aromatase excess syndrome, or familial syndromes associated with

---

Box 8.7 Major causes of gynaecomastia

Physiological

Neonates

Pubertal gynaecomastia

Pathological

Absolute oestrogen excess

Exogenous oestrogens (therapeutic, intentional (e.g. aromatizable androgen abuse), unintentional)

Endogenous oestrogen excess:

- tumours secreting E2, E2 precursors, or hCG:

  testicular Sertoli or Leydig cell tumours

  germ cell tumours

  adrenocortical feminizing tumours

  ectopic hCG-secreting tumours (e.g. lung)

- familial/sporadic aromatase excess syndrome

Relative oestrogen excess

Ageing

Chronic liver disease

Chronic renal disease/dialysis

Starvation/refeeding gynaecomastia

Hyperthyroidism

Testosterone deficiency

Primary or secondary hypogonadism

Androgen insensitivity syndrome

Drugs (see below)

Drugs

Drugs that increase oestrogens/oestrogenic activity:

- oestrogens
- aromatizable androgens
- hCG
- digitalis

Drugs that decrease/antagonism of testosterone:

- GnRH analogues
- ketoconazole
- cimetidine
- spironolactone
- flutamide
- finasteride
- cytotoxic agents
- marijuana
- antipsychotic agents/drugs that raise prolactin

  Drugs whose mechanisms are poorly defined:

  isoniazid

  phenytoin

  antidepressants (e.g. tricyclic antidepressants)

  statins

  antiretroviral therapy in HIV-positive men

  proton-pump inhibitors (e.g. omeprazole)

  calcium channel blockers (e.g. amlodipine, verapamil)

  ACE inhibitors

Other

Idiopathic causes

Abbreviations: E2, estradiol; GnRH, gonadotrophin-releasing hormone; hCG, human chorionic gonadotrophin.

---

testicular Sertoli cell tumours (e.g. Peutz—Jeghers syndrome, Carney complex).

In recent-onset gynaecomastia, the first step is to determine if the breast enlargement is true gynaecomastia or pseudo-gynaecomastia (adipose tissue), by physical examination. Pseudo-gynaecomastia is characterized by increased sub-areolar fat without glandular enlargement. Rapid-onset gynaecomastia requires evaluation to exclude breast carcinoma, which is typically non-tender, unilateral, located outside the nipple-areolar region, and firm/hard upon palpation and can be associated with nipple retraction. In true gynaecomastia, the affected area is concentric to the nipple/areolar region, is soft/elastic to palpate, and is typically bilateral without any skin/nipple abnormality. The physical exam should look for evidence of testosterone deficiency (facial/axillary/pubic hair, muscle bulk/strength, penile size, testicular volume) and signs of chronic liver or renal disease or hyperthyroidism. Once the diagnosis of true gynaecomastia is established, laboratory evaluation should include thyroid, liver and renal function tests along with serum testosterone (total, bioavailable, and free), estradiol, SHBG, LH, FSH, beta-hCG, alpha-fetaprotein, and prolactin measurements. Karyotyping to identify Klinefelter's syndrome should be performed if gonadotrophins are found to be elevated. Evaluation for an underlying adrenal abnormality should be undertaken if indicated, including seum levels of DHEAS and androstenedione; adrenal-protocol CT or MRI; and, increasingly, urine steroid metabolomic profiling. Imaging investigations (testicular sonography, CT/MRI of adrenals, pituitary/sella, etc.) should be guided by physical examination findings and laboratory measurements. The precise underlying aetiology may remain unclear despite extensive evaluation. If breast carcinoma cannot be excluded by physical exam, diagnostic mammography (high sensitivity but poor positive predictive value) and fine-needle aspiration cytology should be considered.

Treatment

Treatment depends on the underlying aetiology of the condition. Long-standing gynaecomastia in asymptomatic men does not require treatment, and reassurance and periodic follow up may be sufficient to allay any associated anxiety. Physiological gynaecomastia of puberty often resolves spontaneously but therapy may be considered in those who have significant psychological distress. Any suspected offending medication should be stoppe, and improvement is usually expected within few months of stopping therapy. Hyperthyroidism, liver disease, and renal disease should be treated appropriately. Gynaecomastia secondary to refeeding/renal dialysis often resolves spontaneously. Testosterone deficiency should be treated with androgen replacement, but may worsen gynaecomastia as androgens can be aromatized to estradiol.

In cases where gynaecomastia fails to respond to correcting the underlying abnormality or in cases where cosmetic appearance creates psychological distress, pharmacotherapy and surgical options may be considered. Response to medical pharmacotherapy is extremely variable and is most likely to be effective during the early proliferative stage (usually <6 months from the onset of gynaecomastia). Oestrogen-receptor antagonists (tamoxifen and raloxifene) and aromatase inhibitors

---

Box 8.8 Treatment of gynaecomastia

Identify and treat underlying cause
Stop any offending medication
Surgical reduction, if desired
Medical therapy:[†]

- tamoxifen
  typical dose: 10–20 mg/day
  side effects: hot flushes, weight gain
- raloxifene
- typical dose: 60 mg/day
- side effects: hot flushes, thrombosis
- anastrozole
  typical dose: 1 mg/day
  side effects: stiff joints, headache

[†] Unapproved indication; not useful in long-standing gynaecomastia.

---

have been used to treat gynaecomastia with variable efficacy. Tamoxifen has also been used successfully to prevent gynaecomastia in men who have prostate cancer and are undergoing androgen deprivation therapy. It is to be noted that none of these drugs are clinically approved to treat gynaecomastia. Medical therapy is unlikely to be effective in long-standing fibrotic gynaecomastia and, in this context or if medical therapy fails, or the breast appearance is disfiguring causing significant psychological distress, surgery to remove breast tissue (with or without liposuction) is the most effective therapy. Surgical results are best in the hands of highly experienced surgeons, and endocrinologists should work in a multidisciplinary setting to achieve acceptable outcomes. A summary of the treatments for gynaecomastia is given in Box 8.8.

Breast carcinoma in men

Male breast cancer is rare (0.1% of all male cancers; 0.5%–1.0% of all breast cancers) but, due to poor awareness, men often present with higher-stage tumours and carry a relatively poorer prognosis than females do. Risk factors include higher age, Afro-Caribbean race, positive family history (*BRCA2* > *BRCA1*), abnormal oestrogen-to-androgen ratio (Klinefelter's syndrome, obesity, liver cirrhosis), and radiation exposure. Gynaecomastia per se is not an established risk factor for male breast cancer. A painless breast lump is the most common presenting feature. Ultrasonography and mammography are imaging investigations of choice, with the former having a better sensitivity and specificity. Cytologic techniques such as fine-needle aspiration provide diagnostic staging information. More than 90% of breast cancers in men are invasive ductal carcinomas. Most patients require modified/radical mastectomy, but simple mastectomy may be sufficient in those with early stage disease. Sentinel node biopsy is recommended to stage axillary disease. As 90% of breast cancers are oestrogen- and progesterone-receptor positive, adjuvant hormonal therapy with tamoxifen, an oestrogen-receptor modulator, has been reported in retrospective reports. Metastatic disease typically requires adjuvant radiotherapy and adjuvant cytotoxic chemotherapy. Prognosis is worse with older age at onset, higher tumour grade, and lymph node involvement.

Further reading

Braunstein GD. Gynecomastia. *N Eng J Med* 2007; 357: 129–37.

Carlson HE. Approach to the patient with gynecomastia. *J Clin Endocrinol Metab* 2013; 96: 15–21.

Karavolos S, Reynolds M, Panagiotopoulou N, et al. Male central hypogonadism secondary to exogenous androgens: A review of the drugs and protocols highlighted by the online community of users for prevention and/or mitigation of adverse effects. *Clin Endocrinol (Oxf)* 2015; 82: 624–32.

Patten DK, Sharifi LK, and Fazel M. New approaches in the management of male breast cancer. *Clin Breast Cancer* 2013; 13: 309–14.

Chapter 9

Disorders of gender and fertility

Chapter contents

9.1 Disorders of sex development

Introduction

Disorders of sex development comprise a wide range of conditions with diverse pathophysiology that most often present in the newborn or the adolescent. Affected newborns usually present with atypical genitalia, whereas adolescents present with atypical sexual development during the pubertal years. Whilst the prevalence of genital anomalies at birth may be as high as 1 in 300 births, the birth prevalence of complex anomalies that may lead to true genital ambiguity may be as low as 1 in 5000 births. Rather than treating every affected individual as a medical emergency, it is paramount that appropriate assessment is performed by an expert with knowledge of the variation in the physical appearance of genitalia, the underlying pathophysiology of disorders of sex development, and the strengths and weaknesses of available tests. This expert should be able to ensure that the parents' and patients' needs for information are comprehensively addressed whilst appropriate investigations are performed in a timely fashion. This expert also needs to have immediate access to the multidisciplinary team. Finally, in the field of rare conditions, it is imperative that the clinician shares with others through national and international clinical and research collaboration.

Terminology

The use of terminology which is clear and easy to use and understand by all health professionals, patients, and their families is fundamental to the understanding, investigation, and management of disorders of sex development. In addition, terminology should respect the individual and avoid terms which might cause offence. Terminology was revised in 2005 following the publication of a consensus statement by the Lawson Wilkins Pediatric Endocrine Society and the European Society for Paediatric Endocrinology. Whilst the new nomenclature (Table 9.1) is easier to use and understand, it will nevertheless evolve over time as our understanding of long-term outcomes, as well as molecular aetiology, improves.

Communication

The initial contact with the parents of a child with a disorder of sex development is important, as first impressions from these encounters often persist. In those cases where there are no doubts about sex assignment, it should not be assumed that the parents' need for information and psychological help are any less; the parents' perception of risk may be quite different from the clinical perception of the severity of illness. In those cases where there is true genital ambiguity, it should be explained to the parents that the best course of action may not initially be clear, but that the healthcare team will work with the family to reach the best possible set of decisions in the circumstances. The healthcare team should discuss with the parents what information to share in the early stages with family members and friends. It is essential that the parents do not register the birth until the sex of rearing is established. Parents need to be informed about sex development; they should be provided written information and directed to internet-based information.

The multidisciplinary team

Optimal care for children with a disorder of sex development requires an experienced multidisciplinary team, generally found in regional centres or a network. Ideally, the team includes paediatric subspecialists in endocrinology; surgery and/or urology; psychology/psychiatry; gynaecology; genetics; neonatology; nursing; and, if possible, social work and medical ethics. Transitional care should be organized with the multidisciplinary team operating in an environment comprising specialists with experience in both paediatric and adult practice. Support groups have an important role to play, and their contact details should be supplied to the parents. It is possible that affected parents may prefer to talk to local families affected in a similar way. The availability of such a local pool of voluntary helpers who had some support from the specialists would complete the composition of the multidisciplinary team.

Rationale in the clinical evaluation of an affected infant

The infant with a suspected disorder of sex development requires evaluation for four broad reasons:
- to determine the sex of rearing
- to address concerns about immediate, life-threatening metabolic conditions (e.g. those associated with adrenal insufficiency)
- to obtain knowledge of the aetiology of the underlying condition (as this may aid in the development of a long-term management plan)
- to help understand issues such as fertility, sexual function, and risk of tumour development
- to help with the explanation of the diagnosis itself

History

Knowledge of what has already been discussed with the parents by health professionals is essential. An adequate history should concentrate particularly on:
- family history (which may suggest the mode of inheritance):
  - parental consanguinity
  - history of an infant with salt losing
  - unexplained infant deaths
  - disorders of sex development in relatives

Table 9.1 Nomenclature for disorders of sex development

Previous term	New nomenclature
Intersex	Disorder of sex development
Male pseudohermaphrodite, under-virilization of XY male, under-masculinization of XY male	46, XY disorder of sex development
Female pseudohermaphrodite, over-virilization of XX female, masculinization of XX female	46, XX disorder of sex development
True hermaphrodite	Ovotesticular disorder of sex development
XX male, XX sex reversal	46, XX testicular disorder of sex development
XY sex reversal	46, XY complete gonadal dysgenesis

- antenatal history:
  - maternal ingestion of drugs which may cause fetal virilization
  - signs of maternal androgen excess
  - exposure to specific environmental factors able to inhibit virilization of the foetus
  - assisted conception
- results of prenatal tests
- social history:
  - families social network
  - parents' understanding of disorders of sex development
  - current concerns.

General examination

A general, systematic physical examination should be performed in all suspected cases, particularly focusing on:
- dysmorphic features and associated malformations
- birth weight and anthropometry
- midline defects
- hydration state and blood pressure
- jaundice
- urine dipstick for protein
- prefeed blood glucose

Which infant should be investigated?

Besides those whose genitalia are truly ambiguous, infants can often be divided into those who are apparently a boy with atypical genitalia, and those who are apparently a girl with atypical genitalia. When evaluating these infants, the clinical features of the external genitalia that require examination include:
- the presence of gonads in the labioscrotal folds
- fusion of the labioscrotal folds
- the size of the phallus
- the site of the urinary meatus on the phallus, although the real site of the urinary meatus may, sometimes, only become clear on surgical exploration

These features can be scored to provide an aggregate score: the external masculinization score (EMS; see Figure 9.1). Infants who have a suspected disorder of sex development and require further clinical evaluation and consideration for investigation by a specialist should include those with isolated perineal hypospadias, isolated micropenis, isolated clitoromegaly, or a combination of genital anomalies with an EMS of less than 11. The coexistence of a metabolic disorder or a positive family history would also lower the threshold.

Normal variants

Clitoral lengths are variable and, when in doubt, should be compared to published norms. In addition, the clitoris may be enlarged in conditions such as neurofibromatosis. In any newborn girl, the labial folds may be very swollen and oedematous immediately after birth and may look like scrotal sacs. In premature babies, the lack of labial adipose tissue may pronounce the relative size of the clitoris so that it is mistaken for clitoromegaly. Labial adhesions and vaginal bleeding in the newborn are signs of the normal oestrogen surge in the newborn period.

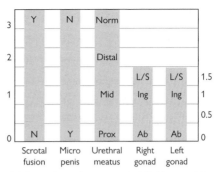

Fig 9.1 External masculinization score; L/S, labioscrotal; Ing, inguinal; Ab, abdominal or absent on examination. Reproduced from Ahmed SF., Achermann JC, Arlt W et al., UK guidance on the initial evaluation of an infant or an adolescent with a suspected disorder of sex development, *Clinical Endocrinology*, Volume 75, pp. 12–26, Copyright (2011) John Wiley and Son, with permission from Blackwell Publishing Ltd.

First-line investigations in infants

In all infants with bilaterally impalpable gonads or ambiguous genitalia, the following first tier of investigations should be undertaken:
- karyotype and PCR or fluorescent in situ hybridization analysis using Y- and X-specific markers to define the sex chromosomes
- pelvic ultrasound to delineate the internal genitalia
- plasma glucose
- serum 17-hydroxyprogesterone (unreliable before 36 hours of age)
- serum electrolytes (unlikely to deteriorate before Day 4 in cases of salt wasting)

These investigations should be sufficient in most cases to exclude a life-threatening condition such as congenital adrenal hyperplasia. In situations where the level of suspicion of congenital adrenal hyperplasia is very high and the infant needs immediate steroid replacement therapy, further serum samples should be collected and stored before starting therapy with a view to assessing testosterone, androstenedione, and renin activity or concentration, in that order of priority. Whilst it is safest to provide salt and mineralocorticoid where salt loss is suspected, it is also important to establish the diagnosis for long-term management. At least one spot or 24-hour urine sample (at least 5 mL) for a urine steroid profile should be collected before starting therapy. These samples can be collected at a later date if treatment is not started immediately.

Typically, in the young infant with a disorder of sex development, gonadal palpability combined with karyotyping (usually available within 48 hours of presentation), ultrasound examination for Müllerian structures, and determination of 17- hydroxyprogesterone should provide a reasonable guide for the initial practical management of the newborn with a disorder of sex development. Results should be interpreted with caution: tissue-dependent mosaicism may be present; the karyotype may not match the prenatal karyotype (in which case it should be repeated); and the ultrasound examination may provide misleading results, especially when the infant is unwell or does not have a full bladder, or the operator lacks experience.

Serial measurements of steroid hormones and gonadotrophins are valuable, as levels fluctuate over the first few weeks of life. This also applies to urea and electrolyte estimations; infants with salt-losing forms of congenital adrenal hyperplasia may start to show a rise in serum potassium as the first biochemical sign of salt loss from Day 4. Monitoring weight is useful in any infant at risk of salt loss but urinary electrolytes are unhelpful. Plasma renin activity prior to treatment can help retrospectively.

Serum testosterone has often been used as a marker of functioning testes and of intact pathways for the synthesis of testosterone. However, many commercially available testosterone assays can cross-react with other conjugated steroids in the early neonatal period, so, for the newborn infant, the level of serum anti-Müllerian hormone may be a more diagnostically reliable marker of the presence of testes than serum testosterone would be.

Second-line investigations

Second-line investigations will be guided by the results of the first-line investigations. In most cases, these tests are performed to investigate the underlying aetiology but are usually not necessary to determine the sex of rearing. In infants with sex chromosomes other than 46, XX, a second tier of investigations is necessary to determine the presence of testes and the adequacy of androgen production and action.

These investigations could include:

- biochemistry:
  - to assess the pituitary, gonadal, and adrenal axes by luteinizing hormone releasing hormone, hCG, and adrenocorticotrophic hormone stimulation, respectively
  - steroid analysis can also be performed by urine gas chromatography–mass spectrometry and baseline measurements of renin and aldosterone
  - serum cholesterol and 7-dehydrocholesterol are indicated in the child who has features consistent with Smith–Lemli–Opitz syndrome
- imaging:
  - MRI
  - genitogram
- internal endoscopic examination:
  - cystourethroscopy
  - laparoscopy
- pathology:
  - gonadal biopsy (although a single biopsy does not represent the whole gonad)
  - the minimum amount of ovarian or testicular tissue that should be present to classify the gonad as an ovotestis is unclear
- genetic:
  - high-resolution karyotype
  - karyotype from different tissues (blood, skin, gonads)
  - DNA for storage and analysis in the clinical genetics department
- functional studies of androgen sensitivity:
  - a functional assessment of androgen sensitivity can be performed by assessing the clinical response of testosterone on the phallus, although there is no consensus on methodology or interpretation

- alternatively, androgen sensitivity can be assessed by measuring changes in SHBG: SHBG levels should fall following androgen exposure, and a failure to show this reduction may be indicative of androgen insensitivity; this test can also be unreliable, as SHBG is very variable in the young infant
- hCG stimulation test:
  - this test detects the presence of functioning testicular tissue and defects in testosterone biosynthesis
  - most protocols in the UK use intramuscular hCG 1000–1500 units on 3 consecutive days for a standard test
  - if there is a poor response, this test can be followed by prolonged hCG stimulation: 1500 units on 3 consecutive days for the first week, followed by 1500 units on 2 days a week for the following 2 weeks, with samples taken on designated days during and after this period
  - besides testosterone, other androgens should be assessed, including dihydrotestosterone and androstenedione, with the Day 4 sample being most informative for these hormones

Aetiology of XX disorders of sex development

The 46, XX disorders of sex development can be divided into the following (also see Table 9.2):

- disorders of gonadal development
- disorders of androgen synthesis
- disorders of Müllerian development
- other conditions affecting sex development

In addition, complex urogenital abnormalities such as cloacal anomalies can affect both sexes and require major reconstructive surgery.

Aetiology of XY disorders of sex development

The 46, XY disorders of sex development can be divided into the following (also see Table 9.3):

- disorders of gonadal development:
  - have a variety of phenotypes
  - often associated with abnormalities in other systems
- disorders of androgen synthesis:
  - the defect involved may be anywhere along the pathway of androgen synthesis
  - biochemical changes depend on the site of the disorder
- disorders of androgen action:
  - the spectrum of disorders ranges from partial to complete androgen insensitivity
  - there is a range of phenotypes
- other conditions affecting sex development

Gender and its development

Unlike the sex categories 'male' and 'female', gender has several aspects: gender assignment, gender role, gender identity, gender attribution, and sexuality. In most societies, gender assignment occurs at birth, long before we have a say in the matter, marking the beginning of the process of gender socialization. The process of gender socialization also includes society's expectations of how males or females should behave, as expressed in their

Table 9.2 Characteristics of 46, XX disorders of sex development

Condition	Inheritance and gene	Genitalia	Wolffian duct	Müllerian duct	Gonads	Typical features	Hormone profile
Disorder of gonadal development							
46, XX ovotesticular DSD	Sporadic. Likely overlap with testicular DSD	Ambiguous	Present, abnormal	Present, abnormal	Lateral type: 1 ovary, 1 testis. Bilateral type: 2 ovotestis. Unilateral type: 1 ovotestis, 1 ovary or testis	Breast development in puberty with menses if ovarian tissue present. Virilization at puberty if testicular tissue not removed	Testosterone response to hCG stimulation if testicular tissue present
46, XX testicular DSD	Usually sporadic. SRY (majority). RSPO1. SOX9. SOX3	Normal male or mild hypospadias	Normal	Absent	Testes	Small testes. Gynaecomastia. Azoospermia following puberty. Pubic hair/phallus length normal	May be age dependent. LH and FSH moderately elevated. Decreased testosterone. Subnormal testosterone response to hCG stimulation
Disorder of androgen excess							
21-alpha-hydroxylase deficiency	Autosomal recessive. CYP21A2	Ambiguous	Absent	Normal	Ovary	Severe adrenal insufficiency in infancy ± salt loss. Moderate-to-severe androgenization at birth	Decreased cortisol and/or mineralocorticoids. Increased 17-OHP, 21-deoxycortisol, androstenedione, testosterone, and/or plasma renin (activity)
11-beta-hydroxylase deficiency	Autosomal recessive. CYP11B1	Ambiguous	Absent	Normal	Ovary	Adrenal insufficiency in infancy. Moderate-to-severe androgenization at birth. Arterial hypertension often developing at different ages	Decreased cortisol, corticosterone, aldosterone, and or plasma renin (activity). Increased 11-deoxycortisol, 11-deoxycorticosterone, 17-OHP (less than in 21-alpha-hydroxylase deficiency), androstenedione, and testosterone
3-beta-hydroxysteroid dehydrogenase 2 deficiency	Autosomal recessive. HSD3B2	Commonly clitoromegaly or mild virilization. Also normal	Absent	Normal	Ovary	Severe adrenal insufficiency in infancy ± salt loss. Androgenization during childhood and puberty. Premature pubarche	Increased concentrations of delta-5 C_{21} and C_{19} steroids, 17-hydroxypregnenolone, and DHEA suppressible by dexamethasone

(continued)

Table 9.2 Continued

Condition	Inheritance and gene	Genitalia	Wolffian duct	Müllerian duct	Gonads	Typical features	Hormone profile
p450 oxidoreductase deficiency	Autosomal recessive POR	Ambiguous or normal female	Absent	Normal	Ovary	Variable androgenization at birth and puberty Glucocorticoid deficiency Features of skeletal malformations Possible maternal androgenization from the second trimester of pregnancy	Combined p450c17 and p450c21 insufficiency Normal or low cortisol with poor response to ACTH stimulation Elevated 17-OHP and testosterone E2 low
p450 aromatase deficiency	Autosomal recessive CYP19A1	Ambiguous	Absent	Normal	Ovary	Delayed bone age Development of ovarian cysts during infancy, childhood, and puberty Maternal androgenization during pregnancy	High androgens in cord blood; androgens may stay elevated or normalize soon after birth
Familial glucocorticoid resistance	Autosomal recessive NR3C1	Ambiguous	Absent	Normal	Ovary	Signs of mineralocorticoid and androgen excess	Increased cortisol Increased 24-hour urinary free cortisol in the absence of clinical hypercortisolism other than mineralocorticoid effects ACTH normal or high
Maternal androgen excess	Not genetic	Ambiguous	Absent	Normal	Ovary	Virilization of female Maternal androgen-secreting tumour Maternal ingestion of androgen/progestogen	Normal

Disorders of Müllerian development

Condition	Inheritance and gene	Genitalia	Wolffian duct	Müllerian duct	Gonads	Typical features	Hormone profile
MRKH Syndrome MURCS	Usually sporadic WNT4	Normal female	Absent	Absent	Ovary	Absence of the uterus and the upper two-thirds of the vagina Associated with Müllerian duct aplasia, renal dysplasia, and cervical somite anomalies in MURCS	Normal

Abbreviations: 17-OHP, 17-hydroxyprogesterone; ACTH, adrenocorticotrophin hormone; DHEA, dehydroepiandrosterone; DHT, dihydrotestosterone; DSD, disorder of sex development; E2, estradiol; FSH, follicle-stimulating hormone; hCG, human chorionic gonadotrophin; LH, luteinizing hormone; MRKH, Mayer–Rokitansky –Kuster-Hauser; MURCS, Müllerian renal cervical spine syndrome;

Table 9.3 Characteristics of 46, XY disorders of sex development

Condition	Inheritance and gene	Genitalia	Wolffian duct	Müllerian duct	Gonads	Typical features	Hormone profile
Disorders of gonadal development							
Gonadal dysgenesis	Usually sporadic SRY SF1/NR5a1 DHH WT1 9p24 del GATA4 MAP3K1 NR0B1/DAX1 SOX9 RSPO1	Spectrum from female to normal male	Absent to normal	May be present	Dysgenetic testes/streak	In complete dysgenesis, female appearance; presents in adolescence with amenorrhoea (Swyer syndrome) In partial gonadal dysgenesis, male infertility; ambiguous genitalia May be associated with WAGR syndrome, Denys–Drash syndrome, Frasier syndrome, cardiac defects, and adrenal failure	Absent/reduced AMH Absent/variable testosterone response to hCG stimulation Low oestrogen
Disorder of androgen synthesis							
Smith–Lemli–Opitz syndrome	Autosomal recessive DHCR7	Female or ambiguous	Absent to normal	Absent	Testes	Facial/bone abnormalities Cardiac and pulmonary defects Renal agenesis Syndactyly of second and third toes Developmental delay Seizures Hypotonia	Low cholesterol Raised 7-dehydrocholesterol Decreased aldosterone-to-renin ratio
Leydig cell hypoplasia	Autosomal recessive LH/HCGR	Female, hypospadias, or micropenis	Hypoplastic	Absent	Testes	Poor androgenization with variable failure of sex hormone production at puberty	Low T and DHT Elevated LH and FSH Exaggerated LH response to LHRH Poor T and DHT response to hCG stimulation
Lipoid CAH	Autosomal recessive StAR	Female; rarely, ambiguous or male	Hypoplastic or normal	Absent	Testes	Severe adrenal insufficiency with salt loss Failure of pubertal development Rarely associated with isolated glucocorticoid deficiency	Usually deficient of glucocorticoids, mineralocorticoids, and sex steroids

(continued)

Table 9.3 Continued

Condition	Inheritance and gene	Genitalia	Wolffian duct	Müllerian duct	Gonads	Typical features	Hormone profile
p450 side deficiency	Autosomal recessive CYP11A1	Female; rarely, ambiguous or hypospadias	Hypoplastic or normal	Absent	Testes or absent	Severe adrenal insufficiency in infancy with salt loss ranging to milder adrenal insufficiency, with onset in childhood	Usually deficient of glucocorticoids, mineralocorticoids, and sex steroids
3-Beta-hydroxysteroid dehydrogenase type 2 deficiency	Autosomal recessive HSD3B2	Ambiguous, hypospadias	Normal	Absent	Testes	Severe adrenal insufficiency in infancy ± salt loss, poor androgenization at puberty with gynaecomastia	High concentrations of delta-5 C_{21} and C_{19} steroids, 17-hydroxypregnenolone, and DHEA suppressible by dexamethasone, low progesterone, and cortisol
Combined 17-alpha-hydroxylase/ 17,20-lyase deficiency	Autosomal recessive CYP17A1	Female, ambiguous, hypospadias, or micropenis	Absent or hypoplastic	Absent	Testes	Absent or poor virilization at puberty Gynaecomastia Hypertension Hypokalaemic alkalosis	Low T Raised LH and FSH Raised plasma deoxycorticosterone, corticosterone, and progesterone Low renin Normal or low cortisol with poor response to ACTH stimulation
Isolated 17,20-lyase deficiency	Autosomal recessive CYP17A1 or CYB5	Female, ambiguous, or hypospadias	Absent or hypoplastic	Absent	Testes	Absent or poor androgenization at puberty Gynaecomastia	Low T Raised LH, FSH, androstenedione, estradiol, and DHEA Increase in plasma 17-OHP and 17-hydroxypregnenolone Increased ratio of C_{21} deoxysteroids to C_{19} steroids after hCG stimulation
p450 oxidoreductase deficiency	Autosomal recessive POR	Ambiguous, hypospadias or micropenis	Absent or hypoplastic	Absent	Testes	Androgenization at birth / puberty Glucocorticoid deficiency Bone abnormalities Maternal virilization in pregnancy	Normal or low cortisol with poor response to ACTH stimulation Elevated 17-OHP T low with poor response to hCG stimulation
17-Beta-hydroxysteroid dehydrogenase type 3 deficiency	Autosomal recessive HSD17B3	Female, blind vaginal pouch, or ambiguous	Present	Absent	Testes	Androgenization at puberty Gynaecomastia	Increased plasma oestrone Decreased ratio of testosterone/androstenedione and estradiol after hCG stimulation Increased FSH and LH

Disorder	Inheritance/Gene	External genitalia	Internal ducts (Wolffian)	Internal ducts (Müllerian)	Gonads	Clinical features	Laboratory findings
5-alpha-reductase type 2 deficiency	Autosomal recessive, SRD5A2	Ambiguous, micropenis, hypospadias, blind vaginal pouch	Normal	Absent	Testes	Decreased facial and body hair; No temporal hair recession; Prostate not palpable; Variable androgenization at puberty	Decreased ratio of 5-alpha/5-beta C$_{21}$ and C$_{19}$ steroids in urine; Increased T/DHT ratio before and after hCG stimulation; Modest increase in LH; Decreased conversion of T to DHT in vitro

Disorder of androgen action

Disorder	Inheritance/Gene	External genitalia	Internal ducts (Wolffian)	Internal ducts (Müllerian)	Gonads	Clinical features	Laboratory findings
CAIS	X-linked recessive, AR	Female with blind vaginal pouch	Often present	Absent or vestigial	Testes	Scant or absent pubic and axillary hair; Breast development and female body habitus at puberty; Primary amenorrhea	Increased LH and T; Increased estradiol; FSH levels normal or slightly increased; Resistance to androgenic and metabolic effects of T
PAIS	X-linked recessive, AR	Ambiguous with blind vaginal pouch, isolated hypospadias, male	Often normal	Absent	Testes	Decreased-to-normal axillary and pubic hair, beard growth, and body hair; Gynaecomastia common at puberty; Normal male with infertility	Increased LH and T; Increased estradiol; FSH levels normal or slightly increased; Partial resistance to androgenic and metabolic effects of T

Other disorders

Disorder	Inheritance/Gene	External genitalia	Internal ducts (Wolffian)	Internal ducts (Müllerian)	Gonads	Clinical features	Laboratory findings
PMDS	Autosomal recessive, AMH or AMHR2	Normal male or cryptorchidism	Present	Present	Testes	Persistence of Müllerian structures; Inguinal hernia containing ipsilateral testus, fallopian tube, and uterus	Normal testosterone response to hCG stimulation; AMH low in AMH defect, high in AMHR2 defect
Disorders of testes maintenance	Sporadic	Cryptorchidism, with ambiguous to male	Present	May be present	Atrophic or absent	Absent or rudimentary testes with male phenotype.	Increased FSH and LH; Low testosterone; Reduced AMH and testosterone response to hCG stimulation

Abbreviations: 17-OHP, 17-hydroxyprogesterone; ACTH, adrenocorticotrophin hormone; AMH, anti-Müllerian hormone; CAH, congenital adrenal hyperplasia; CAIS, Complete androgen insensitivity syndrome; DHEA, dehydroepiandrosterone; DHT, dihydrotestosterone; DSD, disorder of sex development; FSH, follicle-stimulating hormone; hCG, human chorionic gonadotrophin; LH, luteinizing hormone; LHRH, luteinizing hormone releasing hormone; PAIS, partial androgen insensitivity syndrome; PMDS, persistent Müllerian duct syndrome; T, testosterone.

gender role behaviour. Gender identity refers to the individual's perception of one's own gender and how it conforms to the male or female gender role in society. Gender attribution is what we all do when we meet someone and want to decide whether they are a man or a woman. Finally, sexuality refers to erotic desires, sexual practices, or sexual orientation.

For most people, their gender identity, gender role, and the symbolic gender manifestations are congruent and, in addition, they will be sexually attracted to the opposite sex. Some aspects of gender, such as role, assignment, and the symbolic manifestations, as well as the different types of sexuality, may differ markedly from one society to another and continue to evolve within respective societies. In some cultures, the distinction is becoming less absolute and it may be better to consider these aspects as a continuum, with female characteristics at one extreme and male ones at the other. The development of gender identity is the result of a complex interaction between genetic, prenatal, and postnatal endocrine influences, and postnatal psychosocial and environmental experiences. Gender development consists of gender identity formation such as gender knowledge, self-perception, preferences (toy, playmate), and gender role behaviours.

Sex assignment in the affected newborn

Initial gender uncertainty is unsettling and stressful for families as well as the health professionals. Given that gender development is a relatively long-term process, clinical professionals involved in management need to be clear of the distinction between sex assignment and gender assignment; the latter cannot be achieved by the clinical team and should be considered intrinsic to the child's own development. However, expediting a thorough assessment and reaching a decision on sex assignment is desirable. Factors that influence sex assignment include the diagnosis, the genital appearance, the surgical options available, any need for lifelong replacement therapy, the potential for fertility, the age at presentation, the views of the family and, sometimes, circumstances relating to cultural practices.

Surgical management

A clear explanation of the pros and cons of surgery by a surgeon with expertise in the care of children with disorders of sex development is generally valued by parents and affected adults. Emphasis is nowadays placed more on functional outcome, rather than a strictly cosmetic appearance. It is possible that surgery that is performed for cosmetic reasons in the first year of life relieves parental distress and improves attachment between the child and the parents but there is little supporting evidence. It is anticipated that surgical reconstruction in infancy will need to be refined at the time of puberty. An absent or inadequate vagina (with rare exceptions) may require a vaginoplasty or vaginal dilatation in adolescence when the patient is psychologically motivated and a full partner in the procedure. In the case of hypospadias, standard techniques for surgical repair include chordee correction, urethral reconstruction, and the judicious use of testosterone supplementation. Techniques of phalloplasty continue to improve but the complexity of phalloplasty and current results in adulthood should be taken into account during the initial counselling period. Gonadectomy may be required in some conditions, with the decisions on timing of this procedure being guided by the malignant potential of the gonad.

Psychosocial management

Psychosocial care should be an integral part of management in order to promote positive adaptation and allow parents to express and resolve their concerns. Whilst the mental-healthcare staff should have some knowledge about disorders of sex development, in most cases, the early concerns of parents may be less to do with the long-term implications of the condition and more to do with coping and adjustment of the parents during early infancy, and some of these issues are generic to many stressful neonatal situations.

A common issue seems to be related to how the condition should be explained to friends and relatives. This expertise can facilitate team decisions about gender assignment/reassignment, the timing of surgery, and sex hormone replacement. Psychosocial screening tools that identify families at risk for maladaptive coping with a child's medical condition should be considered. It should be explained to the new parents that it is routine practice to involve mental-health staff and that they will have access to these staff throughout the child's development. Once the child is sufficiently developed for a psychological assessment of gender identity, such an evaluation must be included in discussions about gender reassignment.

Atypical gender role behaviour is more common in children with disorders of sex development than in the general population, but should not be taken as an indicator for gender reassignment. It is important to emphasize the separability of sex-typical behaviour, sexual orientation, and gender identity. In the long term, most current studies suggest that affected individuals lead productive lives but a small proportion may have functional problems and may also suffer from gender identity disorders. Medical education and counselling for children as well as the parents shall be a recurrent gradual process of increasing sophistication which is commensurate with changing cognitive and psychological development.

Useful websites

The following websites may be useful:
- The I-DSD Registry: http://www.i-dsd.org
- Scottish Differences in Sex Development Network: http://www.sdsd.scot.nhs.uk
- DSD Families: http://www.dsdfamilies.org
- Living with CAH: http://www.livingwithcah.com
- Androgen Insensitivity Syndrome Support Group: http://www.aissg.org

Further reading

Ahmed SF, Achermann JC, Arlt W, et al. UK guidance on the initial evaluation of an infant or an adolescent with a suspected disorder of sex development. *Clin Endocrinol (Oxf)* 2011; 75: 12–26. Revised 2016: *Clin Endocrinol* 2016; 84: 771–88.

Ahmed SF and O'Toole S. Management of boys and men with disorders of sex development. *Curr Opin Endocrinol Diabetes Obes* 2012; 19: 190–6.

Duguid A, Morrison S, Robertson A, et al. The psychological impact of genital anomalies on the parents of affected children. *Acta Paediatr* 2007; 96: 348–52.

Eggers S and Sinclair A. mammalian sex determination: Insights from humans and mice. *Chromosome Res* 2012: 2015–238.

Hughes IA, Houk C, Ahmed SF, et al. Consensus statement on management of intersex disorders. *Arch Dis Child* 2006; 91: 554–63.

Warne GL. Long term outcome of disorders of sex development. *Sex Dev* 2008; 2: 268–77.

9.2 Gender dysphoria

Definition and pathophysiology

The neuroanatomical origin of gender identity is unknown, but the inner sense of being female or male is almost universally present by the age of 4. A child typically reports a gender concordant with phenotype before he or she knows his or her surname, nationality, religion, or address. Gender identity is distinct from sexual orientation, the only congruity being that people discover rather than choose what they are.

Gender dysphoria is characterized by discomfort with one's phenotypic sex and a wish to have treatment to make one's body correspond to that of the preferred sex.

Epidemiology

Gender dysphoria is self-diagnosed, self-reported, and subjective. It affects approximately 1 in 15,000 males, and 1 in 35,000 females, in all societies and across all social strata.

Fertility

Counselling regarding sperm storage or ovarian cryopreservation should be considered prior to hormonal or surgical treatment.

Name change

A deed poll facilitates a name change on medical records and financial, utility, and insurance documents but not on birth or educational certificates. A gender recognition certificate issued in accordance with the Gender Recognition Act 2004 in Great Britain, however, allows a new birth certificate to be issued in the correct gender. Other nations may have different legal situations.

Drug treatment: Male to female

Oestrogens

The following oestrogen treatments may be used:
- transdermal oestrogen patches: 25–200 µg estradiol per day (Estraderm TTS or MX®)
- transdermal estradiol gel: 2.5 g gel containing 0.06% estradiol (Estrogel® 2 measures) or Sandrena® gel up to maximum 5 mg
- oral estradiol valerate (Progynova®): 2–6 mg daily
- oral estradiol (Zumenon®): 2–6 mg daily

Anti-androgens

The following anti-androgen treatments may be used:
- cyproterone acetate: 50–100 mg daily
- spironolactone: 50–400 mg daily

The following 5-alpha-reductase inhibitors may be used:
- dutasteride: 500 µg daily
- finasteride: 5 mg daily

The following gonadotrophin-releasing hormone superagonists may be used:
- goserelin 3.6 mg subcutaneously every 28 days
- leuprorelin 3.75 mg subcutaneously every month

Physical treatment: Male to female

Facial and body hair removal

The following methods may be used for facial and body hair removal:
- shaving
- electrolysis
- laser hair removal
- ornithine decarboxylase cream

Scalp hair restoration

The following methods may be used for scalp hair restoration:
- implants
- high-tech hairpieces
- minoxidil may be helpful

Surgery

The following surgical procedures may be used:
- face lift to lower hairline and elevate eyebrows
- removal of the supraorbital ridge
- cheek and lip augmentation
- removal of mandibular flare
- rhinoplasty
- chondrolaryngoplasty (a.k.a. tracheal shave)
- chin reduction
- breast augmentation
- penectomy and orchidectomy
- construction of a neovagina and neoclitoris

Modest lactation has been reported in transsexual women who wish to breastfeed their adopted infants. The addition of off-label dopamine antagonists such as domperidone or metoclopramide to oestrogen treatment, with or without oral progestogen (up to 400 mg po daily), together with persistent use of breast pumps over several months may make nursing possible.

Effects of male-to-female treatments

Oestrogens induce subtle physical and psychological feminization and may lighten mood. Muscle bulk and strength diminish, facial hair growth slows, and libido, erections, and fertility are reduced. Testicular atrophy may become irreversible in the longer term. Gynaecomastia begins after 2–3 months and is typically modest, but more pronounced in younger women with a higher body mass index. Most require breast augmentation to achieve the desired profile.

Anti-androgens may discourage further body hair growth by blocking the effects of adrenal as well as gonadal androgens.

5-Alpha-reductase inhibitors may transiently reduce the rate of male pattern baldness progression.

GnRH superagonists are prescribed in highly specialist clinics to reversibly slow pubertal progression pending the establishment of a more secure diagnosis. They are occasionally used in adulthood when high doses of oestrogen appear insufficient to suppress gonadal androgen production.

Progestogens are sometimes taken by transsexual women in the belief that they maintain libido and augment breast growth. There is no rationale or evidence to support this.

Risks of male-to-female treatments

Oestrogen-induced thromboembolic events increase probably about tenfold compared to untreated controls but absolute risks are low (0.5%), particularly after the first 2 years of treatment in non-smokers, and may be further reduced by avoiding ethinylestradiol and using transdermal preparations. Breast cancer is rare. Hyperprolactinaemia and prolactinoma development has been reported. Transient (less than three months) abnormalities of liver function may occur secondary to estrogen treatment, but longer term of liver function typically discloses concurrent alcoholic or non-alcoholic steatohepatitis or viral hepatitis.

Drug treatment: Female to male

See also Chapter 8, Section 8.3. The following drug treatments may be used:

- Sustanon® (licensed)
- Nebido®: 1 g intramuscularly every 3 months
- testosterone enantate: 250 mg every 2–3 weeks intramuscularly
- Testim®, Testogel®, or Tostran® transdermal gel: 50 mg daily

Physical treatment: Female to male

The following physical treatment may be used:

- breast reduction (a.k.a. 'top surgery')
- metoidioplasty (enhancement of clitoral size)
- phalloplasty from free forearm flap
- hysterectomy and salpingo-oophorectomy

Effects of female-to-male treatments

Facial and body hair begins to develop after 6–12 weeks of testosterone treatment and slowly progresses over many years. Genetic predisposition to male pattern baldness is disclosed, the facial appearance becomes more masculine, and the voice pitch descends but may not reach typical male range. Menstrual flow ceases but cramp-like pains sometime persist. Regular ultrasound of the endometrium should be performed to monitor for the development of endometrial hyperplasia. Clitoromegaly is minimal. The rationale for oophorectomy and hysterectomy is tenuous, but transmen may feel more comfortable when the risks of cervical, endometrial, and ovarian neoplasia are eliminated.

Risks of female-to-male treatments

The following risks are associated with female-to-male treatments:

- testosterone side effects; these are limited to polycythaemia and a potential predisposition to osteoporosis
- adverse liver profile
- psychological problems, including depression and increased suicide risk although depression may improve with testosterone treatment

Further reading

Bower H. The gender identity disorder in the DSM-IV classification: A critical evaluation. *Aust N Z J Psychiatry* 2001; 35: 1–8.

Gooren LJ, Gitay EJ, and Bunck MC. Long-term treatment of transsexuals with cross-sex hormones: Extensive personal experience. *J Clin Endocrinol Metab* 2008; 93: 19–25.

Levy A, Crown A, and Reid R. Endocrine intervention for transsexuals. *Clin Endocrinol (Oxf)* 2003; 59: 409–18.

Meriggiola MC and Gava G. Endocrine care of transpeople part I. A review of cross-sex hormonal treatments, outcomes and adverse effects in transmen. *Clin Endocrinol (Oxf)* 2015 Nov;83(5):597–606.

Meriggiola MC and Gava G. Endocrine care of transpeople part II. A review of cross-sex hormonal treatments, outcomes and adverse effects in transwomen. *Clin Endocrinol (Oxf)* 2015; 83: 607–15.

Reisman T and Goldstein Z. Case report: induced lactation in a transgender woman. Transgend Health 2018; 3: 24–26.

van Kesteren PJ, Asscheman H, Megens JA, et al. Mortality and morbidity in transsexual subjects treated with cross-sex hormones. *Clin Endocrinol (Oxf)* 1997; 47: 337–42.

WPATH WPAfTHC. *Standards of Care for the Health of Transsexual, Transgender, and Gender Nonconforming People*, 2001. Available at http://www.wpath.org (accessed 4 January 2018).

9.3 Male and female infertility

Definition
Infertility is defined as an inability to conceive despite regular unprotected intercourse over a specific time course (usually 1–2 years). The spontaneous pregnancy rate for a couple is 20% per cycle, and cumulative rates are 85% after 1 year, and 93% after 2 years.

Epidemiology
Infertility affects 9% of couples. Seventy per cent have never been pregnant, and 30% have secondary infertility, with pregnancy either with a different partner or at an earlier age. This equates to a worldwide rate of infertility of 70 million couples.

Clinical features of female infertility
A female cause of infertility is identified in approximately 35% of couples.

Anovulatory infertility
Anovulation can be classified according to the level of disruption of the hypothalamo-pituitary axis, dividing anovulatory infertility into three main categories: ovarian dysfunction, hypogonadotrophic hypogonadism, and hypergonadotrophic hypogonadism, with other less common causes considered separately.

Ovarian dysfunction
The most common presentation of anovulation is associated with normal gonadotrophin concentrations. Normogonadotrophic anovulation is usually seen in PCOS (see Chapter 7, Section 7.4). In its classic form, it is a combination of anovulation with oligomenorrhoea, and hyperandrogenism. It is estimated to affect 5%–15% of the female population, depending on the definition used to define the disorder. Endocrine and paracrine abnormalities in the early stages of folliculogenesis are the main causes of anovulation in PCOS.

Hypogonadotrophic hypogonadism
When pulsatile secretion of GnRH is slowed or stopped, anovulation ensues due to a lack of pituitary and ovarian stimulation. This is seen in hypothalamic dysfunction commonly secondary to excessive exercise, psychologic stress, weight loss, or anorexia nervosa. There are also a number of disorders of the anterior pituitary gland that lead to failure of production of FSH, including infarction (Sheehan's syndrome), inflammatory reaction in TB infection, and tumours such as non-functioning adenomas or craniopharyngioma. Rarer causes include an intracranial mass, Laurence–Moon–Biedl syndrome, Kallman syndrome or isolated gonadotrophin deficiency, with mutations of the GnRH receptor or kisspeptin. The pituitary may also be affected iatrogenically by cranial irradiation or surgically at the time of hypophysectomy for a pituitary tumour.

Hypergonadotrophic hypogonadism
Hypergonadotrophic hypogonadism occurs as a result of the ovary's failure to respond to gonadotrophic stimulation by the pituitary gland. The absence of negative-feedback hormones (estradiol and inhibin B) from the follicle results in excessive secretion of the gonadotrophic hormones FSH and LH. Hypergonadotrophic hypogonadism is usually due to menopause; if it occurs before the age of 40, it is referred to as premature ovarian failure or primary ovarian insufficiency with the early depletion of the ovarian follicular pool. It is now understood that a number of women with primary ovarian insufficiency have sporadic ovarian function, and 5%–10% are able to conceive despite elevated FSH levels, and biopsy-proven depleted follicular counts. Defects in the FSH receptor have been implicated.

Others
Endocrine disorders such as hyperprolactinaemia and hypothyroidism are also possible causes of anovulation and should be excluded in the infertile female.

Obstruction to the path of sperm and oocyte
Tubal infertility
Tubal damage is the cause for infertility in 40% of infertile women. The fallopian tube is important in sperm and oocyte transport, for the capacitation of sperm, for fertilization, and for the early development of the early zygote and embryo. The main cause of tubal damage is pelvic inflammatory disease, with chlamydia trachomatis being the prime pathogen in the majority of cases. Fallopian tubes may also be damaged iatrogenically in tubal sterilization or inadvertently at the time of pelvic surgery.

Endometriosis
Endometriosis in moderate-to-severe cases may lead to mechanical obstruction of the fallopian tubes. However, even in its mild form, it has been linked to infertility, despite there being no clear understanding of the pathogenesis. Theories include alterations to the ovary and oocyte, or immune dysfunction, with the toxic effects of peritoneal cytokines affecting sperm function, and altered B-cell activity affecting the endometrium, as possible explanations for this established link.

Intrauterine factors
Submucous leiomyomata, congenital uterine anomalies, endometrial polyps, and uterine adhesions are all potential causes of infertility, particularly if the intrauterine pathology forms a mechanical obstruction to sperm and oocyte transportation or to implantation. Uterine septum or distortion to the uterine cavity, such as a T-shaped uterus as a result of in utero exposure of diethylstilbestrol can lead to implantation failure and recurrent miscarriage. Intrauterine adhesions may alter fertility (Asherman's syndrome) and can occur as a result of curettage, caesarean delivery, or myomectomy. Endometritis in the case of TB will cause infertility, although the relationship between other pathogens and implantation is less clear.

Unexplained infertility
Completion of the standard investigations for infertility fails to reveal a cause in 15%–30% of cases. It is likely that the cause is related to undiagnosed problems with the oocyte being of embryo quality, or implantation failure, and these are not able to be tested unless IVF is undertaken.

Investigations
As only 50% of couples who have not conceived after 1 year will do so in the second year, investigations are warranted after 1 year of subfertility or sooner if there is reason to suspect impaired fertility such as irregular menstrual cycles, pelvic surgery, or where there is advanced maternal age (>35 years of age).

The history should include:
- the length of the period of infertility
- the menstrual history, including cycle length and pelvic pain
- past obstetric history
- past medical history
- smoking, alcohol consumption, drugs (prescription and recreational)

The examination should include:
- observation for pubertal staging, acne, hirsutism, acanthosis nigricans, and stigmata of anomalies such as Turner syndrome, or Cushing's disease
- thyroid examination
- abdominal examination, taking note of scars and masses
- vaginal examination using a bimanual speculum, looking for anatomical abnormalities and taking a cervical swab if the history suggests there is a risk of pelvic infection
- bimanual examination of the uterus and ovaries

Investigations should include the following baseline tests:
- antenatal screening bloods
- TFTs
- prolactin
- FSH
- LH
- estradiol
- progesterone

Tests of ovulation

- A history of a regular menstrual period is indicative of ovulation. Historically, tests of the effects of progestogens on the basal body temperature, the endometrium, and the cervical mucous were assessed. However, they are not as accurate as biochemical markers, and are now infrequently used.
- A mid-luteal progesterone rise, usually 8 days after the LH surge, with levels in excess of 30 nmol/L (943 ng/dL) is diagnostic of ovulation.
- The LH surge should be assessed on serum and or urine. Commercially available urinary LH detection kits can detect the LH surge and may be used to time intercourse in natural cycles or in assisted conception with ovulation induction or donor insemination treatments.

Ovarian reserve tests

Women with advanced age, or ovarian surgery are at risk of diminished ovarian reserve or function. Ovarian reserve testing involves:
- measuring FSH
- measuring estradiol
- measuring anti-Müllerian hormone
- ultrasound of the ovaries to assess the antral follicle count.

The results of these tests are not absolute indicators of infertility, but abnormal levels correlate with a decreased response to ovulation induction stimulation, and lowered live birth rates at IVF.

Ultrasound

Ultrasound is an important investigation to assess:
- congenital anomalies of the Müllerian duct
- endometrial polyps
- fibroids

- intrauterine adhesions
- hydrosalpinx
- ovarian cysts such as endometriomas, or multiple follicles suggestive of PCOS

Assessment of tubal patency

- Ultrasound with saline infusion of the endometrial cavity and fallopian tubes (hysterosalpingocontrast sonography) is a good screening test, involving cannulation of the cervix and injecting gas microtubules in galactose microparticles into the endometrial cavity and fallopian tubes. The advantages of this technique are that it requires relatively low levels of intervention, and the ovaries and uterus may be viewed.
- Hystersalpingography carried out in the first 10 days of the cycle has a sensitivity of 65% and a specificity of 83%. It has the added advantage of making it possible to assess the uterine cavity.
- Laparoscopy and hydrotubation with or without dye is the gold-standard diagnostic test. Although more invasive and expensive, the test has the advantage of being able to visualize the fimbrial ends of the fallopian tubes, and pelvic structures for endometriosis.

Assessment of the uterine cavity

The uterine cavity can be assessed via the following methods:
- hysteroscopy: for direct visualization of the endometrial cavity
- pelvic ultrasound: best performed transvaginally in the first half of the cycle
- 3D ultrasound: high sensitivity; used for the diagnosis of intrauterine polyps or intrauterine synechiae
- hystersalpingography

Management

Management of anovulatory infertility

Selection of the most appropriate method for managing anovulatory infertility depends on the cause of anovulation. Such methods include the following:
- normalization of body weight in obese and overweight women to regain ovulation
- ovulation induction in patients with hypogonadotrophic hypogonadism; can be achieved with pulsatile administration of GnRH or by daily injection of gonadotrophins
- medical management of patients with PCOS: includes the use of clomiphene citrate or gonadotrophins; both approaches should include ultrasound monitoring during the cycle to minimize the risk of multiple pregnancy
- surgical methods such as ovarian drilling:
  - offers similar ovulation and pregnancy rates as medical ovulation induction, with reduced multiple pregnancy rates
  - predictors of success include LH >10 I U/L, normal BMI, and shorter duration of infertility
  - concerns about the technique include its invasiveness, which can cause damage to the ovarian tissue and destruction of primordial follicles
- controlled ovarian stimulation with gonadotrophins and intrauterine insemination seems to confer a better pregnancy rate than timed intercourse
- IVF and embryo transfer in unexplained infertility has diagnostic and therapeutic value, as it provides

information about fertilization and egg and embryo quality

Congenital uterine anomalies

- Congenital defects, leiomyomas, and intrauterine adhesions and polyps are the only treatable uterine factors.
- Fibroids may be excised either laparoscopically or hysteroscopically. However, there is only evidence of improved pregnancy rates with excision of submucous fibroids or obstructing fibroids.
- Intrauterine adhesions may be resected to improve pregnancy outcomes.
- Surgical excision of uterine septum may also improve implantation, but only in the group with implantation failure.

Assisted reproduction

The term 'assisted reproductive technology' refer to all forms of infertility treatment which requires laboratory handing of gametes. A typical cycle of such treatment involves initial assessment and counselling; ovarian stimulation and monitoring; oocyte retrieval; IVF; embryo transfer; luteal phase support; a pregnancy test; and confirmation of intrauterine pregnancy via ultrasound. This process may include ICSI, or pre-implantation genetic diagnosis.

Natural conception and ovulation induction regimes rely on monofollicular development, whereas IVF success relies on multifollicular development.

Ovulation induction

The process of ovulation induction is aimed to induce monofollicular development in the ovary, and then ovulation, so that pregnancy occurs with timed intercourse or intrauterine insemination.

Drugs used in ovarian stimulation

Clomifene citrate

Clomifene citrate is a non-steroidal analogue of estradiol; it binds to oestrogen receptors and acts as a competitive oestrogen-receptor antagonist. After administration of clomifene citrate, there are enhanced pituitary gonadotrophins, follicular recruitment, selection, assertion of a dominant follicle, and follicle rupture (ovulation). The most common regime is commencement on Day 5 of the cycle for 5 days, usually at 50 mg/day. Ovulation rates of 70%–92% are expected, and half of the women who ovulate will become pregnant. The discrepancy may be due to:

- anti-oestrogen effects on the endometrium
- anti-oestrogen effects on cervical mucus
- decreased uterine blood flow
- impaired placental protein synthesis
- subclinical pregnancy loss
- effect on tubal transport
- detrimental effects on the oocyte

Clomifene citrate will generally double the couple's chance of pregnancy compared to no treatment.

The side effects include:

- hot flushes
- abdominal discomfort
- breast discomfort
- nausea and vomiting
- visual disturbance and headaches

- multiple pregnancy: mainly twins, although higher order multiples also occur

Aromatase inhibitors

Aromatase inhibitors are competitive inhibitors of the aromatase enzyme system and therefore inhibit conversion of androgens to oestrogens. Their use will decrease levels of oestrone, estradiol, and oestrone sulphate overall, with no change in the levels of corticosteroids, aldosterone, or thyroid hormones. They are useful in patients where high levels of estradiol are to be avoided, such as patients with oestrogen-dependent breast cancer. The main side effects include:

- bone pain
- back pain
- nausea
- dyspnoea

Ovulation rates of 75%, and pregnancy rates of 25% are expected with treatment. Aromatase inhibitors do not have the negative side effect of anti-oestrogen alterations to the endometrium, and may have a lower risk of multiple pregnancies.

Gonadotrophins

Recombinant gonadotrophins administered subcuticularly are now available for use in ovarian stimulation. Daily injection of FSH to stimulate monofollicular development is used in ovulation induction (see Figure 9.2). The dose depends on the women's age, weight, previous cycles, and level of anti-Müllerian hormone, with a standard starting dose of 50–75 IU/day. In general, the addition of LH is not required, unless the patient has hypogonadotrophic hypogonadism.

Side effects include:

- ovarian enlargement
- abdominal distention and pain
- ovarian hyperstimulation syndrome
- ovarian cysts
- vaginal bleeding
- breast tenderness
- urinary tract infection
- febrile reactions and flu-like symptoms (joint pains, malaise, headache, and fatigue)
- local side effects include pain, rash, swelling, and/or irritation at the site of injection

It is useful to track the follicle growth using transvaginal ultrasound and serial estradiol measures. Once the ovary has been stimulated adequately, so that there is a leading follicle >18 mm in diameter, a trigger for ovulation may be used. hCG is commonly used as an LH-surge surrogate, as it is similar to LH in size and structure, with an identical alpha subunit, and high cysteine content. Both induce luteinization, and support the lutein cells. hCG has a longer half-life, compared to LH, and does not inhibit the endogenous LH surge.

When there are preovulatory follicles (when follicles are the right size, and LH receptors are appropriate), hCG injection stimulates:

- granulosa cell luteinization
- the production of progesterone instead of estradiol
- the resumption of meiosis
- maturation of oocytes
- follicle rupture 36–40 hours later

The negative effects of the prolonged half-life and excretion of hCG include:

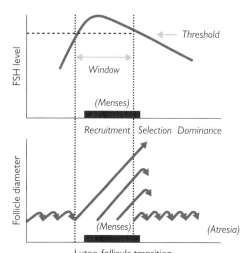

Fig 9.2 Window and threshold for follicle-stimulating hormone stimulation of follicles; FSH, follicle-stimulating hormone. Reproduced from Fauser BC, Van Heusden AM, Manipulation of human ovarian function: physiological concepts and clinical consequences, *Endocrine Reviews*, Volume 18, Issue 1, pp. 71–106. Copyright © 1997 by The Endocrine Society.

- causing the interpretation of pregnancy tests to be problematic
- encouraging increased luteinization for longer
- causing a predisposition for multiple corpora luteum and ovarian hyperstimulation syndrome
- prolonged estradiol and progesterone levels (prolonged estradiol is implicated in implantation failure and early pregnancy loss)
- causing small follicles to subsequently ovulate, increasing the risk of multiple pregnancies in ovulation induction

Once ovulation is triggered, a pregnancy test may be performed 1 week later to assess for pregnancy in the ovulation-induction cycle. If the pregnancy test is positive, an early pelvic ultrasound to assess the viability of the location of the implantation is required. Success rates of up to 15%–40% per cycle are reported.

Multifollicular development in assisted reproductive technology

In IVF and ICSI, multifollicular development is the aim of ovarian stimulation. Controlled ovarian hyperstimulation using high-dose gonadotrophins must be monitored closely with blood tests and ultrasound. A trigger for ovulation is administered when the leading follicles are mature, and oocyte pickup is performed via a transvaginal approach 36 hours later. This process bypasses the fallopian tubes, and has the highest success of pregnancy of all the methods of assisted reproductive technology (see Figure 9.3).

Pituitary downregulation

The advent of GnRH agonists and antagonists has revolutionized the ability to control ovulation in stimulated cycles by suppressing the natural surge of gonadotrophins. These are routinely used in IVF cycles (see Figure 9.4).

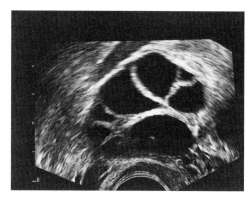

Fig 9.3 Ultrasound image of a hyperstimulated ovary. Courtesy of Genea Ltd.

GnRH agonists

With initial use of GnRH agonists, a flare of gonadotrophin occurs, lasting 7–14 days; however, with prolonged administration, this leads to a downregulation of receptors. The agonist binds to the receptor in the pituitary, the ligand–receptor complex is internalized by endocytosis, and subsequently undergoes dissociation, degradation of the ligand, and then partial recycling of the receptors. Therefore, GnRH agonists are associated with:

- receptor downregulation
- pituitary desensitization
- initial flare up
- slow reversibility

They are generally used from Day 21 of the preceding cycle to suppress endogenous gonadotrophins, and may be administered via nasal spray or injection.

GnRH antagonists

More recently, GnRH antagonists have been used in stimulated cycles. GnRH antagonists have a direct inhibitory effect on gonadotrophin secretion; however, this effect is rapidly reversible. Antagonist molecules compete and occupy the pituitary GnRH receptors, thereby competitively blocking the access of GnRH, and precluding receptor occupation and stimulation. There is no loss of receptors. Therefore, a constant supply and a higher dose range of antagonist is required. There is also no initial flare response. Actions include:

- receptor blockage without receptor activation
- competitive inhibition
- immediate dose-dependent suppression
- rapid reversibility

Use of these antagonists usually commences on Day 5 of the cycle, making the entire length of cycle shorter in this protocol. There is also a reduction of ovarian hyperstimulation syndrome in cycles where GnRH antagonists are used.

Ovarian stimulation

The approach used in ovarian stimulation is similar to that used for ovulation induction; however, the doses used in ovarian stimulation are higher than those used in ovulation induction. For IVF cycles, multifollicular development is the goal. The FSH threshold is not identical for

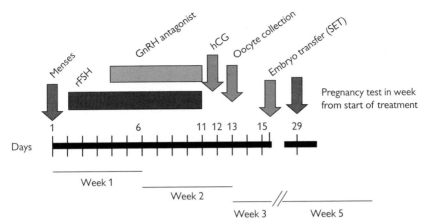

Fig 9.4 IVF antagonist protocol; GnRH, gonadotrophin-releasing hormone; hCG, human chorionic gonadotrophin; rFSH, recombinant follicle-stimulating hormone; SET, single-embryo transfer.
Courtesy of Genea Ltd.

all follicles; therefore, FSH levels need to be well above threshold. Follicular development continues for as long as FSH is administered (reduction of FSH, as per the natural cycle, promotes atresia and the development of a leading follicle). Occasionally, LH supplementation is required, especially in the situation of hypogonadotrophic hypogonadism.

The starting dose of FSH is altered according to predictors of response, such as the patient's age and weight. Baseline anti-Müllerian hormone and FSH levels and ultrasound findings are also taken into consideration.

When the lead follicles are mature, a trigger of ovulation is used in the same way as for ovulation-induction cycles. Following this, oocyte retrieval is planned. During this procedure, which is guided by transvaginal ultrasound, the follicle is punctured via the vaginal wall with a sharp 17-gauge collection needle. Negative pressure is applied to encourage retrieval of the oocyte from within the follicle, with laminar flow to protect the oocyte. The temperature is controlled using warmed tubing, collection racks, and zygote media. All accessible follicles are aspirated for oocytes during the collection.

Luteal phase support

In a normal menstrual cycle, estradiol and progesterone begin to rise after the LH surge (approximately 4 days after ovulation) and continue to rise for 1 week after this time. There is then a rapid fall associated with menstruation unless pregnancy ensues. During IVF cycles, there are supraphysiologic levels of sex steroids (estradiol and progesterone) in the early luteal phase, and a shorter duration of action, with a short luteal phase and early bleeding. The addition of GnRH analogues to suppress the pituitary worsens this effect. Luteal support has been shown to increase pregnancy rates in IVF cycles, and should continue until the foetus is 10 weeks gestation or for 8 weeks after oocyte collection. Common preparations of luteal phase support include:

• progesterone, either intramuscularly 50 mg/day or via the vaginal route such as with progesterone 8%, 90 mg gel, daily or twice daily

• hCG every 3–5 days provides both estradiol and progesterone support; however, this treatment is associated with an increased risk of ovarian hyperstimulation syndrome and should be avoided in high-risk women

On the day of the oocyte collection, the male partner is to produce sperm for IVF or ICSI, or frozen sperm may also be used. In conventional IVF cycles, incubation of the oocyte cumulus complex in a washed sperm suspension of approximately 200,000 spermatozoa is performed, and signs of fertilization and embryo development are reviewed regularly. ICSI involves stripping the oocyte from the cumulus complex and injecting the spermatozoa directly into the oocyte cytoplasm (see Figure 9.5). This is the treatment of choice where there is low sperm number or poor semen parameters.

Embryo transfer

On Day 3 or Day 5 following oocyte collection, the cleavage-stage embryo or blastocyst is transferred back into the uterine cavity via a catheter threaded through the internal os.

Complications and risks

Common complications of assisted reproductive technology include haemorrhage of greater than 100 mL (0.8%), and pelvic inflammatory disease risk (0.2%–0.5%), which most commonly occurs secondary to an endometrioma in the ovary.

Ovarian hyperstimulation syndrome

A risk of ovarian stimulation is ovarian hyperstimulation syndrome, which occurs due to a large number of follicles and granulosa cells under FSH influence. The hallmark of ovarian hyperstimulation syndrome is an increase in capillary permeability resulting in a fluid shift from the intravascular space to the third space compartment; this increase is probably mediated by VEGF. In the severe setting, this syndrome can lead to respiratory distress, pulmonary embolus, or stroke. There are two types of ovarian hyperstimulation syndrome: early (occurring prior to Day 9) and late (occurring after Day 9 (usually due to pregnancy)). Patients present with abdominal pain

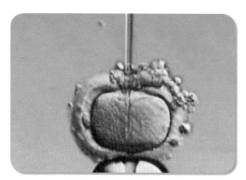

Fig 9.5 ICSI.
Courtesy of Genea Ltd.

and discomfort, shortness of breath, or with neurological symptoms. Risk factors for the development of ovarian hyperstimulation syndrome include:

- young age (<33 years old)
- low body weight
- polycystic ovaries on ultrasound (>12 follicles 2–8 mm)
- PCOS
- increased level of anti-Müllerian hormone
- antral follicle count (>14)
- previous occurrence of ovarian hyperstimulation syndrome
- high numbers of follicles (>20) on the trigger day
- serum estradiol level >20,000 pmol/L (545 ng/dL) on the trigger day
- high luteal progesterone post trigger

Pregnancy will worsen this condition.

Treatment is supportive, with no embryo transfer if the patient is high risk, to avoid pregnancy. Treatment includes the use of oral and intravenous fluids, and minimizing risks of deep vein thrombosis. Occasionally, patients will require admission to the intensive care unit for inotrope support.

Clinical features of male infertility

It has been estimated that 35% of infertility is male related.

Primary testicular disease

Primary testicular disease is the most common cause of male factor infertility, with failure of spermatogenesis. There is no underlying pathology in 50% of cases. Known causes include:

- microdeletions of genes in the Y chromosome
- testicular maldescent, particularly if left uncorrected until puberty
- testicular torsion, trauma, or infection
- testicular neoplasm
- chemotherapy
- haemochromotosis
- chromosomal anomalies including Klinefelter's syndrome (see Chapter 8, Sections 8.2 and 8.3)
- inflammatory conditions include mumps orchitis and severe epididymal orchitis leading to testicular damage

Obstructive pathology

Obstruction can occur at any level of the male reproductive tract, from the rete testis, to the epididymis, to the vas deferens, and may be due to congenital, inflammatory, or iatrogenic causes. Bilateral congenital absence of the vas deferens is associated with cystic fibrosis gene carrier status.

Endocrinological causes of male infertility

Hypogonadotrophic hypogonadism, thyroid disease, and adrenal disease will cause male infertility. Hyperprolactinaemia in men can lead to impotence, with little effect on sperm production.

Autoimmune

Anti-sperm antibodies are commonly found in men (12%), and these may lead to reduced sperm motility and decrease the spermatozoon's ability to bind with the zona pellucida or oocyte, when present in high levels. The exact cause of anti-sperm antibodies is unknown; however, a breach to the sperm testis barrier as a result of trauma or surgery is implicated.

Drugs: Prescribed and recreational

Alcohol, tobacco, opiates, and marijuana can reduce spermatogenesis and sperm function. Anabolic steroids, corticosteroids, antifungal medications, and sulphasalazine can affect spermatogenesis. Largely, these effects are reversible. Chemotherapy (cytostatic agents and alkylating agents) can permanently damage spermatogenesis. Other drugs such as antidepressants, particularly SSRIs, sedatives, and antihypertensives, may cause erectile dysfunction leading to infertility.

Environmental factors

Exposure to ionizing radiation, heat, and chemicals such as organic solvents, lead-based products, and pesticides can damage sperm production. Core temperatures of greater than 38.5 °C may suppress spermatogenesis for up to 6 months and are also associated with DNA damage to sperm. Although epidemiological studies have shown a demonstrable decline in semen parameters in the developed world, it is difficult to extrapolate this data from these studies to individual cases.

Varicocele

Distension of the intrascrotal veins (plexus pampiniformis) leads to varicocele formation. The mechanism by which varicoceles cause infertility is poorly understood and there is no consensus that treatment restores fertility. Theories include increased testicular temperature, toxic and oxidative stress, and decreased blood supply to the testis, as these can impair spermatogenesis (Sertoli cells), and decreased testosterone (Leydig cells). There is no increase in pregnancy rates in couples with treated varicocele when this is the only abnormality found.

Ejaculatory disorders

Ejaculatory disorders are rare causes of male infertility. Retrograde ejaculation can occur in certain neurological conditions, in diabetes, and where there has been surgery on the bladder neck or prostate.

Investigation of the male

The history should include:

- pregnancies with current or previous partners
- sexual function, and difficulties with intercourse
- genitourinary investigations and treatment

- surgery (e.g. vasectomy, inguinal hernia repair, orchidopexy, or transurethral resection of the prostate); testicular maldescent in infancy is associated with oligospermia and an increased risk of testicular malignancy in later life
- neurological disease, including neurological disease associated with diabetes mellitus or multiple sclerosis
- infections such as mumps orchitis
- recent febrile illness prior to semen analysis (as this may affect results)
- smoking, or alcohol consumption
- drugs (prescription and recreational)
- family history of genetic disorders or cystic fibrosis

The physical examination should include:

- height, limb length, and stigmata of chromosomal anomalies
- assessment for gynaecomastia
- degree of masculinization, including sparse hair or signs of hypoandrogenism, or bodybuilders' build, if suspicious of anabolic steroid use
- scrotal assessment: for size, consistency, volume (using an orchidometer), looking for varicoceles, epididymitis, vas deferens problems, and masses. A soft consistency is associated with impaired spermatogenesis. Masses should be assessed using ultrasound.
- groin examination: for surgical scars, a hernia, or the presence of a testis in the inguinal canal
- penile assessment of hypospadias or phimosis

The investigation should also include semen analysis and sperm function tests. A wide biological variation limits the reproducibility of the semen analysis as a test. Semen quality is taken as a surrogate marker for male fecundity, and therefore reference data from a fertile population are used to form a prognosis for fertility or diagnosis of infertility. See Box 9.1.

The function of sperm in vivo is to move through the cervical mucus and through the female reproductive tract into the ampullary part of the fallopian tube in sufficient numbers to undergo capacitation and finally fertilize the egg. Routine semen analysis does not test these functions. Tests of sperm function include:

- objective assessment of motility
- hypo-osmotic swelling test
- nuclear maturity
- the acrosome reaction
- acrosin activity

Box 9.1 The WHO reference range for semen analysis

Volume: 1.5 mL
Total sperm number: 39 million
Sperm concentration: 15×10^6/mL
Total motility: 40%
Progressive motility: 32%
Morphology: >4% (using Krueger strict criteria)

Data from *Human Reproduction Update*, Volume 16, World Health Organization reference values for human semen characteristic, Cooper TG, Noonan E, von Eckardstein S et al., 2010, pp. 231–245.

- human sperm binding
- penetration and sperm selection devices

Largely, these tests are of academic value and have been superseded by the processes of IVF and ICSI, which negate the actual function the sperm requires for fertilization in vivo. The role of these tests in routine fertility investigation is yet to be established.

Tests of anti-sperm antibodies have also been devised, including biochemical analysis of seminal fluid and the detection of anti-sperm antibodies via the immunobead or mixed antibody reaction.

Unexplained sperm abnormality, including azoospermia, merits further investigation, including measurements of:

- FSH
- LH
- testosterone
- prolactin

Genetic testing should be carried out as follows (see Table 9.4):

- karotype if <1 million sperm/mL
- if the vas deferens is absent, check for mutations in *CFTR* (85% of men have 1–2 mutations)
- check for deletions in genes encoding Y-chromosome-binding proteins (e.g. *DAZ, RBM, SPGY*).
- check for deletions in the AZF region of the Y chromosome; three locations are involved (AZFa, AZFb, and AZFc)

The object of conducting all these tests is to identify whether azoospermia is due to a primary testicular disorder or an outflow obstruction. Obstructive azoospermia is associated with a normal serum FSH; in contrast, disorders of spermatogenesis result in interruption of the gonadal–pituitary feedback loop, with elevation of serum FSH. Invasive testing such as testicular biopsy can assess the extent of damage to spermatogenesis and identify whether it is possible to obtain testicular sperm for ICSI, despite the patient being azoospermic on semen analysis.

If there is obstructed azoospermia, ultrasound should be used to assess the vas deferens and the epididymus (scrotal); alternatively, transrectal ultrasound can be used to assess prostatic or vesicle obstruction.

Management

Until recently, men with obstructed azoospermia or testicular dysfunction were unable to reproduce. IVF and ICSI now offer men the opportunity to father children and is the mainstay of treatment in this cohort.

Hypogonadotrophic hypogonadism is often associated with Kallman syndrome, and is successfully treated with pulsatile GnRH or hMG to restore spermatogenesis drive and fertility. Initiation can take several months. Men with idiopathic semen abnormalities should not be offered anti-oestrogens, gonadotrophins, androgens, bromocriptine, or kinin-enhancing drugs, as these drugs have not been shown to be effective.

Management of anti-sperm antibodies includes the use of condoms, corticosteroids, and intrauterine insemination of washed spermatozoa. However, the value of such an approach is controversial, and IVF and ICSI are the treatment of choice presently.

Reversal of vasectomy can be carried out, with up to 80% chance of subsequent pregnancy, with the chance inversely proportional to the length of time since the

Table 9.4 Genetic abnormalities associated with oligospermia or azoospermia

Disorder	Inheritance	Location	Incidence
Cystic fibrosis	AR (*CFTR*)	Ch7q 31.2	1/2500
Kartagener syndrome	AR	Ch 1q35.1	1/30,000
Kallman syndrome	X-linked recessive	*KAL* locus	1/30,000
		Ch Xp22.3	
Myotonic dystrophy	AD (variable penetrance)	Ch 19q13.3	1/8000
Klinefelter's syndrome	Aneuploidy 47, XXY		1/1000
	Mosaic 47, XXY/46, XY		
Noonan syndrome	AD	Ch 12q22ter	1/2000
	Mosaic 46, XY/XO		
Y deletions/Deletion *AZF* locus	Y chromosome	Ch Yq11.21	1/8000

Abbreviations: AD, autosomal dominant; AR, autosomal recessive; Ch, chromosomal location.

initial vasectomy procedure. Although the vas might be patent in the majority of cases, anti-sperm antibodies are common after vasectomy and reversal and probably constitute the main reason for failure to conceive post surgery. In these cases, IVF and ICSI are recommended for treatment.

Assisted reproductive technology

Intrauterine insemination is the first choice when oligospermia is an issue. Motility and morphology are the best predictors. Results worsen if the motile count is <1 million and there are <4% normal forms on semen analysis. Treatment protocols commonly include 3–4 cycles of intrauterine insemination before progressing to IVF and ICSI if pregnancy does not ensue. If the motile count is <1 million and there are <4% normal forms on semen analysis, then the prognosis is poor, and the recommendation is to proceed straight to ICSI. For men with obstructed azoospermia, epididymal sperm may be aspirated and used with ICSI.

Risks

Azoospermic and severely oligospermic men should have chromosomal karyotyping before the sperm is used for ICSI, in order that they may be counselled adequately about the risk of transmission of a chromosomal disorder such as a Y chromosome microdeletion or translocation to potential offspring.

Prognosis

Pregnancy rates with IVF and ICSI cycles differ but range from 25%–40% per cycle, depending on the cause of infertility, maternal age, and cause of infertility.

Patient support groups/useful websites

The following patient support groups and websites may be useful:

NICE Clinical guideline CG11: Fertility: Assessment and treatment for people with fertility problems: http://www.nice.org.uk/nicemedia/pdf/CG011niceguideline.pdf

American Society for Reproductive Medicine: http://www.asrm.org

Endotext: http://www.endotext.com

International Asherman's Association: http://www.ashermans.org

Endometriosis UK: http://www.endometriosis-uk.org

Endometriosis Resolved: http://www.endo-resolved.com

Further reading

Gardner DK, Weissman A, Howeles CM, et al., eds. *Textbook of Assisted Reproductive Technologies, Laboratory and Clinical Perspectives* (3rd edition), 2009. Informa.

Strauss J and Barbieri R, eds. *Yen and Jaffe's Reproductive Endocrinology: Physiology, Pathophysiology, and Clinical Management* (6th edition), 2009. Saunders.

WHO, Department of Reproductive Health and Research. WHO Laboratory Manual for the Examination and Processing of Human Semen (5th edition), 2010. WHO.

Chapter 10

Endocrine disorders in pregnancy

Chapter contents

10.1 Thyroid disorders in pregnancy

Normal thyroid physiology in pregnancy

A series of changes in thyroid hormone economy take place in normal pregnancy (see Table 10.1). As a result of these changes, thyroid hormone levels in pregnancy differ from those in the non-pregnant state.

Thyroid hormones
A rise in total thyroid hormone (T4 and T3) levels is seen from as early as 6 weeks gestation due to oestrogen-mediated increases in TBG concentrations, as well as the thyroid-stimulating actions of hCG. TSH suppression occurs, being maximal at about 10–12 weeks gestation, due to the negative-feedback action of increased thyroid hormone production. FT4 levels fall in the second half of pregnancy but remain within the non-pregnant reference range. Based on studies in healthy pregnant women, the upper limit of normal TSH is estimated at approximately 2.5 mU/L in early pregnancy, and 3.0 mU/L in latter pregnancy, although these thresholds vary more widely, according to the population studied, as well as the assay method employed. The lower limit of normal TSH in pregnancy is also less than the non-pregnant reference range. Thus, the non-pregnant TSH reference range will underestimate hypothyroidism in early pregnancy whilst over-diagnosing hyperthyroidism. It is now recommended that each laboratory derive its own population-based, trimester-specific pregnancy normative data.

Iodine nutrition status
Pregnancy is accompanied by a state of relative iodine deficiency. This results from increased renal iodide clearance as well as losses through the feto-placental unit (see Table 10.1). Furthermore, the increase in thyroid hormone production requires an increased iodide supply, and the thyroid gland responds to these changes with moderate enlargement and increased thyroglobulin

secretion. Iodine deficiency may therefore be precipitated during pregnancy, especially in women with borderline iodine nutrition status. A daily iodine intake of 250 μg is recommended in pregnancy but this is not realized in many parts of the world, including in industrialized countries. Daily antenatal multivitamin preparations containing 150 μg of iodine in the form of potassium iodide are recommended in some countries but policies on iodine supplementation in pregnancy are generally lacking.

Immunological changes
Local and systemic immune mechanisms operate to maintain the immune-tolerant state of pregnancy, presumably to prevent rejection of the feto-placental allograft (see Table 10.2). At the local level, there is trophoblast expression of non-classic MHC preventing NK cytotoxicity. The trophoblast also produces immune-suppressing complement regulatory proteins and pro-apoptotic Fas ligands. Increased maternal production of catecholamines, glucocorticoids, progesterone, and 1,25-dihydroxyvitamin D further promote the expression of cytokines from type 2 T helper cells, and this suppresses cellular immunity. Autoantibody production is reduced by the direct effects of oestrogens and progesterone on B cells.

Thyroid disorders specific to pregnancy

Gestational transient thyrotoxicosis
Gestational transient thyrotoxicosis (GTT) results from physiological stimulation of the thyroid gland by elevated hCG levels in early pregnancy. GTT is typically transient and does not require specific treatment with anti-thyroid drugs. It should be distinguished from hyperthyroidism, which usually necessitates anti-thyroid therapy (see Table 10.3).

Table 10.1 Summary of physiological changes that take place in normal pregnancy, and their clinical implications

Physiological change	Clinical or laboratory implications
↑ thyroid binding globulin levels	↑ serum total thyroid hormones (T3 and T4)
↑ HCG levels with ↑ thyroid stimulation	↑ serum total thyroid hormones (T3 and T4)
Negative feedback action of raised thyroid hormones	↓ serum TSH concentration
↑ plasma volume	↑ circulating T3 and T4 pool
↑ type III 5-deiodinase in placenta	↑ degradation of T3 and T4, and ↑ T4 requirements
↑ renal iodide clearance, ↑ placental iodide losses	Iodine deficiency in women with borderline iodine nutrition
↑ thyroid size	↑ serum thyroglobulin levels

Abbreviations: HCG, human chorionic gonadotrophin; T3, triiodothyronine; T4, thyroxine; TSH, thyroid-stimulating hormone.

Adapted from Brent G., Maternal Thyroid Function: Interpretation of Thyroid Function Tests in Pregnancy, *Clinical Obstetrics and Gynecology*, Volume 40, Issue 1, pp. 3–15. Copyright (1997), with permission from Wolters Kluwer Health, Inc.

Table 10.2 Mechanisms of immune tolerance in normal pregnancy

Mechanisms	Effects
Local mechanisms	
Trophoblast expression of non-classic MHC molecules	Protection of foetus from natural-killer-cell-mediated cytotoxicity
Trophoblast expression of Fas ligands	Induction of apoptosis in Fas-expressing maternal immune cells
Trophoblast production of complement regulatory proteins	Prevention of complement mediated cellular damage
Placental production of Th2 cytokines	Suppression of Th1 cytokines
Systemic mechanisms	
Increased maternal production of catecholamines, glucocorticoids, progesterone, and 1,25-dihydroxyvitamin D	Switch from Th1 to Th2 cytokine phenotype
Increased maternal production of progesterone and oestrogen	Reduction in antibody production

Abbreviations: Th1, Type 1 T helper; Th2, Type 2 T helper cell.

Pathophysiology

hCG and TSH have marked structural homology, so high hCG levels may stimulate the thyroid gland to cause the transient thyrotoxic state of GTT. Free thyroid hormones are elevated, with ensuing blunting of the pituitary–thyroid axis and suppressed TSH levels. hCG secretion begins in early pregnancy and peaks by about 8–10 weeks gestation. Serial measurements of TSH and hCG levels in early pregnancy show an inverse relationship with peak hCG levels, corresponding to suppressed TSH concentrations. GTT may coexist with hyperemesis gravidarum. High concentrations of circulating asialo-hCG with high thyrotrophic bioactivity have been demonstrated in women with both conditions. A mutant TSH receptor that is hypersensitive to hCG has also been reported in a family with gestational hyperthyroidism.

Epidemiology

GTT occurs in 2%–3% of all pregnancies but prevalence rates vary according to geography and ethnicity. GTT is present in up to two-thirds of patients with hyperemesis gravidarum.

Clinical features

GTT may be clinically silent and is frequently detected on routine laboratory testing. Some patients may show mild thyrotoxic features such as anxiety, palpitations, and excessive sweating, all of which may be difficult to distinguish from the features of normal pregnancy. Severe clinical presentations with prominent thyrotoxic features may occur but the absence of goitre or eye signs distinguish such patients from women with Graves' disease (see Table 10.3). Patients may also present with hyperemesis gravidarum, the severity of which is proportional to the degree of thyroid dysfunction.

Investigations

The thyroid hormone profile shows elevated free thyroid hormones (FT4 and FT3) and suppressed TSH concentrations. Subclinical hyperthyroidism (i.e. normal thyroid hormones but suppressed TSH) may also be seen. Anti-thyroid-receptor antibodies are not present, unlike the case in Graves' hyperthyroidism, where these antibodies are present.

Table 10.3 Features that distinguish gestational transient thyrotoxicosis from Graves' hyperthyroidism in pregnancy

Gestational transient thyrotoxicosis	Graves' hyperthyroidism in pregnancy
Common; occurs in 2%–3% of pregnancies	Less common: occurs in 0.2–0.4% of pregnancies
Occurs in early pregnancy	May occur at any stage of pregnancy
Transient	Persistent
Symptoms are mild	Symptoms may be severe
No goitre	Diffuse goitre may be present
No proptosis	May have proptosis
Patient is negative for anti-thyroid antibodies	Patient is positive for anti-thyroid antibodies
Does not require anti-thyroid drugs	Usually requires anti-thyroid drug treatments
No association with adverse pregnancy outcomes	Associated with adverse pregnancy outcomes

Management

The treatment of GTT is supportive and, in most cases, symptoms will subside without specific anti-thyroid treatment. Beta-blocking agents may be helpful in patients with prominent symptoms; in severe cases, anti-thyroid drugs may be used for short periods.

Complications and prognosis

In contrast to hyperthyroidism, GTT is not associated with adverse pregnancy outcomes, and symptoms usually resolve within weeks.

Hyperemesis gravidarum

Hyperemesis gravidarum is defined as vomiting that occurs in early pregnancy and is severe enough to lead to dehydration, electrolyte imbalance, acid–base imbalance, and loss of 5% of body weight. Hospitalization and treatment with intravenous fluids is required in most cases. The onset is usually between 6–10 weeks gestation, and symptoms typically resolve by 20 weeks. Although self-limiting, serious life-threatening metabolic complications can occur. Furthermore, patients suffer considerable morbidity and incur significant time away from work and family, due to illness.

Pathogenesis

A number of pathogenic mechanisms have been proposed for hyperemesis gravidarum, although the aetiology remains uncertain. An array of maternal hormones has been implicated, including hCG, progesterone, oestrogen, prolactin, cortisol, and thyroid hormones. hCG is widely believed to play a key causative role, since the development of symptoms coincides with peak secretions of the hormone. In addition, hyperemesis gravidarum is common in women with conditions associated with elevated hCG levels, such as multiple or molar pregnancies. Most studies report that hCG levels in the serum of women with hyperemesis gravidarum are higher than those in pregnant controls without hyperemesis. However, other factors may be involved, since some other studies have not demonstrated these differences. It has been proposed that discrepancies in hCG levels in women with hyperemesis may be explained by pathogenic hCG isoforms that are undetectable in routine assays.

Epidemiology

Most pregnant women experience nausea and vomiting but these are typically mild. The incidence of hyperemesis gravidarum is estimated at 0.3%–1.5% of all live births, and about 30%–60% of patients with hyperemesis gravidarum have GTT.

Clinical features

The clinical features of hyperemesis gravidarum are those of the metabolic complications of vomiting, including metabolic alkalosis, ketoacidosis, hypokalaemia, and prerenal failure. Severe vomiting may be complicated by oesophageal tear (Mallory–Weiss syndrome) or rupture. Some patients develop liver dysfunction, and severe cases may rarely result in serious neurological complications such as Wernicke's encephalopathy and central pontine myelinolysis. Other causes of vomiting, such as peptic ulcer disease, pancreatitis, gallstones, and pyelonephritis, should be excluded. Endocrine disorders such as Addison's disease and hyperthyroidism should also be considered in the differential diagnosis.

Management

Hospital admission for correction of metabolic abnormalities with intravenous fluid rehydration is usually required. Dietary modification towards smaller and more frequent meals, and avoidance of precipitating foods, may be helpful. In severe cases, all food intake may need to be stopped and nutrition maintained through nasogastric tube or parenteral feeding. Anti-emetic medications like metoclopramide and ondansetron may be used judiciously. Alternative therapies such as acupuncture and ginger have been tried, with variable degrees of success. Psychological support may be necessary in women with a strong psychological impact of the illness.

Post-partum thyroiditis

Post-partum thyroiditis is a syndrome of destructive thyroiditis occurring within the first 12 months of delivery. If unrecognized, patients suffer significant morbidity, which may be misattributed to other common conditions encountered in the post-partum period, such as depression and anxiety states.

Pathogenesis

Like Hashimoto's disease, post-partum thyroiditis is mediated by both cellular and humoral immunopathogenic mechanisms. There is increased production of thyroid reactive antibodies, namely, anti-thyroglobulin antibody and anti-thyroid-peroxidase antibody. Circulating complementing-fixing anti-thyroid-peroxidase antibodies are found in the serum of patients but the extent of complement-mediated thyroid cell destruction is unclear. T-cell abnormalities have also been demonstrated. The net effect of these changes is a destructive thyroiditis marked with increased urinary iodine excretion and elevated serum thyroglobulin levels in the active disease phase.

Epidemiology

The reported prevalence of post-partum thyroiditis is highly variable, with figures ranging from 1.1% to 16.7% of pregnant women. Most studies report an occurrence of 5%–9% of unselected pregnant women. About 10% of all pregnant women are positive for anti-thyroid-peroxidase antibodies in early pregnancy; of these, 50% develop post-partum thyroiditis.

Clinical features

Patients may present with a transient hyperthyroid phase which typically starts at about 8–16 weeks gestation, followed by a transient hypothyroid phase several weeks later. Hyperthyroidism may pass unnoticed, whilst the hypothyroid phase is typically more pronounced. Although the condition is self-limiting, permanent hypothyroidism may occur in 30%–50% of women. Some studies have suggested an association between post-partum thyroiditis and depression.

Investigations

Thyroid function may show a hyperthyroid, euthyroid, or hypothyroid picture, depending on the stage of the disease. Most cases are positive for anti-thyroid-peroxidase antibodies.

Management

The hyperthyroid phase is self-limiting, and treatment is usually not required. Beta-blocking drugs are indicated for short periods in severe symptomatic cases. Although the hypothyroid phase is reversible, most women are symptomatic and require treatment with synthetic levothyroxine at regular dose ranges of 75–150 µg daily. Thyroid function should be monitored in the long term, due to the risk of permanent hypothyroidism.

Thyroid disorders concurrent with pregnancy

Because thyroid disorders are common in women of childbearing age, they feature frequently in pregnancy. Hyperthyroidism and hypothyroidism may be diagnosed for the first time in pregnancy but thyroid dysfunction in pregnancy is more commonly encountered in women who have pre-existing disease and become pregnant. Careful management of these conditions is essential for optimal maternal and fetal outcomes.

Hyperthyroidism

Epidemiology

The prevalence of hyperthyroidism is 0.2%–0.4% of all pregnancies in the UK. The majority of cases in iodine-sufficient countries are due to Graves' disease, whilst other causes include GTT (see 'Gestational transient thyrotoxicosis'), solitary or multiple autonomous nodules, and subacute thyroiditis.

Clinical features

Hyperthyroidism may mimic the features of normal pregnancy. Discriminatory features of Graves' disease include ophthalmopathy, diffuse goitre, or pretibial myxoedema. The course of hyperthyroidism in pregnancy is variable. Disease exacerbation may be seen in the first trimester, possibly due to a rise in the titres of anti-thyroid-receptor antibodies, as well as the thyroid-stimulatory effects of hCG. Poor medication compliance and hyperemesis may also contribute to poor disease control in early pregnancy. Graves' disease tends to remit in latter pregnancy but may recur in the post-partum period, in keeping with the immune tolerance of pregnancy and the ensuing immunologic rebound seen in the post-partum period.

Investigations

TFTs will show hyperthyroidism (raised FT4 or FT3 and suppressed TSH). The presence of thyroid-receptor antibodies, the hallmark of Graves' disease, will confirm the aetiology of hyperthyroidism as due to Graves' disease.

Management

The approach to management will depend on disease activity during pregnancy (see Box 10.1). Women in remission following previous therapy for Graves' disease before pregnancy will need careful monitoring since there is a risk of relapse in the first trimester or in the post-partum period. Maternal levels of anti-thyroid-receptor antibodies should be checked, due to the risk of neonatal thyrotoxicosis from transplacental transfer of antibodies. Levels of anti-thyroid-receptor antibodies are more likely to remain elevated in women who were treated with surgery or radioiodine rather than those treated with anti-thyroid drugs, and it is unnecessary to check for anti-thyroid-receptor antibodies in the latter group of women. Levels of anti-thyroid-receptor antibodies should be measured in early pregnancy, and women with positive titres should be monitored closely with serial fetal ultrasonography. Levels of anti-thyroid-receptor antibodies may be rechecked in the third trimester of pregnancy.

Patients with newly diagnosed hyperthyroidism in pregnancy should be treated promptly in order to optimize fetal and maternal outcomes. Medical therapy with anti-thyroid medications is the preferred therapeutic option

---

Box 10.1 Management of Graves' hyperthyroidism in pregnancy

Previous hyperthyroidism: Treated with anti-thyroid drugs
- Check thyroid function in early pregnancy: if normal, recheck again at 6 weeks post partum.

Previous hyperthyroidism: Treated with radioiodine or surgery
Check thyroid function in early pregnancy; treat hypothyroidism if present.
   Check for anti-thyroid-receptor antibodies in early pregnancy; if they are present, monitor the foetus with serial ultrasound.
   Recheck for anti-thyroid-receptor antibodies in late pregnancy; if they are present, continue fetal monitoring and inform paediatricians.

Current hyperthyroidism
Use the following approach in the first trimester:
- use propylthiouracil at the lowest effective dose (100–200 mg daily)
- give propranolol only in severe cases
- monitor thyroid functions monthly: aim for free T4 at the upper end of normal
- check for anti-thyroid-receptor antibodies
- monitor the foetus with serial ultrasound

Second and third trimesters
Use the following approach in the second and third trimesters:
- switch to carbimazole at the lowest effective dose
- monitor thyroid functions monthly: aim for free T4 at the upper end of normal range
- treatment may need to be stopped before delivery
- check for anti-thyroid-receptor antibodies; if they are present, monitor the foetus with serial ultrasound and inform paediatricians

At delivery
Check the baby's thyroid function at delivery; if normal, recheck at Days 4–7.

In the post-partum period
Use the following approach in the post-partum period:
- continue carbimazole at the lowest effective dose
- if the patient is breastfeeding, carbimazole should be taken after feeds
- check thyroid function at 6 weeks post partum

---

in pregnancy. Radioiodine is absolutely contraindicated, and surgery is reserved for exceptional cases of serious medication reactions, in which case it is best performed in the second trimester. The consequences of inadvertent exposure to radioiodine treatment in pregnancy are unclear. Exposure in late pregnancy carries a risk of fetal hypothyroidism, attention-deficit disorder, and cognitive impairment but exposure in the first trimester is unlikely to have significant adverse effects, since the fetal thyroid only begins to concentrate iodine after the twelfth week of gestation. Pregnancy should be excluded in women of childbearing age who undergo radioiodine treatment, and all cases of accidental exposure should be discussed sensitively with the mother, who may be given the option of pregnancy termination.

Anti-thyroid drug therapy
The thionamides, propylthiouracil, methimazole, and its pro-drug derivative, carbimazole, are the drugs of choice. These compounds inhibit thyroid hormone synthesis by inhibition of the thyroid-peroxidase-catalysed iodination of thyroglobulin, and coupling of tyrosine residues. In addition, they exhibit immunosuppressant properties, and propylthiouracil also blocks the peripheral conversion of T4 to T3. Due to its longer half-life (6–8 hours), carbimazole may be administered in a single daily dose, whereas propylthiouracil has a short half-life (1–2

hours) and is administered twice or thrice daily. Both drugs have similar transplacental transfer kinetics and effects on neonatal thyroid function. It is recommended that carbimazole be avoided in the first trimester of pregnancy, due to the small risk of aplasia cutis in the babies of mothers exposed to carbimazole. There have also been a growing number of reports of serious and occasionally fatal propylthiouracil-induced liver failure. Thus, it is now recommended that propylthiouracil is used in the first trimester only and then switched to carbimazole from the second trimester onwards. The smallest dose of these compounds that renders the patient euthyroid should be administered, and the T4 level should be maintained in the upper third of the normal reference range. The combined use of carbimazole with levothyroxine, the 'block-and-replace' regimen, is not recommended in pregnancy, as this approach increases the risk of fetal hypothyroidism and goitre by exposing the foetus to unduly high levels of anti-thyroid drugs in utero. Both drugs are secreted in breast milk but at small, clinically insignificant amounts. Nonetheless, lactating mothers should time their medications to follow the breastfeeds.

Adverse effects of hyperthyroidism on fetal and maternal well-being
Hyperthyroidism has the following adverse effects on fetal and maternal well-being:

Table 10.4 Adverse fetal and maternal effects
of hyperthyroidism

Maternal	Fetal
Preeclampsia	Early fetal loss
Abruptio placenta	Preterm delivery
Congestive cardiac failure	Intrauterine growth restriction
Arrhythmias	Low birth weight
Hypertension	Stillbirth
	Hydrops foetalis
	Fetal goitre
	Neonatal goitre
	Neonatal hyperthyroidism
	Neonatal hypothyroidism

- uncorrected hyperthyroidism:
  - carries a risk of adverse fetal and maternal outcomes (see Table 10.4)
  - pregnant women with hyperthyroidism show reversible haemodynamic abnormalities, including elevations in heart rate, blood pressure, and cardiac output, and reduction in peripheral vascular resistance
- fetal hyperthyroidism:
  - may occur from the transplacental transfer of thyroid-stimulating maternal anti-thyroid-receptor antibodies
  - in such cases, fetal goitre, fetal tachycardia, and hydrops foetalis may be detected on fetal ultrasound
- neonatal hyperthyroidism:
  - seen in about 1% of infants born to mothers with Graves' disease
  - the presentation may be delayed for several days after birth, due to the residual effects of anti-thyroid drugs from the maternal circulation
  - affected neonates may present with tachycardia, heart failure, accelerated bone maturation, and a range of neurodevelopmental abnormalities
  - treatment is with anti-thyroid drugs but beta blockers, iodine, and glucocorticoids may be used in severe cases
- neonatal hypothyroidism:
  - neonatal hypothyroidism and goitre may occur from the transfer of maternal anti-thyroid drugs, from suppression of the fetal pituitary–thyroid axis as a result of transplacental transfer of maternal T4, or, rarely, from transfer of maternal blocking antibodies
  - prompt treatment with levothyroxine is essential to prevent permanent neurodevelopmental abnormalities in the infant

Subclinical hyperthyroidism
Treatment of subclinical hyperthyroidism (low TSH and normal FT4 and FT3) is not advised. In some cases, a low TSH may be normal for pregnancy and may be a transient phenomenon. Furthermore, there is no evidence that subclinical hyperthyroidism has adverse feto-maternal consequences. Rather, the use of anti-thyroid drugs in this circumstance exposes the foetus to these drugs and increases the risk of fetal hypothyroidism and goitre.

Hypothyroidism
Epidemiology
Hypothyroidism is common in pregnancy, with an estimated prevalence of 0.3%–0.5% for overt hypothyroidism, and 2%–3% for subclinical hypothyroidism. Most cases in iodine-replete populations are due to Hashimoto's thyroiditis, although iodine deficiency remains a common aetiology worldwide. Other causes of hypothyroidism are surgery and radioactive iodine therapy for benign and malignant thyroid diseases, and secondary hypothyroidism due to pituitary disease.

Clinical features
Some women present with classic features like cold intolerance and constipation but these symptoms can be difficult to distinguish from normal pregnancy. A high index of suspicion is required in women with a personal or family history of thyroid disease, goitre, or coexistent autoimmune condition like type 1 diabetes.

Investigations
Thyroid hormone tests confirm the diagnosis (low FT4 and elevated TSH). Anti-thyroid-peroxidase antibodies and, less commonly, anti-thyroglobulin antibodies are present in patients with Hashimoto's thyroiditis.

Management
Synthetic levothyroxine is the treatment of choice. Levothyroxine is metabolized to the biologically active T3 in target tissues and has good oral bioavailability, with about 70%–80% of the administered dose absorbed, mostly from the small intestine. It is better absorbed in the fasting state and should be administered first thing in the morning without food or, alternatively, at bedtime. A series of physiological changes, including plasma volume expansion, thyroid hormone deactivation by placental deiodinase, and an increase in plasma TBG, reduces levothyroxine availability in pregnancy. Poor medication compliance and hyperemesis may also reduce levothyroxine availability. Patients should be advised to avoid taking levothyroxine at the same time as iron preparations and antacids, as these reduce levothyroxine absorption.

TSH targets in pregnancy
T4 requirements increase in pregnancy, and most hypothyroid women require an increase in levothyroxine dose in pregnancy. Optimal correction of hypothyroidism in early pregnancy is crucial, since the developing foetus wholly depends on maternal T4 sources up until about 14 weeks of gestation, when the fetal thyroid gland attains full maturation and can then meet its own T4 requirements. Hypothyroid women contemplating pregnancy should have preconception levothyroxine dose adjustments to attain a TSH <2.5 mU/L (Box 10.2). Additional titrations on conception should aim to maintain TSH <2.5 mU/L in the first trimester, and <3.0 mU/L in later pregnancy. In newly detected cases in pregnancy, the recommended daily levothyroxine dose is approximately 1.0–2.0 µg/kg. Much higher starting doses, double the anticipated dose, may be administered initially to rapidly restore euthyroidism in severe cases. Dose increases may be required in latter pregnancy and, following delivery, some women return to their pre-pregnancy dosage. Thyroid function can be monitored every 4 weeks if abnormal and then every 6 weeks if stable.

Box 10.2 Management of hypothyroidism in pregnancy

Preconception

Inform hypothyroid women of childbearing age of the need for optimal preconception and gestational thyroid hormone replacement.
  Optimize levothyroxine dose preconception to achieve TSH <2.5 mU/L.

At conception

Increase levothyroxine dose by 30%–50% once pregnancy confirmed.
  Check thyroid function tests and adjust levothyroxine dose to maintain TSH <2.5 mU/L.

During the first trimester

Maintain TSH <2.5 mU/L.
  Monitor thyroid function tests every 4 weeks.

During the second and third trimester

Maintain TSH <3.0 mU/L.
  Monitor thyroid function tests every 6 weeks if TSH is stable, or more frequently if dose adjustments are required.
  Further dose increases may be needed in later pregnancy.

In the post-partum period

Check thyroid function tests at 6 weeks post partum.
  Reduction of the levothyroxine dose to the pre-pregnancy level may be indicated.

Adverse effects of hypothyroidism on fetal and maternal well-being

Uncorrected maternal hypothyroidism has adverse feto-maternal consequences (see Table 10.5). These complications are reported in mothers with subclinical as well as overt hypothyroidism and there is also evidence that women who are positive for anti-thyroid-peroxidase antibodies in pregnancy suffer adverse outcomes, regardless of thyroid function. The effects of hypothyroidism may also extend beyond pregnancy to affect the subsequent neurointellectual development of the offspring. Observational studies show that children born to mothers with hypothyroidism have lower IQs than children of euthyroid mothers do. However, a large randomized controlled trial, the Controlled Antenatal Trial Study (CATS) showed that early correction of maternal hypothyroidism did not have any benefit on childhood cognitive function.

Subclinical hypothyroidism

Some studies have shown an increased risk of adverse fetal and maternal outcomes in women with subclinical hypothyroidism (TSH level above the pregnancy reference range and normal FT4). Levothyroxine treatment prevented adverse obstetric events in some trials but had no effect on offspring cognitive

function in the CATS trial. Women with subclinical hypothyroidism should be treated with levothyroxine if they are positive for anti-thyroid peroxidase antibodies or if TSH >10.0 mU/L. Women who are not treated should be monitored closely for progression to overt hypothyroidism.

Isolated hypothyroxinaemia

Isolated hypothyroxinaemia (low FT4 and normal TSH) is frequently seen in pregnancy but its impact on feto-maternal outcomes is unclear. This biochemical pattern may also be seen in the setting of acute illness, anti-thyroid drug therapy, and central hypothyroidism. Most cases are discovered routinely, and patients are rarely symptomatic. Isolated low FT4 is particularly common in iodine-deficient pregnant women, and such women are negative for anti-thyroid antibodies. A consensus on whether these patients should be treated has not been reached.

Euthyroid women who are positive for anti-thyroid antibodies

Euthyroid women who are positive for anti-thyroid antibodies in early pregnancy have a risk of thyroid dysfunction in later pregnancy or in the post-partum period. Whether they should be treated with levothyroxine is unsettled. Some studies have shown that women who are positive for anti-thyroid-peroxidase antibodies carry an increased risk of fetal loss and that levothyroxine treatment reduces this risk. However, current guidelines do not recommend treatment and, pending further data, euthyroid women who are positive for anti-thyroid-peroxidase antibodies should be monitored closely, with treatment initiated if TSH rises above the trimester-specific reference range.

Screening for hypothyroidism in pregnancy

The question of routine screening for hypothyroidism in pregnancy is controversial and has continued to divide opinion among endocrinologists and obstetricians. The case for screening rests upon the high prevalence of gestational hypothyroidism, its deleterious effects on

Table 10.5 Adverse effects of hypothyroidism on fetal and maternal outcomes

Maternal outcomes	Fetal outcomes
Anaemia in pregnancy	Early fetal loss
Pre-eclampsia	Preterm delivery
Abruptio placenta	Stillbirth
Increased frequency of caesarean sections	Low birth weight
	Neonatal distress
Post-partum haemorrhage	Neurointellectual impairment

Box 10.3 Indications for thyroid screening in pregnancy

Personal or family history of thyroid disease
Autoimmune disorders (e.g. type 1 diabetes, coeliac disease, Addison's disease)
History of head and neck irradiation
History of infertility
History of adverse pregnancy outcomes (e.g. preterm delivery, stillbirths, low birthweight)
Suggestive symptoms and signs of thyroid disease
Other suggestive features of thyroid disease (e.g. anaemia, dyslipidaemia, hyponatraemia)
Goitre
Being positive for anti-thyroid antibodies

---

pregnancy outcomes, the availability of simple diagnostic tests of thyroid dysfunction, and the cost-effectiveness of levothyroxine therapy. The opposing argument, however, is that evidence for adverse feto-maternal effects is limited to overt hypothyroidism but remains unclear for subclinical disease. Furthermore, a benefit for maternal levothyroxine treatment on child cognitive function was not proven in two large randomized controlled trials. Current international guidelines do not support routine gestational thyroid screening but recommend a case-finding approach in high-risk individuals (Box 10.3). This targeted screening strategy offers a reasonable compromise but will still miss a significant proportion of women with gestational hypothyroidism. Further studies are required to clarify the full extent of thyroid dysfunction on fetal and maternal outcomes.

Thyroid nodules and cancer
Thyroid nodules are present in about 10% of pregnant women. Some studies suggest that pregnancy predisposes to new nodular formation as well as increase in size of pre-existing nodules. Thyroid nodules detected in pregnancy should be confirmed on ultrasound. The workup for lesions with benign ultrasound characteristics can be postponed until after delivery. Lesions with suspicious ultrasound features should be subjected to fine-needle aspiration biopsy, which can be safely performed in pregnancy. If the biopsy is suspicious of malignancy, surgery can usually be deferred until after delivery, according to patient preference. The decision to delay treatment until after pregnancy should be discussed with the patient, who may be reassured by the fact that most thyroid cancers are slow-growing.

Thyroid surgery should, however, not be deferred if there are ominous features such as lymph-node involvement, large primary size, or histological characteristics of anaplastic or medullary cancer. Women who defer surgery should undergo serial thyroid ultrasound scans and be offered early surgery if there is rapid nodule growth. Thyroidectomy can be safely undertaken in the second trimester of pregnancy. Radioactive iodine treatment is absolutely contraindicated in pregnancy and the postpartum period. There is no evidence that pregnant patients with thyroid cancer have less favourable outcomes than non-pregnant individuals. Furthermore, women who become pregnant after they have completed treatment for thyroid cancer do not appear to have an additional risk of progression, provided they are disease-free at conception. Such women should continue levothyroxine therapy in pregnancy, with the aim of maintaining a suppressed but detectable TSH level.

Patient support groups/useful websites
The following website may be useful:
- British Thyroid Foundation: http://www.btf-thyroid.org

Further reading
Abalovich M, Amino N, Barbour LA, et al. Management of thyroid dysfunction during pregnancy and postpartum: An Endocrine Society Clinical Practice Guideline. *J Clin Endocrinol Metab* 2007; 92: S1–47.

Alexander EK, Pearce EN, Brent GA, et al. 2017 Guidelines of the American Thyroid Association for the diagnosis and management of thyroid disease during pregnancy and postpartum. *Thyroid* 2017; 27: 315–89.

Brent GA. Maternal thyroid function: Interpretation of thyroid function tests in pregnancy. *Clin Obstet Gynecol* 1997; 40: 3–15.

De Groot L, Abalovich M, Alexander EK, et al. Management of thyroid dysfunction during pregnancy and postpartum: An Endocrine Society clinical practice guideline. *J Clin Endocrinol Metab* 2012; 97: 2543–65.

Glinoer D, de Nayer P, Bourdoux P, et al. Regulation of maternal thyroid during pregnancy. *J Clin Endocrinol Metab* 1990; 71: 276–87.

Glinoer D. The regulation of thyroid function in pregnancy: Pathways of endocrine adaptation from physiology to pathology. *Endocr Rev* 1997; 18: 871–87.

Jueckstock JK, Kaestner R, and Mylonas I. Managing hyperemesis gravidarum: A multimodal challenge. *BMC Med* 2010; 8: 46.

Krassas GE, Poppe K, and Glinoer D. Thyroid function and human reproductive health. *Endocr Rev* 2010; 31: 702–5.

Lazarus JH, Bestwick JP, Channon S, et al. Antenatal thyroid screening and childhood cognitive function. *N Engl J Med* 2012; 366: 493–501.

Lazarus JH, Parkes AB, and Premawardhana LD. Postpartum thyroiditis. *Autoimmunity* 2002; 35: 169–73.

Okosieme OE, Marx H, and Lazarus JH. Medical management of thyroid dysfunction in pregnancy and the postpartum. *Expert Opin Pharmacother* 2008; 9: 2281–93.

Stagnaro-Green A, Abalovich M, Alexander E, et al. Guidelines of the American Thyroid Association for the diagnosis and management of thyroid disease during pregnancy and postpartum. *Thyroid* 2011; 21: 1081–125.

Stagnaro-Green A. Approach to the patient with postpartum thyroiditis. *J Clin Endocrinol Metab* 2012; 97: 334–42.

Wegrzyniak LJ, Repke JT, and Ural SH. Treatment of hyperemesis gravidarum. *Rev Obstet Gynecol* 2012; 5: 78–84.

10.2 Adrenal disease in pregnancy

Introduction

The presentation and management of adrenal disease in pregnancy differs from the non-pregnant state for several reasons. Normal pregnancy may mimic the symptoms of both adrenal insufficiency and Cushing's syndrome, making clinical assessment more difficult. The endocrine changes which occur during normal pregnancy have a significant effect on the physiology of the maternal HPA axis. It is important to consider the impact of both the disease and the potential treatments on the mother and the feto-placental unit. In all cases of adrenal disease in pregnancy, the endocrinologist should work closely with the obstetrician, the obstetric anaesthetist, and the appropriate surgeon at each stage of pregnancy.

Changes in the HPA axis in normal pregnancy

Maternal HPA axis

Both bound and unbound cortisol levels are higher in pregnancy than in the non-pregnant state. The increased oestrogen levels in pregnancy cause an elevation in CBG, which leads to higher values in routine cortisol assays, which measure total rather than free cortisol levels. This elevation affects the interpretation of basal and dynamic assessments of the maternal HPA axis, and may lead to false-negative interpretation of suspected adrenal insufficiency, and false positives in suspected Cushing's syndrome.

Later in pregnancy, increasing progesterone levels displace bound cortisol from CBG, thus leading to increased free cortisol biological action on tissues. The feto-placental unit produces increasing amounts of CRH and adrenocorticotrophic hormone throughout pregnancy, and placental CRH stimulates the maternal HPA system. This means that adrenocorticotrophic hormone levels may be unsuppressed in situations where they normally would be low, such as in adrenal Cushing's syndrome and secondary adrenal failure.

Fetal HPA axis

The fetal adrenal gland is roughly the same size as the adult gland, with all three layers of the cortex functional, and is controlled by its own HPA axis and renin–angiotensin system. The placental unit protects the foetus from maternal changes in the HPA axis to a certain extent by the presence of aromatase enzymes (to protect from high maternal androgens) and 11-beta-hydroxysteroid dehydrogenase (to protect from high maternal corticosteroids). Dexamethasone crosses the placenta without oxidation of the 11-hydroxyl group and therefore can suppress the fetal adrenal gland; this can be of use in the management of fetal congenital adrenal hyperplasia during pregnancy (see 'Congenital adrenal hyperplasia and pregnancy').

Key points for adrenal disease in pregnancy

- Symptoms of adrenal disease are similar to those of normal pregnancy.
- Pregnancy alters the normal HPA axis and may make standard biochemical tests difficult to interpret.
- The impact of any investigation and treatment on the pregnancy must be considered.
- The obstetrician plays as important a role as the endocrinologist in the management of adrenal disease in pregnancy.

Cushing's syndrome in pregnancy

Clinical features

Normal pregnancy is not uncommonly associated with weight gain, emotional disturbance, hypertension, abdominal striae, and diabetes, so it can be difficult to clinically distinguish Cushing's syndrome from the history alone. Discriminatory clinical features such as bruising and proximal myopathy can be useful to distinguish genuine Cushing's syndrome presentation from normal pregnancy.

Cushing's syndrome in pregnancy is usually initiated or exacerbated by pregnancy. Pre-existing untreated Cushing's syndrome is rare because of the reduced fertility associated with active hypercortisolaemia, particularly in situations of androgen excess such as adrenocorticotrophic-hormone-dependent Cushing's and adrenal carcinoma, where high androgen levels will inhibit the gonadotrophin axis. It is probably for this reason that there is a disproportionately high preponderance of adrenocorticotrophic-hormone-*independent* Cushing's syndrome, due to benign adrenal adenoma (40%), unlike the case outside pregnancy, as there 80% cases are due to adrenocorticotrophic-hormone-secreting pituitary tumours.

If there is a high index of clinical suspicion of Cushing's syndrome, investigation should be initiated because of the significantly increased maternal and fetal morbidity associated with untreated disease. Untreated Cushing's syndrome in the mother leads to increased hypertension, pre-eclampsia, cardiac failure, and post-intervention sepsis. There is also a significant increase in premature labour, intrauterine growth retardation, and fetal death.

Investigation of suspected Cushing's in pregnancy
Confirmation of Cushing's syndrome

Because of the physiological changes in the HPA axis during pregnancy, biochemical confirmation of disease may be challenging. As with Cushing's syndrome outside pregnancy, demonstration of loss of the diurnal variation in cortisol may be useful. UFC and low-dose DSTs are used to aid confirmation of Cushing's syndrome in pregnancy but results should be interpreted with less confidence than when outside pregnancy because of the lack of trimester-specific cortisol ranges. Demonstration of a loss of the circadian rhythm of cortisol may be helpful. Salivary free cortisol may play a role in the future.

Differential diagnosis

The differential diagnosis of Cushing's syndrome is made more difficult because the lack of adrenocorticotrophic-hormone suppression from placental CRH production makes the different response to low- and high-dose dexamethasone less reliable. MRI is safe in pregnancy (without gadolinium), and it is appropriate to image the adrenal glands in pregnancy if adrenocorticotrophic-hormone-independent Cushing's syndrome is suspected (although it would be advisable to avoid the first trimester, if possible).

Although CRH tests are helpful in the differential diagnosis of Cushing's syndrome outside pregnancy, the effect of placental CRH makes the exaggerated rise in adrenocorticotrophic hormone after CRH injection less obvious during pregnancy. Venous catheter sampling using the internal jugular rather than petrosal approach has been used, although it is not routinely recommended.

Management

Because of the increased maternal and fetal morbidity associated with Cushing's syndrome in pregnancy, simple observation without treatment is not justifiable unless the condition is diagnosed at the end of pregnancy, when safe delivery of the foetus may allow for rapid treatment of the disease afterwards.

In adrenal Cushing's syndrome, the optimum timing for adrenalectomy is the second trimester, because, later on in pregnancy, the gravid uterus makes surgical access more difficult. Pregnancy may cause enlargement of an adrenocorticotrophic-hormone-secreting pituitary tumour, and trans-sphenoidal surgery should be considered if there are is worsening vision or other local compressive symptoms. Medical treatments, including ketoconazole and metyrapone, have been used safely in pregnancy but there are insufficient data to comment on their safety.

Women who were previously treated for Cushing's syndrome and are in remission should be watched closely in a joint antenatal clinic setting to look for signs of clinical recurrence and to ensure there are no signs of adrenal insufficiency, as these may not have been clinically apparent before pregnancy.

Key points for Cushing's syndrome in pregnancy

- Adrenal adenomas are the cause of a higher proportion of Cushing's syndrome cases in pregnancy than in the non-pregnant state.
- Adrenocorticotrophic-hormone levels may be unsuppressed due to placental CRH secretion.
- A new diagnosis of Cushing's syndrome in pregnancy should prompt action rather than simple observation.

Addison's disease and pregnancy

The outlook for pregnancy in patients with treated primary adrenal failure is very good. There are reports of increased rates of caesarean section, preterm delivery, and low birthweight in women with Addison's disease, but not all studies have shown this. The reasons for the association between preterm delivery and low birthweight with Addison's disease are unknown, but explanations include coexisting autoimmune endocrine disease, and downregulation of placental 11-beta-hydroxysteroid dehydrogenase activity, which may paradoxically expose the foetus to excessive steroid due to reduced inactivation of maternal corticosteroid.

The most common clinical situation is the patient who has known pre-existing Addison's disease and becomes pregnant. The key management consideration is adequate corticosteroid replacement during the first trimester, particularly if there is severe morning sickness or frank hyperemesis gravidarum. Mothers should be taught how to self-administer intramuscular hydrocortisone injections, although the threshold for admitting a patient with Addison's disease and frank hyperemesis is low.

Clinical features and investigation

Because the symptoms of early pregnancy are very similar to those of subtle adrenal corticosteroid deficiency, it is very difficult to distinguish mild under-replacement from normal pregnancy. Many patients feel tired, nauseous, and dizzy in the first trimester, and pigmentation may be part of normal pregnancy. Patients who have had previous pregnancies can often distinguish between adrenal under-replacement and normal pregnancy symptoms themselves.

Increased pigmentation in the buccal mucosa, knuckles, and palmar creases, together with 'addisonian' electrolytes and postural hypotension, may specifically point to under-replacement and indicate that an increase in steroid dose is required.

Measurement of serum cortisol is relatively unhelpful during pregnancy because of the falsely reassuring levels arising from raised CBG, and sensible clinical assessment is probably the most helpful guide to management. However, several cut-offs have been suggested (see Table 10.6).

Management

Women do not usually require an increase in corticosteroid dose during early pregnancy. In the second and third trimesters, some groups advocate a 20%–40% increase in corticosteroid dose (e.g. 5–10 mg hydrocortisone), although patients may remain asymptomatic on an unchanged dose. Before term, a coordinated management plan should be made regarding the administration of hydrocortisone and preferred mode of delivery, and this plan should be readily available in the mothers' handheld records.

Because labour is a major physiological stress, women should have parenteral hydrocortisone 100 mg at the onset, followed by 6-hourly hydrocortisone for the duration of labour. With a caesarean section, 100 mg hydrocortisone should be given at the onset of the procedure, followed by double-dose oral hydrocortisone for 24–48 hours.

Mineralocorticoid replacement does not usually require any adjustment during pregnancy. Pregnancy-induced hypertension may occur in patients with Addison's disease and should be treated on its own merits rather than by reducing the dose of fludrocortisone. Only specific electrolyte suggestions of under- or over-replacement should lead to changes in mineralocorticoid dose. Because of the altered volume distribution in pregnancy, maternal renin levels are not a helpful guide to mineralocorticoid replacement, and renin is itself subject to

Table 10.6 Serum cortisol cut-offs for diagnosis of adrenal insufficiency in pregnancy (DPC Bierman assay)

Trimester	Baseline serum cortisol	Peak cortisol 30 minutes after Synacthen®
1	<300 nmol/L (11 µg/dL)	<700 nmol/L (25 µg/dL)
2	<450 nmol/L (16 µg/dL)	<800 nmol/L (29 µg/dL)
3	<600 nmol/L (22 µg/dL)	<900 nmol/L (33 µg/dL)

oestrogen modification, so usual reference ranges are inappropriate.

Making a new diagnosis of Addison's disease in pregnancy is very uncommon, but untreated primary adrenal failure previously had a maternal mortality of up to 40% so it is important not to miss. Patients who have an autoimmune endocrine disease, such as type 1 diabetes and hypothyroidism, and have suggestive symptoms should have a lower threshold for investigation.

Secondary adrenal disease in pregnancy

Adrenocorticotrophic-hormone deficiency due to pituitary disease or exogenous steroid administration is not uncommon in pregnancy. Monitoring corticosteroid replacement is the same as for primary adrenal failure, without the need to consider mineralocorticoid replacement. Patients with known pituitary disease or lymphocytic hypophysitis will normally already be in an endocrine clinic milieu, but patients on long-term steroids for non-endocrine disease may not be aware of the importance of increasing the dose at the time of labour.

Key points for Addison's disease in pregnancy

- Clinical judgement is as good as biochemical assessment of steroid replacement in pregnancy.
- Adrenal insufficiency may occur in the first trimester if there is significant pregnancy-associated nausea and vomiting.
- A planned regime of parenteral steroid administration should be documented and readily available at the time of delivery.

Congenital adrenal hyperplasia and pregnancy

The commonest enzyme defect in congenital adrenal hyperplasia is 21-hydroxylase deficiency, with the majority of remaining cases (5%) being due to 11-beta-hydroxylase deficiency. Women with non-classical congenital adrenal hyperplasia may have a mild presentation of disease presenting in a similar way to PCOS. Uncontrolled congenital adrenal hyperplasia reduces fertility because of androgen-induced suppression of gonadotrophins. Previously uncontrolled disease in early life may cause anatomical abnormalities in the female genital tract, and suboptimal reconstructive surgery can also cause reproductive problems due to physical or psychological sequelae; there are also reports of an increased number of same-sex relationships in women with congenital adrenal hyperplasia. Mechanical problems during delivery in women with an android pelvis may increase the risk of cephalo-pelvic proportion.

Management

Pregnancy in a mother with known congenital adrenal hyperplasia

Control of maternal hyperandrogenaemia is important to prevent potential virilization of a female foetus. The exogenous steroids routinely used to treat congenital adrenal hyperplasia (such as hydrocortisone and prednisolone) are safe in pregnancy because they are inactivated by placental 11-beta-hydroxysteroid dehydrogenase, which protects the foetus against adrenal suppression.

Patients with congenital adrenal hyperplasia should be seen antenatally every 4–6 weeks to ensure adequate control of androgens, as well as to assess appropriate corticosteroid and mineralocorticoid replacement, in the same way as described for hypoadrenalism.

If antenatal scanning shows clear evidence of a male foetus, repeated measurement of androgen levels and tight monitoring of corticosteroid dose is less important than in the female because maternal androgen excess has little effect on male fetal development.

As with adrenal failure, a coordinated plan of delivery should be arranged, with a documented regime for the administration of parenteral corticosteroids at the time of labour or caesarean section. The mode of delivery is an obstetric decision and may be influenced by the effect on early circulating androgens on the patient's reproductive anatomy.

Known increased risk of congenital adrenal hyperplasia in pregnancy

In situations where there is an increased risk of congenital adrenal hyperplasia in the child, such as when the father is a known genetic carrier or if there has previously been a child with congenital adrenal hyperplasia, genetic counselling plays an important role in the run up to pregnancy. Genetic confirmation of congenital adrenal hyperplasia in a foetus is now possible using prenatal diagnostic investigations such as amniocentesis and, later on, chorionic villous sampling, both of which have concomitant risks.

If the mother has had a previous child with congenital adrenal hyperplasia, or if the father is known to be a carrier, the administration of dexamethasone in early pregnancy may be considered in order to suppress adrenocorticotrophic-hormone-driven hyperandrogenaemia in the early female foetus with suspected congenital adrenal hyperplasia. Dexamethasone is not inactivated by placental 11-beta-hydroxysteroid dehydrogenase, and will therefore pass the placenta in its active form and suppress the fetal adrenal axis. The use of dexamethasone in this situation can only be justified if there is known to be an increased risk of congenital adrenal hyperplasia in this pregnancy. In this situation, the potential benefits of early androgen suppression should be balanced against the risks of maternal hypercortisolaemia.

The dilemma for the clinician and parents is that the clinical manifestations of congenital adrenal hyperplasia can vary widely within families, and seven out of eight pregnancies may not develop any signs of virilization. In patients where dexamethasone is deemed appropriate, a suggested regime is 20 µg/kg per day in three divided doses until the sex of the foetus has been determined. Non-invasive fetal sex determination may allow for the identification of male foetuses as early as 37 days after conception. This early sex determination would restrict the need for chorionic villous sampling to female foetuses only, after which dexamethasone could be stopped if classical congenital adrenal hyperplasia is absent.

Although there are reassuring data that dexamethasone administration is safe in terms of rates of stillbirth, spontaneous abortions, fetal malformations, and developmental/neuropsychological outcomes, long-term follow-up studies are lacking. Pregnant mothers treated with dexamethasone commonly develop cushingoid side effects, including weight gain, hypertension, and glucose intolerance. It is therefore important to counsel parents with a family history of congenital adrenal hyperplasia about the 'pros and cons' of antenatal testing and treatment, and this should be done together with a clinical geneticist and an obstetrician so that patients can make an informed decision about their preferred approach. The paediatrician also plays a key role in the assessment of the neonate, to ensure there is no clinical or biochemical evidence of classical congenital adrenal hyperplasia after delivery.

Key points for congenital adrenal hyperplasia in pregnancy

- Control of maternal androgens is important to prevent virilization of a female foetus.
- Dexamethasone may be considered during an at-risk pregnancy for congenital adrenal hyperplasia, to suppress fetal androgens.
- Early confirmation of fetal sex and prenatal genotyping may prevent the unnecessary use of dexamethasone.

Phaeochromocytomas and paragangliomas in pregnancy

The increased recognition that phaeochromocytomas and paragangliomas have a genetic basis has led to improved prenatal diagnosis. This is important, because an undiagnosed phaeochromocytoma in pregnancy may have catastrophic consequences for both the mother and the foetus.

There has been a dramatic improvement in the management of phaeochromocytoma in pregnancy, with the maternal mortality having dropped since the 1970s from 50% to the current estimate of 4%. The high mortality associated with an untreated phaeochromocytoma in pregnancy is due to the massive catecholamine release that occurs during a crisis and which may lead to critical vasoconstriction of the utero-placental circulation. In addition, a maternal crisis may be associated with uncontrolled swings in blood pressure and vascular collapse, and this may not be compatible with fetal survival.

Clinical features

Because pregnancy-induced hypertension is very common, a high index of clinical suspicion is required to make the diagnosis of a phaeochromocytoma during pregnancy. If there is hypertension in the absence of proteinuria, oedema, and hyperuricaemia, a diagnosis other than pre-eclampsia should be considered. The symptoms of a catecholamine crisis are no different to those outside pregnancy and are typically characterized by paroxysms of sympathetic symptoms that usually last less than 1 hour.

With the increasingly gravid uterus, pressure from fetal movements and mechanical irritation of the tumour may cause increased susceptibility to a crisis. The onset of uterine contractions and established labour in an untreated phaeochromocytoma is a significant risk of sudden death.

Investigations

Pregnancy does not alter maternal catecholamine secretion, and the biochemical diagnostic approach is the same as outside pregnancy: 24-hour urine collection for catecholamine and metanephrine levels usually shows a significant elevation in the presence of a phaeochromocytoma. Plasma metanephrines may have a role to play in the diagnosis, as they are a sensitive marker of catecholamine excess. MRI is the preferred imaging modality in pregnancy, and MIBG nuclear medicine scans are contraindicated.

Management

Management issues depend upon the stage of pregnancy and the clinical situation. The ideal time for surgical removal is early in the second trimester, when anaesthesia is safe and the anatomy will not be distorted by the gravid uterus. As soon as a phaeochromocytoma is diagnosed, alpha-adrenoceptor blockade should be started in order to prevent the effects of catecholamine excess and to control blood pressure.

Both phenoxybenzamine (a non-competitive alpha antagonist) and doxazosin (a competitive antagonist) have been used safely and effectively in pregnancy. Beta blockade should be added after alpha blockade later in pregnancy, due to the potential for growth retardation with beta blockers early in pregnancy.

The timing and appropriateness of surgery should be determined by the degree of medical control of symptoms and blood pressure, and after discussion with the endocrine surgeon, the obstetrician, the anaesthetist, and the patient. Elective caesarean section may be preferred to vaginal delivery, with adrenal exploration occurring either immediately after the caesarean delivery or at a later stage.

Key points for phaeochromocytoma in pregnancy

- Undiagnosed phaeochromocytoma has a high maternal and fetal mortality.
- The diagnosis should be considered in atypical pregnancy-induced hypertension.
- Alpha-adrenoceptor blockade should be started during pregnancy once a phaeochromocytoma has been detected.
- The ideal time for surgical removal is early in the second trimester.

Further reading

Bjornsdottir S, Cnattingius S, Brandt L, et al. Addison's disease in women is a risk factor for an adverse pregnancy outcome. *J Clin Endocrinol Metab* 2010; 95: 5249–57.

Cox ME, Williams LL, and Lien LF. Pheochromocytoma in pregnancy. *Endocr Pract* 2010; 16: 337–8.

Lebbe M and Arlt W. What is the best diagnostic and therapeutic management strategy for an Addison patient during pregnancy? *Clin Endocrinol (Oxf)* 2013; 78: 497–502.

Lekarev O and New MI. Adrenal disease in pregnancy. *Best Pract Res Clin Endocrinol Metab* 2011; 25: 959–73.

Lindsay JR, Jonklaas J, Oldfield EH, et al. Cushing's syndrome during pregnancy: Personal experience and review of the literature. *J Clin Endocrinol Metab* 2005; 90: 3077–83.

Merce Fernandez-Balsells M, Muthusamy K, Smushkin G, et al. Prenatal dexamethasone use for the prevention of virilization in pregnancies at risk for classical congenital adrenal hyperplasia because of 21-hydroxylase (CYP21A2) deficiency: A systematic review and meta-analyses. *Clin Endocrinol (Oxf)* 2010; 73: 436–44.

10.3 Pituitary adenomas in pregnancy

Introduction

Pituitary adenomas cause problems because of hormone hypersecretion as well as by causing hypopituitarism.

Prolactinoma

Bromocriptine and cabergoline are the primary modes of therapy, restoring ovulatory menses in about 80% and 90% of women with prolactinomas, respectively. In addition, macroadenoma size can be reduced by >50% in 50%–75% of patients with bromocriptine and in >90% with cabergoline. Trans-sphenoidal surgery is usually done only in patients not responding to medical therapy.

The stimulatory effect of the hormonal milieu of pregnancy and the withdrawal of the dopamine agonist may result in significant tumour enlargement in 2.7% of patients with microadenomas, and 23% of those with macroadenomas. In almost all cases, such enlargement can be successfully treated with reinstitution of a dopamine agonist. If the pregnancy is sufficiently advanced, another approach is to deliver the baby. Surgical decompression is only resorted to if these other approaches fail.

Usually, the dopamine agonist is stopped once pregnancy is diagnosed, to limit fetal exposure. No increase in spontaneous abortions, ectopic pregnancies, trophoblastic disease, multiple pregnancies, or malformations has been found with either bromocriptine or cabergoline but the safety database for bromocriptine is about eightfold larger than that for cabergoline. Patients with large macroadenomas should be assessed monthly for symptoms of tumour enlargement, and visual fields should be tested each trimester. Prolactin levels may rise without tumour enlargement and not rise with tumour enlargement during pregnancy; therefore, levels are often misleading and should not be obtained.

Acromegaly

Most patients with acromegaly are treated with surgery as primary therapy; those not cured are usually treated medically with the somatostatin analogues octreotide and lanreotide. Only a few patients with tumours secreting growth hormone have been reported to have enlargement of their tumours during pregnancy. Therefore, those with macroadenomas with suprasellar extension should be monitored for symptoms and visual field testing. Gestational diabetes and hypertension are increased in acromegalic patients but cardiac disease is not.

Fewer than 50 pregnant patients treated with somatostatin analogues have been reported; no malformations were found in their children. However, the analogues cross the placenta and can bind to somatostatin receptors in the brain and other tissues. Therefore, some recommend that somatostatin analogues be discontinued if pregnancy is considered unless they are needed to control tumour growth. Bromocriptine is licensed for conception, whilst cabergoline is not but has been used in the context of patients with prolactinomas (see 'Prolactinoma'). Pegvisomant, a growth-hormone-receptor antagonist, has been given to three patients with acromegaly during pregnancy, without harm, but the safety of this is certainly not established.

Cushing's syndrome

Less than 150 cases of Cushing's syndrome in pregnancy have been reported and less than half of these had pituitary adenomas. Diagnosing Cushing's syndrome during pregnancy may be difficult, as both conditions may be associated with weight gain in a central distribution; fatigue; oedema; emotional upset; glucose intolerance; and hypertension. The striae associated with normal pregnancy are usually pale but are red or purple in Cushing's syndrome.

Elevated total and free serum cortisol, levels of adrenocorticotrophic hormone, and UFC excretion are compatible with normal pregnancy as well as Cushing's disease. The overnight dexamethasone test usually demonstrates inadequate suppression during normal pregnancy. Adrenocorticotrophic hormone levels are normal to elevated, even with adrenal adenomas, perhaps due to the production of adrenocorticotrophic hormone by the placenta or from the non-suppressible stimulation of pituitary adrenocorticotrophic hormone by placental CRH. A persistent diurnal variation in the elevated levels of serum cortisol during normal pregnancy may be most helpful in distinguishing the hypercortisolism of pregnancy from Cushing's syndrome, where diurnal variation is characteristically absent. Little experience has been reported with CRH stimulation testing or petrosal venous sinus sampling during pregnancy.

Cushing's syndrome is associated with a pregnancy loss rate of 25% due to spontaneous abortion, stillbirth, and early neonatal death because of extreme prematurity. Hypertension, diabetes, and myopathy may complicate the pregnancy. Post-operative wound infection and dehiscence are common after caesarean section.

Treatment of the Cushing's disease during the pregnancy is recommended because it increases the frequency of live births and decreases prematurity. Trans-sphenoidal surgery has been carried out successfully in many patients. Although any surgery poses risks for the mother and foetus, the risks of not operating are considerably higher than those of proceeding with surgery. Medical therapy for Cushing's syndrome during pregnancy is not very effective.

TSH-secreting adenomas

Only three cases of pregnancy occurring in women with TSH-secreting tumours have been reported. In two, octreotide was needed to control tumour size. The most pressing issue with such tumours is the need to control hyperthyroidism during pregnancy and that can usually be done with standard anti-thyroid drugs.

Clinically non-functioning adenomas

Pregnancy would not expected to influence tumour size in patients with clinically non-functioning adenomas and only two cases have been reported with tumour enlargement during pregnancy. In one, the patient responded rapidly to bromocriptine treatment, probably due to shrinkage of the lactotroph hyperplasia with decompression of the chiasm and probably with little or no direct effect on the tumour itself.

Hypopituitarism

Hypopituitarism may be partial or complete. A variety of techniques have been used for ovulation induction, including administration of hCG and FSH, pulsatile GnRH, and IVF. Although the malformation rate is not increased in such pregnancies, there seems to be an increased frequency of caesarean sections, miscarriages, and small-for-gestational age babies.

The average increase in the need for T4 in hypothyroid patients during pregnancy is about 0.05 mg/day. Because patients with hypopituitarism do not elevate their TSH levels normally in the face of an increased need for T4, it is reasonable to increase the T4 supplementation by 0.025 mg after the first and second trimesters.

The dose of glucocorticoid replacement does not usually need to be increased during pregnancy, with the usual dose being 12–15 mg/m^2, given in two or three doses. Additional glucocorticoids are needed for the stress of labour and delivery.

There are few data on the use of growth hormone during pregnancy in hypopituitary individuals and, in most series, growth-hormone therapy has been stopped at conception without adverse effects.

Hypopituitarism developing during pregnancy may be due to lymphocytic hypophysitis, enlargement of a preexisting tumor, or pituitary infarction. Rapid diagnosis and HRT are necessary for a good outcome.

Further reading

Cheng S, Grasso L, Martinez-Orozco JA, et al. Pregnancy in acromegaly: Experience from two referral centers and systematic review of the literature. *Clin Endocrinol* 2012; 76: 264–71.

Karaca Z, Tanriverdi F, Unluhizarci K, et al. Pregnancy and pituitary disorders. *Eur J Endocrinol* 2010; 162: 453–75.

Kübler K, Klingmüller D, Gembruch U, et al. High-risk pregnancy management in women with hypopituitarism. *J Perinatol* 2009; 29: 89–95.

Lindsay JR, Jonklaas J, Oldfield EH, et al. Cushing's syndrome during pregnancy: Personal experience and review of the literature. *J Clin Endocrinol Metab* 2005; 90: 3077–83.

Molitch ME. Prolactinoma in pregnancy. *Best Pract Res Clin Endocrinol Metab* 2011; 25: 885–96.

Mineral metabolism

Chapter contents

11.1 Anatomy and physiology

Introduction

The skeleton functions as a major store for several minerals, including calcium, phosphate, and magnesium; 99% of calcium (about 1 kg) in the human body is retained within the skeleton, combined with phosphate in the form of hydroxyapatite crystals contained within and between type 1 collagen fibres. Hydroxyapatite attachment and the calcification of bone are partly controlled by glycoproteins and proteoglycans with a high ion-binding capacity. The most abundant protein in bone is type 1 collagen, which is formed from a triple helix of amino acid chains that orientate in fibres with a high density per unit volume and are packed in layers to give the microscopic lamellar structure. A process of collagen maturation with post-translational modifications results in the formation of intra- and intermolecular pyridinoline and pyrrole crosslinks that contribute to the elasticity and strength of bone as well as to matrix mineralization. This complex molecular structure and intricate microarchitecture enable bone to function as the body's reservoir of calcium.

Osteoblasts are responsible for the production of the organic matrix of bone; this matrix is known as osteoid and is mineralized by two main mechanisms.

* In the first mechanism, plasma-membrane (chondrocyte)-derived matrix vesicles act as a focus for calcium and phosphate deposition, with hydroxyapatite crystals forming on the lipid-rich inner membrane. Osteoblasts also secrete matrix proteins, which allow rapid mineralization within the matrix spaces, and alkaline phosphatase, which can destroy inhibitors of this process contained within the matrix environment, such as pyrophosphate.

* In the second mechanism, where tightly packed lamellar bone is present, matrix vesicles are rarely observed and mineralization is in association with matrix fibrils. Non-collagenous proteoglycans and osteonectin control the mineralization taking place in the spaces between collagen molecules.

It is essential that calcium and phosphate are readily available to allow mineralization and normal bone formation to take place. When there is a reduced supply of these minerals, the percentage of osteoid increases, resulting in the clinical condition of osteomalacia.

Bone is constantly undergoing remodelling with a coupled process of resorption and breakdown of matrix by osteoclasts (multinucleated giant cells), and formation and mineralization by osteoblasts. During these processes, minerals are exchanged between bone and the extracellular fluid, with a relative balance of calcium maintained between newly formed bone and older, resorbed bone. Increased resorption of bone by osteoclasts can result in the release of calcium to the extracellular fluid from the bone matrix, to maintain calcium homeostasis when demand for calcium is high. Deposition of calcium within bone can result in increased storage when a plentiful supply of calcium exists.

Organ and cell functions are dependent on tight control of the calcium concentration in extracellular fluid, and it is essential that the body also has the physiological mechanisms to make calcium readily available for several important processes such as cell proliferation; neural conduction; cellular production and secretion of multiple molecules; muscle contraction; clotting of blood; maintenance of cell stability; and permeability. The concentration of calcium circulating in the plasma is tightly regulated between 2.2 and 2.6 mmol/L (8.8 and 10.4 mg/dL) with the calcium present in three major forms:

* 50% as calcium ions, the physiologically active form
* 40% protein bound, mainly to albumin
* 10% complexed to anions such as phosphate, sulphate, and citrate

The majority of laboratory measurements of plasma calcium estimate total calcium and this can be significantly affected by the prevailing protein concentration. When plasma proteins increase, such as in dehydration or after prolonged venous stasis, increased protein-bound calcium, and therefore increased total calcium, are observed. In diseases or conditions resulting in decreased plasma proteins (e.g. liver disease, nephrotic syndrome, sepsis, malnutrition), there are decreased amounts of protein-bound calcium and total calcium. In many of these circumstances, the concentration of calcium ions can be maintained within the reference range (1.1–1.3 mmol/L (4.4–5.2 mg/dL)) by the physiological control processes. Plasma albumin can be altered by acute and chronic diseases and, as a result, total calcium can be misleading. In clinical practice, it is important to adjust the calcium for the patient's albumin concentration so that the reported value better reflects the level of calcium ions. A simple formula to adjust for a patient's albumin concentration has been devised that utilizes the population mean albumin concentration of 40 g/L (see Section 11.2). This is particularly useful in situations where a chronic low albumin level, such as in a patient with cancer, can mask hypercalcaemia.

Regulating plasma calcium

Regulation of plasma calcium is achieved by the actions of the three calcitrophic hormones PTH, 1,25-dihydroxyvitamin D, and calcitonin and their interactions on the kidneys, the bones, and the gastrointestinal tract. Figure 11.1 outlines the important responses that take place when circulating calcium is decreased.

* The calcium-sensing receptor (CaSr) on the chief cells of the parathyroid gland responds to the decreased level of calcium ions by stimulating PTH synthesis, encapsulating PTH in vesicles, and, in the presence of normal intracellular magnesium concentrations, fusing the vesicles to the cell surface and releasing PTH into the circulation.

* PTH stimulates calcium reabsorption via the kidney to increase plasma calcium and phosphate excretion, decreasing plasma phosphate.

* PTH stimulates osteoclast resorption of bone, releasing calcium and phosphate and thus increasing the levels of both in plasma.

* PTH stimulates 1-hydroxylation of 25-hydroxyvitamin D in the kidney to produce 1,25-dihydroxyvitamin D.

* 1,25-Dihydroxyvitamin D acts on the gastrointestinal tract to stimulate calcium absorption, increasing plasma calcium.

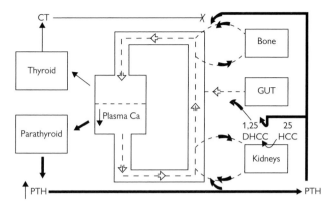

Fig 11.1 Regulation of plasma calcium by PTH and calcitonin via kidneys, gut, and bone; 1,25 DHCC, 1,25-dihydroxycholecalciferol; 25 HCC, 25-hydroxycholecalciferol.
Reprinted from *The Lancet*, Volume 374, Fraser WD, Hyperparathyroidism, pp. 145–158, Copyright (2009) with permission from Elsevier.

- As the calcium concentration increases, a classical feedback loop is observed, with the CaSr responding to the increasing level of calcium ions by switching off the PTH release from the chief cells.

CaSR

The CaSR is a 120 kDa GPCR with a large extracellular domain (612 amino acids) seven transmembrane-spanning domains (250 amino acids), and a C-terminal intracellular tail (216 amino acids) that plays a major role in calcium homeostasis. Dimerization and glycosylation of the receptor is essential for receptor function. The receptor is activated by divalent and trivalent cations, principally calcium ions, as well as by polyamines, aminoglycoside antibiotics (neomycin), L-isomers of amino acids (phenylalanine), and synthetic phenylalkylamines (calcimimetics). The CaSR is a multifunction receptor expressed in many tissues throughout the body but its particular importance is in calcium metabolism via its expression in parathyroid cells, controlling PTH secretion; in renal tubular cells, directly regulating calcium reabsorption; in C cells of the thyroid, controlling calcitonin secretion; in the placenta, regulating calcium transport from the mother to the foetus; and in bone, where it can influence osteoblast, osteoclast, and chondrocyte function/survival, thus significantly affecting bone metabolism.

The structural complexity of the CaSR predisposes to several important inherited disorders of calcium homeostasis that involve *CaSr* in both activating and inactivating mutations (Box 11.1). Seventy different *CaSr* mutations have been identified, leading to autosomal-dominant hypocalcaemic hypercalciuria (ADHH), autosomal-dominant hypocalcaemia hypercalcuria, and neonatal severe hyperparathyroidism. Manipulation of CaSR by both calcimimetics (stimulatory) and calcilytics (inhibitory) is becoming a very important therapeutic intervention. Calcimimetics are playing a significant role in the treatment of bone and cardiovascular complications related to chronic kidney disease. The widespread distribution of the CaSR and its functional diversity is liable to lead to increased association with diseases in future.

Box 11.1 Inherited disorders of calcium homeostasis involving the calcium-sensing receptor

Activating
Familial hypoparathyroidism
Autosomal dominant hypocalcaemia hypercalcuria
Type 5 Bartter syndrome

Inactivating
Familial benign hypocalciuric hypercalcaemia
Neonatal severe hyperparathyroidism

PTH

PTH is expressed almost exclusively by the chief cells of the parathyroid gland, with minor expression in the thymus and hypothalamus. The PTH gene is located on the short arm of Chromosome 11, and the primary translational product is pre-pro-PTH, with a 25-amino acid presequence, a 6-amino-acid prosequence, and the 84-amino-acid mature sequence. Transport and processing within the chief cell is controlled by the pre-pro sequence, which allows the PTH (1–84) molecule to be incorporated into secretory vesicles which can enable either secretion of this mature peptide or enzyme cleavage to produce peptide fragments that lack the N-terminal sequence and therefore are unable to fully interact with the PTH 1 receptor (PTH1R). Secretion from the chief cell is by classical exocytosis, and biologically active PTH normally circulates in plasma as the single-chain 84-amino-acid polypeptide. Cleavage of PTH into N-terminal and C-terminal fragments can happen both in the kidneys and in the liver. Figure 11.2 shows the metabolism and known common circulating forms of PTH.

The classical biological actions of PTH require the presence of the N-terminal region in order to fully activate the PTH1R. Some of these effects are shown in Figure 11.1. In addition, PTH can:

- activate adenylyl cyclase increasing cAMP excretion
- activate several other signal transduction pathways, including those involving:
  - protein kinase C

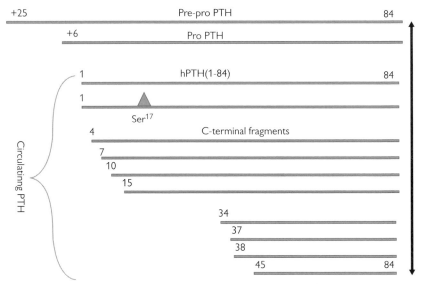

Fig 11.2 PTH metabolism and molecular forms circulating in blood. The hPTH (1–84) and Ser[17] modified PTH (1–84) fragments account for 20% of the circulating PTH, and the C-terminal fragments account for 80% of the circulating PTH.

- phospholipase A_2, C, and D
- cytosolic calcium ions
- MAP kinases
- stimulate bone formation (intermittent administration)
- stimulate bone resorption (continuous administration)
- cause proliferation of blood and liver cells

In plasma, PTH (1–34) has a half-life of 2–3 minutes, PTH (1–84) has a half-life of 15–20 minutes, and C-terminal fragments of PTH can have a half-life of 30–60 minutes. In chronic kidney disease, PTH (1–84) has an increased half-life, and some C-terminal fragments can remain in plasma with a half-life of hours. The concentration of the PTH (7–84) fragment is increased in patients with chronic kidney disease, and this plus other C-terminal PTH molecules are now thought to have some biological activity and may act to block N-terminal PTH activity at PTH1R and directly act through putative PTH 2 receptors (PTH2Rs). PTH (7–84) can antagonize the calcaemic and phosphaturic actions of PTH (1–84) when administered in high concentrations and when abnormal molar ratios exist in animal and cell models. There is evidence that PTH (7–84) can act via PTH2R and result in hypocalcaemia, inhibit formation of tartrate-resistant acid-phosphatase-positive bone cells, and interfere with PTH (1–84) and (1–34) effects both in vivo and in vitro.

The development of 'sandwich'-type immunoassays (second generation; immunometric assays) that allow the measurement of PTH (1–84) and are termed 'intact PTH' assays was a significant advance in diagnosing and treating diseases affecting bone and calcium homeostasis. It is now known that the C-terminal of PTH is detected in intact PTH assays, resulting in an overestimation of PTH (1–84) when PTH (7–84) is present. 'Whole' PTH assays have been developed (third generation) that do not react with PTH (7–84) and, by measuring intact PTH and then subtracting whole PTH, an estimate of PTH (7–84) can be made. The percentage of PTH (7–84) within each patient sample remains relatively constant but increases in chronic kidney disease and so intelligent application of current PTH assays is advisable.

Vitamin D

The synthesis and metabolism of vitamin D and its main metabolites are shown in Figure 11.3. There are two major sources of vitamin D in humans, with approximately 80%–90% produced by the action of sunlight (UVB) on the skin converting 7-dehydrocholesterol to cholecalciferol (vitamin D_3). The other 10%–20% is derived from dietary sources and is either animal-derived cholecalciferol or plant-derived ergocalciferol (vitamin D_2). Vitamin D and its hydroxylated metabolites are transported in plasma bound to a specific globulin called vitamin D-binding protein. Differing binding affinities for this protein ensures the movement of cholecalciferol from the skin to the liver, and dietary vitamin D is transported to the liver in chylomicrons. 25-Hydroxylation is carried out by a liver microsomal enzyme and is the rate-limiting step in the conversion of vitamin D to its active metabolites. 25-Hydroxyvitamin D is the major storage (liver) and circulating form of vitamin D, with a half-life of 25–30 days, and measurement of 25-hydroxyvitamin D is felt to be the best reflection of vitamin D status. 25-Hydroxyvitamin D is subject to enterohepatic circulation and is excreted in bile and then reabsorbed in the small bowel. Disruption of this pathway can result in significant vitamin D deficiency.

The metabolite with greatest biological activity is 1,25-dihydroxyvitamin D, with the 1-hydroxylation taking place mainly in mitochondria of the renal tubules but also in bone, skin, placenta, and granuloma tissue (e.g. in sarcoidosis, TB). 1-Alpha-hydroxylase activity is stimulated by PTH, low plasma phosphate concentration, low calcium concentration, vitamin D deficiency, calcitonin, growth

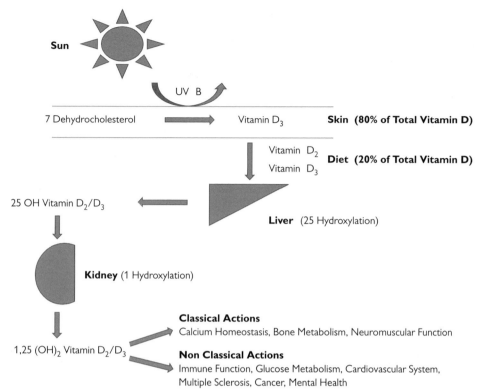

Sun

UV B

7 Dehydrocholesterol ➡️ Vitamin D$_3$ **Skin (80% of Total Vitamin D)**

Vitamin D$_2$
Vitamin D$_3$ **Diet (20% of Total Vitamin D)**

25 OH Vitamin D$_2$/D$_3$

Liver (25 Hydroxylation)

Kidney (1 Hydroxylation)

1,25 (OH)$_2$ Vitamin D$_2$/D$_3$

Classical Actions
Calcium Homeostasis, Bone Metabolism, Neuromuscular Function

Non Classical Actions
Immune Function, Glucose Metabolism, Cardiovascular System,
Multiple Sclerosis, Cancer, Mental Health

Fig 11.3 Vitamin D production and metabolism.
Reproduced from Gosney M, Harper A, and Conroy S, *Oxford Desk Reference: Geriatric Medicine*, Fig. 8.6, Copyright © 2012, with permission from Oxford University Press.

hormone, prolactin, and oestrogen and is inhibited by 1,25-dihydroxyvitamin D, high calcium, high fibroblast growth factor 23 (FGF23), high phosphate, and low PTH.

Calcitonin

Calcitonin is a 32-amino acid peptide synthesized and secreted by the parafollicular cells of the thyroid gland (the C cells). Secretion of calcitonin is regulated via the CaSr ,with an increase in plasma calcium ions stimulating a proportional increase in calcitonin, and a decrease resulting in a corresponding reduction in calcitonin. Chronic repeated stimulation of the CaSr results in exhaustion of the secretory reserve of the C cells. Calcitonin acts on osteoclasts to inhibit bone resorption by causing osteoclasts to shrink and retract from the bone surface ultimately decreasing calcium release from bone. Renal reabsorption of phosphate is inhibited by calcitonin, which can also cause sodium excretion in the urine, thus contributing to urinary calcium loss and lowering plasma calcium. Pharmacological doses of calcitonin have been used to treat hypercalcaemia, osteoporosis, and Paget's disease of bone.

Calcitonin can be detected in the plasma in high concentrations in patients with medullary carcinoma of the thyroid. It can be used in such circumstances as a tumour marker.

Gastrointestinal absorption and excretion of calcium

The main site of calcium absorption in the gastrointestinal tract is the proximal small intestine. Regulation is firstly through the quantity of calcium ingested in the diet (see Table 11.1 for major dietary sources) and then by two cellular transport processes:
- active saturable transcellular absorption stimulated by 1,25-dihydroxyvitamin D

Table 11.1 Major dietary sources of calcium

Food	Milligrams per average serving
Yoghurt (8 oz)	415
Cheese (1.5 oz)	300–340
Sardines (3 oz)	325
Milk (8 oz, depending on fat content)	275–300
Salmon (3 oz)	180
Cereals (ready to eat, 1 cup, various)	100–1000
Green vegetables (1 cup)	40–100
Wholewheat bread (1 slice)	30

- non-saturable paracellular absorption controlled by the concentration of calcium in the lumen relative to the plasma calcium concentration

Normal adults ingesting a Western diet are in calcium balance, where the amount of dietary calcium consumed and the deposition in bone are matched by the calcium excreted in faeces and urine. Increased or reduced calcium absorption happens when there are changes in dietary calcium intake or alterations in intestinal calcium solubility or in the metabolism of vitamin D. When kidney function is normal, variation in urinary calcium excretion tends to directly reflect changing plasma calcium, with increasing urinary calcium as plasma calcium increases, and reduced calcium excretion as plasma calcium decreases, mainly as a result of the changing filtered load of calcium.

Regulation of phosphate

Regulation of phosphate is a complex process involving the kidneys, the intestines, and the skeleton. Plasma phosphate in adults is maintained between 0.7 and 1.4 mmol/L. In a 24-hour cycle, plasma phosphate demonstrates a diurnal variation, with a significant increase after the evening meal to a peak in the early hours of the morning and then falling to a nadir later in the morning. This circadian rhythm is almost completely removed by fasting, demonstrating the importance of dietary intake on the daily changes in phosphate. 1,25-Dihydroxyvitamin D can promote calcium and phosphate absorption via the intestine and can increase phosphate mobilization from the bone by stimulating osteoclastic resorption of bone mineral containing hydroxyapatite as the storage form of phosphate. PTH can have effects on phosphate via the kidney by increasing the expression of the type 2a sodium–phosphate cotransporter (NPT2a) in the proximal tubule, and downregulating NPT2a by decreasing the time the transporter remains in the apical membrane of the tubule. PTH action at the tubule promotes phosphaturia and will lower circulating phosphate indirectly. PTH can act via the osteoclast to stimulate both bone resorption and bone formation, depending on the fluctuation in PTH, and so can either release or deposit phosphate in bone, depending on the PTH signal. An increase in plasma phosphate will stimulate PTH synthesis and secretion from the parathyroid chief cells and also inhibit 1-alpha-hydroxylase, decreasing 1,25-dihydroxyvitamin D production. It is clear that the variations observed in PTH and 1,25-dihydroxyvitamin D in health and disease do not fully explain the changes in phosphate homeostasis and so the existence of 'phosphatonins' has been suspected for some time.

The term 'phosphatonin' refers to a class of molecules that regulate phosphate metabolism acting in an autocrine, paracrine, or hormonal (humoral) manner, mainly via bone, intestine, and renal metabolism. There is a growing list of phosphatonins that are being identified in association with disorders of phosphate metabolism (see Box 11.2) and it is likely that combined actions of these molecules are required in phosphaturic diseases (see Section 14.1, p. 394).

Plasma inorganic phosphate is freely filtered at the glomerulus, and 80% of reabsorption takes place through specific cotransporters, particularly sodium-dependent phosphate cotransporter 2a (NPT2a) in the proximal tubule. The factors increasing and decreasing phosphate

---

Box 11.2 Phosphatonins involved in phosphate regulation

Fibroblast growth factor 23
Matrix extracellular phosphoglycoprotein
Secreted frizzled-related protein 4
Fibroblast growth factor 7

---

reabsorption are listed in Table 11.2. Increased reabsorption is often associated with increasing NPT2a present on the surface of brush border membranes; decreased NPT2a expression is associated with reduced reabsorption. The phosphatonins are phosphaturic factors and decrease NPT2a expression.

FGF23 is the best known phosphatonin and is a 251-amino acid secretory hormone with two functional domains: the N-terminal domain, which contains the fibroblast growth factor homology region, and the unique C-terminal domain. There is one recognized proteolytic cleavage site (RXXR, 176RHTR179) and several glycosylation sites, enabling post-translational modification, which can alter function leading to disease. Intact FGF23 is biologically active in terms of effects on phosphate and vitamin D metabolism; the N- and C-terminal fragments are currently believed to be inactive, although inhibitory functions of these fragments have been described.

Although FGF23 transcripts are present in many tissues (e.g. the brain, the thymus, the small intestine, the heart, the liver, and the thyroid/parathyroid), the only physiologically important source is the skeleton, in particular via production by osteocytes and osteoblasts. FGF23 is known to have its main effects on phosphate and vitamin D metabolism but several other effects have been reported (Table 11.3).

FGF23 action is mediated by binding to cell-surface fibroblast growth factor receptors types 1 (FGFR1), 3c (FGFR3c), and FGFR4. The specificity of FGF23 action is dependent on the co-expression of the membrane protein alpha Klotho in the kidneys, the parathyroid, and the pituitary. Binding of alpha Klotho to FGFR1, FGFR3c, and FGFR4 specifically increases their affinity for FGF23 and is essential for subsequent FGF23 actions. The

---

Table 11.2 Factors involved in renal tubular phosphate transport

Increasing tubular phosphate reabsorption	Decreasing tubular phosphate reabsorption
Phosphate depletion	Phosphate repletion/loading
Hypoparathyroid/low PTH	Hyperparathyroid/high PTH
Hypocalcaemia	Hypercalcaemia
Plasma volume contraction	Plasma volume expansion
Hypocapnia	Hypercapnia
Increased 1,25-dihydroxyvitamin D	Decreased 1,25-dihydroxyvitamin D
Growth hormone	Glucose
Insulin-like growth factors	Increased bicarbonate
	Carbonic anhydrase inhibitors
	Phosphotonins

Table 11.3 Actions of fibroblast growth factor 23

Target organ	Effects
Kidney	Decreased phosphate reabsorption, increased plasma phosphate
	Decreased synthesis of 1-alpha-hydroxylase, decreased plasma 1,25-dihydroxyvitamin D
	Increased expression of 25-hydroxylase, decreased plasma 1,25-dihydroxyvitamin D
Parathyroid gland	Inhibition of PTH synthesis, subsequent decreased plasma 1,25-dihydroxyvitamin D
Heart/vascular	Left ventricular hypertrophy
	Atherosclerosis
Whole body	Anti-ageing factor

organ-specific expression of alpha Klotho helps restrict the major activity of FGF23 to a limited number of target organs in the body, although some direct cellular effects of FGF23 are being recognized.

FGF23 does not respond directly to rapid changes in circulating phosphate. Oral phosphate loading will increase and restriction decrease FGF23 secretion but the phosphate-sensing mechanism is unknown. 1,25-Dihydroxyvitamin D at an appropriate concentration will stimulate FGF23 synthesis by activating the *FGF23* promoter in bone cells. PTH stimulates FGF23 expression and secretion in bone; parathyroidectomy, despite increasing plasma phosphate, results in a significant reduction in FGF23. Alpha Klotho expression in the kidney is also decreased following parathyroidectomy, resulting in a reduced FGF23 response.

Further reading

Seeman E (ed), 'Mineral homeostasis', in Rosen CJ, Bouillon R, Compston JE, et al., eds., *Primer on the Metabolic Bone Diseases and Disorders of Mineral Metabolism* (8th edition), 2013. Wiley-Blackwell, pp. 171–248.

11.2 Investigations

Genetics

Introduction

A precise genetic diagnosis is often of major importance in order to choose the right treatment, inform on prognosis, implement prenatal diagnostics, and provide correct genetic counselling. Suggestions for genetic tests and providers of the tests can be found on the Online Mendelian Inheritance in Man (OMIM) website (http://www.ncbi.nlm.nih.gov/omim), http://www.eddnal.com (EU), and http://www.genetests.org (USA). Genetic testing is most important in familial hyper- and hypocalcaemic patients, in patients with chronic hypophosphataemia, and in patients with osteogenesis imperfecta.

Inherited hypercalcaemia

Genetic testing is indicated in selected patients with primary hyperparathyroidism to diagnose multiple endocrine neoplasia type 1 or type 2b, hyperparathyroidism–jaw tumour syndrome, other cases of familial primary hyperparathyroidism (see Chapter 12), and familial hypocalciuric (benign) hypercalcaemia.

Familial hypocalciuric hypercalcaemia

Familial hypocalciuric hypercalcaemia is a group of benign, autosomal-dominant conditions caused by inactivating mutations in CASR (familial hypocalciuric hypercalcaemia type 1; OMIM #145980), GNA11 (familial hypocalciuric hypercalcaemia type 2; OMIM #145981), or AP2S1 (familial hypocalciuric hypercalcaemia type 3, OMIM #602242), leading to reduced sensitivity for plasma calcium in target tissues, including the parathyroids and the renal tubules. The prevalence is around 1:10,000. It is associated with mild to moderate usually asymptomatic equilibrium hypercalcaemia and low-normal renal calcium excretion in spite of hypercalcaemia. Plasma PTH is increased in 20%–30% and inappropriately high normal in the remaining. Plasma 25-hydroxyvitamin D is normal but plasma 1,25-dihydroxyvitamin D and bone turnover markers tend to be slightly increased. The bone mineral density is normal, and there is no increased risk of fractures. Muscle function, renal function, and quality of life are all normal and there is no increased risk of renal stones. Most patients with familial hypocalciuric hypercalcaemia have a calcium-to-creatinine clearance ratio <0.01 (see 'Biochemistry'), whereas the majority of patients with primary hyperparathyroidism have values >0.02. The interpretation of levels between 0.01 and 0.02 is uncertain without mutational analysis. Levels <0.01 may also be seen in patients who have primary hyperparathyroidism and impaired renal function or severe vitamin D deficiency. Autoantibodies targeting the CaSR, or lithium therapy, may lead to acquired hypocalciuric hypercalcaemia.

It is recommended that the following patients be tested for mutations in CASR: (1) hypercalcaemic patients with inappropriately high-normal or elevated PTH and a calcium-to-creatinine clearance ratio <0.02, (2) patients with a family history of hypercalcaemia, (3) hypercalcaemic patients diagnosed before the age of 30, and (4) patients with persistent hypercalcaemia following otherwise successful parathyroid exploration. This strategy will diagnose 98% of patients with familial hypocalciuric hypercalcaemia. The different CASR point mutations reflect different phenotypes with respect to degree of hypercalcaemia and plasma PTH levels. Patients with familial hypocalciuric hypercalcaemia should not be operated on, since the disease appears to be asymptomatic and parathyroidectomy is ineffective.

Hypocalcaemia

Most cases of chronic hypocalcaemia are caused by hypoparathyroidism following neck surgery, but some are inherited, caused by either familial hypoparathyroidism, with decreased PTH secretion, or pseudohypoparathyroidism, with increased peripheral resistance to PTH.

Inherited hypoparathyroidism

All non-acquired cases of inherited hypoparathyroidism should be tested for mutations. When resources are limited, the focus should be on autosomal-dominant hypocalcaemia, DiGeorge syndrome, and autoimmune polyendocrine insufficiency type 1, as, for these disorders, the diagnosis has major implications for supplementary investigations, clinical follow-up, and therapy.

Familial isolated hypoparathyroidism

Familial isolated hypoparathyroidism is caused by mutations in PTH (OMIM # 146200) or GCMB (OMIM #146200), both with autosomal-recessive or autosomal-dominant inheritance. X-linked hypoparathyroidism (OMIM #307700; X-linked recessive) is caused by a deletion–insertion mutation in SOX3. Only males are affected.

Autosomal-dominant hypocalcaemia

Autosomal-dominant hypocalcaemia (OMIM #601198), is caused by an activating mutation in CASR. It is characterized by oligosymptomatic hypocalcaemia with functional hypoparathyroidism and reduced renal tubular reabsorption of calcium. The phenotype may be similar to that seen in Bartter syndrome. There is an increased risk of nephrocalcinosis and renal stones in response to calcium and vitamin D treatment.

DiGeorge syndrome

DiGeorge syndrome (OMIM #188400; autosomal dominant, sporadic), also known as CATCH 22 syndrome (for cardiac abnormality, abnormal facies, T-cell deficit, cleft palate, and hypocalcaemia), is the most common (13/100,000 live births) familial hypoparathyroidism and can be complicated with other clinical findings. It is caused by a microdeletion involving TBX1 on Chromosome 22.

Autoimmune polyendocrine insufficiency type 1

Autoimmune polyendocrine insufficiency type 1 (OMIM #240300; autosomal recessive or autosomal dominant), also known as APECED syndrome (for autoimmune, polyendocrinopathy, candidiasis, and ectodermal dystrophy), is caused by mutations in the autoimmune regulator gene AIRE1. The syndrome includes hypoparathyroidism (79%), chronic mucocutaneous candidiasis (70%), Addison's disease (60%), primary hypogonadism (female: 60%; male: 14%), and other autoimmune diseases. A few cases may have CaSR-activating antibodies. This disease is most common in Finns, Sardinians, and Iranian Jews.

*Hypoparathyroidism sensoneuronal deafness
and renal dysplasia*

Hypoparathyroidism sensoneuronal deafness and renal dysplasia (OMIM #146255; autosomal dominant) is caused by a microdeletion in *GATA3*. There is a progressive deterioration of renal function.

Sanjad–Sakati syndrome and Kenny–Caffey syndrome

Both Sanjad–Sakati syndrome (OMIM #241410; autosomal recessive) and Kenny–Caffey syndrome (OMIM #244460; autosomal recessive) are caused by mutations in *TBCE*. These syndromes are characterized by reduced height, eye abnormalities, and mental retardation; in addition, there is medullary stenosis of the long bones in Kenney–Caffey syndrome.

Mitochondrial dysfunctions

Mitochondrial dysfunctions are rare syndromes (OMIM #530000). They include Kearns–Sayre syndrome, MELAS syndrome, and mitochondrial trifunctional protein deficiency syndrome.

Pseudohypoparathyroidism

Pseudohypoparathyroidism is characterized by an increased tissue resistance to circulating PTH and is typically caused by a mutation in *GNAS1*.

Pseudohypoparathyroidism type 1a

Pseudohypoparathyroidism type 1a (OMIM #103580; autosomal dominant) is caused by a loss-of-function mutation (frameshift mutation, missense mutation, abnormal splicing, deletion, or inversion) in the maternal copy of *GNAS1*, so that expression of the protein only comes from the paternal allele. This leads to impaired expression of the Gs alpha protein in the proximal renal tubule, and resistance to PTH, as demonstrated by impaired urine cAMP and renal phosphate response (determined by the maximal renal tubular reabsorption capacity for phosphate per litre glomerular filtrate (TmP/GFR)) to exogenous PTH. Resistance to TSH, gonadotrophins, and GHRH may lead to hypothyroidism, hypogonadism, and impaired growth. Albright's hereditary osteodystrophy may be caused by decreased expression of Gs alpha in other tissues. Paternally inherited *GNAS* mutations may lead to pseudopseudohypoparathyroidism (OMIM #612463).

Pseudohypoparathyroidism types 1b and 1c

Pseudohypoparathyroidism type 1b (OMIM #603233) is caused by maternally inherited heterozygous microdeletions in *STX16*; these mutations prevent methylation of *GNAS*, thus leading to renal tubular PTH resistance, as demonstrated by impaired urine cAMP and renal phosphate response (as TmP/GFR) to exogenous PTH. Sporadic cases are seen. Pseudohypoparathyroidism type 1c (OMIM #103580) is a variant of pseudohypoparathyroidism type 1a with the same phenotype. Probably for technical reasons, Gs-alpha deficiency cannot be demonstrated.

Pseudohypoparathyroidism 2

Pseudohypoparathyroidism 2 (OMIM #203330) is a variant with no clear genetic background, and some cases may be acquired. The condition is characterized by partial renal resistance to PTH as demonstrated by normal urine cAMP response but impaired renal phosphate response (as TmP/GFR) to exogenous PTH. There is a normal phenotype and no signs of multiple hormone resistance.

Hypophosphataemic rickets

FGF23 is a skeletal hormone produced by osteocytes that decrease renal phosphate reabsorption and impair renal 1,25-dihydroxyvitamin D production, leading to hypophosphataemic rickets. Mutational analysis can be used to separate the familial diseases caused by abnormal FGF23 metabolism from acquired tubular renal disorders (acquired Fanconi's syndrome) and from tumour-induced osteomalacia, which is caused by small mesenchymal tumours that produce FGF23. Furthermore, such analysis is important for prenatal or early postnatal diagnosis and, thereby, genetic counselling and early treatment of diseased offspring. Cases of hypophosphataemic rickets can be subdivided into those with increased plasma FGF23, and those with normal values.

Hypophosphataemic rickets with increased serum FGF23

X-linked hypophosphataemic rickets (OMIM #307800; X-linked dominant) is caused by a loss-of-function mutation (point mutation, deletion, or duplication) in *PHEX*, leading to decreased degradation of FGF23. This is the most common form (~4/100,000 live births). The patients have renal phosphate loss from birth and a characteristic phenotype, with bowing of lower weight-bearing extremities, and growth impairment.

Autosomal-dominant hypophosphataemic rickets (OMIM #193100; autosomal dominant) is caused by an *FGF23* mutation that makes FGF23 resistant to degradation by PHEX and therefore biologically more active. The phenotype is like that for X-linked hypophosphataemic rickets but often occurs with later onset.

Autosomal-dominant hypophosphataemic rickets with hyperparathyroidism (OMIM #612089; autosomal dominant) with rickets and hypercalcaemic hyperparathyroidism is caused by a balanced 9;13 translocation in *KL*, with increased plasma levels of alpha Klotho and FGF23.

Autosomal-recessive hypophosphataemic rickets type 1 (OMIM #241520; autosomal recessive) is caused by loss-of-function mutations in the gene coding for dentin matrix protein 1 (DMP1). DMP1 inhibits osteocyte differentiation and increases skeletal secretion of FGF23.

Autosomal-recessive hypophosphataemic rickets type 2 (OMIM #613312; autosomal recessive) is caused by loss-of-function mutations in *ENPP1*. FGF23 is increased. The phenotype is the same as that for X-linked hypophosphataemic rickets.

Hypophosphataemic rickets with normal FGF23 concentrations

Hereditary hypophosphataemic rickets with hypercalciuria (OMIM #609826; autosomal recessive) is caused by a mutation in *SLC34A3*. The phenotype is characterized by renal phosphate wasting, elevated plasma 1,25-dihydroxyvitamin D, and hypercalciuria, with risk of renal calcifications and nephrolithiasis.

Osteogenesis imperfecta

Osteogenesis imperfecta is a hereditary connective tissue disease characterized primarily by low-energy fractures, which may start already in fetal life. In most cases, this is a consequence of deficient or abnormal production of procollagen type 1, due to mutations in *COL1A1* and *COL1A2*. However, other genes regulating the post-translational modification of collagen type 1 (e.g. *CRTAP*, *LEPRE1*, *PPIB*, *SERPINH1*, and *FKBP10*) may be important in some cases. The prevalence of osteogenesis imperfecta has been estimated as 22/100,000 live births. Ninety per cent of cases are due to autosomal-dominant mutations, whilst the remaining 10% are autosomal recessive or of unknown cause. Based on clinical signs, symptoms, and radiology, cases have been divided into up to nine phenotypes. However, relations between phenotypes and genotypes have not been sufficiently clarified. Positive mutational analyses are especially helpful in (1) distinguishing osteogenesis imperfecta from phenotypically similar diseases, (2) distinguishing osteogenesis imperfecta from battered-child syndrome, and (3) prenatal diagnosis and counselling. Quantitative protein analysis based on skin biopsy may be helpful in specific cases.

Biochemistry

Introduction

In the clinic, plasma concentrations of calcium, phosphate, magnesium, creatinine, PTH, alkaline phosphatase, and sometimes 25-hydroxyvitamin D are primarily used to screen for disturbed mineral homeostasis. If specific symptoms, signs, or biochemical abnormalities indicate it, supplementary investigations of plasma 1,25-dihydroxyvitamin D, PTH-related protein (PTHrP), bone markers, and renal excretions of calcium and phosphate may be indicated. Finally, computed variables may be used for specific diagnostic purposes.

Biochemical quantities

Plasma calcium

Plasma calcium is determined as the level of calcium ions, total calcium, or albumin-adjusted calcium, the latter of which takes into account changes in total calcium due to variations in plasma albumin levels caused by disease, physical activity, or venous stasis during blood sampling. Falsely elevated total calcium levels may be seen in hyperalbuminaemia (e.g. from dehydration) or in dysproteinaemia (e.g. from Waldenström macroglobulinaemia, multiple myeloma). Falsely reduced values are seen in hypoalbuminaemia (e.g. from liver disease or gastroenteral or renal losses). To compensate for the effect of acid–base disturbances on the plasma calcium level, plasma calcium may be measured by using a calcium-ion selective electrode at the actual pH and at a pH adjusted to the normal 7.4.

Urinary calcium

Urinary calcium can be measured as 24-hour calcium excretion on a calcium-free or calcium-standardized diet, or via a spot urine as the calcium-to-creatinine excretion ratio. The 24-hour calcium excretion reflects the amount of calcium absorbed from the intestine and the net amount of calcium released from the skeleton. In the case of skeletal balance between resorption and formation, the 24-hour calcium excretion reflects intestinal absorbed calcium. The usual range is 2.5–6.25 mmol/day in women, and 2.5–7.5 mmol/day in men.

Plasma phosphate

Plasma phosphate levels show diurnal variations and decrease following food intake. They are best measured fasting in the morning. Reference values are higher in childhood than in adults. Haemolysis will give falsely elevated values.

Plasma magnesium

Plasma magnesium is usually not corrected for plasma albumin, since it is less protein bound than calcium. It is an insufficient indicator of total body magnesium, which is mainly found in the intracellular compartment. To diagnose magnesium deficiency, it may be necessary to measure erythrocyte magnesium or muscle magnesium or to perform a magnesium infusion test (described in 'Derived biochemical variables').

Plasma intact PTH

Plasma intact PTH (PTH (1–84)) is usually measured by immunoradiometric or electrochemiluminescent immunoassays, where the intact hormone bridges two antibodies directed against separate C- or N-terminal binding sites in the molecule. There are three generations of assays, differentiated by their ability to measure the intact hormone without measuring fragments.

Plasma PTHrP

Plasma PTHrP is determined via an immunoradiometric assay. Elevated values are seen in hypercalcaemic patients with solid tumours and in malignant haematological disorders.

Plasma calcitonin

Plasma calcitonin is not used in the diagnosis of calcium metabolic disorders.

Plasma 25-hydroxyvitamin D

Plasma 25-hydroxyvitamin D is determined by radioimmunoassay, ELISA, high-performance liquid chromatography, or liquid-phase chromatography–tandem mass spectrometry. The last two methods distinguish plasma 25-hydroxyvitamin D_2 from plasma 25-hydroxyvitamin D_3. Plasma 25-hydroxyvitamin D is used to estimate vitamin D status and to diagnose vitamin D insufficiency and deficiency. The usual cut-off points for deficiency and insufficiency are 30 nmol/L (12 ng/mL) and 50 nmol/L (20 ng/mL), respectively.

Plasma 1,25-dihydroxyvitamin D

Plasma 1,25-dihydroxyvitamin D is usually determined by radioimmunoassay, ELISA, or radioreceptor assay. In vitamin D deficiency, variable levels are found because of secondary homeostatic changes in the renal synthesis. Measurements may be indicated in renal osteodystrophy and 1-alpha-hydroxylase deficiency, revealing low values, and in vitamin D-receptor defect, sarcoidosis with hypercalcaemia, and intoxication with 1-alpha-hydroxylated vitamin D metabolites, where elevated values are found.

Bone markers

Bone markers in plasma and urine may also be examined (see Chapter 10).

Derived biochemical variables

Calcium-to-creatinine clearance ratio

The calcium-to-creatinine clearance ratio is determined from 24-hour excretions in urine and plasma collected the same day (or on fasting, second-morning-void urine samples) and calculated as follows:

$$\frac{\text{24-hour urinary calcium (mmol)} \times \text{plasma creatinine (mmol/L)}}{\text{plasma calcium, total (mmol/L)} \times \text{24-hour urinary creatinine (mmol)}}.$$

Indication: The calcium-to-creatinine clearance ratio is used to distinguish familial hypocalciuric hypercalcaemia (calcium-to-creatinine clearance ratio <0.01) from primary hyperparathyroidism (calcium-to-creatinine clearance ratio >0.02). In the interval spanning 0.01–0.02, both diseases may be found. Familial hypocalciuric hypercalcaemia should be confirmed by genetic testing if the calcium-to-creatinine clearance ratio is <0.02. Falsely low values can be seen in cases with reduced renal function, low dietary calcium intake, vitamin D deficiency, and malabsorption.

TmP/GFR

TmP/GFR, expressed in mmoles per litre, is derived from fasting plasma levels and 24-hour excretions of phosphate and creatinine, according to the following equations, where Cl_p/Cl_{Cr} is the phosphate-to-creatinine clearance ratio, which can be determined by using the formula given for calculating the calcium/creatinine clearance ratio but substituting 24-hour urinary phosphate and plasma phosphate values for the 24-hour urinary calcium and plasma calcium values, respectively:

if $Cl_p/Cl_{Cr} > 0.2$,

$$TmP/GFR = \left(1 - Cl_p/Cl_{Cr}\right) \times \text{plasma phosphate;}$$

if $Cl_p/Cl_{Cr} < 0.2$,

$$TmP/GFR = \text{plasma phosphate} \times e^x,$$

where $x = 10.3(Cl_p/Cl_{Cr})^2 - 5.2(Cl_p/Cl_{Cr}) + 0.4$. The mean of three separate determinations are often used. A nomogram for calculation is also available. The reference interval for adults is 0.80–1.35 mmol/L; for children aged 1–4 years, it is 1.32–1.66 mmol/L.

Indication: TmP/GFR is used for diagnostic investigations in chronic hypophosphatemia. It is reduced in primary and secondary hyperparathyroidism and in congenital or acquired renal tubular reabsorption defects, but increased in hypoparathyroidism, pseudohypoparathyroidism, and phosphate depletion caused by inanition and use of phosphate binders.

The modified Ellsworth–Howard test

The modified Ellsworth–Howard test evaluates the effect of exogenous PTH (1–34) on the renal excretion of cAMP and phosphate. The fasting patient is kept well hydrated with 250 mL water orally per hour from 6:00 h to 12:00 h. Urine is collected from 7:00 to 8:00 h, 8:00 to 9:00 h, 9:00 to 9:30 h, 9:30 to 10:00 h, 10:00 to 11:00 h, and 11:00 to12:00 h, for measurements of urinary cAMP, phosphate, and creatinine. Plasma phosphate and plasma creatinine are measured at 9:00 h and 11:00 h. At 9:00–9:15 h, 0.625 μg/kg (maximally 25 μg total) PTH (1–34) is given intravenously. Results are expressed as urinary cAMP and TmP/GFR).

Indication: The modified Ellsworth–Howard test is used for diagnosing pseudohypoparathyroidism and differentiating between subtypes.

The magnesium retention test

In the magnesium retention test, first, a baseline 24-hour urinary magnesium level is measured. The bladder is then emptied. Then, 0.5 mmol of magnesium sulfate per kilogram of bodyweight, in 1000 mL isotonic glucose, is infused over 6 hours. Next, a second 24-hour urinary magnesium measurement is taken. The percentage of retained magnesium is calculated using the following equation:

$$\left[1 - \left(dU\text{-}Mg(2) - dU\text{-}Mg(1)\right)/ \, Mg \, \text{infused}\right] \times 100,$$

where dU-Mg(1) is the first urinary magnesium measurement, dU-Mg(2) is the second urinary magnesium measurement. This test is used when there is suspicion of magnesium depletion in spite of there being normal plasma magnesium levels. Retention >50% is diagnostic for magnesium depletion. Retention >20% suggests magnesium deficiency However, in inherited renal tubular reabsorption defects with obligate renal magnesium loss, retention will be low.

Imaging and localization

99mTc-Sestamibi scintigraphy

99mTc-Sestamibi scintigraphy is based on the preferential uptake of sestamibi in the mitochondria-rich parathyroid adenoma cells. Physiological uptake is also seen in the thyroid gland, the salivary glands, thymus (in young individuals), liver, mammary glands (during lactation), and, to some extent, in bone marrow and brown adipose tissue. There are several technical options.

Washout scintigraphy using a single isotope is based on the observation that there is faster washout of 99mTc-sestamibi from thyroid tissue than from parathyroid adenoma. Anteroposterior scans are performed early (10–15 minutes) and following washout (90–120 minutes). A well-defined area with delayed washout is classified as a parathyroid adenoma.

Subtraction scintigraphy uses two isotopes to distinguish between the uptake in the thyroid gland (99mTc-pertecnetate) and in both the thyroid and the parathyroids (99mTc-sestamibi; see Figure 11.4). Subtraction of the images may be visual or digital. A parathyroid adenoma

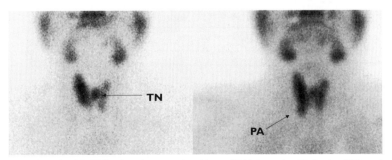

Fig 11.4 (*Left*) A hot thyroid nodule (TN) in the isthmus on a thyroid scan. (*Right*) A parathyroid adenoma (PA) on subtraction 99mTc-sestamibi scintigraphy as a new, upcoming configuration change.

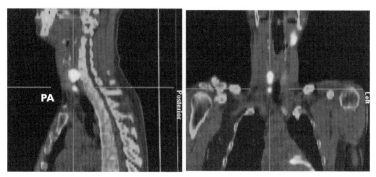

Fig 11.5 Parathyroid adenoma (PA) at crossing lines on subtraction 99mTc-sestamibi scintigraphy with low-dose CT.

may show as an area with increased uptake or as a new upcoming configuration change on 99mTc-sestamibi scintigraphy.

Both techniques can be improved by adding a supplementary SPECT investigation in combination with a low-dose CT study without contrast. A subsequent tomographic 3D reconstruction permits a better separation between the activity in the thyroid gland and the activity in a parathyroid adenoma situated behind the thyroid. The CT scan gives a more exact anatomical location of the adenoma (see Figure 11.5). These techniques are especially helpful when planning a reoperation.

Sources of error
A small parathyroid adenoma is the most frequent cause of a false-negative scintigraphy. The diagnostic sensitivity also depends on parathyroid adenoma vascularity and perfusion and on its cellular density. Often, there is no uptake in parathyroid hyperplasia. Sestamibi retention in

cold or warm thyroid adenomas may lead to false positive interpretations. Multinodular thyroid goitres pose a special problem. Moreover sestamibi is taken up in both benign (reactive lymphoid nodes, sarcoidosis) and malignant tissues (primary tumours and metastases).

Indication
Combined 99mTc-sestamibi and 99mTc scintigraphy with SPECT is now a preoperative routine investigation in most situations and especially in case of previous neck surgery in the region. For detection of parathyroid adenomas, this technique has a sensitivity of 79% (95% confidence interval 64%–91%) and a positive predicative value of 91% (95% confidence interval 84%–96%).

Ultrasound of parathyroid glands
On ultrasound, a parathyroid adenoma is typically presented as a round, oval, or lengthy well-defined, hypoechogenic structure (see Figure 11.6) delineated by

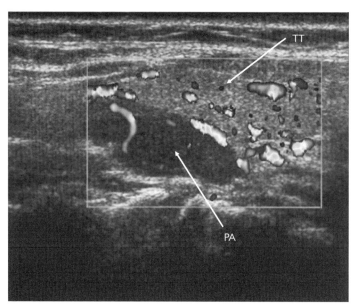

Fig 11.6 A parathyroid adenoma (PA) and normal thyroid tissue (TT), demonstrated by ultrasound. Vessels demonstrated by Doppler technique.

an echogenic line and contrasting the overlying hyper-echogenic thyroid tissue. Calcifications and cysts may be found in larger parathyroid adenomas. Normal parathyroid glands with the size of rice grains usually cannot be detected. Ultrasound is best qualified for adenomas localized in the proximity of the thyroid gland or in relation to the upper cervical part of the thymus. It is less suitable for parathyroid adenomas situated behind the trachea and the oesophagus or behind the oesophagus and cannot be used to detect ectopic glands in the thorax. For detection of parathyroid adenoma, the ultrasound technique has a sensitivity of 76% (95% CI 70%–81%) and a positive predicative value of 93% (95% CI 91%–95%). However, the method is highly observer dependent. Furthermore, the quality is reduced in patients with short, plump necks.

Indication
An ultrasound investigation is recommended as a routine investigation to confirm the localization of a parathyroid adenoma found by ^{99m}Sestamibi scintigraphy.

^{11}C-Methionine PET/CT parathyroid scintigraphy
^{11}C-Methionine PET/CT parathyroid scintigraphy utilizes the fact that the essential amino acid methionine is taken up in parathyroid tissue and used for PTH synthesis. This technique may have a high sensitivity even in patients where conventional investigations have failed.

Indication
^{11}C-Methionine PET/CT parathyroid scintigraphy is mainly used to detect ectopic parathyroid adenomas located in the mediastinum and the thorax before reoperation in cases where 99mTc-sestamibi scintigraphy is inconclusive.

MRI scanning of parathyroid glands
With MRI scanning of parathyroid glands, parathyroid adenoma appears as a soft tissue mass with high signal intensity on T2-weighted frames but low-to-moderate signal intensity in T1-weighted frames. Parathyroid adenoma signal intensity is enhanced after gadolinium injection on T1-weighted frames, compared with thyroid tissue. The sensitivity is around 65%–80%. Lymph nodes may have the same appearance.

Indication
MRI scanning of parathyroid glands is mainly used to detect ectopic parathyroid adenomas located in the mediastinum and the thorax before reoperation in cases where 99mTc-sestamibi scintigraphy is inconclusive.

Conventional CT
Conventional CT in the arterial phase after contrast injection may be considered to exclude an ectopic parathyroid adenoma in the mediastinum. The sensitivity is around 46%–87%, being lowest in patients with previous surgery. Due to radiation and use of contrast, the method is not used for routine purposes.

Indication
Conventional CT is mainly used to detect ectopic parathyroid adenomas located in the mediastinum and the thorax before reoperation in cases where 99mTc-sestamibi scintigraphy is inconclusive.

Preoperative venous sampling
Preoperative venous sampling may, in rare cases, give further information regarding the localization of parathyroid adenomas, especially if ectopic localization is expected.

Indication
Preoperative venous sampling is mainly used to detect ectopic parathyroid adenomas located in the mediastinum and the thorax before reoperation in cases where 99mTc-sestamibi scintigraphy is inconclusive.

Further reading
Bastepe M. The GNAS locus in pseudohypoparathyroidism. *Adv Exp Med Biol* 2008; 626: 27–40.

Bergwitz C, Jüppner H. FGF23 and syndromes of abnormal renal phosphate handling. *Adv Exp Med Biol* 2012; 728: 41–64.

Bijvoet OL. The assessment of phosphate reabsorption. *Clin Sci* 1969; 37: 23–36.

Bilezikian JP, Khan A, Potts JT Jr, et al. Hypoparathyroidism in the adult: Epidemiology, diagnosis, pathophysiology, target-organ involvement, treatment, and challenges for future research. *J Bone Miner Res* 2011; 26: 2317–37.

Carpenter TO. The expanding family of hypophosphatemic syndromes. *J Bone Miner Metab* 2012; 30: 1–9.

Cheung K, Wang T, Farrokhyar F, et al. A meta-analysis of preoperative localization techniques for patients with primary hyperparathyroidism. *Ann Surg Oncol* 2012; 19: 577–83.

Christensen SE, Nissen PH, Vestergaard P, et al. Familial hypocalciuric hypercalcaemia: A review. *Curr Opin Endocrinol Diabetes Obes* 2011; 18: 359–70.

Gagel FR. 'Dynamic tests', in: Favus MJ, ed., *Primer on the Metabolic Bone Diseases And Disorders of Mineral Metabolism* (2nd edition), 1993. Raven Press, pp. 418–22.

Hindié E, Ugur Ö, Fuster D, et al. 2009 EANM parathyroid guidelines. *Eur J Nucl Med Mol Imaging* 2009; 36: 1201–16.

Holm CN, Jepsen JM, Sjøgaard G, et al. A magnesium load test in the diagnosis of magnesium deficiency. *Hum Nutr Clin Nutr* 1987; 41: 301–6.

Krakow D, Rimoin DL, Cohn DH, et al. CRTAP and LEPRE1 mutations in recessive osteogenesis imperfecta. *Hum Mutat* 2008; 29: 1435–42.

Malette LE, Kirkland JL, Gagel RF, et al. Synthetic human parathyroid hormone (1–34) for the study of pseudohypoparathyroidism. *J Clin Endocrinol Metab* 1988; 67; 964–72.

Pidasheva S, D'Souza-Li L, Canaff L, et al. CASRdb: Calcium-sensing receptor locus-specific database for mutations causing familial (benign) hypocalciuric hypercalcemia, neonatal severe hyperparathyroidism, and autosomal dominant hypocalcemia. *Hum Mutat* 2004; 24: 107–11.

Roach PJ, Schembri GP, Ho SI, et al. SPECT/CT imaging using a spiral CT scanner for anatomical localization: Impact on diagnostic accuracy and reporter confidence in clinical practice. *Nucl Med Commun* 2006; 27: 977–87.

Tang BN-T, Moreno-Reyes R, Blocklet D, et al. Accurate preoperative localization of pathological parathyroid glands using 11Cmethionine PET/CT. *Contrast Media Mol Imaging* 2008; 3: 157–63.

Shoback D. Clinical practice. Hypoparathyroidism. *N Engl J Med* 2008; 359: 391–403.

Underberg L, Sikjaer T, Mosekilde L, et al. The epidemiology of non-surgical hypoparathyroidism in Denmark: A nationwide case finding study. *Bone Miner Res* 2015; 30: 1738–44.

Venturi G, Tedeschi E, Mottes M, et al. Osteogenesis imperfecta: Clinical, biochemical and molecular findings. *Clin Genet* 2006; 70: 131–9.

Vieira JG. PTH assays: Understanding what we have and forecasting what we will have. *J Osteoporos* 2012; 2012: 523246.

Walton RJ and Bijvoet OL. Nomogram for derivation on renal threshold phosphate concentration. *Lancet* 1975; 2: 309–10.

Zhang ZL, Zhang H, Ke YH, et al. The identification of novel mutations in COL1A1, COL1A2, and LEPRE1 genes in Chinese patients with osteogenesis imperfecta. *J Bone Miner Metab* 2012; 30: 69–77.

11.3 Hypercalcaemia

Introduction

Hypercalcaemia is an important and common medical problem. It can range from a mild asymptomatic abnormality to a life-threatening emergency. The most common causes of hypercalcaemia are primary hyperparathyroidism and hypercalcaemia of malignancy but there are many other less common causes (Table 11.4). The treatment of mild hypercalcaemia is dependent on its cause, whereas the initial treatment of severe hypercalcaemia is similar for all causes. In general, a level of total calcium (adjusted for serum albumin) above 2.9 mmol/L (11.6 mg/dL) should be considered as severe, as the risk of symptoms and disequilibrium hypercalcaemia (a sudden rapid increase in serum calcium levels) increases above this level.

Epidemiology

It is estimated that about 1% of people have persistent hypercalcaemia but, in the vast majority of people, this is asymptomatic and of questionable clinical significance. The prevalence depends on the frequency of testing and the way in which the normal range is defined. The prevalence is much higher in patients in hospital (around 3%) and undergoing critical care. Hypercalcaemia is less common in children than in adults.

Pathophysiology

In general, hypercalcaemia develops when the amount of calcium entering the circulation exceeds the amount leaving. Calcium levels are normally regulated by the parathyroid glands. In primary hyperparathyroidism, abnormal parathyroid gland overactivity and increased serum PTH levels results in hypercalcaemia through increased resorption of bone, reduced renal clearance of calcium, and increased production of 1,25-dihydroxyvitamin D. In other causes of hypercalcaemia, the level of PTH is generally suppressed through negative feedback. However, since asymptomatic primary hyperparathyroidism is relatively common, occasional patients will present with dual pathology due to PTH-dependent and PTH-independent disease. In hypercalcaemia of malignancy, hypercalcaemia is most commonly due to the secretion of PTHrP by the tumour. Less commonly, hypercalcaemia of malignancy is due to excessive bone resorption by osteolytic metastases. Myeloma and some other haematological malignancies are also associated with hypercalcaemia due to local bone resorption. Sarcoidosis and related granulomatous conditions can cause hypercalcaemia through the extra-renal production of 1,25-dihydroxyvitamin D, thus leading to excessive absorption of calcium through the gastrointestinal tract.

In severe hypercalcaemia, the kidneys are particularly important in that this is the primary route by which calcium can leave the circulation. If renal function is compromised by dehydration secondary to nausea and vomiting, then calcium levels in the circulation can increase rapidly (disequilibrium hypercalcaemia).

Clinical features

Classical features of hypercalcaemia are nausea, thirst, polyuria, confusion, and abdominal pain. Abdominal pain is most commonly due to severe constipation but sometimes gastric ulceration, kidney stones, or pancreatitis. In long-standing hypercalcaemia, renal stones or nephrocalcinosis can occur. Pancreatitis is an uncommon but important complication of hypercalcaemia. Fractures can occur in patients with primary hyperparathyroidism or metastatic cancer involving bone. The main ECG change seen in severe hypercalcaemia is shortening of the QT interval. However, many people with hypercalcaemia are asymptomatic.

The approach to the underlying diagnosis of hypercalcaemia is outlined in Figure 11.7.

Treatment

A schedule for treatment is outlined in Figure 11.8. Severe symptomatic hypercalcaemia is a medical emergency. Patients are frequently dehydrated, often with a fluid deficit of many litres. The most important treatment in this situation is fluid resuscitation with normal saline. A typical level of fluid replacement is 1 litre of normal saline every 6–8 hours. Fluid resuscitation alone will significantly decrease calcium levels by up to 0.5 mmol/L (2 mg/dL) through a dilutional effect. It will additionally increase glomerular filtration and will encourage urinary excretion of calcium. Urinary calcium excretion is a sodium-dependent process; this fact emphasizes the importance of sodium in the rehydration regimen. More controversial is whether loop diuretics (e.g. furosemide) should be given at the same time as sodium rehydration. The original reports that suggested an effect used massive doses of furosemide but there is very little high-quality evidence to support this treatment and there is a significant risk of aggravating hypovolaemia. Current advice is to only use furosemide as an adjunct to fluid management in patients at risk of fluid overload.

Intravenous bisphosphonates represent an important treatment for controlling hypercalcaemia in the long term, particularly in patients with hypercalcaemia of malignancy. Both pamidronate and zoledronic acid can be used. Zoledronic acid results in a slightly quicker and more sustained decrease in serum calcium but the clinical significance of the difference is relatively small. It is more important that these drugs are not administered until fluid resuscitation has commenced. This will typically be a few hours after admission. It takes 2–3 days for

Table 11.4 Differential diagnosis of hypercalcaemia

Frequency	Condition
Common	Primary hyperparathyroidism
	Malignancy
	Renal failure
Uncommon	Familial hypocalciuric hypercalcaemia
	Sarcoidosis
	Other granulomatous diseases
	Immobilization
	Vitamin D intoxication
	Milk–alkali syndrome
Rare	Thyrotoxicosis
	Addison's disease

Hypercalcaemia

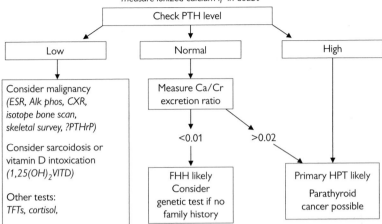

Ensure genuine elevated calcium level—adjust for albumin and measure ionized calcium if in doubt

Fig 11.7 Outline for the determination of the cause of hypercalcaemia; 1,25(OH)2VITD, 1,25-dihydroxyvitamin D; Alk phos, alkaline phosphatase; CXR, chest X-ray; ESR, erythrocyte sedimentation rate; FHH, familial hypocalciuric hypercalcemia; HPT, hyperparathyroidism; PTHrP, parathyroid hormone-related protein; TFT, thyroid function test.

these drugs to begin to act. Longer-term management of hypercalcaemia will depend on the underlying causes.

Primary hyperparathyroidism

Introduction
Primary hyperparathyroidism is the most common cause of hypercalcaemia. In its severe form, the condition can present with life-threatening hypercalcaemia, renal stones, and bone disease (osteitis fibrosa cystica). However, these presentations are now uncommon, with

most people presenting with either no or minimal symptoms. The treatment of symptomatic primary hyperparathyroidism is almost always surgical. The management of asymptomatic primary hyperparathyroidism depends on the risk of progression of disease and of development of end-organ damage.

Epidemiology
Primary hyperparathyroidism is common, with a prevalence of around 0.4% in the general population and rising to 2% in women between the ages of 55 and 75.

Serum calcium (mmol/L)

2.60–2.90*	>2.90†
Check if dehydrated	Rehydration with normal saline, 3–4 L/24 hours
Stop medications that might increase serum calcium e.g. thiazides	Stop medications that might increase serum calcium e.g. thiazides
Encourage oral fluid intake ~3 L/day	If malignancy likely, give intravenous pamidronate (60–90 mg over 2 hours) or zoledronic acid (4 mg over 30 minutes)
Observe calcium level (can often be as outpatient)	
Determine cause of hypercalcaemia	Determine cause of hypercalcaemia

Fig 11.8 Outline for the emergency treatment of hypercalcaemia.
* 10.4–11.6 mg/dL.
† >11.6 mg/dL; some patients with primary hyperparathyroidism may have stable levels of calcium in excess of 3.0 mmol/L (12.0 mg/dL) and can be managed as an outpatient whilst awaiting surgery.

It most commonly occurs in a sporadic form but can also be part of a genetic syndrome. The sporadic form is more common in women, with a 3:1 ratio compared to men. Since many people have asymptomatic disease, the number of patients diagnosed with primary hyperparathyroidism is heavily dependent on whether serum calcium is checked for other reasons. Although sporadic primary hyperparathyroidism can occur at any age, the development of primary hyperparathyroidism, particularly multigland hyperplasia, in adolescence and young adulthood increases the likelihood that the condition is secondary to an underlying genetic condition. For example, primary hyperparathyroidism in multiple endocrine neoplasia type 1 usually becomes clinically apparent before the age of 40.

Pathophysiology
Hypercalcaemia results from a primary abnormality in one or more parathyroid glands. This leads to an increase in the set point for parathyroid-gland sensing of serum calcium. This results in an increased, but usually stable, level of calcium in the blood. The condition is caused by a single adenoma in around 85% of cases, with multiple adenomas or multiglandular hyperplasia occurring in around 15% of cases. Parathyroid cancer is the underlying pathology in less than 1% of patients presenting with primary hyperparathyroidism. Parathyroid cancer can be sporadic or associated with germ-line mutations in HRPT2.

Clinical features
The classical features of long-standing primary hyperparathyroidism are kidney and bone disease. Kidney disease most commonly takes the form of nephrolithiasis but nephrocalcinosis can also occur. These pathologies in association with dehydration increase the risk of renal failure. Bone disease comprises osteitis fibrosa cystica, brown tumours, and osteoporosis. Bone loss with osteoporosis preferentially occurs in sites of cortical bone. Increased clearance of 25-hydroxyvitamin D by high PTH levels commonly causes vitamin D deficiency and thus bone disease can be complicated by vitamin D deficiency. This can lead to a myopathy that is difficult to distinguish from a myopathy associated with hypercalcaemia. Clinical features can also relate directly to the high level of calcium (see 'Clinical features').

The classical features, with the exception of nephrolithiasis, are now uncommon. Most patients with primary hyperparathyroidism either are asymptomatic or have minimal symptoms. There is considerable debate about a possible impact of long-standing hyperparathyroidism on quality of life, cardiovascular health, and cognitive function. Although some evidence supports an adverse impact of primary hyperparathyroidism on these features, randomized trials have not suggested major benefits in these measures following parathyroidectomy. Some patients with otherwise mild hyperparathyroidism display neuropsychiatric abnormalities. Resolution of these abnormalities has been reported in many instances but there is no way of predicting prior to surgery whether these features will resolve.

Investigations
The diagnosis of primary hyperparathyroidism is usually straightforward, with both serum calcium and PTH levels being elevated. In a minority of patients, PTH levels will be in the upper part of the normal range. This high level is still inappropriate for hypercalcaemia

and, in the absence of features suggesting familial hypocalciuric hypercalcaemia (see 'Familial hypocalciuric hypercalcaemia'), is also indicative of primary hyperparathyroidism. Additional investigations to help clarify the diagnosis and determine the presence of end-organ damage include the estimated glomerular filtration rate (eGFR); serum 25-hydroxyvitamin D levels; urinary calcium excretion and the calcium-to-creatinine clearance ratio; bone densitometry by DXA at the hip, the spine, and the wrist; and ultrasound or plain radiography of the kidneys, the ureters, and the bladder.

Imaging of parathyroid tissue is not normally required for the diagnosis of primary hyperparathyroidism. However, sestamibi scanning and ultrasound are important investigations if minimally invasive parathyroidectomy is being considered. These tests are also important in localizing parathyroid tissue in patients who have not been cured by initial parathyroidectomy.

Genetic testing should be considered in patients where a familial syndrome is possible. The important syndromes are multiple endocrine neoplasia type 1, multiple endocrine neoplasia type 2, familial isolated hyperparathyroidism, CASR mutations, and hyperparathyroidism–jaw tumour syndrome. Multiple endocrine neoplasia type 1 is suggested by early onset of hypercalcaemia and the presence of other endocrine tumours within the family. Familial primary hyperparathyroidism is likely to be a subtype of multiple endocrine neoplasia type 1, and thus the possibility of other endocrine tumours developing needs to be considered. Primary hyperparathyroidism is not normally the presenting feature of multiple endocrine neoplasia type 2. Parathyroid jaw tumour syndrome is caused by germ-line mutations in HRPT2. The importance of making this diagnosis is that parathyroid cancer is common in this condition. A good case can also be made for genetic testing in all patients with parathyroid cancer to determine whether a germ-line mutation of HRPT2 is present. This would allow identification of other family members at risk.

Treatment
Treatment of primary hyperparathyroidism is outlined in Figure 11.9. The treatment for symptomatic primary hyperparathyroidism is surgical parathyroidectomy. Traditionally, the first-line operation of choice was a full examination of all four glands. Increasingly, this operation is being replaced by minimally invasive parathyroidectomy. Suitability for minimally invasive surgery depends on the accurate preoperative localization of abnormal parathyroid tissue by sestamibi and ultrasound scanning. Minimally invasive parathyroidectomy is also unsuitable in patients with genetic syndromes where the risk of multigland disease is high.

In patients who have symptomatic hyperparathyroidism but are unfit for surgery, medical treatment with cinacalcet should be considered. This drug works through binding to CaSR, with a calcimimetic activity. It decreases serum PTH and calcium levels in the majority of patients. Unlike parathyroidectomy, this medication has little impact on urinary calcium excretion and does not increase bone mineral density.

Parathyroidectomy is also recommended for younger patients (e.g. those under the age of 50), since the risk of progression of disease appears greater in younger individuals. In other patients with asymptomatic primary hyperparathyroidism, surgery is still a very reasonable

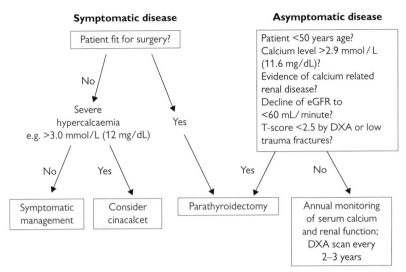

Fig 11.9 Outline of the treatment of primary hyperparathyroidism; DXA, dual-energy x-ray absorptiometry; eGFR, estimated glomerular filtration rate.

option, since the chance of cure is very high (around 98%) and the operation itself carries little morbidity. However, consensus guidelines suggest that many patients can be managed with medical follow-up as long as they have a calcium level that is minimally elevated, have no decrease in renal function, and have no evidence of bone damage (see Figure 11.9). In patients with isolated low bone mass, an alternative to surgery is the use of a bisphosphonate. A recently recognized and important aspect of management of patients with primary hyperparathyroidism is to ensure that vitamin D levels are sufficient. Patients with low levels of vitamin D are exposed to higher levels of PTH and are at a greater risk of bone disease.

Vitamin D replacement was previously considered to be dangerous since it had the potential to increase serum calcium levels. However, clinical trials have suggested that vitamin D replacement is safe in the majority of patients. Treatment should aim to achieve a vitamin D level of 50 nmol/L (2000 ng/dL) and could be achieved with either 800 units of vitamin D per day initially or higher-strength preparations (e.g. 50,000 units) once monthly. Calcium levels should be monitored during supplementation.

Special situations
Hyperparathyroidism in pregnancy is a rare but difficult situation. Primary hyperparathyroidism is associated with adverse outcomes for both the foetus and the mother. The risk of complications appears to be limited with calcium levels of up to around 2.85 mmol/L (11.4 mg/dL) but they increase substantially with calcium levels above this. Parathyroidectomy during the first trimester is associated with a high risk of fetal loss and, in the third trimester, with premature labour. As such, surgery is generally recommended in the second trimester. There is currently little data relating to the use of cinacalcet in pregnancy, and its use in pregnancy should be avoided if possible. In patients managed conservatively,

parathyroidectomy is mandatory after delivery and before further pregnancies.

Primary hyperparathyroidism appears to be more common in patients taking lithium. A possible explanation for this is interference with the normal functioning of CaSR. Where possible, lithium should be stopped to see if serum levels of calcium decrease. However, in the majority of patients, this medication needs to be continued due to the original indication for its use. In the majority of patients operated on for primary hyperparathyroidism in this setting, parathyroid gland abnormalities are found and the condition can usually be cured.

Patients with severe hyperparathyroidism are at risk of 'hungry bones syndrome' post parathyroidectomy. This syndrome manifests as severe and prolonged hypocalcaemia post-operatively and is due to the movement of calcium from the circulation into unmineralized bone. The risk of hungry bone syndrome increases with serum calcium and in particular with the presence of overt bone disease (e.g. substantially raised alkaline phosphatase). Treatment is with prolonged calcium supplementation, often for many weeks, with or without active vitamin D metabolites.

Familial hypocalciuric hypercalcaemia
Familial hypocalciuric hypercalcaemia is an autosomal-dominant genetic disorder due to mutations that reduce the sensitivity of the CaSR to calcium. As such, a higher level of extracellular calcium is needed for an equivalent effect on PTH secretion. Patients usually have mildly elevated calcium in the presence of a normal or slightly raised PTH level. In addition to being expressed on parathyroid cells, the CaSR is also expressed in the kidneys, with the result that urinary calcium excretion is low for the degree of hypercalcaemia. The condition is usually asymptomatic, treatment is rarely needed, and attempts at parathyroidectomy should be avoided. The condition is suggested by a low excretion of calcium into the urine relative to creatinine. Care must be taken to ensure that

patients are vitamin D replete, since patients with primary hyperparathyroidism and coexisting vitamin D deficiency can have low urinary calcium excretion leading to a false-positive result supporting familial hypocalciuric hypercalcaemia. The presence of mild hypercalcaemia in other family members is often sufficient to make a definitive diagnosis but genetic testing can now be carried out if doubt persists.

Hypercalcaemia of malignancy

Introduction

Hypercalcaemia secondary to malignancy is a common diagnosis in patients presenting with hypercalcaemia. Hypercalcaemia occurs in up to 30% of patients with cancer at some stage of their disease, although the presence of an underlying cancer is usually known. Except in the situation where primary hyperparathyroidism coexists with malignancy, the PTH level will be low. Production of ectopic PTH by tumours appears to be extremely rare. Where hypercalcaemia is the presenting feature, the prognosis is often very poor, with a mortality of 50% within 30 days in historical series.

Pathophysiology

It is now clear that, in the majority (~80%) of patients with hypercalcaemia of malignancy, the cause is production of PTHrP by the tumour. PTHrP has similar effects to PTH but is not detected in the PTH assay. PTHrP can be measured specifically, although the diagnosis is usually achieved without the need for this test. In a minority of patients, hypercalcaemia is caused by osteolytic metastases. These patients normally have bone pain and are at additional risk of fracture. In multiple myeloma, hypercalcaemia is due to bone lysis by disease within the bone marrow.

Clinical features

The clinical features of hypercalcaemia of malignancy are those of hypercalcaemia plus symptoms relating to the underlying disease. Patients are generally more unwell than patients with primary hyperparathyroidism, and the level of calcium in the circulation can be more extreme. The presence of bone pain is suggestive of hypercalcaemia of malignancy rather than primary hyperparathyroidism.

Treatment

The initial treatment of severe hypercalcaemia is outlined in 'Treatment'. In these patients, bisphosphonates are particularly useful, since these can reduce the release of calcium from bone. As discussed in 'Treatment', intravenous pamidronate (90 mg) or zoledronic acid (4 mg) can be used. The long-term treatment of hypercalcaemia will depend on the underlying malignancy and, in many patients, the prognosis will be poor. Where cure is not possible, continued treatment with either intravenous bisphosphonates or oral bisphosphonates (e.g.

sodium clodronate) can be given. In myeloma, the hypercalcaemia normally responds to successful anti-tumour therapy. In patients with other haematological diagnoses, the hypercalcaemia is often responsive to treatment with glucocorticoids.

Other causes

Hypercalcaemia can occur in renal failure through a range of mechanisms complicated by the common use of calcium supplements and active vitamin D analogues in this setting. Although the list of other causes of hypercalcaemia is relatively long, most are not commonly encountered. Hypercalcaemia can occur in patients who ingest excessive amounts of vitamin D. In general, the doses needed to produce hypercalcaemia are in excess of 10,000 units per day. Hypercalcaemia can occur in sarcoidosis. In this situation, the hypercalcaemia is caused by extra-renal production of 1,25-dihydroxyvitamin D by the granuloma tissue. Often, other features of sarcoidosis will be present. Although not diagnostic of sarcoidosis, a raised level of serum angiotensin-converting enzyme is commonly seen in this setting. The hypercalcaemia of sarcoidosis normally responds rapidly to oral glucocorticoids. Immobilization can occasionally cause hypercalcaemia, since it stimulates bone resorption and reduces bone formation. However, to cause significant hypercalcaemia, there usually needs to be a state of high bone turnover (e.g. as seen in patients with untreated Paget's disease). Milk–alkali syndrome was a major problem before the development of modern drugs to treat indigestion. Alkali can interfere with urinary excretion of calcium, so the combination of alkali with calcium could lead to hypercalcaemia. This condition is now most commonly seen in patients who had pre-existing renal impairment and are taking oral calcium supplements. Although thyrotoxicosis has been reported to commonly cause hypercalcaemia, this is usually mild. Severe hypercalcaemia in this setting can, however, be seen if Addison's disease coexists.

Further reading

Bilezikian JP, Brandi ML, Eastell R, et al. Guidelines for the management of asymptomatic primary hyperparathyroidism: Summary statement from the Fourth International Workshop. *J Clin Endocrinol Metab* 2014; 99: 3561–9.

Cooper MS. Disorders of calcium metabolism and parathyroid disease. *Best Pract Res Clin Endocrinol Metab* 2011; 25: 975–83.

Endres DB. Investigation of hypercalcemia. *Clin Biochem* 2012 45: 954–63.

Joshi D, Center JR, and Eisman JA. Investigation of incidental hypercalcaemia. *BMJ* 2009; 339: b4613.

Marcocci C and Cetani F. Primary hyperparathyroidism. *N Engl J Med* 2011; 365: 2389–97.

Stewart AF. Hypercalcemia associated with cancer. *N Engl J Med* 2005 352: 373–9.

11.4 Inherited primary hyperparathyroidism

Introduction

Whilst primary hyperparathyroidism is encountered most frequently as a non-familial entity, ~10% of cases occur as part of a hereditary disorder, either in isolation or in association with other clinical manifestations. In contrast to sporadic primary hyperparathyroidism, which typically presents in patients >50 years of age, with a 3F:1M predominance, familial forms of parathyroid disease often present at a younger age (<50 years), with an equal sex distribution. The identification of such familial cases is important as it allows the optimum management of parathyroid disease; the identification of associated co-morbidities; and the evaluation of family members. Thus, it is important to establish the presence or absence of a family history of parathyroid disease or associated conditions in all individuals with primary hyperparathyroidism. However, the absence of a family history does not exclude a hereditary aetiology as affected family members may be asymptomatic, associated disorders may have a variable clinical penetrance, and family members may be geographically and/or socially separated. Therefore, even in the absence of a family history, a genetic diagnosis should be considered in those with any of the following features: young age at presentation (<50 years), evidence of multigland parathyroid disease, or the presence of clinical features of an associated disorder.

The following disorders are associated with inherited primary hyperparathyroidism: multiple endocrine neoplasia types 1, 2, and 4; hyperparathyroidism–jaw tumour syndrome; familial isolated hyperparathyroidism; and neonatal severe hyperparathyroidism. In addition, familial hypocalciuric hypercalcaemia should be considered in the differential diagnosis, as this diagnosis has important management implications.

Clinical features, diagnosis, and management

The clinical features and diagnosis of hyperparathyroidism do not differ from those of sporadic cases, although patients are frequently asymptomatic in association with mild disease. Evidence of end-organ involvement (e.g. renal calculi, osteoporosis) should be established. Parathyroid tumour localization should be performed in those in whom surgery is considered, although disease-specific considerations are required. The main differences between the investigation of familial and sporadic forms of hyperparathyroidism include an evaluation for multigland versus single-gland involvement; screening for any associated clinical features; the establishment of a genetic diagnosis; and, where appropriate, the identification and screening of first-degree relatives. An outline of the management of suspected familial hyperparathyroidism is shown in Figure 11.10.

Multiple endocrine neoplasia type 1

Clinical and genetic features

Multiple endocrine neoplasia type 1 is the most common cause of familial hyperparathyroidism. Primary hyperparathyroidism occurs with almost complete penetrance, and is typically the first manifestation of the disorder. The majority (~90%) of affected individuals present at <50 years of age (M = F), with a mean age of onset of 20 years. Multiple glands are typically involved. Multiple endocrine neoplasia type 1 is inherited as an autosomal-dominant disorder, with ~90% of families harbouring a heterozygous mutation of *MEN1*. No clear genotype/phenotype correlation exists. Genetic testing of *MEN1* should be considered in individuals with a clinical diagnosis of multiple endocrine neoplasia type 1(i.e. the combined occurrence of parathyroid, pituitary, and/or pancreatic islet tumours); symptomatic and asymptomatic first-degree relatives of confirmed *MEN1* mutation carriers; and individuals with multigland parathyroid disease or atypical presentation of multiple endocrine neoplasia type 1 (e.g. parathyroid plus adrenal adenoma).

Management

The management of parathyroid disease in multiple endocrine neoplasia type 1 remains controversial. Symptomatic individuals or those with end-organ damage should be offered surgery. The optimum timing of surgery for asymptomatic individuals has not been established. Preoperative localization of parathyroid glands is of limited value due to multigland involvement. Minimally invasive parathyroidectomy is not typically recommended. The preferred surgical options include subtotal parathyroidectomy (at least 3.5 glands) or total parathyroidectomy with autotransplantation. Concurrent transcervical thymectomy should be considered at the time of surgery. Patients with multiple endocrine neoplasia type 1 require life-long biochemical and radiological screening for associated conditions. First-degree relatives should be identified and screened with appropriate counselling.

Multiple endocrine neoplasia type 2

Clinical and genetic features

Primary hyperparathyroidism occurs in 20%–30% of individuals with multiple endocrine neoplasia type 2A, which is less frequent than medullary thyroid cancer (~95%) and phaeochromocytoma (50%). Hyperparathyroidism typically occurs at <40 years of age, and the majority of patients are asymptomatic at diagnosis. Pathological evaluation of parathyroid glands may reveal single or multigland involvement with hyperplasia or adenoma formation. Multiple endocrine neoplasia type 2 is inherited as an autosomal-dominant disorder due to heterozygous *RET* mutations. Multiple endocrine neoplasia type 2A is most frequently associated with mutations affecting five cysteine residues (codons 609, 611, 618, 620, and 634). A genotype/phenotype correlation is observed, with the majority of patients with multiple endocrine neoplasia type 2A and primary hyperparathyroidism harbouring codon 634 mutations.

Management

Indications for surgery are similar to those for sporadic disease. The surgical approach should be tailored to the extent of parathyroid involvement. Minimally invasive parathyroid surgery may be effective for single-gland disease. More extensive approaches (e.g. subtotal/total parathyroidectomy) have been employed for multigland involvement. Exploration of parathyroid glands may be undertaken at the time of thyroidectomy.

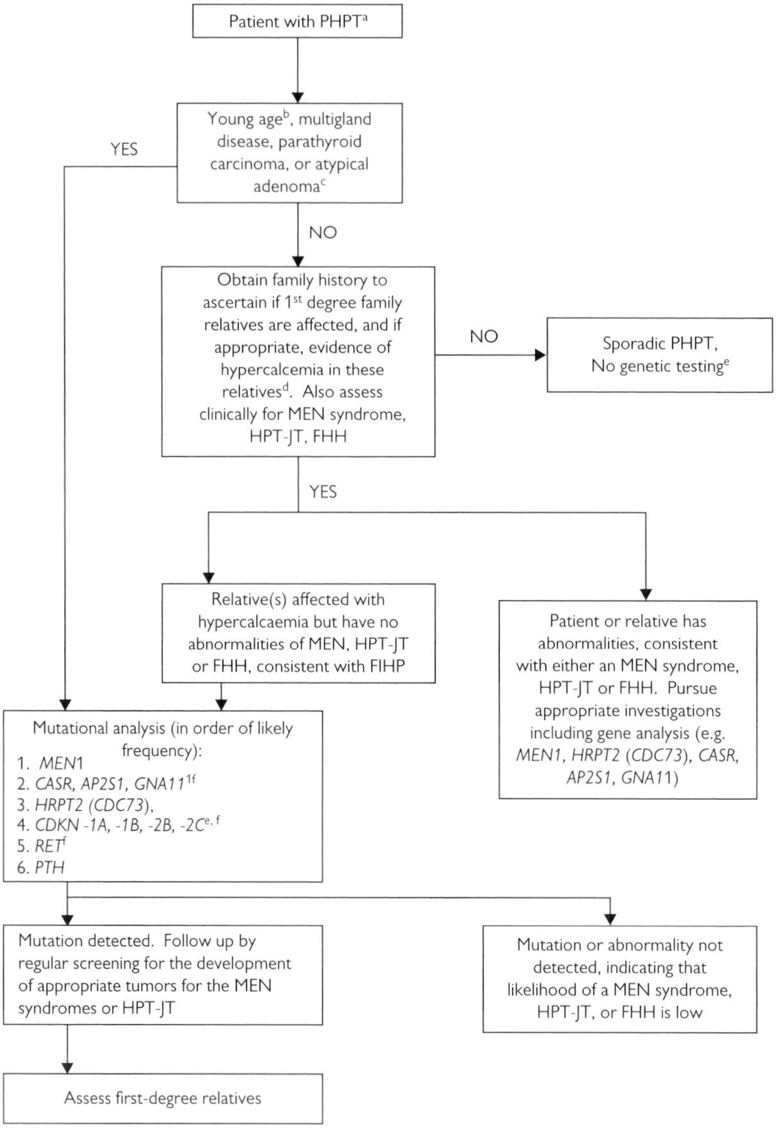

Fig 11.10 Management of suspected familial hyperparathyroidism; FHH, familial hypocalciuric hypercalcaemia; FIHP, familial isolated hyperparathyroidism; HPT-JT, hyperparathyroidism–jaw tumour syndrome; MEN, multiple endocrine neoplasia; PHPT, primary hyperparathyroidism.

[a] PHPT presenting without manifestations of MEN-associated tumours, or tumours associated with HPT-JT.

[b] Guidelines for MEN1 recommend *MEN1* mutational analysis in patients with PHPT occurring before age of 30 years, and ~10% of PHPT patients below the age of 45 years have been reported to have a germline mutation involving the *MEN1, CASR,* or *HRPT2* (*CDC73*) genes.

[c] Atypical parathyroid adenoma may have cysts or fibrous bands.

[d] PHPT may be the first manifestation of MEN1 and HPT-JT in ~90% and ~95% of patients, respectively, with these disorders.

[e] <5% of patients presenting with non-familial (sporadic) and non-syndromic PHPT, due to solitary parathyroid adenomas in the sixth to the ninth decades of life may have rare variants/mutations of *CDKN1A, CDKN2B,* or *CDKN2C.*

[f] *CASR, AP2S1, GNA11, HRPT2* (*CDC73*), *CDKN1B,* and *RET* mutations are associated with FHH1, FHH3, FHH2, HPT-JT, MEN4, and MEN2, respectively.

Multiple endocrine neoplasia type 4

Clinical features, genetic features, and management
Multiple endocrine neoplasia type 4 is an autosomal-dominant disorder which is similar to multiple endocrine neoplasia type 1 but in which parathyroid and pituitary tumours predominate. The majority of cases to date have included primary hyperparathyroidism, although the precise clinical expression of this disorder has not been defined. Multiple endocrine neoplasia type 4 is due to mutations in *CDKN1B*. A management approach similar to that used for multiple endocrine neoplasia type 1 is likely to be appropriate.

Hyperparathyroidism–jaw tumour syndrome

Clinical and genetic features
Hyperparathyroidism–jaw tumour syndrome is an autosomal-dominant disorder characterized by the occurrence of parathyroid tumours in association with ossifying fibromas of the maxilla and/or mandible. In addition, patients may develop other manifestations, including benign, and less commonly, malignant tumours of the renal and uterine tracts. Parathyroid tumours are typically the first manifestation of disease and usually occur as single adenomas with cystic enlargement, and notably, there is a high incidence (~15%) of parathyroid carcinoma. The age-related penetrance of the disorder has not been fully defined, although parathyroid disease may occur in children and adolescents. Ossifying fibromas occur in 25%–50% of patients. Hyperparathyroidism–jaw tumour syndrome is associated with heterozygous mutations in *CDC73*. No clear genotype/phenotype correlation is observed. A proportion of individuals with apparent sporadic parathyroid cancer will have germline *CDC73* mutations.

Management
The increased risk of parathyroid carcinoma should lower the threshold for surgical intervention. Current practice typically involves removal of any grossly enlarged parathyroid gland(s). More extensive surgery may be indicated if multiple glands are involved or there are any features suspicious for parathyroid carcinoma at the time of surgery. Patients require follow up to detect recurrent hyperparathyroidism or associated clinical manifestations

Familial isolated hyperparathyroidism

Clinical and genetic features
Familial hyperparathyroidism occurring in isolation has been reported in >100 families. However, the distinction between familial isolated hyperparathyroidism and other hereditary parathyroid disorders may be challenging, particularly as hyperparathyroidism is often the first manifestation of disease (e.g. multiple endocrine neoplasia type 1 and hyperparathyroidism–jaw tumour syndrome), whilst incomplete penetrance may result in misclassification of associated disorders. Familial isolated hyperparathyroidism is inherited in an autosomal-dominant manner and likely represents a genetically heterogeneous condition. Mutations in *MEN1* and *CDC73* have been reported in kindreds with familial isolated hyperparathyroidism, although the finding of such a mutation should lead to a revised diagnosis of multiple endocrine neoplasia type 1 or hyperparathyroidism–jaw tumour syndrome, respectively. Although loss-of-function *CASR* mutations are most commonly associated with familial hypocalciuric hypercalcaemia, such mutations have also been reported in kindreds with familial isolated hyperparathyroidism. The genetic aetiology of the remaining ~70% of cases of familial isolated hyperparathyroidism has not been established.

Management
Management of parathyroid disease will be context specific. Surgical management is indicated as for sporadic disease. Determining the presence of single-gland versus multigland disease will determine the surgical approach. Management of kindreds with apparent familial isolated hyperparathyroidism and *MEN1* or *CDC73* mutations should follow the recommendations given for multiple endocrine neoplasia type 1 and hyperparathyroidism–jaw tumour syndrome, respectively.

Neonatal severe hyperparathyroidism

Rarely, severe hyperparathyroidism may present in the neonatal period due to homozygous or compound heterozygote loss-of-function *CASR* mutations. Hyperplasia of all four glands is typically observed, and urgent total parathyroidectomy is required and may be life-saving.

Familial hypocalciuric hypercalcaemia

It is important to distinguish familial forms of primary hyperparathyroidism from familial hypocalciuric hypercalcaemia, as a failure to do so may result in unnecessary investigation and treatment. Familial hypocalciuric hypercalcaemia is inherited in an autosomal-dominant manner and typically presents with lifelong mild asymptomatic hypercalcaemia in association with an inappropriately normal or mildly raised PTH concentration. It is differentiated from primary hyperparathyroidism by the presence of a low urinary calcium-to-creatinine clearance ratio (<0.01). Familial hypocalciuric hypercalcaemia requires no specific treatment. Approximately 65% of individuals with familial hypocalciuric hypercalcaemia have a loss-of-function *CASR* mutation (familial hypocalciuric hypercalcaemia type 1), whilst mutations in *GNA11* and *AP2S1* have been reported in association with familial hypocalciuric hypercalcaemia types 2 and 3, respectively. Establishing a genetic diagnosis may aid identification of family members and avoid unnecessary investigation and treatment.

Genetic testing

Information regarding approved clinical genetic testing centres may be found at http://www.orpha.net/consor/cgi-bin/index.php and https://www.ncbi.nlm.nih.gov/gtr/.

Patient support groups

The patient support group Association for Multiple Endocrine Neoplasia Disorders (AMEND) may be useful.

Future developments

The advent of affordable high-throughput DNA sequencing technologies is likely to further define the genetic landscape of hereditary parathyroid disorders and establish the extent of genotype/phenotype correlations. The main clinical goal remains defining the optimal surgical approach with the aim of achieving long-term biochemical remission, whilst minimizing risks of hypoparathyroidism.

Further reading

Fraser WD. Hyperparathyroidism. *Lancet* 2009: 374; 145–58.

Hannan FM, Nesbit MA, Christie PT, et al. Familial isolated primary hyperparathyroidism caused by mutations of the MEN1 gene. *Nat Clin Pract Endocrinol Metab* 2008; 4: 53–8.

Hendy GN, Cole DEC. Genetic defects associated with familial and sporadic hyperparathyroidism. *Front Horm Res* 2013; 41: 149–65.

Newey PJ, Bowl MR, Cranston T, et al. Cell division cycle protein 73 homolog *(CDC73)* mutations in the hyperparathyroidism-jaw tumour syndrome (HPT-JT) and parathyroid tumours. *Hum Mutat* 2010: 31; 295–307.

Stalberg P and Carling T. Familial parathyroid tumors: Diagnosis and management. *World J Surg* 2009; 33: 2234–43.

Thakker RV, Newey PJ, Walls GV, et al. Clinical practice guidelines for multiple endocrine neoplasia type 1 (MEN1). *J Clin Endocrinol Metab* 2012; 97: 2990–3011.

11.5 Hypocalcaemia

Introduction

Hypocalcaemia is a potentially life-threatening electrolyte disturbance that carries risks for serious errors in diagnosis and management. The overall prevalence of hypocalcaemia in hospitalized patients is 18%, increasing to 85% in critically ill patients. Hypocalcaemia may be an asymptomatic laboratory finding or a life-threatening metabolic disturbance. Acute hypocalcaemia can result in severe symptoms necessitating urgent intravenous correction. In contrast, when hypocalcaemia develops slowly, even if quantitatively severe, patients may be surprisingly free of symptoms.

Pathophysiology

Calcium ions are critical for many fundamental cellular functions, including secretion, neuromuscular function, and haemostasis; thus, there is tight physiological regulation of extracellular calcium concentrations. Calcium sensing occurs via the calcium sensing receptor (CaSR) on parathyroid cells, which modulates PTH synthesis and secretion, which in turn triggers downstream-effector events.

Hypocalcaemia can be broadly categorized into conditions associated with a quantitative deficiency of PTH (hypoparathyroidism), conditions where there is secondary hyperparathyroidism, and conditions due to other causes (see Box 11.3).

Hypocalcaemia with hypoparathyroidism

Destruction of parathyroid glands

Hypocalcaemia due to hypoparathyroidism is most frequently encountered as a consequence of parathyroid damage during thyroid or parathyroid surgery, particularly following repeated neck explorations or surgery for parathyroid hyperplasia. Reduced PTH concentrations lead to excessive renal calcium loss and reduced intestinal calcium absorption secondary to decreased renal production of 1,25-dihydroxyvitamin D.

Hypoparathyroidism may also occur as an isolated autoimmune condition and less commonly as part of autoimmune polyglandular syndrome type 1. This autosomal recessive disorder affecting the autoimmune regulator gene *AIRE-1* is also associated with mucocutaneous candidiasis and other autoimmune manifestations, particularly adrenal insufficiency. Antibodies directed at parathyroid tissue may be found in some cases of autoimmune hypoparathyroidism.

Developmental parathyroid disorders

Isolated hypoparathyroidism may have X-linked, autosomal-dominant, or autosomal-recessive patterns of inheritance. Hypoparathyroidism also features as part of a number of syndromes including DiGeorge syndrome, which occurs due to developmental anomalies of the third and fourth branchial pouches and is associated with cardiac defects, cleft palate, thymic aplasia, immunodeficiency, and abnormal facies with hypoparathyroidism. A phenotype that is milder than that for DiGeorge syndrome is seen in the hypoparathyroidism, sensorineural deafness, and renal dysplasia syndrome.

Reduced PTH secretion

Mild hypocalcaemia with hypoparathyroidism is seen in autosomal dominant hypercalciuric hypocalcaemia

---

Box 11.3 Causes of hypocalcaemia

Hypocalcaemia with inappropriately low serum PTH

Destruction of parathyroid glands
Surgery
Autoimmune destruction
Radiation
Infiltration

Developmental parathyroid disorders
  Isolated hypoparathyroidism (autosomal recessive, autosomal dominant, or X linked)
  Syndromes of hypoparathyroidism associated with complex developmental anomalies (e.g. DiGeorge syndrome)
  Reduced PTH secretion/function, due to:
- constitutively activating *CASR* mutations
- autoimmune activation of CaSR
- hypomagnesaemia
- hungry bone disease following parathyroidectomy

Hypocalcaemia with secondary hyperparathyroidism

Vitamin D deficiency
Inadequate UV exposure
Poor diet
Malabsorption
Chronic renal disease
Enzyme-inducing drugs

Resistance to PTH
Pseudohypoparathyroidism
Hypomagnesaemia

Resistance to vitamin D
Mutations in the vitamin D receptor gene
(Mutations in 1-alpha hydroxylase)

Miscellaneous causes

Following drug treatment
  Intravenous bisphosphonates (and other drugs that inhibit bone turnover) in untreated vitamin D deficiency
    Gadolinium salts used in MRI
    Foscarnet

Other causes
  Osteoblastic metastases
  Hyperphosphataemia
  Acute pancreatitis
  Acute rhabdomyolysis
  Acute severe illness
  Tumour lysis
  Hyperventilation
  Post massive transfusion

Abbreviations: CaSR, calcium-sensing receptor; PTH, parathyroid hormone.

(ADHH), which is caused by constitutively activating *CASR* mutations that lower the set point for extracellular calcium sensing. The hallmark feature of ADHH is hypercalciuria that can be exacerbated by inappropriate attempts to normalize serum calcium by prescribing calcium salts and vitamin D. An acquired form of hypocalcaemia with low PTH secretion and hypercalciuria has also been described that occurs as a result of autoimmune activation of the parathyroid and renal CaSRs.

Hypocalcaemia with hyperparathyroidism

Vitamin D deficiency

Reduced exposure to UV light, especially in the presence of pigmented skin and poor dietary intake of vitamin D, may cause vitamin D deficiency (osteomalacia) and, occasionally, associated hypocalcaemia. Frankly low serum calcium occurs with severe and chronically low vitamin D concentrations; mild vitamin D deficiency/insufficiency does not usually cause hypocalcaemia. Vitamin D requirements increase during and after pregnancy, and low maternal vitamin D levels are associated with hypocalcaemia in breastfed children.

Hypocalcaemia due to vitamin D deficiency may be seen in some patients taking anti-epileptic therapy, since these drugs induce enzymes that can increase vitamin D metabolism.

Patients with small-intestinal diseases such as Crohn's disease or coeliac disease may have suboptimal absorption of dietary calcium and vitamin D and are thus at particular risk of hypocalcaemia. Occasionally, hypocalcaemia is seen in patients with profoundly deficient dietary calcium intake/absorption despite adequate vitamin D concentrations. Severe hypocalcaemia has also been reported in patients who have pre-existing vitamin D deficiency and receive intravenous bisphosphonates, caused by the reduced ability of the elevated PTH levels to stimulate bone resorption.

Resistance to PTH

A biochemical pattern similar to hypoparathyroidism occurs in the presence of high PTH levels and is due to tissue resistance to PTH. This is termed pseudohypoparathyroidism and is due to the failure of PTH to activate its signalling pathways. Pseudohypoparathyroidism is a genetically heterogeneous condition, with some patients having skeletal abnormalities (e.g. those with Albright's hereditary osteodystrophy; see the next paragraph) that can occur in other family members independent of any abnormality of serum calcium. The presence of these features and normal calcium biochemistry is termed pseudopseudohypoparathyroidism.

The most common variant of pseudohypoparathyroidism is pseudohypoparathyroidism type 1a, which is characterized by short stature, round facies, brachydactyly, mild learning problems, subcutaneous ossifications (in Albright's hereditary osteodystrophy), and obesity. In this variant, heterozygous mutations of *GNAS* reduce expression/function of the G-alpha subunit, which makes up part of the transmembrane signalling protein which couples the PTH receptor to stimulation of adenylate cyclase. Many hormones signal through the G-alpha subunit, and thus resistance to other hormones (e.g. thyrotrophin, gonadotrophins, GHRH, and calcitonin) may be seen. Patients with pseudohypoparathyroidism type 1b lack the clinical features of Albright's hereditary osteodystrophy but may have identifiable brachydactyly as well as biochemical features of pseudohypoparathyroidism. Patients with Albright's hereditary osteodystrophy but no classical biochemical features of pseudohypoparathyroidism have pseudopseudohypoparathyroidism due to haploinsufficiency of *GNAS* and inheritance of the inactivating mutation on the paternal *GNAS* allele.

'Resistance' to vitamin D

The identification of rare cases of rickets 'resistant' to vitamin D treatment has led to the finding of very rare anomalies of vitamin D metabolism and of the vitamin D receptor. Inactivating mutations of the 1-alpha-hydroxylase gene, inherited in an autosomal recessive pattern, result in deficient activation of 25-hydroxyvitamin D to the active form 1,25-dihydroxyvitamin D; this is not a true resistance state but rather 'pseudovitamin D' deficiency. True vitamin D resistance occurs in the setting of mutations in the vitamin D receptor, again inherited as autosomal recessive traits. The clinical presentation of both conditions is early in life, with hypocalcaemia and rickets.

Hypocalcaemia due to other causes

For other causes of hypocalcaemia, see Box 11.3.

Clinical features of hypocalcaemia

Extracellular calcium is important for normal muscle and nerve function. Thus, the classical symptoms of hypocalcaemia are driven by neuromuscular excitability in the form of muscle twitching, spasms, tingling, and numbness. The development of neuromuscular excitability depends on both the absolute level of calcium and how rapidly it falls. Precipitous falls in serum calcium (e.g. after surgical removal of the parathyroid glands) are frequently associated with symptoms, whereas patients who develop hypocalcaemia gradually can be surprisingly free of symptoms and the diagnosis may only become evident as an incidental biochemical finding.

Carpopedal spasm is characteristic of hypocalcaemia that, in severe cases, can progress to tetany, laryngo-, or brochospasm, seizures, and cardiac dysrhythmias. Prolongation of the QT-c interval may also be observed on ECG. In patients without overt signs, underlying neuromuscular excitability can become evident with provocation (e.g. tapping the parotid gland over the facial nerve can induce facial muscle spasm (Chvostek's sign)). However, 10% of normal subjects have a positive Chvostek's sign; conversely, in confirmed hypocalcaemia, 29% of patients have a negative Chvostek's sign, making this a poor clinical discriminator.

Mild hypoxia induced by inflation of a blood pressure cuff can precipitate carpopedal spasm (Trousseau's sign). Trousseau's sign appears more specific for hypocalcaemia, with 94% of hypocalcaemic patients displaying a positive sign, compared to 1% in normocalcaemic subjects.

Long-standing hypocalcaemia, even without neuromuscular symptoms, is associated with the development of neuropsychiatric symptoms, cataract formation, and, occasionally, raised intracranial pressure and reversible cardiac failure.

Investigation of hypocalcaemia

Where the cause of hypocalcaemia is not clinically obvious, the most important investigation is measurement of serum intact PTH. In most cases, a standard biochemical profile and a PTH measurement in association with the clinical history will provide the likely cause of hypocalcaemia. A suggested algorithm for the investigation of hypocalcaemia is given in Figure 11.11.

In hypocalcaemia where there is intact and appropriate negative feedback, PTH is elevated; a low

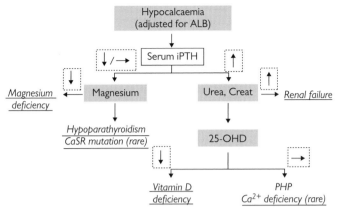

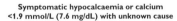

Fig 11.11 Diagnostic algorithm for hypocalcaemia; 25OHD, 25-hydroxyvitamin D; ALB, serum albumin; CaSR, calcium-sensing receptor; Creat, creatinine; iPTH, intact PTH; PHP, pseudohypoparathyroidism.

serum PTH signifies that the parathyroids are causally linked to the hypocalcaemia. PTH concentrations within the reference range in the setting of hypocalcaemia are inappropriate and thus are regarded as 'abnormal'. A high PTH in the presence of normal renal function suggests deficiency of vitamin D or calcium malabsorption; pseudohypoparathyroidism is also a rare consideration. A low PTH usually indicates hypoparathyroidism. A normal PTH is sometimes seen in hypoparathyroidism but usually within the lower reaches of the reference range. PTH may be inappropriately normal in hypomagnesaemia (discussed below) or in ADHH.

Serum alkaline phosphatase, if raised, suggests osteomalacia due to vitamin D deficiency. Metastatic cancer with sclerotic metastases causing rapid absorption of calcium into the skeleton should also be considered. Measurement of serum phosphate indicates PTH action since PTH stimulates renal phosphate clearance, so phosphate is low in vitamin D deficiency with secondary hyperparathyroidism, and high in hypoparathyroidism and pseudohypoparathyroidism. The usefulness of phosphate measurement is limited by its variation in a diurnal rhythm and with food intake. Renal function should be measured, since the kidney is central to several aspects of calcium homeostasis.

Direct measurement of serum 25-hydroxyvitamin D is useful in confirming vitamin D deficiency and should be assessed in patients with possible pseudohypoparathyroidism. Serum magnesium is important for PTH synthesis and release. This becomes apparent in hypomagnesaemia where PTH release is inhibited, leading to (potentially severe) hypocalcaemia. Poor nutrition associated with chronic alcohol excess, prolonged diarrhoea, and treatment with proton-pump inhibitors, diuretics, and certain chemotherapeutic drugs (e.g. cisplatin) are recognized causes of hypomagnesaemia. Recognition of hypomagnesaemia is important, since hypocalcaemia secondary to hypomagnesaemia is difficult to reverse without magnesium repletion.

24-Hour urinary calcium measurements are helpful when considering the possibility of ADHH when hypercalciuria is observed in the context of hypocalcaemia.

Treatment of hypocalcaemia

Optimal management of hypocalcaemia has not been examined in rigorous clinical trials. There is however a core of accepted practice. The approach to treatment depends on the clinical context, which in turn is determined by the speed of onset and biochemical severity of hypocalcaemia.

Acutely presenting hypocalcaemia
Neuromuscular irritability with hypocalcaemia indicates the requirement for prompt management within a hospital environment and treatment with intravenous calcium. In asymptomatic patients with adjusted serum calcium <1.9 mmol/L (7.6 mg/dL), there is a risk of developing serious complications, and inpatient management should be considered. An algorithm for managing acute hypocalcaemia in adults based on clinical experience and expert recommendations is suggested in Figure 11.12.

Calcium gluconate is the preferred form of intravenous calcium, as calcium chloride is more likely to cause local irritation. One to two 10 mL ampoules of 10% calcium gluconate should be diluted in 50–100 mL of 5% glucose and infused slowly over 10 minutes. ECG monitoring is recommended, since over-rapid correction can

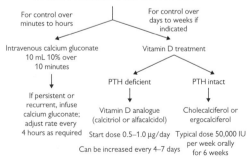

Fig 11.12 Treatment algorithm for acute hypocalcaemia.

cause dysrhythmias. This can be repeated until symptoms have abated. Often, this will only offer temporary relief and, to prevent recurrence of hypocalcaemia, continuous administration of a dilute solution of calcium is usually necessary. A regimen using ten ampoules of 10 mL of 10% calcium gluconate in 1 L of 5% glucose or 0.9% saline may be used at an initial infusion rate of 50 mL/hour, aiming to maintain serum calcium at the lower end of the reference range. An infusion of 10 mL/kg of this solution over 4–6 hours will increase serum calcium ~0.3–0.5 mmol/L (1.2–2.0 mg/dL). Oral calcium supplementation is initiated concurrently and, if PTH is deficient or non-functional, calcitriol given (e.g. 1 μg/day).

Patients taking digoxin have increased cardiac sensitivity to fluctuations in serum calcium, so intravenous calcium administration should be more cautious in this setting, with careful ECG monitoring. In patients with hypomagnesaemia-related hypocalcaemia, magnesium replacement will be required.

Persistent hypocalcaemia
With milder degrees of hypocalcaemia, treatment depends on the underlying cause. In vitamin D deficiency, treatment should be with vitamin D, either colecalciferol (vitamin D_3) or ergocalciferol (vitamin D_2). Lower-dose vitamin D preparations often include calcium. Typically, two tablets of calcium/vitamin D, each containing 400 IU vitamin D, are given daily. This dose of vitamin D is relatively low, and patients with symptomatic vitamin D deficiency or who fail to respond can effectively be treated in the short term with higher loading doses (e.g. 50,000 IU orally once per week for 6 weeks).

In patients with hypoparathyroidism (and pseudohypoparathyroidism), vitamin D is ineffective at these doses, since PTH is required for conversion to 1,25-dihydroxyvitamin D. Thus, calcitriol or alfacalcidol is required. Starting doses are typically 0.5 μg (calcitriol) or 1 μg (alfacalcidol) per day, with doses increased every 4–7 days to achieve a serum calcium in the lower part of the reference range (supplemental oral calcium salts are also usually used in divided doses). Once a stable calcium concentration is achieved, levels should be monitored every 3–6 months. The main long-term risk is the development of nephrocalcinosis due to hypercalciuria. Urinary calcium excretion should be monitored and, if high, may require a reduction in dose of vitamin D. Thiazide diuretics may also be of value in reducing renal calcium excretion and promoting calcium retention. Interval imaging for nephrocalcinosis and renal stone formation should also be considered. Replacement PTH therapy has recently become available as a form of adjuvant therapy for managing hypoparathyroidism.

In hypocalcaemia due to malabsorption, the underlying pathology should be treated where possible. Patients with coeliac disease should receive calcium/vitamin D orally as well as complying with a gluten-free diet. If hypocalcaemia is secondary to hypomagnesaemia, the latter must be fully addressed by correcting the serum (and body stores of) magnesium, as simply administering calcium will not achieve a sustainable resolution of hypocalcaemia.

Further reading

Alimohammadi M, Bjorklund P, Hallgren A, et al. Autoimmune polyendocrine syndrome type 1 and NALP5, a parathyroid autoantigen. *N Engl J Med* 2008; 358: 1018–28.

Ayuk J and Gittoes NJ. How should hypomagnesaemia be investigated and treated? *Clin Endocrinol* 2011; 75: 743–6.

Brandi ML and Brown EM (eds). *Hypoparathyroidism*, 2015. Springer Verlag Italia.

Brandi ML. Genetics of hypoparathyroidism and pseudohypoparathyroidism. *J Endocrinol Invest* 2011; 34: 13–7.

Cooper MS and Gittoes NJL. Diagnosis and management of hypocalcaemia. *BMJ* 2008; 336: 1298–302.

Eisenbarth G and Gottlieb PA. Autoimmune polyendocrinopathy syndromes. *N Engl J Med* 2004; 350: 2068–79.

Gavalas NG, Kemp EH, Krohn KJ, et al. The calcium-sensing receptor is a target of autoimmune polyendocrine syndrome type 1. *J Clin Endocrinol Metab* 2007; 92: 2107–14.

Liamis G, Milionis HJ, and Elisaf M. A review of drug-induced hypocalcemia. *J Bone Miner Metab* 2009; 27: 635–42.

Malloy PJ and Feldman D. Genetic disorders and defects in vitamin D action. *Endocrinol Metab Clin North Am* 2010; 39: 333–46.

Shaw N. A practical approach to hypocalcaemia in children. *Endocr Dev* 2009; 16: 73–92.

Shoback D. Clinical practice. Hypoparathyroidism. *N Engl J Med* 2008; 359: 391–403.

11.6 Disorders of phosphate homeostasis: Hypophosphataemia, including X-linked hypophosphataemic rickets

Definition

The serum phosphate level in healthy adults is maintained between 0.8 and 1.4 mmol/L (2.5 and 4.5 mg/dL). However, serum phosphate levels change with age. Phosphate levels in children are higher than those in adults. Therefore, it is necessary to consider the reference ranges appropriate for the patients when evaluating phosphate levels. Hypophosphataemia is defined as a serum phosphate level less than the lower limit of the reference range.

Pathophysiology

Serum phosphate levels are regulated by intestinal phosphate absorption, phosphate handling in kidneys, and equilibrium between extracellular phosphate and intracellular phosphate or phosphate in bone (see Figure 11.13).

Therefore, hypophosphataemia is caused by impaired intestinal phosphate absorption, a urinary phosphate leak, or a shift of extracellular phosphate into intracellular phosphate or bone (see Box 11.4).

Renal phosphate handling is the primary regulator of chronic phosphate level. Most phosphate filtered from glomeruli is reabsorbed in proximal tubules. This proximal tubular phosphate reabsorption is suppressed by signals through PTH1R. In addition, FGF23 and glucocorticoids also suppress proximal tubular phosphate reabsorption. FGF23 is produced by bone and works by binding to a complex of FGF receptor and Klotho. In addition to suppressing proximal tubular phosphate reabsorption, FGF23 reduces levels of serum 1,25-dihydroxyvitamin D and thereby intestinal phosphate absorption.

Clinical features

Phosphate is a component of DNA, RNA, ATP, and various intracellular metabolites. Therefore, phosphate is necessary for virtually all cells. Tissue hypoxia is induced by severe hypophosphataemia because of decreased levels of 2,3-diphosphoglycerate in erythrocytes. Hypophosphataemia causes several symptoms. Muscle weakness is the most common manifestation of hypophosphataemia. In severe cases, rhabdomyolysis can be observed. Cardiac and respiratory functions may be also affected. Several neurological manifestations,

including confusion, seizures, coma, and peripheral neuropathy, are reported in patients with hypophosphataemia. Hypophosphataemia can cause haemolysis and impaired leukocyte function.

In addition to these symptoms, chronic hypophosphataemia is the major cause of rickets and osteomalacia. Rickets and osteomalacia are diseases characterized by impaired mineralization of bone matrix, making bone soften. Whilst impaired mineralization of bone is often considered to be caused by calcium

---

Box 11.4 Causes of hypophosphataemia

Impaired phosphate absorption
  Phosphate depletion
  Malabsorption
  Impaired actions of vitamin D metabolites
    Vitamin D deficiency
    Vitamin D-dependent rickets types 1 and 2
    Drugs (e.g. diphenylhydantoin, rifampicin)
Urinary phosphate leak
  Enhanced signalling through PTH1R, due to:
    primary hyperparathyroidism
    familial hypocalciuric hypercalcaemia
    Humoral hypercalcaemia of malignancy
    Ectopic PTH-producing tumour
    Jansen-type metaphyseal chondrodysplasia
  Excessive activities of FGF23
    X-linked hypophosphatemic rickets
    Autosomal dominant hypophosphatemic rickets
    Autosomal recessive hypophosphatemic rickets 1, 2
    Hypophosphatemic disease with dental anomalies and ectopic calcification
    Osteoglophonic dysplasia
    Hypophosphataemic disease associated with McCune-Albright syndrome
    Hypophosphataemia, skin and bone lesions
    Tumour-induced rickets/osteomalacia
    Hypophosphataemia induced by iron polymaltose or saccharated ferric oxide
  Proximal tubular damage
    Hereditary hypophosphataemic rickets with hypercalciuria
    Fanconi's syndrome
    Dent's disease
    Renal tubular acidosis
    Drugs (e.g. ifosphamide, adefovir dipivoxil)
  Cushing's syndrome
Shift into intracellular pool or bone
  Hungry bone syndrome
  Osteoblastic bone metastases
  Refeeding
  Recovery phase of ketoacidosis
  Alkalosis

Abbreviations: FGF23, fibroblast growth factor 23; PTH, parathyroid hormone; PTH1R, parathyroid hormone 1 receptor.

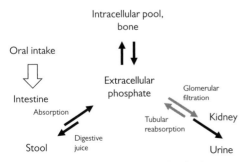

Fig 11.13 Regulation of extracellular phosphate levels.

deficiency or hypocalcaemia, it is actually rare that rickets and osteomalacia are caused by abnormal calcium metabolism. Rickets develops before the closure of growth plates. Bone deformities such as genu varum and valgum, curvature of the spine, craniotabes, bulging anterior fontanelle, and rachitic rosary are characteristic signs of rickets. In addition, X-ray findings such as irregular widened epiphyseal plates, fraying/cupping of metaphysis, and the delayed appearance of a mineralized epiphyseal centre are typical for rickets. On the other hand, muscle weakness and bone pain are major symptoms of patients with osteomalacia, and X-ray findings of pseudofractures (Looser's zones) may be observed.

Epidemiology of rickets and osteomalacia

Historically, vitamin D-deficient rickets was a big social problem. Whilst there still are patients with vitamin D-deficient rickets, especially children who avoid sunburn or artificial milk, vitamin D deficiency can be cured by the administration of vitamin D. On the other hand, several causes of vitamin D-resistant rickets have been recently clarified. In vitamin D-resistant rickets, the disease cannot be cured by usual dose of vitamin D used in vitamin D deficiency. However, the term 'vitamin D-resistant rickets' has been sometimes used as a synonym for X-linked hypophosphataemic rickets (OMIM #307800), partly because no other diseases with similar phenotypes were known. It is now clear that there are several causes of rickets and osteomalacia that cannot be cured by the usual dose of vitamin D. Most of these cases are caused by excessive actions of FGF23 (see Box 11.4). The genes responsible for X-linked hypophosphataemic rickets, autosomal-dominant hypophosphataemic rickets (OMIM #193100), autosomal-recessive hypophosphataemic rickets types 1 and 2 (OMIM #241520 and #613312) are *PHEX*, *FGF23*, *DMP1*, and *ENPP1*, respectively. In addition, hypophosphataemic disease with dental anomalies and ectopic calcification is caused by mutations in *FAM20C*, and osteoglophonic dysplasia (OMIM #166250) is caused by mutations in *FGFR1*. Whilst inactivating mutations in *PHEX*, *DMP1*, *ENPP1*, and *FAM20C* are considered to result in overproduction of FGF23 in bone, the precise functions of these gene products are not clear.

Hypophosphataemia usually enhances 1,25-dihydroxyvitamin D production. In contrast, in patients with FGF23-related or FGF23-dependent hypophosphataemic rickets/osteomalacia, serum 1,25-dihydroxyvitamin D remains low to low normal because FGF23 works to reduce 1,25-dihydroxyvitamin D levels. Excessive FGF23 activity also causes acquired hypophosphataemic rickets/osteomalacia. Tumour-induced rickets/osteomalacia is a paraneoplastic syndrome usually caused by a slow-growing mesenchymal tumour. Hypophosphataemia induced by intravenous administration of iron polymaltose or saccharated ferric oxide is associated with high FGF23 levels.

Vitamin D-dependent rickets type 1 is caused by mutations in *CYP27B1*, which encodes 25-hydroxyvitamin D-1-alpha-hydroxylase, and vitamin D-dependent rickets type 2 is caused by mutations in *VDR*, which encodes the vitamin D receptor. 25-Hydroxyvitamin D-1-alpha-hydroxylase is an enzyme that produces 1,25-dihydroxyvitamin D. Hereditary hypophosphataemic rickets with hypercalciuria is caused by mutations in *SLC34A3*. This gene encodes the type 2c sodium–phosphate cotransporter, which is expressed in proximal tubules. Patients with these diseases do not respond to physiological doses of vitamin D.

Investigations

Various causes of hypophosphataemia can be differentiated by assessing serum and urinary biochemical parameters (see Table 11.5). The best indicator of renal handling of phosphate is TmP/GFR. TmP/GFR is low in hypophosphataemic patients with urinary phosphate leak. On the other hand, TmP/GFR is not low in hypophosphataemic patients with impaired phosphate absorption or phosphate shift if secondary hyperparathyroidism, which can be observed in some patients with impaired actions of vitamin D metabolites, is not present.

25-Hydroxyvitamin D is a marker for the vitamin D supply, and a clearly low level indicates the presence of vitamin D deficiency. FGF23 is reported to be high in patients with FGF23-related hypophosphataemic diseases and rather low in other patients with chronic hypophosphataemia. Therefore, FGF23 measurement is useful for the differential diagnosis of hypophosphataemic diseases. However, this assay is not always available in clinical medicine.

Table 11.5 Biochemical parameters in patients with various causes of rickets/osteomalacia

	Serum calcium	Serum phosphate	TmP/GFR	Bone-type alkaline phosphatase	1,25(OH)₂D	25(OH)D	FGF23
FGF23-related hypophosphataemia	↓→	↓	↓	↑	↓→	→	↑
Phosphate depletion	→	↓	↑	↑	→↑	→	↓→
Fanconi's syndrome	→	↓	↓	↑	↓→	→	↓→
Vitamin D-dependent rickets type 1	↓	↓	↓	↑	↓	→	↓→
Vitamin D-dependent rickets type 2	↓	↓	↓	↑	↑	→	↓→
Hereditary hypophosphataemic rickets with hypercalciuria	→	↓	↓	↑	↑	→	↓→
Vitamin D deficiency	↓→	↓→	↓→	↑	→↑↓	↓	↓→

Abbreviations: 1,25(OH)₂D, 1,25-dihydroxyvitamin D; 25(OH)D, 25-hydroxyvitamin D; FGF23, fibroblast growth factor 23; TmP/GFR, maximal renal tubular reabsorption capacity for phosphate per litre glomerular filtrate.

High bone-type alkaline phosphatase is characteristic of rickets and osteomalacia. Bone mineral density is low in patients with osteomalacia because radiologic measurement of bone density detects calcium content in bone.

Management

In addition to the treatment of underlying diseases, hypophosphataemia can be treated by either intravenous or oral phosphate. On the other hand, treatment of hypophosphataemic rickets/osteomalacia differs depending on the causes.

Vitamin D deficiency is treated with native vitamin D. Vitamin D-dependent rickets type 1 can be managed with physiological doses of active vitamin D. In contrast, treatment of vitamin D-dependent rickets type 2 is difficult. Large doses of calcium and active vitamin D are usually used. The effectiveness of active vitamin D depends on the residual function of the mutated vitamin D receptor.

FGF23-related hypophosphataemic diseases are generally treated by oral phosphate and active vitamin D. Surgery may be necessary to correct bone deformities in patients with genetic hypophosphataemic rickets. However, tumour-induced rickets/osteomalacia can be cured by complete removal of the responsible tumour, and hypophosphataemia recovers after cessation of intravenous iron polymaltose or saccharated ferric oxide. Hereditary hypophosphataemic rickets with hypercalciuria is treated by phosphate alone. Hypophosphataemia caused by drugs can be reversible after stopping the medications.

Complications

Oral phosphate administration can cause gastrointestinal symptoms, including nausea, vomiting, stomach pain, and diarrhoea. In addition, chronic administration of phosphate can induce secondary or tertiary hyperparathyroidism. It is necessary to evaluate the presence of hypercalcaemia, hypercalciuria, and nephrolithiasis when active vitamin D is used.

Prognosis

The prognosis of hypophosphataemic patients depends on the cause. Several diseases, such as those due to phosphate depletion, those due to vitamin D deficiency, and tumour-induced rickets/osteomalacia, can be completely cured. In contrast, even with treatment with phosphate and active vitamin D, the adult height of patients with X-linked hypophosphataemic rickets is usually shorter than that of controls.

Patient support

The XLH network website (http://xlhnetwork.org/) summarizes important information about patients with X-linked hypophosphataemic rickets.

Further reading

Carpenter TO, Imel EA, Holm IA, et al. A clinician's guide to X-linked hypophosphatemia. *J Bone Miner Res* 2011; 26: 1381–8.

Endo I, Fukumoto S, Ozono K, et al. Clinical userfulness of measurement of fibroblast growth factor 23 (FGF23) in hypophosphatemic patients: Proposal of diagnostic criteria using FGF23 measurement. *Bone* 2008; 42: 1235–9.

Fukumoto S and Martin TJ. Bone as an endocrine organ. *Trends Endocrinol Metab* 2009; 20: 230–6.

Schouten BJ, Hunt PJ, Livesey JH, et al. FGF23 elevation and hypophosphatemia after intravenous iron polymaltose: A prospective study. *J Clin Endocrinol Metab* 2009; 94: 2332–7.

Walton RJ and Bijvoet OL. Nomogram for the derivation of renal tubular threshold phosphate concentration. *Lancet* 1975; 2: 309–10.

11.7 Disorders of phosphate homeostasis: Hyperphosphataemia, including tumoural calcinosis

Definition
Serum phosphate levels need to be assessed considering the ages of the patients, as mentioned in Section 11.6. Hyperphosphataemia is defined as a serum phosphate level higher than the upper limit of the reference range.

Pathophysiology
Serum phosphate is maintained by intestinal phosphate absorption, phosphate handling in kidneys, and equilibrium between extracellular phosphate and intracellular phosphate or phosphate in bone (Figure 11.13). Therefore, hyperphosphataemia is caused by enhanced intestinal phosphate absorption, impaired urinary phosphate excretion, or a shift of phosphate from the intracellular pool or bone (see Box 11.5).

Clinically, chronic kidney disease, as described in Section 11.8, is by far the most frequent cause of hyperphosphataemia. In addition to chronic kidney disease, impaired actions of PTH and FGF23, and the effect of growth hormone, cause hyperphosphataemia by enhancing proximal tubular phosphate reabsorption. Deficient PTH action derives from either reduced secretion of PTH from parathyroid glands or peripheral resistance to PTH. The latter is called pseudohypoparathyroidism. Furthermore, hypomagnesaemia also causes impaired PTH action by inhibiting both PTH secretion and function.

Deficient actions of FGF23 cause a rare inherited disease called hyperphosphataemic familial tumoral calcinosis (HFTC: OMIM #211900). Tumoral calcinosis is characterized by ectopic coarse calcification, especially around the large joints. This disease is most often observed in patients with end-stage renal disease undergoing dialysis. In contrast, patients with HFTC show normal renal function. The genes GALNT3, FGF23, and KL have been identified as being responsible for HFTC. GALNT3 encodes an enzyme that attaches N-acetylgalactosamine to serine or threonine residue as an initial sugar of mucin-type O-linked glycosylation. Part of FGF23 is proteolytically cleaved into inactive fragments before or during the process of secretion. The GALNT3 gene product initiates O-linked glycosylation of a threonine residue near the processing site in FGF23, thus preventing the processing. Therefore, in patients with homozygous inactivating mutations in GALNT3, FGF23 is susceptible to processing into inactive fragments (Figure 11.14). Secretion of full-length FGF23 is also suppressed in patients with mutations in FGF23. On the other hand, resistance to FGF23 seems to be the cause of impaired FGF23 action in a patient with a mutation in KL, which encodes Klotho, because Klotho is a co-receptor for FGF23.

Clinical features
Patients with hyperphosphataemia are usually asymptomatic. However, some patients present symptoms from underlying diseases. These include muscle cramp; tetany and numbness from hypocalcaemia; and nausea, anorexia, fatigue, and pruritus from uraemia. In addition, chronic hyperphosphataemia is a risk factor for ectopic calcification, including in vascular tissue. In addition to tumoral calcinosis, some patients with mutations in GALNT3 present hyperostosis–hyperphosphataemia syndrome, which is characterized by cortical hyperostosis and painful swellings of the long bones.

Investigations
Several biochemical measurements including calcium and renal function clarify the causes of hyperphosphataemia in most patients (see Table 11.6). Patients with impaired urinary phosphate excretion show high TmP/GFR. Whilst patients who are hypophosphataemic due to excessive FGF23 activity show low TmP/GFR and low to low-normal levels of 1,25-dihydroxyvitamin D, patients with HFTC exhibit high TmP/GFR and high levels of 1,25-dihydroxyvitamin D, indicating that these diseases are mirror images. FGF23-knockout mice also show hyperphosphataemia and high levels of 1,25-dihydroxyvitamin D, indicating that HFTC is caused by impaired actions of FGF23.

Box 11.5 Causes of hyperphosphataemia

Increased phosphate intake
  Excessive phosphate intake
  Phosphate enema
  Excessive parenteral phosphate administration
  Vitamin D intoxication
Impaired urinary phosphate excretion
  Chronic kidney disease
  Hypoparathyroidism
    impaired secretion of parathyroid hormone
    pseudohypoparathyroidism
    hypomagnesaemia
  Hyperphosphataemic familial tumoral calcinosis
  Acromegaly
Shift from intracellular pool or bone
  Local osteolytic hypercalcaemia
  Immobilization
  Thyrotoxicosis
  Tumour lysis syndrome
  Rhabdomyolysis
  Hemolytic anaemia
  Acidosis

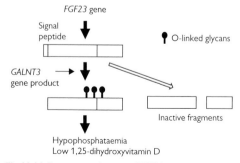

Fig 11.14 Processing and actions of FGF23.

Table 11.6 Biochemical parameters in patients with various hyperphosphatemic diseases

	Serum calcium	Serum phosphate	Creatinine	PTH	1,25(OH)$_2$D
Hypoparathyroidism	↓	↑	→	↓↑	↓→
Hyperphosphataemic familial tumoral calcinosis	→	↑	→	→	→↑
Chronic kidney disease	↓→	↑	↑	↑	↓→

Abbreviations: 1,25(OH)$_2$D, 1,25-dihydroxyvitamin D; PTH, parathyroid hormone.

Management

The management of hyperphosphataemia in patients with chronic kidney disease is described in Section 11.8. The causes of hyperphosphataemia, such as excessive intake of phosphate and vitamin D intoxication, should be addressed, if possible. In patients with preserved renal function, hyperphosphataemia can be treated by volume expansion by saline and loop diuretics. Patients with hypoparathyroidism are treated by active vitamin D with or without calcium. This treatment increases serum calcium and usually ameliorates hyperphosphataemia. Treatment for HFTC has not been established.

Complications

Active vitamin D with or without calcium in patients with hypoparathyroidism can cause hypercalcaemia, hypercalciuria, and nephrolithiasis.

Further reading

Benet-Pages A, Orlik P, Strom TM, et al. An FGF23 missense mutation causes familial tumoral calcinosis with hyperphosphatemia. *Hum Mol Genet* 2005; 14: 385–90.

Frishberg Y, Topaz O, Bergman R, et al. Identification of a recurrent mutation in GALNT3 demonstrates that hyperostosis–hyperphosphatemia syndrome and familial tumoral calcinosis are allelic disorders. *J Mol Med* 2005; 83: 33–8.

Ichikawa S, Imel EA, Kreiter ML, et al. A homozygous missense mutation in human KLOTHO causes severe tumoral calcinosis. *J Clin Invest* 2007; 117: 2684–91.

Shimada T, Kakitani M, Yamazaki Y, et al. Targeted ablation of Ffg23 demonstrates an essential physiological role of FGF23 in phosphate and vitamin D metabolism. *J Clin Invest* 2004; 113: 671–8.

Urakawa I, Yamazaki Y, Shimada T, et al. Klotho converts canonical FGF receptor into a specific receptor for FGF23. *Nature* 2006; 444: 770–4.

11.8 Disorders of phosphate homeostasis: Chronic kidney disease–mineral and bone disorder

Definition
Kidney Disease: Improving Global Outcomes (KDIGO) defined chronic kidney disease–mineral and bone disorder (CKD–MBD) as a systemic disorder of mineral and bone metabolism due to chronic kidney disease manifested by either one or a combination of the following:

* abnormalities of calcium, phosphorus, PTH, or vitamin D metabolism
* abnormalities in bone turnover, mineralization, volume, linear growth, or strength
* vascular or other soft-tissue calcification

Pathophysiology
Several abnormalities of mineral metabolism develop as the eGFR declines (see Figure 11.15). Cross-sectional studies indicated that the increase in FGF23 and the decrease of 1,25-dihydroxyvitamin D start at Stage G2 before the increment of PTH. Hyperphosphataemia and/or hypocalcaemia develop later in Stages G4 or G5. In addition, the fractional excretion of phosphate increases with the decline of eGFR in patients with pre-dialysis chronic kidney disease. It was shown that this increase is associated with FGF23 and PTH, and the decrease of 1,25-dihydroxyvitamin D with FGF23. Furthermore, animal experiments have shown that inhibition of FGF23 activity enhances tubular phosphate reabsorption and increases 1,25-dihydroxyvitamin D in a model of early chronic kidney disease. These results indicate that FGF23 suppresses proximal tubular phosphate reabsorption and prevents the development of hyperphosphataemia. At the same time, FGF23 contributes to the pathogenesis of secondary hyperparathyroidism by decreasing 1,25-dihydroxyvitamin D. It is also possible that FGF23 inhibits PTH production and secretion by binding to the Klotho–FGF receptor complex on parathyroid cells.

Further progression of chronic kidney disease induces decreased expression of Klotho both in the kidney and in the parathyroid, thus causing resistance to FGF23.

Together with severely decreased nephron mass, hyperphosphataemia and hypocalcaemia develop and work to stimulate PTH release.

Renal osteodystrophy is now defined as an alteration of bone morphology in patients with chronic kidney disease and is one component of CKD–MBD. There are several types of bone diseases in patients with chronic kidney disease. Secondary hyperparathyroidism causes the high-turnover bone disease osteitis fibrosa. In contrast, low-turnover bone diseases such as osteomalacia and adynamic bone can be present in patients with chronic kidney disease. Whilst the precise mechanism of adynamic bone is not clear, risk factors such as low PTH, bisphosphonate use, high calcium in dialysates, calcium-containing phosphate binders with vitamin D analogues, and diabetes mellitus have been reported. Aluminium was the main cause of osteomalacia in patients with chronic kidney disease. Vitamin D insufficiency or deficiency can contribute to the development of secondary hyperparathyroidism.

Vascular calcification is one of risks of mortality in patients with chronic kidney disease. Ectopic calcification, including that in vascular tissue, can be caused by increased calcium–phosphate product. In addition, phosphate was shown to induce osteoblastic genes in vascular smooth muscle cells. Whilst medial calcification may be more frequent in patients with chronic kidney disease, it is not uncommon that these patients show both medial and intimal calcification.

Clinical features
Patients with Stage G5 disease can present with hypocalcaemia. However, it is not common that these patients present with symptoms such as tetany and convulsion, because the concomitant metabolic acidosis works to increase the amount of calcium ions present. Bone diseases in patients with CKD–MBD cause abnormal quality and quantity of bones and result in fragility fractures.

Investigations
There may be different guidelines and drugs in the management of patients with CKD–MBD, depending on the country the patients are in. The KDIGO guideline recommends measurement of serum calcium, phosphate, PTH, and alkaline phosphatase, starting at Stage G3a. The guideline also suggests the measurement of 25-hydroxyvitamin D in patients with Stage G3a–G5D disease, for the evaluation of vitamin D insufficiency or deficiency. As far as bone diseases are concerned, the guideline indicates that it is reasonable to perform a bone biopsy if knowledge of the type of renal osteodystrophy will impact treatment decisions. It also suggests the measurement of PTH or bone-specific alkaline phosphatase for the evaluation of bone turnover in patients with Stage G3a–G5D disease. Furthermore, bone mineral density is suggested to assess fracture risk in patients with Stage G3a–G5D disease with evidence of CKD–MBD and/or risk factors for osteoporosis. Renal function affects the levels of some bone turnover markers, so only bone-specific alkaline phosphatase is recommended. Whilst the reference standard in the detection of cardiovascular calcification is a CT-based coronary artery calcification

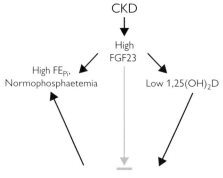

Fig 11.15 Pathogenesis of disordered mineral metabolism in early chronic kidney disease; 1,25(OH)₂D, 1,25-dihydroxyvitamin D; CKD, chronic kidney disease; FEPi, fractional excretion of phosphate.

score, the KDIGO guideline suggests a lateral abdominal radiograph and an echocardiogram for the evaluation of vascular and valvular calcification, respectively.

Management

The KDIGO guideline suggests lowering elevated phosphate levels towards the normal range in patients with Stage G3a–G5D disease. It also suggested to avoid hypercalcaemia in adult patients with Stage G3a–G5D disease. Hyperphosphataemia is usually treated with dietary phosphate restriction and phosphate binders. These are two classes of phosphate binders: calcium-based phosphate binders and non-calcium-based phosphate binders (such as sevelamer). Hypocalcaemia in patients with CKD–MBD can be treated with active vitamin D.

The KDIGO guideline suggests evaluating for the presence of hyperphosphataemia, hypocalcaemia, high phosphate intake, and vitamin D deficiency in patients who have Stage G3a–G5 disease, are not on dialysis, and have high PTH levels. The guideline also suggests maintaining intact PTH levels in the range of approximately 2–9 times the upper normal limit in patients with Stage G5D disease. This is due to the resistance to PTH in patients with chronic kidney disease. There are several ways to reduce PTH levels in patients with secondary hyperparathyroidism (see Figure 11.16). Calcimimetics (e.g. cinecalcet 30–90 mg/day) suppress PTH release from parathyroid glands by mimicking the effects of extracellular calcium on CaSR. Active vitamin D inhibits the transcription of *PTH* and suppresses PTH production. In addition, active vitamin D increases serum calcium and inhibits PTH release through CaSR. Furthermore, hyperphosphataemia stimulates PTH production by stabilizing *PTH* mRNA. Therefore, correction of hyperphosphataemia also contributes to lower PTH levels.

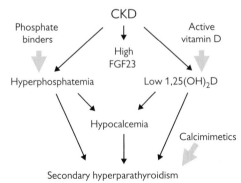

Fig 11.16 Pathogenesis and treatment of disordered mineral metabolism in advanced chronic kidney disease; 1,25(OH)$_2$D, 1,25-dihydroxyvitamin D; CKD, chronic kidney disease.

It is not uncommon that patients with chronic kidney disease have osteoporosis. In patients with chronic kidney disease up to Stage G3 but without evidence of secondary hyperparathyroidism, the same management of osteoporosis as used for the general population is suggested by the KDIGO guideline. However, the treatment of bone disease in patients who have Stage G3 disease and high PTH levels and in patients with Stage G4–G5 disease has not been established.

Complications

Non-calcium-based phosphate binders may cause gastrointestinal complications, including perforation and ileus. Calcium-based phosphate binders and active vitamin D can cause hypercalcaemia, hypercalciuria, and nephrolithiasis. Hypocalcaemia is reported as one of complications of calcimimetics.

Prognosis

Several observational studies indicate that abnormal mineral metabolism and fracture are risks for mortality and suggest that treatment of CKD–MBD by phosphate binders, active vitamin D, or calcimimetics improves patient outcomes. However, this is not confirmed by randomized clinical trials.

Further reading

Ben-Dov IZ, Galitzer H, Lavi-Moshayoff V, et al. The parathyroid is a target organ for FGF23 in rats. *J Clin Invest* 2007; 117: 4003–8.

Block GA. Therapeutic interventions for chronic kidney disease–mineral and bone disorders: focus on mortality. *Curr Opin Nephrol Hypertens* 2011; 20: 376–81.

Gutierrez O, Isakova T, Rhee E, et al. Fibroblast growth factor-23 mitigates hyperphosphatemia but accentuates calcitriol deficiency in chronic kidney disease. *J Am Soc Nephrol* 2005; 16: 2205–15.

Hasegawa H, Nagano N, Urakawa I, et al. Direct evidence for a causative role of FGF23 in the abnormal renal phosphate handling and vitamin D metabolism in rats with early-stage chronic kidney disease. *Kidney Int* 2010; 78: 975–80.

Komaba H, Goto S, Fujii H, et al. Depressed expression of Klotho and FGF receptor 1 in hyperplastic parathyroid glands from uremic patients. *Kidney Int* 2010; 77: 232–8.

Mathew S, Tustison KS, Sugatani T, et al. The mechanism of phosphorus as a cardiovascular risk factor in CKD. *J Am Soc Nephrol* 2008; 19: 1092–105.

Moe S, Drueke T, Cunningham J, et al. Definition, evaluation, and classification of renal osteodystrophy: A position statement from Kidney Disease: Improving Global Outcomes (KDIGO). *Kidney Int* 2006; 69: 1945–53.

Wheeler DC and Winkelmayer WC. KDIGO 2017 clinical practice guideline update for the diagnosis, evaluation, prevention, and treatment of chronic kidney disease–mineral and bone disorder (CKD–MBD). *Kidney Int* 2017; 7: 1–59.

Wolf M. Forging forward with 10 burning questions on FGF23 in kidney disease. *J Am Soc Nephrol* 2010; 21: 1427–35.

Chapter 12

Bone

Chapter contents

12.1 Anatomy and physiology

Introduction

Bone is a dynamic organ that provides both a structural framework and a source of ions for metabolic purposes. Bones are shaped by modelling during growth, from the in utero period to adolescence, with chondrocyte differentiation, matrix synthesis, and calcium deposition. In adults, bone is remodelled, with resorption of old bone and formation of new bone.

Anatomy and macroscopic organization of bone

The skeleton is made of two parts: the axial skeleton including the vertebrae, the pelvis, and other flat bones such as the skull and sternum; and the appendicular skeleton, including all the long bones.

Long bones

Long bones (e.g. the femur and the humerus) include the diaphysis, with the epiphyses at their extremities (Figure 12.1). In the diaphysis, the cortical bone (cortex) surrounds the medullary canal. Epiphyses have a thinner cortex, and the central area of the bone is filled with trabecular (cancellous) bone. The outer bone envelope is the periosteum, including nerve fibres, blood vessels, and lymph vessels. The internal surface of cortical bone is called the endosteal surface. The metaphysis is the boundary between the diaphysis and the epiphysis, where the growth plate is located in growing children. Although bone length growth stops with growth plate fusion, a slow process of increase in bone width continues throughout life, as a mechanical adaptation to cortical thinning due to ageing.

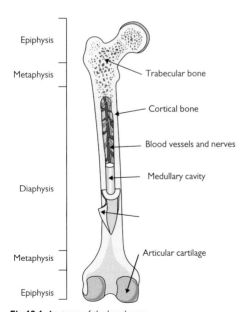

Fig 12.1 Anatomy of the long bones.
Courtesy of Dr Y Bala, INSERM UMR 1033.

Epiphysis

Metaphysis

Trabecular bone

Cortical bone

Blood vessels and nerves

Medullary cavity

Diaphysis

Articular cartilage

Metaphysis

Epiphysis

Short, flat, and irregular bones

In these bones, cortical bone surrounds trabecular bone, embedding bone marrow. The periosteal and endosteal surfaces are comparable to those of long bones.

Cortical and trabecular bone

Cortical bone is the outer layer of the bone, made of dense mineralized tissue, surrounding trabecular bone, which forms a tridimensional network of anastomosed bone trabeculae. Bone trabeculae are arranged in plates and rods, and their proportions differ according to the bone site and the individual age. For example, at the lumbar spine, rods are more common, whereas plates are predominant at the femoral neck. The organization and the orientation of bone trabeculae are key for bone strength and stem from mechanical strains applied to the bone. In adults, 80% of the total bone mass is cortical bone, although this proportion may vary across different bone sites.

Microscopic organization of bone

Bone texture

We can distinguish two types of bone texture: woven and lamellar. Woven bone includes disorganized big collagen fibres and is found in fetal bone, ear ossicles, transiently in fracture callus, and in some conditions like Paget's disease of bone and dense bone metastasis. In contrast, in lamellar bone, collagen fibres are organized in lamellae. Within each lamella, fibres are parallel, but form angles around 90° with adjacent lamellae, which is responsible for bone resistance. This disposition can be observed under polarized light microscopy as birefringence.

Organization of cortical bone

Bone structural units correspond to concentric lamellae, surrounding the Haversian canal, which contains blood vessels. These canals communicate with transverse canaliculae, the Volkmann's canals. This cylindrical structure including the Haversian canal, with its lamellae, is also called an osteon. It lies within interstitial bone, resulting from partial osteon remodelling.

Organization of trabecular bone

Trabecular bone is a dense tridimensional network (Figure 12.2). Bone remodelling produces bone packets, reminiscent of the cortical osteon structure, but open to the bone marrow.

Bone remodelling

The bone cells

Osteoblasts are the bone-forming cells: they produce the organic matrix, including collagen and non-collagenous proteins, before it starts mineralizing.

Osteocytes are the most abundant cells in the bone (90%). They differentiate from mature osteoblasts which are embedded within the bone matrix during the bone-formation process and acquire the essential role of mechanosensors, to regulate bone remodelling, through cytokine secretion.

Osteoclasts are the bone-resorbing cells. They are multinucleated cells adhering to the bone matrix. They

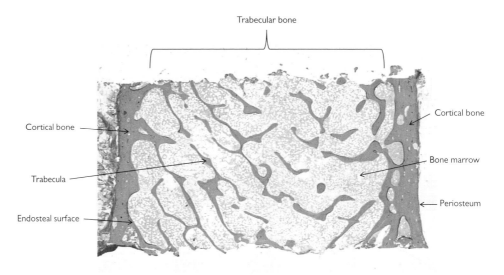

Fig 12.2 Bone microarchitecture.
Courtesy of Dr Chavassieux, INSERM UMR 1033.

acidify the bone to dissolve the mineral and they produce various enzymes to digest the proteins.

Lining cells are osteoblasts which can be observed at the surface of inactive bone. They form the bone-remodelling compartment, which separates the bone remodelling site from the bone marrow and they may play a role in the coupling of bone resorption and formation.

The different steps of bone remodelling

Older bone is periodically resorbed by osteoclasts, and newer bone is deposited in the resulting cavities by osteoblasts. This is bone remodelling. All the bone cells will cooperate within the basic multicellular unit (BMU), in four steps. First, osteoclasts resorb bone; this is followed by a second phase, which is called 'inversion'; third, osteoblasts form new bone; and fourth, these cells enter into a quiescent phase.

The role of bone remodelling

Bone remodelling alters the balance of minerals by increasing or decreasing their concentration in serum. It also allows the skeleton to adapt to its mechanical environment, by repairing the damage created in bone by mechanical loading.

Bone remodelling in cortical and trabecular bone

In cortical bone, the BMU moves along the Haversian canal, from the inner to the outer part of the osteon, thus forming a cutting cone. Thereafter, osteoblasts form new bone, in a closing cone. The new bone matrix will mineralize from the outer part to the inner part of the osteon.

In trabecular bone, osteoclasts dig resorption lacunae, which will be filled by osteoblasts. This new matrix will be mineralized later on. The number of active BMUs is much greater in the trabecular bone than in the cortical bone, so that 25% of trabecular bone is renewed each year, compared with only 4% of cortical bone.

Regulation of bone remodelling

Osteoclasts differentiate due to the effect of the cytokine receptor activator of nuclear factor kappa-B ligand (RANKL), in presence of macrophage-colony stimulating factor. RANKL is essentially produced by osteocytes, which, thereby, are the essential regulators of bone remodelling. Osteocytes, by their numerous cellular projections, extend throughout the bone matrix, to connect to other cells at the bone surface, so that membrane-bound RANKL expressed by osteocytes may interact with osteoclast progenitors.

There are two types of bone remodelling: stochastic bone remodelling, which is not site-dependent; and targeted remodelling, which is targeted towards specific bone sites. Osteocytes undergo apoptosis when bone microdamage crosses their canaliculae, which provide the stimulus to start remodelling targeted towards removing the damaged zone. Stochastic remodelling may be under the influence of systemic hormones and cytokines.

Mineralization

The mineralization process occurs after the bone matrix (osteoid tissue) is secreted by osteoblasts, consisting in the deposition of calcium phosphate (as calcium apatite) in the osteoid tissue.

The crystal nucleation takes place in holes at the surface of collagen fibres. Crystal growth occurs through ion addition to a single crystal or proliferation of other crystals. In the early phases of development, when woven bone is produced, mineralization also occurs in matrix vesicles. These vesicles also contain an essential enzyme for mineralization—alkaline phosphatase—and other proteins, such as bone sialoprotein. The first phase is primary mineralization, accounting for 50%–60% of the maximal mineral amount of bone tissue; this phase lasts for less than 3 months. The mineralization front can be identified using specific fluorescent dyes (e.g. tetracyclines administered prior to bone biopsies) to calculate the mineral apposition rate. The secondary mineralization is a slower process to increase the number, size, and perfection of crystals, during 6–24 months. Crystal size plays an important role in bone mechanical properties. Crystal size and homogeneity in individual trabeculae are associated with ageing, and bone fragility reflects increased crystal maturity.

Further reading

Bouxsein ML and Seeman E. Quantifying the material and structural determinants of bone strength. *Best Pract Res Clin Rheumatol* 2009; 23: 741–53.

Xiong J, Onal M, Jilka RL, et al. Matrix-embedded cells control osteoclast formation. *Nature Med* 2011; 17: 1235–41.

12.2 Investigation of metabolic bone disease: Biochemical markers of bone turnover

Introduction

Bone turnover markers are products of the bone remodelling cycle; they can be measured in blood or urine and used to estimate the level of bone resorption or formation. Many of the markers are derived from the synthesis or breakdown of the collagen matrix (see Table 12.1).

Type 1 collagen in bone matrix is derived from procollagen, and products of procollagen cleavage are used as markers of bone formation.

Bone matrix collagen is a triple helix stabilized with intra- and intermolecular crosslinks, and circulating crosslinks are used as a measure of bone resorption.

An international working group has recommended that procollagen type 1 N-terminal propeptide (P1NP) and the beta form of the C-terminal cross-linking telopeptide of type 1 collagen (CTX) be adopted as the reference markers for use in research and clinical practice, to allow standardization of assays and the development of reference ranges, meta-analyses, and comparison of clinical trial results.

Measurement of bone turnover markers

Levels of bone turnover markers are high in children and adolescents, decrease in adulthood, and increase again with ageing. They are higher in men than in women during young adulthood, but higher in postmenopausal women than in older men, so it is important that reference ranges are gender and age appropriate. Measurement of bone turnover markers is subject to pre-analytical variability. Bone turnover markers have a circadian rhythm: they are higher at night and lower during the day, mostly driven by the effects of feeding. Resorption markers are more affected by circadian rhythms and feeding than formation markers, and so it is particularly important that sampling of resorption markers is controlled for these factors. Urinary N-terminal cross-linking telopeptide of type 1 collagen (NTX) should ideally be measured on a fasted, second-morning void sample. The precision of the more variable markers can be improved by using a pooled sample (e.g. from two or three consecutive second-morning voids). Markers with less of a circadian and feeding/fasting response, such as P1NP, may be preferable for widespread use in clinical practice. Levels of bone turnover markers vary with season and with menstrual cycle, but these variations are probably not significant at an individual level. Pregnancy and lactation significantly increase levels of bone turnover markers, with levels returning to baseline 6–12 months after the end of lactation. Immobility and exercise both affect levels of bone turnover markers. Markers rise acutely after a fracture and remain increased for up to 12 months, depending on the size of the bone fractured. This is particularly import to consider if using bone turnover markers to monitor response to osteoporosis treatment.

Abnormal bone turnover markers

In postmenopausal osteoporosis, resorption and formation markers are increased.

Pathological causes of high bone turnover include:

- Paget's disease of bone
- fibrous dysplasia

Table 12.1 Biochemical markers of bone turnover

Abbreviation	Name	Origin	Assay
Formation markers			
P1NP	Procollagen type 1 N-terminal propeptide	Cleaved from procollagen	Serum
P1CP	Procollagen type 1 C-terminal propeptide	Cleaved from procollagen	Serum
BALP	Bone-specific alkaline phosphatase	Osteoblast enzyme	Serum
OC	Osteocalcin	Osteoblast hydroxyapatite-binding product	Serum/urine
Resorption markers			
NTX	N-terminal cross-linking telopeptide of type 1 collagen	Breakdown of bone matrix collagen	Serum/urine
Beta CTX	Beta C-terminal cross-linking telopeptide of type 1 collagen	Breakdown of bone matrix collagen (mature bone)	Serum
Alpha CTX	Alpha C-terminal cross-linking telopeptide of type 1 collagen	Breakdown of bone matrix collagen (new bone)	Serum/urine
1CTP or CTX-MMP	C-terminal cross-linking telopeptide of type 1 collagen	Breakdown of bone matrix collagen	Serum
DPD	Deoxypyridinoline	Breakdown of bone matrix collagen	Urine
PYD	Pyridinoline	Breakdown of bone matrix collagen (and cartilage, tendon, blood vessels)	Urine
TRACP5b	Serum tartrate-resistant acid phosphatase	Osteoclast enzyme	Serum

- osteomalacia
- chronic kidney disease
- bone metastases
- myeloma
- primary hyperparathyroidism
- thyrotoxicosis
- acromegaly

In glucocorticoid excess, there is dissociation of bone turnover, with increased resorption and decreased formation. This pattern is also seen in restrictive eating disorders (possibly due to the combination of oestrogen deficiency, high cortisol, lack of skeletal loading, low IGF-1, and low leptin).

Bone turnover markers in osteoporosis

Higher levels of bone turnover markers are associated with lower bone mineral density, worse microarchitectural properties, and greater bone loss in older adults. They may have value in fracture prediction, as high levels of bone turnover markers are associated with increased fracture risk independently of bone mineral density. As yet, they are not used in fracture prediction, but with standardization of assays and further study, it is possible that they may be incorporated into future fracture risk algorithms.

Very high or low levels of bone turnover markers may be an indication to consider further investigation (similarly to a low bone mineral density for age). As yet, there is insufficient evidence to justify the use of bone turnover markers in making treatment choices in osteoporosis (e.g. between an antiresorptive and an anabolic agent).

Currently, the main use of bone turnover markers in clinical practice is in monitoring response to treatment. The size and rate of the response of bone mineral density to antiresorptive treatment is such that it is not reliably measureable by DXA until about 18 months after the initiation of treatment. Bone turnover markers reach their maximal response after about 6 months of treatment, and so allow an earlier evaluation of adherence and response. Results of clinical trials suggest that a decrease in the levels of bone turnover markers of more than 30%, or into the lower half of the premenopausal reference range, with antiresorptive treatment is associated with reduced fracture risk. Decrease in the levels of formation or resorption markers can be used to monitor the response to antiresorptive treatment, and an increase in the level of formation markers can be used to monitor response to anabolic treatment.

One of the uncertainties in bisphosphonate treatment is the optimum duration of treatment and, in patients in whom bisphosphonates have been stopped, when they should be restarted. The use of bone turnover markers in monitoring the offset of bisphosphonate effects is not yet well established, but this may be a future development.

Bone turnover markers in Paget's disease

Bone turnover markers are useful in the diagnosis of active Paget's disease, in monitoring the response to bisphosphonate treatment, and in judging when repeat treatments may be necessary. Bone-specific (or total) alkaline phosphatase is often used to diagnose and monitor Paget's disease because it is widely available and has been well evaluated in Paget's disease. P1NP has also been shown to perform well in diagnosis and monitoring.

Further reading

Shankar S and Hosking DJ. Biochemical assessment of Paget's disease of bone. *J Bone Miner Res* 2007; 21(Supp2): P22–7.

Vasikaran S, Eastell R, Bruyère O, et al. Markers of bone turnover for the prediction of fracture risk and monitoring of osteoporosis treatment: A need for international reference standards. *Osteoporos Int* 2011; 22: 391–420.

12.3 Investigation of metabolic bone disease: Bone densitometry

DXA

Introduction

The gold standard for diagnosis of osteoporosis and most commonly used densitometry method is dual-energy X-ray absorptiometry (DXA). DXA densitometry is based on the differential attenuation of incident X-ray beams by bone mineral and soft tissue. The outputs from the measurement are bone area (expressed in square centimetres), bone mineral content (expressed in grams), and bone mineral density (expressed in grams per square centimetre). The scanner software calculates standard deviation and percentage scores for bone mineral density against a population reference range (see Table 12.2).

The usually measured sites (and the sites at which a diagnosis of osteoporosis can be made, according to the WHO definition; see Table 12.3) are the lumbar spine, the hip, and the forearm (see Figure 12.3). Whole-body scans are more commonly used in children or in the assessment of body composition.

The short-term precision (expressed as the coefficient of variation) of lumbar spine and total hip measurements is 1%–2%. The radiation dose from DXA is low, at about 2–5 μSv at the spine and hip (the average natural background radiation in the UK is about 7 μSv per day).

DXA manufacturers use different image acquisition and processing algorithms, and there is variability in measurement even between scanners of the same manufacturer and model. It is therefore important that measurements from different scanners are not compared, and patients should be measured longitudinally on the same scanner wherever possible.

DXA measurement may be unreliable in patients with osteoarthritis, degenerative changes, or vertebral fractures in the region of measurement; when there is overlying soft tissue calcification (particularly aortic calcification at the lumbar spine); and in patients with a high BMI, or who have had a large weight change between measurements. Because DXA is based on a two-dimensional image, it measures areal bone mineral density (in grams per square centimetre) rather than true or volumetric bone mineral density (which is expressed in grams per cubic centimetre). As a result, it underestimates bone mineral density in patients with small skeletal size,

Table 12.2 Dual-energy X-ray absorptiometry population-referenced scores

Score	Reference population
T-score	Standard deviations from gender-matched young adult mean
PR% (peak referenced)	Percentage of gender-matched young adult mean
Z-score	Standard deviations from gender- and age-matched mean
AM% (age-matched)	Percentage of gender- and age-matched mean

Table 12.3 WHO T-score definition of osteoporosis

T-score	Grade
≥−1.0	Normal
−1.0 to −2.5	Osteopenia
≤−2.5	Osteoporosis
≤−2.5 plus fracture	Established osteoporosis

Data from *WHO Technical Report Series*, 921, Prevention and management of osteoporosis: report of a WHO scientific group, 2004.

and overestimates bone mineral density in patients with large skeletal size. This is particularly important in children, for whom it may be appropriate to consider bone mineral density normalized for body size rather than for age. For the same reason, variability in positioning (particularly the hip rotation) can affect the measurement.

DXA only measures bone mineral, and so does not distinguish between osteoporosis (reduced amount of bone) and osteomalacia (reduced mineralization of bone).

Indications for DXA

Bone densitometry should be considered in low-trauma fracture or in patients with risk factors for osteoporosis and fracture. It may also be useful in the assessment and monitoring of other bone diseases such as osteomalacia and osteogenesis imperfecta.

Interpretation

DXA bone mineral density is a good predictor of fracture risk; the gradient of risk is approximately 1.5- to 2-fold for each standard deviation decrease in bone mineral density. The WHO operational definition of osteoporosis is based on DXA T-scores (see Table 12.3). However, bone mineral density should be considered in the context of other clinical risk factors when making treatment decisions.

The use of T-scores (and the terms 'osteopenia' and 'osteoporosis') is inappropriate before the age of peak bone mass (at about age 25), when bone mineral density should be described as within or outside the expected range for age (Z-score: −2.0 to + 2.0). Low bone mineral density for age may be an indication to investigate for underlying causes.

Monitoring

In most situations, the magnitude and rate of change in DXA are relatively small—for example, a typical response to bisphosphonate treatment may be 4%–5% over the first 18 months.

The least significant change, signifying a change that is greater than the variability of the measurement, is calculated as 2.77 multiplied by the coefficient of variation and is approximately 4%–5% at the lumbar spine and the total hip.

It is therefore important to make follow-up measurements at a long-enough time interval that the expected change is at least the least significant change, and this is usually 18–24 months. In a few situations where more rapid change is expected (e.g. remineralization in the

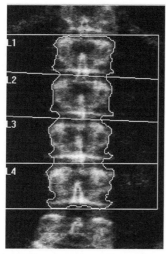
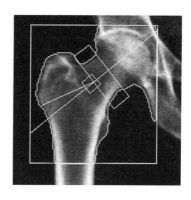

Fig 12.3 Dual-energy X-ray absorptiometry images of the lumbar spine and hip.

case of osteomalacia or high fracture risk due to high-dose glucocorticoid treatment), a shorter interval between measurements may be appropriate.

There is current debate over the utility of monitoring with DXA, particularly in the context of response to and offset of osteoporosis treatments and, in the future, biochemical markers of bone turnover may be used more widely for this purpose.

Vertebral fracture assessment

Vertebral fracture assessment (VFA) is increasingly used in clinical practice. DXA machines are used to obtain low-dose lateral and anteroposterior images of the thoracic and lumbar spine to screen for vertebral fractures. Prevalent and incident vertebral fractures are associated with a significant increase in fracture risk (see

Figure 12.4), independent of bone mineral density, and often do not present clinically, so VFA is helpful in identifying patients who are at high risk of further fracture and who may benefit from treatment.

VFA is added to densitometry in groups at increased risk of vertebral fracture (older age, low bone mineral density for age, height loss, glucocorticoid treatment). Plain radiographs can be used to confirm suspected vertebral fractures.

There are different approaches to the radiological definition of vertebral fracture. In the semi-quantitative method, the defining characteristic of a vertebral fracture is height loss. In the algorithm-based qualitative method, the defining characteristic is end-plate deformity. There are also automated morphometric methods that can be applied to VFA images.

Quantitative CT

Quantitative CT can be performed on purpose-built scanners for peripheral sites (forearm and leg; see

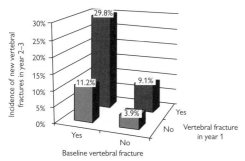

Fig 12.4 Graph from the HORIZON study showing the incidence of new vertebral fracture in the last 2 years of the study, as stratified by risk factors, compared to baseline vertebral fracture and incident vertebral fracture in the first year of the study.
Reproduced from *Osteoporosis International*, Predictors of new and severe vertebral fractures: results from the HORIZON Pivotal Fracture Trial, 23, 1, 2011, pp. 53–58. Copyright © 2011, International Osteoporosis Foundation and National Osteoporosis Foundation, with permission of Springer.

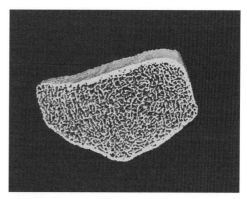

Fig 12.5 High-resolution peripheral quantitative CT image of the distal radius.

Figure 12.5). For spine and hip measurement, a calibration phantom is placed within the field of a conventional CT scanner to convert Hounsfield units to densitometric units (expressed in grams per cubic centimetre). The first advantage of CT over DXA is that it is a three-dimensional technique, giving a volumetric measurement, and so is not influenced by bone size. The second advantage is that cortical and trabecular compartments can be separated and analysed individually to give measurements of bone geometry and distribution of bone mass, as these are important in the estimation of bone strength. New, high-resolution techniques can also quantify microarchitectural properties (e.g. cortical porosity, trabecular number, and trabecular thickness), and images can be used in finite-element analysis models to estimate bone strength under loading conditions that simulate typical falls. However, the higher-radiation dose of spine and hip quantitative CT is a limiting factor. At present, quantitative CT is mainly a research tool.

Quantitative ultrasound

Ultrasound assessment of bone density is usually performed at the calcaneus or fingers. It has the advantage of not using ionizing radiation, and can discriminate between people with osteoporotic fractures and those without. However, there are no clear diagnostic thresholds as there are with DXA, so applicability in clinical practice is limited.

Further reading

Blake GM, Fogelman I. The clinical role of dual energy X-ray absorptiometry. *Eur J Radiol* 2009; 71: 406–14.

International Society for Clinical Densitometry. International Society for Clinical Densitometry 2007 Position Statement, 2007. Available at http://www.iscd.org/official-positions/2007-iscd-official-positions-adult/ (accessed 8 Jan 2017).

Kanis JA, Melton LJ 3rd, Christiansen C, et al. The diagnosis of osteoporosis. *J Bone Miner Res* 1994; 9: 1137–41.

Griffith JF, Genant HK. New imaging modalities in bone. *Curr Rheumatol Rep* 2011; 13: 241–50.

12.4 Investigation of metabolic bone disease: Bone imaging

Plain radiography

Plain radiographs are used in the diagnosis of fracture, and the confirmation of vertebral fracture from VFA (see Figure 12.6). Skeletal dysplasias such as osteopetrosis can be diagnosed based on characteristic appearances on plain radiographs. Radiographs are also useful in the differentiation of causes of increased uptake on isotope imaging. Radiographs in Paget's disease show deformity, cortical thickening, bony expansion, and coarse trabecular architecture. In contrast, radiographs in fibrous dysplasia usually show well-circumscribed medullary cystic or sclerotic lesions with cortical thinning.

Radiographs in osteomalacia may demonstrate bony deformity, areas of demineralization, or the classical Looser's zone or pseudofracture: linear lucency with surrounding sclerosis.

Isotope bone imaging

99mTc-bisphosphonate-labelled uptake imaging is useful in the investigation of osteoporosis and other metabolic bone diseases.

In osteoporosis, the main usage of isotope bone imaging is in the confirmation and dating of vertebral fractures. It can be particularly useful in distinguishing between vertebral fracture other active pathology, and old deformities

or developmental anomalies. If the timing of a vertebral fracture would affect decisions to initiate or change osteoporosis treatment, then an isotope scan can be helpful. Increased tracer uptake persists for about 12 months after a fracture. Isotope imaging cannot distinguish between benign osteoporotic and pathological fracture, but uptake in other skeletal sites can identify skeletal metastases.

Isotope bone imaging is valuable in making a diagnosis and describing the extent of diseases such as Paget's disease of bone, and fibrous dysplasia. In Paget's disease, the characteristic distribution is in the pelvis, the vertebrae, the scapulae, the skull, and the ends of the long bones (See Figure 12.7). The main differential diagnosis of Paget's disease isotope appearances is fibrous dysplasia.

In osteomalacia, there is generally increased isotope uptake, and focal areas of increased uptake may indicate pseudofractures or insufficiency fractures.

MRI

MRI can be helpful in the exclusion of malignancy when abnormalities are identified on plain radiographs. It is also used in the assessment of vertebral fractures that may be suitable for vertebroplasty or kyphoplasty, in the diagnosis of stress fractures, and in other conditions associated with bone marrow oedema, such as transient osteoporosis of the hip.

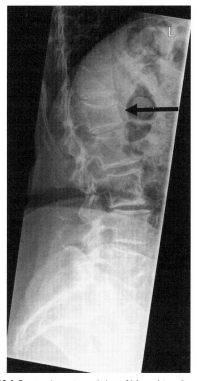

Fig 12.6 Fractured superior end plate of L1 on plain radiograph.

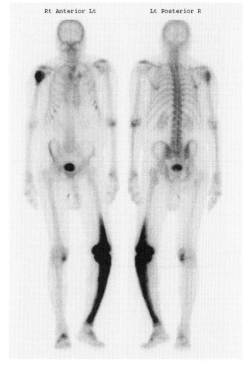

Fig 12.7 Isotope bone scan showing increased uptake in the humerus, the femur, and the tibia in Paget's disease.

High-resolution MRI of bone structure is still limited to research applications. It offers the advantage of fine structural measurement without the use of ionizing radiation, so in the future it may be particularly useful in longitudinal studies and studies of children.

Further reading

Link TM, Guglielmi G, van Kuijk C, et al. Radiologic assessment of osteoporotic vertebral fractures: Diagnostic and prognostic implications. *Eur Radiol* 2005; 15: 1521–32.

Sundaram M. Imaging of Paget's disease and fibrous dysplasia of bone. *J Bone Miner Res* 2006; 21(Suppl 2): P28–30.

12.5 Investigation of metabolic bone disease: Bone biopsy

Indications

Bone biopsy is not usually required in the management of osteoporosis and common metabolic bone diseases. It may be helpful in the assessment of very low bone density or recurrent low trauma fracture when other investigations have not identified an underlying cause, or if there is diagnostic uncertainty and a rare metabolic bone disease is a possibility. Also, if treatment with antiresorptives or parathyroidectomy is being considered in patients with renal bone disease, bone biopsy can be a useful addition to biochemical investigations to exclude adynamic bone disease. The biopsy should be taken before treatment is started, to obtain a meaningful result.

Method

Biopsies are usually obtained at the superior anterior iliac crest, with a core sample including both cortices. A large core of about 7 mm diameter is usually obtained under general or local anaesthesia, but smaller cores of (diameter 3–4 mm) obtained under local anaesthesia have been shown to give accurate results, and may be more acceptable to patients.

Tetracycline or doxycycline labelling is administered to allow evaluation of bone mineral apposition rates. A typical protocol would be 3 days' dose of the label, 10 days off, then 3 more days' dose of the label.

Microscopy and histomorphometric analysis of bone biopsy specimens gives information on the number of osteoclasts, osteoblasts, and osteocytes; microstructural properties; resorption activity; bone mineral apposition rate; and the amount of unmineralized osteoid (see Figure 12.8).

Typical findings in metabolic bone disease

In postmenopausal osteoporosis, histomorphometry shows loss of cortical width, trabecularization of the inner cortical surface, and reduced trabecular number and trabecular connectivity.

In osteomalacia, there is an increased amount of osteoid, and poor double labelling.

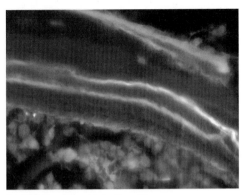

Fig 12.8 Fluorescent-labelled bone biopsy.
Image kindly provided by Dr David Hughes, Sheffield.

High-turnover renal bone disease shows high resorption activity, loss of trabecular structure, and an increased osteoid-to-mineralized bone ratio. Adynamic bone disease is typified by low remodelling activity, and a reduced osteoid-to-mineralized bone ratio.

Further reading

Barger-Lux JM and Recker RR. Toward understanding bone quality. Transilial bone biopsy and bone histomorphometry. *Clin Rev Bone Miner Metab* 2006; 4: 167–76.

Dempster DW. 'Histomorphometric analysis of bone remodeling', in Bilezikian JP, Raisz, LG, and John Martin, TJ, eds, *Principles of Bone Biology* (3rd edition), 2008: Elsevier, pp. 447–63.

Ott SM. Histomorphometric measurements of bone turnover, mineralization, and volume. *Clin J Am Soc Nephrol* 2008; 3: S151–6.

12.6 Osteoporosis

Definition

Osteoporosis is a systemic skeletal disease which is characterized by low bone mass and microarchitectural deterioration of bone tissue and leads to increased bone fragility and a consequent increase in fracture risk. The WHO has defined osteoporosis as bone mineral density, as measured by DXA, less than 2.5 standard deviations below the average sex-specific peak bone mass (T-score ≤ −2.5) at the spine, hip, or forearm. In practice, bone mineral density of the lumbar spine and the hip (either total hip or femoral neck) is used for diagnosis and monitoring of osteoporosis. Patients with prevalent vertebral or hip fractures are considered to have osteoporosis regardless of their bone mineral density, because the fracture is a sign of poor bone quality and is associated with increased future fracture risk.

Epidemiology

The prevalence of osteoporosis varies considerably between individuals of different races and between individuals of the same race living in different parts of the world and even within the same continent.

The incidence of osteoporotic fractures is very low before menopause in women and before the age of 60 in men. The incidence of the three most prevalent osteoporotic fractures—forearm, vertebral, and hip fractures—increases after the age of 55, 65, and 75 years in women, respectively. Forearm fractures are uncommon in men, and the incidence of vertebral and hip fractures is approximately half of the incidence seen among women of the same age. One in two women and one in five men at the age of 50 will suffer an osteoporotic fracture in their remaining lifetime. Other osteoporosis-related fractures are proximal humerus, pelvis, and ankle fractures.

Pathophysiology

Osteoporosis is often multifactorial. Genetics explains approximately 50% of the inter-individual variance in bone mineral density and fracture risk in young and middle-aged individuals, but less in older individuals. Environmental factors, such as diet, calcium intake, vitamin D intake, physical activity, smoking, and alcohol consumption are also important factors. Co-morbidity and some medical treatments may also increase the risk of osteoporosis.

Osteoporosis (i.e. low bone mass and deteriorated architecture of the bone) is caused, in principle, by insufficient bone growth during childhood and adolescence, inappropriate loss of bone after attaining peak bone mass, or a combination of the two mechanisms. Bone gain can be affected by genetics, environmental factors (e.g. smoking), or diseases such as juvenile rheumatic diseases or anorexia nervosa. Healthy individuals lose bone after the age of 40–50 years. There are several reasons for this change. In women the loss of endogenous oestrogen at menopause leads to increased osteoclast activity. Vitamin D insufficiency or deficiency is more common with increasing age, and leads to secondary hyperparathyroidism and increased osteoclast activity. The level of physical activity usually goes down with increasing age, and the bone adapts with increased resorption and decreased bone formation. Individuals that develop osteoporosis may elicit an exaggerated response to these physiological changes; however, postmenopausal and age-related bone loss may also be influenced by genetics, environmental factors, diseases, and treatment thereof, such as hyperthyroidism and glucocorticoid treatment.

Osteoporosis can be divided into two subtypes: primary or idiopathic osteoporosis, and secondary osteoporosis. In primary osteoporosis, no obvious cause of the condition can be identified. Primary osteoporosis can again be divided into postmenopausal, senile, and rare forms of osteoporosis, including pregnancy-associated and juvenile osteoporosis. Postmenopausal osteoporosis (occurring in postmenopausal women aged <65–70 years) is mainly caused by oestrogen deficiency. Senile osteoporosis (occurring in men and women aged >70 years) is mainly caused by age-related secondary hyperparathyroidism.

Osteoporosis is secondary to other conditions, diseases, or medical treatments in one-third of women and two-thirds of men with osteoporosis. The list of secondary causes of osteoporosis is long and includes:

- immobilization (e.g. paresis, multiple sclerosis, rheumatoid diseases)
- nutritional (e.g. anorexia nervosa, malabsorption, vitamin D deficiency)
- toxins (e.g. tobacco, alcohol)
- endocrine disorders (e.g. thyrotoxicosis, Cushing's syndrome, primary hyperparathyroidism, diabetes, menopause at <45 years, male hypogonadism)
- renal insufficiency
- rheumatological diseases (e.g. rheumatoid arthritis, ankylosing spondylosis)
- chronic obstructive lung disease
- drugs (e.g. glucocorticoids, aromatase inhibitors, anti-androgen treatment)

Glucocorticoid-induced osteoporosis is the most common form of secondary osteoporosis. Glucocorticoid treatment is characterized by a rapid phase of increased bone resorption and a prolonged phase of decreased bone formation. Patients treated with glucocorticoids have a pronounced and rapid increase in the risk of vertebral as well as non-vertebral fractures, and studies indicate that these patients fracture at a higher bone mineral density than non-glucocorticoid-treated individuals. It is therefore recommended that patients receiving glucocorticoids undergo anti-osteoporotic treatments at a higher bone mineral density (T-score ≤−1 or −1.5) than patients with other forms of osteoporosis.

Clinical features

Most patients with osteoporosis are without any symptoms because they have been identified by DXA before the first fracture. There is no evidence to suggest that low bone mass, deteriorated architecture, or high bone turnover without a prevalent fracture causes bone pain.

Patients who have suffered non-vertebral fractures may have sequelae. Patients with vertebral fractures may suffer chronic pain. Other signs of prevalent vertebral fractures are height loss, thoracic kyphosis, and reduced distance from the ribs to the iliac crest.

Investigations

Individuals at risk of developing osteoporosis can be identified on the basis of clinical risk factors and algorithms that can estimate the absolute fracture risk based on clinical risk factors, such as FRAX[a] and the fracture risk calculator from the Garvan Institute. The clinical risk factors are:

- family history of osteoporotic fracture (especially hip fracture)
- low body weight
- prevalent fragility fracture
- causes of secondary osteoporosis (listed in 'Pathophysiology')

Once clinical risk factors have been identified, the next step will be DXA of the spine and hip. If DXA reveals osteoporosis, the diagnostic workup should comprise the following:

- medical history and physical examination in order to characterize the severity of the disease, identify secondary causes of osteoporosis, and collect information on the basis of which the optimal choice of treatment can be made
- imaging (X-ray or VFA) of the thoracic and lumbar spine, in order to identify and characterize any vertebral fractures (number and severity)
- biochemical investigation of secondary causes of osteoporosis and contraindications for medical treatment:
  - CRP
  - haemoglobin
  - white blood cells
  - platelets
  - serum 25-hydroxyvitamin D_3
  - serum PTH
  - serum TSH
  - serum creatinine
  - serum sodium
  - serum potassium
  - serum calcium ions
  - serum phosphate
  - serum (bone-specific) alkaline phosphatase
  - in men: serum testosterone
  - in patients with vertebral fractures: serum protein electrophoresis

Patients diagnosed with osteoporosis based on a prevalent hip or vertebral fracture should go through the same diagnostic workup in order to further characterize the severity of the disease.

Future risk of fractures can be estimated using different algorithms, including FRAX® (http://www.shef.ac.uk/FRAX) and the fracture risk calculator from the Garvan Institute (http://www.garvan.org.au/bone-fracture-risk). These algorithms have limitations; therefore, the decision regarding treatment should not be based on these algorithms alone.

Management

The purpose of medical treatment of patients with osteoporosis is to reduce the incidence of future fractures—vertebral as well as non-vertebral fractures. Medical treatment of osteoporosis can be divided into antiresorptive and anabolic therapies based on their mode of action. Antiresorptive therapies primarily inhibit osteoclasts and bone resorption; anabolic therapies primarily stimulate osteoblasts and bone formation.

Calcium and vitamin D

Calcium and vitamin D have weak antiresorptive effects through suppression of the secretion of PTH and stimulation of the mineralization of the bone. Calcium and vitamin D have been demonstrated to have antifracture efficacy and are considered to be basic elements of the treatment of osteoporosis.

Antiresorptive therapies

Antiresorptive therapies comprise bisphosphonates, anti-RANKL antibody, selective oestrogen-receptor modulators, and strontium ranelate. The common feature of these drugs is inhibition of bone resorption, but the underlying mechanisms of action and pharmacodynamics are very different.

Bisphosphonates

Bisphosphonates inhibit bone resorption by inhibiting the mevalonate pathway and thereby the production of isoprenoid lipids that are needed for modification of small GTP-binding proteins that are essential for osteoclast function and survival (Black et al., 2006).

The bisphosphonates available for the prevention and treatment of osteoporosis differ by their affinity for bone and by way of administration. The orally administrated bisphosphonates should be taken daily, weekly, or monthly, whereas the intravenously administrated bisphosphonates are given every 3 months or yearly. The absorption of orally administered bisphosphonates is poor (<1%). It is therefore very important that the patients take the drugs after fasting in the morning, with nothing but plain water, and do not eat breakfast for 30–60 minutes thereafter.

The evidence for antifracture efficacy differs among the different bisphosphonates (Table 12.4). Alendronic acid has demonstrated efficacy against vertebral fractures in men and postmenopausal women; glucocorticoid-induced osteoporosis; and non-vertebral and hip fractures. Zoledronic acid has demonstrated efficacy against vertebral fractures in men, pre- and postmenopausal women; glucocorticoid-induced osteoporosis; and non-vertebral and hip fractures. Risedronate has demonstrated efficacy against vertebral fractures in postmenopausal women; glucocorticoid-induced osteoporosis; and non-vertebral and hip fractures. Ibandronic acid has demonstrated efficacy against vertebral fractures in postmenopausal women.

The side effects of orally administrated bisphosphonates are primarily related to upper gastrointestinal discomfort, nausea, and gastric ulcer. Flu-like symptoms can occur after the first administrations of intravenously as well as orally administrated bisphosphonates. Other rare side effects are muscle and joint pain and uveitis. Very rarely are seen osteonecrosis of the jaw (estimated prevalence between 1 in 10,000 and 1 in 100,000 patients) and atypical femoral fractures (prevalence 3–5 per 10,000 patient years). Bisphosphonates are excreted by the kidneys and should not be administrated to patients with reduced kidney function (glomerular filtration rate (GFR) < 30 mL/minute).

RANKL antibody

Denosumab is a fully human antibody against RANKL. It is administered as a subcutaneous injection every 6 months. The mechanism of action is inhibition of the interaction between RANKL and RANK, which is the receptor for RANKL on preosteoclasts and mature osteoclasts. This results in inhibition of osteoclast activity.

Table 12.4 Antifracture efficacy of the most used drugs for the primary and secondary prevention of osteoporotic fractures

Drug		Antifracture efficacy				
		Vertebral fracture	Hip fracture	Non-vertebral fracture	Glucocorticoid-induced osteoporosis	Male osteoporosis
Antiresorptive modalities	Alendronic acid	A	A	A	A	A
	Zoledronic acid	A	A	A	B	A†
	Risedronate	A	A	A	A	—
	Denosumab	A	A	A	—	—
	Strontium ranelate	A	C	A	—	—
	Ibandronic acid	A	—	C	—	—
	Raloxifene	A	—	—	—	—
Anabolic modalities	Teriparatide	A	—	A	A	—

Note: A: antifracture efficacy demonstrated in randomized, controlled, clinical trials; A†: antifracture efficacy demonstrated in a study including women and men; B: antifracture efficacy demonstrated in a non-inferiority randomized, controlled, clinical trial; C: Antifracture efficacy demonstrated only in a subset of patients (pos thoc analysis) from a randomized, controlled, clinical trial.

The effect of denosumab is very rapid, and a pronounced reduction in osteoclast activity is seen already within the first 24 hours after administration. Denosumab has demonstrated efficacy against vertebral, non-vertebral, and hip fractures in postmenopausal women (Table 12.4). Side effects include skin rashes; respiratory, skin, and urinary tract infections; cataract; and, very rarely, osteonecrosis of the jaw and atypical femur fractures.

Strontium ranelate

Strontium ranelate has demonstrated efficacy against vertebral fractures and non-vertebral fractures in postmenopausal women. The underlying mechanism of action is not completely understood. Strontium can replace calcium in bone and suppress bone resorption, perhaps through the CaSR. It has also been suggested that strontium ranelate increases the ratio of osteoprotegerin to RANKL and thereby inhibits osteoclast recruitment and activity. Strontium ranelate is administered orally as a powder dissolved in plain water every day. Side effects are nausea, loose stools, venous thromboembolism, cardiovascular disease, dermatitis, headache, impaired memory, and, very rarely, allergic reactions, including the DRESS syndrome. Strontium is excreted by the kidneys and should therefore not be administrated to patients with severely reduced renal function (GFR <30 mL/ minute). The European Medicine Agency recommends limiting the use of strontium ranelate to patients who have severe osteoporosis but cannot be treated with any other anti-osteoporotic drugs, because of the risk of cardiovascular disease associated with strontium ranelate.

Selective oestrogen-receptor modulators

Selective oestrogen-receptor modulators are drugs that bind to the two oestrogen receptors in a different way than oestrogen does and thereby confer some effects that are similar to those provided by oestrogen, such as protection against bone loss and osteoporosis; some effects that are unlike those provided by oestrogen, such as protection against breast cancer; and apparently no or only minor effects on other organs known to respond to oestrogen, such as the uterus.

Raloxifene is the only selective oestrogen-receptor modulator marketed for the prevention and treatment of postmenopausal osteoporosis. The underlying mechanism of action is similar to that of oestrogen in postmenopausal women: inhibition of osteoclast recruitment and activity through reduced production of RANKL by the osteoblasts, leading to reduced bone resorption. Raloxifene is administered orally as a daily tablet. It has demonstrated efficacy against vertebral fractures in postmenopausal women and reduces the risk of breast cancer by more than 60%. Side effects include hot flushes; restless legs; peripheral oedema; gallstones; rarely, venous thromboembolism; and, very rarely, a fatal outcome of stroke in women with ischaemic heart disease. Raloxifene is metabolized in the liver and is not recommended in patients with severely impaired renal and hepatic functions.

Duration of antiresorptive treatment

Osteoporosis is a chronic disease and, in this perspective, it is counterintuitive to discuss duration of treatment. However, unlike other drugs used for the treatment of chronic diseases, bisphosphonates have a prolonged effect. Bisphosphonates attach strongly to bone and are retained in the bone for many years, depending on the affinity of the individual bisphosphonate. The best examined bisphosphonates with respect to treatment duration are alendronic acid and zoledronic acid. The FLEX study has demonstrated that it is safe to treat for 10 years with alendronic acid, as bone biopsies showed intact remodelling activity. The study also demonstrated that postmenopausal women without vertebral fractures and non-osteoporotic hip bone mineral density (T-score > −2.5) after 5 years of treatment with alendronate can stop the treatment and still be protected against new fractures. Women with existing vertebral fractures and osteoporotic hip bone mineral density, on the other hand, should continue treatment in order to stay protected against fractures. Very similar results have been obtained with respect to zoledronic acid from an extension of the HORIZON study. Women with low risk (no existing vertebral fractures and non-osteoporotic bone mineral density at the hip) can stop treatment with zoledronic acid after 3 years, whereas women with higher risk benefit from continuing treatment for up to 6 years. Data is not available for risedronate and ibandronic acid, and a similar conclusion about off-treatment effects can therefore not be made with certainty.

The other antiresorptive treatments do not have prolonged duration of the effect and therefore only have antifracture efficacy as long as the patient stays adherent to the therapy. Stopping denosumab treatment leads to rebound activation of bone resorption and very rapid bone loss. This seems to be associated with an increased risk of vertebral fractures.

Bone anabolic therapies

The only bone anabolic therapy currently available is the parathyroid analogue teriparatide. The underlying mechanism of action is not completely known. Studies have demonstrated that the duration of elevated levels of PTH in the circulation is critical for the actions of PTH. Short-term elevation predominately stimulates osteoblasts, whereas continuously elevated levels stimulate both osteoclasts and osteoblasts, resulting in a high-bone-turnover condition similar to that seen in primary hyperparathyroidism characterized by bone loss.

Teriparatide comprises the first 34 amino acids of intact PTH. Teriparatide has demonstrated efficacy against vertebral and non-vertebral fractures in postmenopausal women and against vertebral fractures in glucocorticoid-induced osteoporosis (Table 12.4). The treatment is approved for 24 months. Side effects include nausea, fatigue, perspiration, palpitations, hypercalcaemia, depression, urinary incontinence, and bone pain.

The duration of treatment with teriparatide may be important for the efficacy against non-vertebral fractures, as a positive correlation between duration of treatment and antifracture efficacy has been demonstrated in a post hoc analysis. The effect of treatment with PTH on bone mineral density is rapidly lost when the treatment is stopped. This can be prevented by treatment with antiresorptive therapy, but not with calcium and vitamin D alone. It is, therefore, very important that patients treated with PTH be followed closely and prescribed an antiresorptive drug when treatment with PTH treatment is completed.

Adherence

Evidence-based antiresorptive and anabolic treatments are available for the treatment of postmenopausal osteoporosis. There is also good evidence for the efficacy of at least some of the treatments in male osteoporosis and in glucocorticoid-induced osteoporosis (Table 12.4). However, successful prevention of osteoporotic fractures is dependent on adherence to the therapy. Unfortunately, many studies have demonstrated insufficient adherence with osteoporosis therapies and that the outcome of the treatment is attenuated by poor adherence. A very important way of improving fracture prevention is therefore to improve adherence to treatment. Many factors are important for adherence and therefore need consideration:

- the disease and the patient's perception of the disease
- the fact that adherence to treatment of a symptomatic disease is higher than that for a non-symptomatic disease
- the patient's perception of the treatment with respect to efficacy
- dosing frequencies, dosing procedures, and formulation of the drug
- side effects: patients should be informed about the existence of other treatment options if they experience side effects with the chosen treatment

- the cost and the possibilities for reimbursement
- co-morbidities

In order to improve adherence, all patients should be considered as patients with potentially poor adherence. This knowledge should therefore be included when planning the treatment of the individual patient.

Clinical practice

The first obstacle to treatment of patients with osteoporosis is the identification of the patients. Many patients with fragility non-vertebral fractures are not referred for DXA and osteoporosis treatment. Several initiatives have demonstrated that the way to improve this lack of diagnosis and treatment is establishing fracture liaison services. Similarly, patients with vertebral fractures are not diagnosed either because they are not examined or because vertebral fractures detectable in X-rays for other indications are not mentioned in the radiology report. A relatively new tool that may help diagnosing patients with vertebral fractures is the 'VFA' modality on DXA machines. With this tool, it has become possible, with reduced cost and with exposing patients to a minimum of radiation, to reliably detect at least moderate or severe vertebral fractures.

Once a patient has been diagnosed with osteoporosis, the patient needs to undergo further examinations to clarify the type and severity of the disease. The severity of osteoporosis can be further investigated by collecting information about non-vertebral fractures, measuring bone mineral density, and determining the rate of bone turnover by measuring biochemical markers of bone resorption and formation. If non-vertebral fractures have occurred, a drug that prevents non-vertebral fractures should be preferred; if the bone mineral density is very low, a bone anabolic drug would often be preferred; and, if bone turnover is very high, a drug that reduces bone turnover quickly would often be preferred. Finally, the investigation of the patients should include information about whether the disease is secondary to other diseases or medical treatments and if these are modifiable. For example, if a patient is being treated with glucocorticoids, reduction in the dose should be considered and a drug that has proven efficacy against glucocorticoid-induced osteoporosis should be preferred. Biochemical workup can unravel secondary causes of osteoporosis, such as vitamin D deficiency or subclinical hyperthyroidism, as well as contraindications for some of the treatments, such as renal insufficiency.

Once the type and severity of osteoporosis have been worked out, the physician and the patient should discuss treatment options. In most patients, weekly alendronate will be the first drug of choice because alendronate has well-documented antifracture efficacy and safety, and is cheap. However, in some patients, other treatments should be considered. If osteoporosis is severe with very low bone mineral density or multiple vertebral fractures, bone anabolic treatment with PTH should be considered. If the patient previously has suffered non-vertebral fractures or a hip fracture, treatments with documented antifracture efficacy against these types of fractures should be preferred; again, weekly alendronate would be the first choice. If the patient is treated with glucocorticoids, treatments with documented antifracture efficacy in glucocorticoid-induced osteoporosis should be preferred. If the patient is a man, treatments with documented antifracture efficacy in men should be preferred.

On top of these considerations, co-morbidity and the lifestyle of the patient should be taken into account. If the patient has a recent history of peptic ulcer or difficulties swallowing, oral bisphosphonates should be avoided. If the patient has a history of venous thromboembolism, selective oestrogen-receptor modulators and strontium ranelate should be avoided. If the patient needs to take medication before being able to get out of bed, for example pain killers, oral bisphosphonates are not going to work. If the patient has dementia or just difficulties remembering the days of the week, oral bisphosphonates are not going to work, unless a family member or a home nurse can help.

When a choice of treatment has been made and the patient has been properly instructed, long-term adherence to the treatment should be secured. This could involve education of the patient with respect to the disease and the treatment. A follow-up visit at the clinic within the first 3 months after starting treatment with or without measuring biochemical markers of bone turnover has been demonstrated to improve adherence. The patient should be informed that there are other treatments available if the patient experiences symptoms believed to be side effects. The long-term follow-up of these patients often involves regular consultations, and in some situations, DXA to monitor the response to the treatment and, for patients treated with alendronic acid or zoledronic acid, to identify patients for whom a treatment break can be considered (see Section 12.7 and Chapter 20, Figure 20.6).

Conclusion

Both anabolic and antiresorptive treatments with proven antifracture- efficacy and acceptable safety and tolerability are available for the prevention of the next fracture in patients with osteoporosis. However, osteoporosis is often overlooked and therefore the patients are far too often not offered these treatments. The patient with osteoporosis needs a thorough examination in order to characterize the type and severity of osteoporosis. On basis of this and information about co-morbidities and the patient's preferences, the right treatment for the individual patient should be chosen. Once treatment has been initiated, an effort should be made to ensure adherence to the treatment.

References and further reading

Bischoff-Ferrari HA, Willett WC, Wong JB, et al. Prevention of nonvertebral fractures with oral vitamin D and dose dependency: A meta-analysis of randomized controlled trials. *Arch Intern Med* 9009; 169: 551–61.

Black DM, Schwartz AV, Ensrud KE, et al. Effects of continuing or stopping alendronate after 5 years of treatment: The Fracture Intervention Trial Long-term Extension (FLEX): A randomized trial. *JAMA* 2006; 296: 2927–38.

Cummings SR, San Martin J, McCLung MR, et al. (2009) Denosumab for prevention of fractures in postmenopausal women with osteoporosis. *N Engl J Med* 2009; 361: 756–65.

Kanis JA, Melton LJ 3rd, Christiansen C, et al. The diagnosis of osteoporosis. *J Bone Miner Res* 1994; 9: 1137–41.

Klotzbuecher CM, Ross PD, Landsman PB, et al. Patients with prior fractures have an increased risk of future fractures: A summary of the literature and statistical synthesis. *J Bone Miner Res* 2000; 15: 721–39.

Michaelsson K, Melhus H, Ferm H, et al. Genetic liability to fractures in the elderly. *Arch Intern Med* 2005; 165: 1825–30.

Miller, PD and Papapoulos SE, eds. 'Osteoporosis', in Rosen CJ, Bouillon R, Compston JE, et al., eds, *Primer on the Metabolic Bone Diseases and Disorders of Mineral Metabolism* (8th edition), 2013. Wiley-Blackwell, pp. 343–534.

Neer RM, Arnaud CD, Zanchetta JR, et al. Effect of parathyroid hormone (1–34) on fractures and bone mineral density in postmenopausal women with osteoporosis. *N Engl J Med* 2001; 344: 1434–41.

Russell RG, Watts NB, Ebetino FH, et al. Mechanisms of action of bisphosphonates: Similarities and differences and their potential influence on clinical efficacy. *Osteoporos Int* 2008; 19: 733–59.

Siris ES, Harris ST, Rosen CJ, et al. Adherence to bisphosphonate therapy and fracture rates in osteoporotic women: Relationship to vertebral and nonvertebral fractures from 2 US claims databases. *Mayo Clin Proc* 2006; 81: 1013–22.

Tsourdi E, Langdahl BL, Cohen-Solal M, et al. Discontinuation of denosumab therapy for osteoporosis: A systematic review and position statement by ECTS. *Bone* 2017; 105: 11–17.

12.7 Focal bone disorders

Paget's disease of bone

Paget's disease of bone is a focal disorder of bone remodelling that progresses slowly and leads to changes in the shape and size of affected bones and to skeletal, articular, and vascular complications. In some parts of the world, it is the second most common bone disorder after osteoporosis. The disease is easily diagnosed and effectively treated but its pathogenesis remains incompletely understood.

Epidemiology of Paget's disease

Paget's disease affects typically the elderly, slightly more men than women, and seldom presents before the age of 35 years. Its prevalence increases with age and it affects 1%–5% of those above 50 years of age. There is a distinct geographical distribution and there may also be significant variations in its prevalence in regions of the same country. In recent years, a decline in the prevalence of the disease has been reported in some, but not all, countries and it appears that the clinical severity of the disease has been attenuated. These changes in prevalence and severity of the disease strongly suggest that environmental factors are involved in its pathogenesis.

Pathophysiology of Paget's disease

Paget's disease of bone is characterized by an increase in the number and size of osteoclasts in affected sites whilst the rest of the skeleton remains normal. The typically large multinucleated osteoclasts induce excessive bone resorption associated with increased recruitment of osteoblasts to the remodelling sites, resulting in increased bone formation. This accelerated rate of bone turnover is responsible for the deposition of bone with disorganized architecture and structural weakness. Osteoclasts and their precursors and marrow stromal cells from patients with the disease express high levels of the bone-resorbing factors interleukin 6 and RANKL, respectively, which contribute to the upregulation of osteoclastogenesis. In addition, bone marrow and peripheral cells from patients are hypersensitive to the action of RANKL and calcitriol. The precise mechanism(s) that trigger these changes remain to be elucidated.

Several, hypotheses have been proposed to explain the pathology of the disease, the most relevant being the viral and the genetic. An infection by a slow virus of the paramyxovirus family was supported by some studies but a search for viral presence in pagetic osteoclasts provided conflicting results. There is good evidence, however, that paramyxoviruses and viral proteins can promote the formation of osteoclasts with features similar to those of pagetic osteoclasts. The risk that first-degree relatives of patients with Paget's disease develop the disorder is seven to ten times greater than that for age- and sex-matched controls, and a positive family history has been reported in up to 40% of patients. Familial Paget's disease is inherited as an autosomal-dominant trait but initial analyses indicated genetic heterogeneity. Studies in different parts of the world have identified mutations in *SQSTM1*, which is located at chromosomal position 5q35, in up to 40% of patients with familial Paget's disease and in up to 10% of those with sporadic disease. *SQSTM1* mutations activate the nuclear factor kappa B pathway and increase osteoclast formation. Recent large genetic studies of patients with Paget's disease and no mutations in *SQSTM1* identified seven loci that contribute substantially to the risk of developing the disease. These genetic variants include genes that are known to play important roles in regulating osteoclast differentiation and function but also include genes not previously implicated in the regulation of bone metabolism. The functional significance of these polymorphisms is still unknown. The current view is, therefore, that the disease is caused by interactions between environmental and genetic factors, the nature of which remains to be determined.

Clinical features of Paget's disease

In Paget's disease, the most commonly affected bones are the pelvis, the spine, the femora, and the skull but practically any bone of the skeleton may be affected. About one-third of patients have only one lesion but the frequency of single lesions varies among series, reflecting probably referral patterns, and is higher in asymptomatic patients. The anatomical spread of the disease is not related to age or gender, shows no particular symmetry in the body, and remains largely unchanged throughout life. The disease progresses slowly within an affected bone but does not generally appear in other bones. Patients with limited bone involvement should, therefore, be reassured that the disease will not progress to other bones with time.

The majority of patients are asymptomatic, and the disease may be diagnosed incidentally by skeletal radiographs during the investigation of an unrelated complaint or by the finding of an unexplained elevation of serum alkaline phosphatase activity. Pain is the presenting complaint in the majority of symptomatic patients. It is related to the extent and site of the disease, is usually persistent and present at rest, but is not specific. Pain due to secondary osteoarthritis is common and may hamper assessment of the relative contribution of bone and joint pains to the patient's disability. The origin of such pain can be assessed only retrospectively after treatment which reduces mainly the disease-related pain. Deformities are present in about 15% of patients at the time of diagnosis and affect mainly weight-bearing bones (Figure 12.9a). About 9% of patients present with fractures that can be complete or fissure fractures (Figure 12.9b). The skin overlying an affected bone may be warm as a result of increased blood flow and bone turnover locally, and hypervascularity of affected bones may cause ischaemia of adjacent structures (steal syndrome). Irreversible hearing loss is the most common neurological complication, occurring in about one-third of patients with skull involvement. Malignant transformation of pagetic bone and development of osteosarcoma is a rare (less than 1%) but extremely serious complication.

Investigations for Paget's disease

Radiographic changes are characteristic of the pathophysiology of Paget's disease. Increased bone resorption may be detected as a decrease in the density of affected bones; sometimes, a wedge- or flame-shaped segment of bone resorption may be seen in the long bones, and there may be extensive osteolytic areas in the skull (osteoporosis circumscripta). Older lesions usually have a mixed sclerotic and lytic appearance and, in the last stage of the disease, sclerotic lesions predominate. The involved parts of the skeleton are enlarged and deformed, and the

(a)   (b)

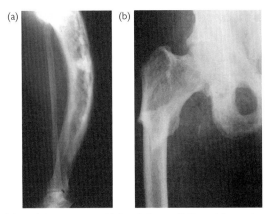

Fig 12.9 (a) Radiograph of a deformed tibia in a patient with Paget's disease. (b) Femoral fracture in a patient with Paget's disease of the pelvis and the hip.

cortex can be thickened and dense. Bone scintigraphy is used to assess the extent of the disease but is not specific. Bone scintigraphy should always be included in the investigation of patients with Paget's disease, and radiographs of the areas of increased radioisotope uptake should be subsequently made to confirm the diagnosis (see Figure 12.10).

The pathology of Paget's disease is reflected in the proportional increase in biochemical markers of bone resorption and formation. These can be markedly increased in patients with extensive disease but can also be within the reference range in patients with limited bone involvement. The most sensitive biochemical markers of bone formation are bone-specific alkaline phosphatase and P1NP; the most sensitive biochemical markers of bone resorption are peptides of the cross-linking domains of collagen type 1, such as NTX or CTX. In clinical practice, total serum alkaline phosphatase activity in the presence of normal levels of liver enzymes is still an adequate marker for assessing the biochemical activity of the disease. Hypercalcaemia may develop in immobilized patients with active, extensive disease or may be due to concurrent primary hyperparathyroidism, the incidence of which is thought to be higher in Paget's disease. Hypercalciuria and renal stone disease occur more frequently in patients with Paget's disease, and secondary hyperparathyroidism is present in about 20% of patients.

Management of Paget's disease

Bisphosphonates are currently the treatment of choice of Paget's disease. Treatment with potent bisphosphonates relieves symptoms, restores bone abnormalities, and improves radiological appearances. Moreover, complications can be prevented if bone turnover is adequately suppressed. However, firm evidence from prospective randomized controlled trials is lacking. Changes of bone remodelling after bisphosphonate treatment of patients with Paget's disease follow a predictable pattern, with an early decrease in the rate of bone resorption followed by a slower decrease in the rate of bone formation due to the coupling between these two processes. It is, therefore, unnecessary to prolong treatment until the lowest level of serum alkaline phosphatase is reached, and short courses of bisphosphonates are sufficient to achieve biochemical remission assessed in practice by measurements of serum alkaline phosphatase activity. Nowadays, efficacy of treatment is assessed only by its ability to decrease serum alkaline phosphatase values to the normal range (see Figure 12.11). In clinical practice, there is no need to measure serum alkaline phosphatase activity earlier than 3 months after the start of treatment, with 6 months being the optimal time.

Clinical responses to treatment include the disappearance or clear improvement of pain in more than 80% of treated patients, when the pain is due to the activity of the disease. A decrease of bone pain is generally observed 1–3 months after the start of treatment, and the effect is maximal after 6 months and is maintained for as long as biochemical markers of bone turnover remain within the normal range. Soon after the start of therapy with a potent bisphosphonate, there may be a transient increase in pain at affected sites, and patients should be reassured. Pain due to osteoarthritis is unresponsive to treatment in about 75% of patients; NSAIDs can then be used. If the hip joint is affected, hip arthroplasty may be required to control the symptoms. Back pain resulting from involvement of lumbar vertebrae is frequently not relieved by treatment. About half of the patients with pain-associated deformity of the femur or the tibia will respond favourably to bisphosphonate therapy, but pain may persist and a corrective osteotomy may be necessary. Deafness is usually not affected but its progression appears to be arrested. Fracture frequency of pagetic bones appears to decrease with treatment and there have been reports of improvement of spinal cord compression with bisphosphonate therapy.

Improvement in bone histology and formation of bone with normal lamellar structure has been reported with currently used bisphosphonates. Radiologically, an arrest of the progression of the disease is usually seen. Radiological improvement can be, however, dramatic if lesions are lytic and are localized in the long bones or in the skull. These clinical, histological, and radiological responses emphasize the need for an intervention with a bisphosphonate before the development of

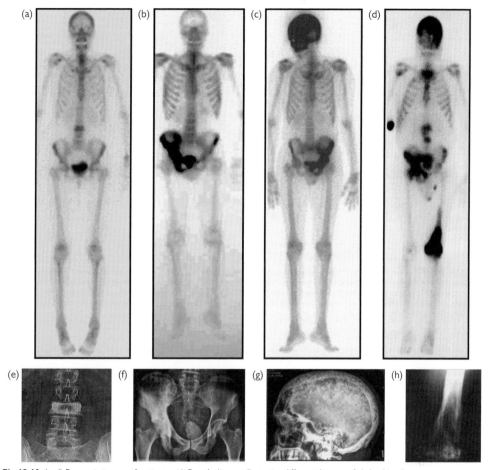

Fig 12.10 (a–d) Bone scintigrams of patients with Paget's disease, illustrating different degrees of skeletal involvement. (e–h) Radiographs of patients with Paget's diseases illustrating the typical changes of the disease. These correspond to the bone scintigrams shown in Panels a–d. Note the flame-shaped lesion in the distal femur in Panel h.

complications. The following treatment indications are currently recommended:

- symptomatic disease
- preoperatively, in preparation for an orthopaedic procedure on pagetic bone, to reduce increased blood flow and excessive bleeding
- asymptomatic patients with skeletal localizations at higher risk of complications, such as those adjacent to large joints, in the skull, the spine, and weight-bearing bones
- young patients

All bisphosphonates given to patients with Paget's disease significantly decrease biochemical markers of bone turnover but there are considerable differences in their ability to induce remission. Generally, potent bisphosphonates induce better responses. Of these, a single, short, intravenous infusion of zoledronic acid, 5 mg, is currently considered the treatment of choice because it induces biochemical remission in nearly all treated patients, it improves certain aspects of the quality of life of patients, and its effect persists for

many years. Oral risedronate, 30 mg/day for 2 months, is a less effective alternative.

Remissions can be long, and recurrences occur slowly; follow-up of patients in remission is, therefore, indicated every 12 months. The duration of remission is determined by the degree of suppression of serum alkaline phosphatase activity and the number of affected bones. The lower the serum alkaline phosphatase activity reached with treatment, the longer is the period of remission. Suppression of serum alkaline phosphatase activity well within the normal range is a prerequisite for long-term remission and should be an aim of treatment.

Risks of treatment for Paget's disease

Impaired mineralization of newly formed bone, osteomalacia, is relevant only for etidronate, which is not used any more. Impaired bone mineralization has also been reported in a few patients treated with high doses intravenous pamidronate and is reversible. Hypocalcaemia may develop, particularly in elderly

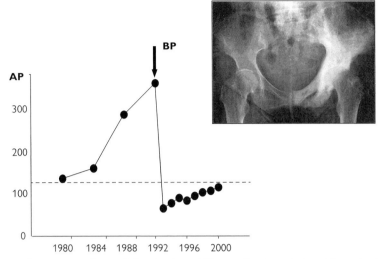

Fig 12.11 Sequential measurements of serum alkaline phosphatase (AP) activity (in units per litre) over 20 years in a 51-year-old woman with Paget's disease of the pelvis. Note the slow progression of the disease when left untreated, and the rapid and sustained decrease in serum AP after treatment with bisphosphonate (BP). At the time of intervention, the patient had already developed secondary osteoarthritis (see inset) and required total hip replacement to control her symptoms. The interrupted line depicts the upper limit of the reference range of AP.
Reproduced from John A.H. Wass, Paul M. Stewart, Stephanie A. Amiel et al, *Oxford Textbook of Endocrinology and Diabetes, Second edition*, Fig. 4.9.1, Copyright © 2011 with permission from Oxford University Press.

patients with high rates of bone turnover and who are frequently vitamin D deficient. Adequate supplementation with vitamin D and calcium should, therefore, be given to all patients.

In some patients treated for the first time with nitrogen-containing bisphosphonates, there is a rise in body temperature and flu-like symptoms during the first 3 days of treatment. These symptoms are transient and subside with no specific measures, even when treatment is continued. This response is dose-dependent and is associated more frequently with intravenous treatment than wth oral treatment. Moreover, it does not generally appear upon retreatment and, if it does, it is of lower intensity. Previous exposure to another nitrogen-containing bisphosphonate, but not to etidronate, generally precludes the development of this response. Laboratory findings are consistent with an acute-phase reaction related to the mechanism of action of nitrogen-containing bisphosphonates. Rarely, high doses of such bisphosphonates may induce ophthalmic reactions such as conjunctivitis, iritis, or uveitis. There are case reports of ototoxicity and central nervous toxicity after intravenous pamidronate. Allergic skin reactions have been occasionally observed with most of the bisphosphonates. Osteonecrosis of the jaw is extremely rare in patients with Paget's disease treated with either oral or intravenous bisphosphonates.

Future developments for Paget's disease
Because of the efficacy and tolerability of bisphosphonate treatment, and the long-term persistence of the effect without need for additional treatment, there is no need for new medications for the treatment of patients with Paget's disease. However, bisphosphonates, particularly zoledronic acid, are not indicated in patients with renal impairment (creatinine clearance less than 35 mL/minute). In such patients, anecdotal evidence suggests that treatment with an inhibitor of RANKL, denosumab, may be effective.

Fibrous dysplasia
Fibrous dysplasia of bone is a rare skeletal disorder with a broad clinical spectrum and severity, sometimes associated with extraskeletal manifestations. The disease may involve one skeletal site and be asymptomatic, or it may involve multiple sites and be associated with severe disability. It is caused by activating mutations of *GNAS*, which encodes the alpha subunit of the stimulatory G protein.

Epidemiology of fibrous dysplasia
The prevalence of fibrous dysplasia is unknown but it has been estimated that it affects 1 in 30,000 individuals and there is no geographic variation. It presents in childhood in about 80% of patients but it can be recognized at any age, and men and women are equally affected.

Pathophysiology of fibrous dysplasia
Fibrous dysplasia is characterized by the abnormal proliferation and differentiation of bone-marrow stromal cells, leading to an accumulation of fibrous tissue in the bone marrow. The tissue is highly vascularized and prone to bleeding. The disease is due to activating mutations in *GNAS*; these lead to the overproduction of cAMP and to abnormal cellular responses such as potentiation of the canonical Wnt signalling pathway in osteoblast progenitors, and an increased production of the bone-resorbing factors interleukin 6 and RANKL. Broader distribution of the mutation leads to a genetic, non-inheritable disease which also involves other organs.

Clinical features of fibrous dysplasia

Fibrous dysplasia is often asymptomatic, involves only one bone in about 60% of patients, and may be discovered incidentally in radiographs performed for other reasons. The skull and the proximal femur are most frequently affected but the disease may localize in any bone of the skeleton. Polyostotic disease is usually unilateral and, like Paget's disease, may progress within an affected bone but not to other bones with time. Bone pain, deformity, and fractures are the most common clinical features. In the skull, fibrous dysplasia involves the skull base and facial bones, leading to facial asymmetry in childhood; this may progress to significant disfiguration, especially when the disease is accompanied by growth hormone excess, and entrapment of cranial nerves. In about 5% of patients, fibrous dysplasia may be associated with extraskeletal lesions or dysfunctions. The combination of fibrous dysplasia, café-au-lait lesions with jagged 'coast of Maine' borders, precocious puberty, and hyperthyroidism was originally termed McCune–Albright syndrome. With time, a number of other manifestations were added to the spectrum of disorders that could be associated with fibrous dysplasia. These include growth hormone excess, hypercortisolism, hypophosphataemia/osteomalacia, testicular hypertrophy, gastrointestinal polyps in unusual locations, and hepatic and cardiac abnormalities. Rarely, fibrous dysplasia may be associated with myxomas of skeletal muscle (Mazabraud's syndrome). Malignant transformation of bone lesions is rare (<1%).

Investigations for of fibrous dysplasia

Fibrous dysplasia is diagnosed radiographically. Appearances vary according to age and degree of sclerosis of the lesions. Typical lesions expand from the medulla to the cortex, which is considerably thinned. Some lesions are radiolucent, whilst others have a ground-glass appearance (see Figure 12.12). Vertebral localizations often present as lytic lesions mimicking malignant tumours or angiomatous conditions, whilst skull lesions are usually sclerotic, resembling those of Paget's disease. Bone scintigraphy is the most sensitive technique for detecting fibrous dysplasia lesions. Biochemical markers of bone turnover are usually increased in patients with polyostotic disease. Endocrine investigations are essential in patients with suspected McCune–Albright syndrome. In some patients, the disease may be accompanied by hypophosphataemia, which is occasionally associated with osteomalacia. This is due to renal phosphate loss resulting from excessive production of FGF23 by the lesions.

Management of fibrous dysplasia

The management of fibrous dysplasia consists of pain treatment and medical and surgical interventions. Pain, independent of fracture, can be severe, and NSAIDs and opiates are required. Intravenous pamidronate has been reported in uncontrolled studies to have a significant effect on pain in a substantial proportion of patients. However, patients unresponsive to this treatment have also been reported. Similar results have been obtained with intravenous zoledronic acid and oral alendronic acid. Bisphosphonates reduce biochemical markers of bone turnover and have also been reported to improve the radiographic appearance of lytic lesions in some patients. The use of calcium and vitamin D supplements is essential in patients with deficiencies, whilst phosphate supplements (with calcitriol) have been recommended for patients with hypophosphatemia treated with bisphosphonates. Coexistent endocrinopathies are treated as indicated. Notably, administration of oestrogen-containing contraceptives can lead to exacerbation of bone symptoms, and exacerbation of bone symptoms is also reported during pregnancy in some patients. Young women with fibrous dysplasia should be advised to use other means of contraception.

Risks of treatment for fibrous dysplasia

The risks of bisphosphonate treatment are described in 'Risks of treatment for Paget's disease'.

Future developments for fibrous dysplasia

The lack of controlled studies with bisphosphonates and their limited efficacy in a subset of patients, combined with the severity of symptoms, disability, and

(a)
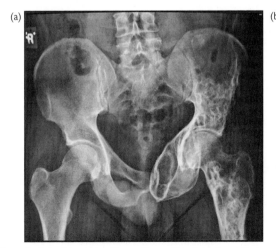
(b)
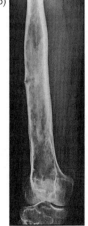

Fig 12.12 (a) Fibrous dysplasia of the pelvis and upper femur, with typical radiographic changes. (b) Radiograph of the femur of a patient with fibrous dysplasia, showing the expansion of the medullary space, thinning of the cortex, and a diaphyseal insufficiency fracture.

poor quality of life of some patients, have led to an exploration of more specific treatments for fibrous dysplasia. Such treatments include inhibitors of interleukin 6 and RANKL.

Osteonecrosis

Osteonecrosis, (also called avascular, ischaemic, or aseptic necrosis) is a focal bone disease affecting most commonly the hip and associated with pain, disability, bone collapse, and osteoarthritis. It is due to interruption of the blood supply and local cellular death.

Epidemiology of osteonecrosis

Osteonecrosis has been earlier reported to affect 10,000–20,000 new individuals annually in the US and most commonly follows trauma such as displaced subcapital fractures of the hip. Atraumatic osteonecrosis affects men more often than women; it can be bilateral and occurs primarily in patients aged 30–50 years. Osteonecrosis of the femoral head in children is known as Legg–Calve–Perthes disease.

Pathophysiology of osteonecrosis

Fracture or dislocation may cause osteonecrosis by interrupting the blood supply, leading to bone death and collapse. If it affects bones in a joint, such as the hip, it often leads to destruction of the joint articular surface. A number of risk factors contribute to atraumatic osteonecrosis, such as excessive alcohol consumption, clotting disorders, sickle cell disease, Gaucher's disease, organ transplantation, and deep diving. Mechanisms implicated in the pathogenesis of osteonecrosis include intravascular thrombosis, arterial embolism, fatigue fractures, and osteocyte apoptosis. In about 20% of patients with atraumatic osteonecrosis, no risk factors are identified (idiopathic). Of special interest to endocrinologists is osteonecrosis associated with the use of glucocorticoids; this condition is related to the dose and length of treatment and is attributed to apoptosis of osteocytes by glucocorticoids. Intra-articular glucocorticoids have also been implicated in the pathogenesis of the disease. The term osteonecrosis is also used to describe a disorder that is specific to the jaw and differs from that occurring in other bones: osteonecrosis of the jaw, which is defined as the presence of exposed bone in the mandible, maxilla, or both, persisting for at least 8 weeks, in the absence of previous irradiation or metastases in the jaw. It has been reported mainly in patients who have a malignant disease and are receiving high intravenous doses of bisphosphonates, denosumab, or antiangiogenic agents but the background incidence in the population and its pathogenesis are poorly defined. In patients with osteoporosis treated with bisphosphonates, osteonecrosis of the jaw is rare, with an estimated incidence ranging from 1/10,000 to <1/100,000 patient years, although this appears to increase with increasing duration of treatment. Recently, cases of osteonecrosis of the jaw were reported in patients with osteoporosis treated with denosumab.

Clinical features of osteonecrosis

The main symptom of osteonecrosis is pain, especially with joint movement, tenderness, and restricted motion; the pain is relieved by rest. The intensity of pain increases with the progressive collapse of the bone. Osteonecrosis of the humeral head often causes less pain and disability than that of the hip or the knee.

Investigations for osteonecrosis

Plain radiographs of patients with osteonecrosis are unremarkable in the early stages of the disease. Late radiographic signs include sclerotic and radiolucent areas following the collapse of subchondral bone (Figure 12.13a). Bone scintigraphy shows increased uptake of the isotope at early stages of the disease but is not specific. MRI is the most sensitive technique for diagnosing the disease, showing bone-marrow oedema at the initial stage of the disease and demonstrating necrosis before any detectable changes of the shape of the bone. The presence of bone-marrow oedema is, however, not specific and, in the absence of risk factors, hip osteonecrosis should be differentiated from transient osteoporosis of the hip. This presents usually in middle-aged men and has symptoms similar to those of osteonecrosis; its pathogenesis is unknown. Measurements of bone mineral density can be diagnostic. In transient osteoporosis of the hip, there is a significant decrease of the bone mineral density of the affected hip compared

(a)

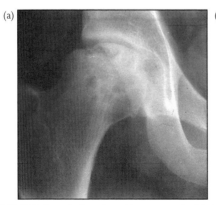

(b)

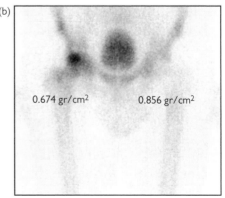

0.674 gr/cm^2 0.856 gr/cm^2

Fig 12.13 (a) Radiograph of a patient with osteonecrosis of the hip, following renal transplantation, with lytic and sclerotic areas and collapse of the head of the femur. (b) Three-phase bone scintigram of a man with severe pain of the right loin, showing increased uptake of the isotope in the right hip. Bone mineral density values of the femoral neck, also depicted in the figure, show marked differences which are diagnostic of transient osteoporosis of the hip.

to the unaffected one whereas, in osteonecrosis, there is no difference between the bone mineral densities of the two hips (Figure 12.13b). Biochemical markers of bone turnover are generally within the reference range in patients with osteonecrosis.

Management of osteonecrosis
Depending on the stage of the disease, management of osteonecrosis includes conservative measures (e.g. rest, physical therapy, NSAIDs), surgical decompression to promote healing, and total hip replacement or other surgical interventions. Osteonecrosis of the hip is the most common cause of total hip replacement in young adults. Bisphosphonates, particularly when administered at early stages of the disease, may improve symptoms and reduce the need for total hip replacement. Progression of the disease could possibly be halted by autologous transplantation of bone-marrow-derived mesenchymal stem cells, a procedure which is currently under investigation.

Further reading

Albagha OME, Wani S, Visconti MR, et al. Genome-wide association identifies three new susceptibility loci for Paget's disease of bone. *Nature Gen* 2011; 43: 685–9.

Chapurlat RD and Orcel P. Fibrous dysplasia of bone and McCune-Albright syndrome *Best Pract Res Clin Rheum*, 2008; 22: 55–69.

Collins MT, Riminucci M, Bianco. 'Fibrous dysplasia', in Rosen CJ, ed., *Primer on Metabolic Bone Diseases and Disorders of Mineral Metabolism* (7th edition), 2008. Wiley–Blackwell, pp. 423–27.

Collins MT, Singer FR, and Eugster E. McCune-Albright syndrome and the extraskeletal manifestations of fibrous dysplasia. 2012. *Orphanet J Rare Dis* 2012; 7: S4.

Emad Y, Ragab Y, El-Shaarawy N, et al. Transient osteoporosis of the hip, complete resolution after treatment with alendronate as observed by MRI description of eight cases and review of the literature. *Clin Rheumatol* 2012; 31: 1641–7.

Kaushik AP, Das A, Quanjun C. Osteonecrosis of the femoral head: An update in year 2012. *World J Orthop* 2012; 18: 49–57.

Papapoulos SE. 'Paget's disease of bone', in Wasss AH and Stewart P, eds, *Oxford Textbook of Endocrinology and Diabetes* (2nd edition), 2011. Oxford University Press, pp. 721–30.

Reid IR, Lyles K, Su G, et al. A single infusion of zoledronic acid produces sustained remissions in Paget disease: Data to 6.5 years. *J Bone Miner Res* 2011; 26: 2261–70.

Rizzoli R, Burlet N, Cahall D, et al. The risk of developing osteonecrosis of the jaw in patients with osteoporosis treated with bisphosphonates: A report from ESCEO. *Bone* 2008; 42: 841–7.

Weinstein RS. Glucocorticoid-induced osteoporosis and osteonecrosis. *Endocrinol Metab Clin N Am* 2012; 41: 595–611.

12.8 Osteogenesis imperfecta

Definitions

Osteogenesis imperfecta is a heritable connective tissue disorder characterized by low bone mass and bone fragility due to defects in type 1 collagen production. The condition encompasses a wide clinical spectrum from antenatal lethality to ostensibly 'normal' individuals with small numbers of fractures. There is debate as to the extent to which the underlying genetic defect should be taken into account in the classification of osteogenesis imperfecta. However, nosology has generally been based on clinical or histological features (see Table 12.5).

Pathophysiology and genetics

The vast majority of cases of osteogenesis imperfecta (85%–90%) are due to mutations in COL1A1 and COL1A2, which are expressed in osteoblasts and chondrocytes. These genes code for the collagen 1 alpha 1 and collagen 1 alpha 2 propeptides, respectively, which combine in a 2:1 ratio to form a triple helix. This type 1 procollagen molecule is exported from the cell and further processed before its association with other type 1 collagen molecules in a staggered arrangement to form fibrils. Defects in COL1A1 or COL1A2 can result in quantitative and qualitative defects of type 1 collagen, depending on the nature of the mutation. Quantitative defects arise from a null mutation and typically result in the phenotype of type 1 osteogenesis imperfecta. Qualitative or structural defects, most commonly due to a glycine substitution (80%), result in post-translational overmodification of procollagen. The incorporation of these affected molecules into collagen fibrils in the extracellular matrix tends to result in moderate to severe osteogenesis imperfecta phenotypes. Various molecules are involved in the post-translational folding, modification, and processing of type 1 procollagen, including the components of the prolyl 3-hydroxylase complex (prolyl 3-hydroxylase 1 (encoded by P3H1), cartilage-associated protein (encoded by CRTAP), cyclophilin B (encoded by PPIB)) and other chaperone proteins (e.g. serpin H1 (encoded by SERPINH1), and FK506-binding protein 10 (encoded by FKBP10)). Over the last few years, mutations in the genes coding for these and other molecules have been identified in a

Table 12.5 Classification and genetic origin of the commonest types of osteogenesis imperfecta

Condition	Phenotype in childhood	Genetic origin
Osteogenesis imperfecta type 1	Mild motor delay	Null allele of COL1A1, resulting from stop, frameshift, or splice-site mutations
	Ligamentous laxity	
	Hernias	
	Deafness	
	Blue sclerae	
	Bowing of long bones and vertebral crush fractures variable	
Osteogenesis imperfecta type 2	Lethal	Missense mutations in COL1A1 or COL1A2
	Subdivided by appearance of ribs	Complete loss of CRTAP, PPIB, or LEPRE1
Osteogenesis imperfecta type 3	Severe	Missense mutations in COL1A1 or COL1A2
	Progressively deforming	Null allele of COL1A2
	Typically fractures in utero	Mutations in CRTAP, PPIB, LEPRE1, SERPINH1, or FKBP10
	Very poor growth/short stature	
	Characteristic facies with small mid-face and pointed chin	
	Very delayed motor development	
	All have dentinogenesis imperfecta	
Osteogenesis imperfecta type 4	Moderately severe	Missense mutations in COL1A1, COL1A2
	May have fractures in utero, but better postnatal growth than in osteogenesis imperfecta type 3	
	Blue sclerae; these fade with age	
	May have dentinogenesis imperfecta	
Osteogenesis imperfecta type 5	Moderately severe	Mutation in 5′-untranslated region of IFITM5
	Metaphyseal sclerosis and calcification of interosseous membranes in the forearm and lower leg	
	Characteristic bowing of the forearms	
	Hypertrophic callus formation	
Osteogenesis imperfecta type 6	Severe	SERPINF1
	Progressively deforming	
	Osteomalacic appearance on bone biopsy	

Data from: Sillence DO, Senn A, Danks DM, Genetic heterogeneity in osteogenesis imperfecta, Journal of Medical Genetics, 1979, Volume 16, Issue 2, pp. 101–116; Rauch F, Glorieux FH, Osteogenesis imperfecta, Lancet, 2004, Volume 363, pp. 1377–85.

variety of rare cases of recessively inherited (typically severe) cases of osteogenesis imperfecta. Other molecular mechanisms for osteogenesis imperfecta include defects in osteoblast function and other aspects of bone formation. The genetic defect in the autosomal-dominant osteogenesis imperfecta type 5 has been identified as a mutation in the 5′-untranslated region of *IFITM5*, which encodes interferon-induced transmembrane protein 5. Osteogenesis imperfecta type 6 is caused by mutations in *SERPINF1*, which encodes the secreted protein pigment epithelium-derived factor (PEDF), an inhibitor of angiogenesis. This has opened up the prospect of a biochemical diagnosis by measurement of reduced serum PEDF concentrations and future treatment with a recombinant protein. It is important to realize that, in general, the bone fragility in osteogenesis imperfecta derives not only from the primary structural or quantitative defects in type 1 collagen but multiple other features of the condition, including high bone turnover, osteoblast dysfunction, matrix abnormalities, and abnormal mineralization.

Epidemiology and clinical features

Osteogenesis imperfecta is a rare condition, estimated to have a prevalence of around 1 in 10,000–20,000 in the general population and is found in all races. The majority of cases, perhaps two-thirds, have a 'mild' phenotype, although such a description belies the impact that the condition can have on individuals. The main features of various types of osteogenesis imperfecta are summarized in Table 12.5. Bony deformities can be obvious or may be more subtle (e.g. minor anterior femoral bowing).

Hypermobility is common and can contribute significantly to delayed motor development. Children with type 1 osteogenesis imperfecta are often relatively late to walk and may need orthotics to support 'flat feet'. In more severe cases, motor development is often largely dependent on fractures, bony deformities, and timing of surgery. Pain is another significant feature of osteogenesis imperfecta and commonly limits mobility. The degree of pain and related limitation are sometimes only evident after medical treatment has provided relief from long-standing discomfort. Hypermobility and the effect of osteogenesis imperfecta on other soft tissues can result in joint dislocations and hernias. Sclerae commonly have a bluish tinge in type 1 osteogenesis imperfecta but this is not pathognomic, especially in infants <6 months old, in whom bluish sclera are common. Dentinogenesis imperfecta is caused by the presence of abnormal collagen in the dentin and is variably present, the frequency depending on the type of osteogenesis imperfecta. Even in the absence of obvious dentinogenesis imperfecta, teeth may chip or crack easily. Hearing impairment is common in osteogenesis imperfecta, as a result of both conductive and sensorineural deficits, and there is an increased incidence of ocular problems. Thus, from the second decade, both audiological screening and regular review by an optician are prudent.

Important skeletal complications include scoliosis and deformity of the skull base. Regular monitoring of the spine is a key role for the responsible physician. Scoliosis is likely to progress once it reaches a Cobb angle of 40°. This has implications for cardiopulmonary health, an important determinant of mortality and morbidity in osteogenesis imperfecta. Abnormalities of the skull can include widely patent fontanelles and sutural diastasis in infancy but, additionally, hydrocephalus is a recognized complication. Skull-base deformities, including platybasia and basilar invagination (the migration of the upper cervical vertebrae into the depression left by the elevated floor of the posterior cranial fossa), can result in compression of the cervical cord and disturbance of CSF flow. The clinician must therefore be on guard for suggestive symptoms, and radiological screening may be justified.

Features of certain types of osteogenesis imperfecta types can direct towards a particular diagnosis (e.g. long phalanges in *LEPRE1* mutations). Osteogenesis imperfecta type 5 is characterized by disordered control of endochondral bone formation. A rachitic appearance of the metaphyses has been observed in early infancy and, later, interosseous membrane calcification and hypertrophic callus formation at fracture and osteotomy sites. Surgeons need to be aware of this, since therapy with indomethacin either post-operatively or after fracture can reduce the risk of massive hyperplastic callus formation. It is important not to mistake hyperplastic callus for a malignancy, in order to avoid unnecessary investigation or even surgery. Histologic bone samples from patients with osteogenesis imperfecta type 6 show a 'fish-scale' pattern under polarized light, with accumulation of osteoid. Individuals with this type of osteogenesis imperfecta often respond relatively poorly to bisphosphonates.

Investigations

The diagnosis of osteogenesis imperfecta is generally based on clinical findings. Radiology can be diagnostic in severe cases and can provide supportive information in milder cases (e.g. Wormian bones) in infancy. DXA scanning has limited value as an aid to diagnosis; bone mineral density can be normal in type 1 osteogenesis imperfecta. However, DXA provides important data for monitoring the effect of medical therapy. The value of biochemical tests is similar, with elevated measures of bone formation and resorption sometimes providing useful supportive data. Confirmatory diagnostic testing for osteogenesis imperfecta is either by analysis of genomic DNA or RNA, or by analysis of type 1 procollagen expression in fibroblasts. DNA analysis can be done on samples of blood or saliva, whilst RNA and collagen analyses require culture of fibroblasts obtained by skin biopsy. Presently, no single test is sufficient to meet all clinical needs. Direct sequencing is now available for all recognized types of osteogenesis imperfecta. However, the process of sequencing *COL1A1* and *COL1A2* remains costly. This is likely to change with the increasing availability of next-generation sequencing technology. Percutaneous transiliac bone biopsy with tetracycline double labelling can provide useful diagnostic information but is invasive.

Management

In general, a multidisciplinary team approach, incorporating at least nurses, therapists, surgeons, and physicians, is essential to achieve optimal outcomes for individuals with osteogenesis imperfecta. In many cases of type 1 osteogenesis imperfecta, specific medical treatment of the bone disease is not necessary, and management is directed towards problems arising from hypermobility, for example the need for orthotics and physiotherapy. Regarding physical activity, whilst a degree of caution is warranted in terms of avoiding contact sports and activities that risk damaging vertebrae, activity is to be encouraged for the benefits that accrue regarding muscle strength, balance, and psychosocial well-being. With greater degrees of severity of osteogenesis imperfecta, the problems of mobility, seating, and self-care become more pronounced, and the input of experienced physiotherapists and occupational therapists becomes invaluable. Medical treatment should be considered in cases that are moderately or severely affected or cases of type 1 osteogenesis imperfecta with changes in vertebral morphology, repeated lower limb fractures, or significant chronic pain not relieved by simple analgesia.

Bisphosphonates

Bisphosphonates are now widely recognized as the medical standard of care in osteogenesis imperfecta. They have been shown to increase bone mass, reduce bone pain, and improve vertebral size and shape and may improve growth. To realize the maximum benefits of bisphosphonates, it is important that they are used alongside the multidisciplinary approach outlined above. Intravenous bisphosphonates used in osteogenesis imperfecta include zoledronic acid and neridronic acid but the most widely used bisphosphonate in childhood osteogenesis imperfecta has been pamidronate. Recently, ease of administration has led to the increased use of oral bisphosphonates, particularly in less severe cases, but the data on effectiveness with regard to pain relief and improvement of vertebral morphology has not been as strong as for intravenous bisphosphonates. However, oral therapy in mild osteogenesis imperfecta with risedronate appears to be safe and effective at reducing the risk of fracture, and a dose of 1 mg/kg per week can increase bone mass in line with age, although higher doses may be required in more severe cases. Zoledronic acid has become the first-choice bisphosphonate in many centres, due to the convenience of infrequent and short infusions, despite some concerns about its relatively high mineral affinity. Apart from type of bisphosphonate, there is no clear consensus on dose, frequency of dosing, dose adjustment, and when to discontinue treatment. There are data

to suggest that the greatest gains in bone mineral density have taken place by 2–4 years of treatment but the tendency to increased bone turnover and fracture does not disappear after this time, and discontinuation may lead to increased pain or fracture at the interface of treated and untreated bone. In paediatric practice, it must be borne in mind that growth is a unique opportunity to optimize skeletal health and vertebral shape. The dose of pamidronate currently being used in different paediatric centres ranges from 4 to 12 mg/kg per year, and duration of treatment varies from 2 years to the completion of growth and beyond. Common acute effects of bisphosphonate administration include an acute-phase reaction with the first cycle of infusions, and transient, usually mild and asymptomatic, hypocalcaemia. There are other idiosyncratic adverse events reported, such as scleritis and nephritis. The residency of bisphosphonates in the skeleton has given rise to concerns about long-term effects such as undertubulation of bones, retention of calcified cartilage, increased risk of osteonecrosis of the jaw, 'atypical' femoral fractures, and poor healing of osteotomies. It is likely that cumulative dose is a key determinant of both benefit and risk of certain long-term adverse outcomes. Female patients should be cautioned against becoming pregnant on bisphosphonates. Vitamin D homeostasis and adequacy should be monitored, as insufficiency may impair the skeletal response to bisphosphonate therapy.

Surgery

Although the majority of individuals with osteogenesis imperfecta can be managed conservatively, often surgery is required to attain reduction of a deformity and improved function. Correction of long-bone deformities has traditionally been achieved with osteotomies and intramedullary rodding (see Figure 12.14) but distraction

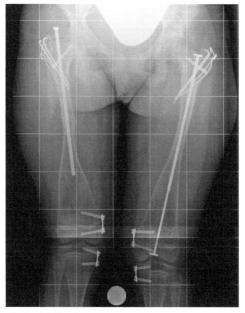

Fig 12.14 Radiograph of the lower limbs of child with osteogenesis imperfecta, showing intramedullary rodding and '8' plates for deformity correction. The undertubulation is due to bisphosphonate therapy.

osteogenesis has been used to correct limb-length discrepancies and deformity. Various devices are employed to stabilize long bones, including Sheffield and Fassier–Duval rods. Upper limb surgery is increasingly being contemplated in light of the potential functional advantages, including self-transfer and wheelchair use. Surgery for scoliosis is generally intended to prevent progression or reduce pain but can be successful in achieving some degree of correction. Surgery for basilar invagination is undertaken to relieve pressure on the cervical cord and to slow progression of the deformity. Unfortunately, even with apparently successful surgery, basilar invagination may continue to progress in up to 80% of cases. In general, both untreated and bisphosphonate-treated bone in osteogenesis imperfecta present difficulties to the surgeon, and it is important that surgery is planned and conducted in consultation with a surgeon with experience of osteogenesis imperfecta wherever possible. Consideration of anaesthetic risks is an important element of preoperative planning.

Monitoring of therapy and complications

Administration and monitoring of the effects of bisphosphonate therapy should be conducted in liaison with those with expertise in managing the condition. In general, biochemical testing and bone densitometry (lumbar spine and total body-less-head measurements) should be undertaken at 6-month intervals in children on treatment, in order to guide treatment. Biochemical monitoring may include measurement of serum concentrations of calcium, phosphate, alkaline phosphatase (total and bone specific), PTH, 25-hydroxyvitamin D, creatinine, and bone turnover markers. Regular plain radiography, including lateral and anteroposterior spine, lateral foramen magnum-centred skull, and selected long-bone images, can be used to monitor deformities and the evolution of complications such as vertebral fractures. Lateral-spine imaging using DXA offers an alternative means of imaging vertebral morphology with lower doses of radiation.

Transition from childhood to adult care

During adolescence, scoliosis can worsen; weight gain, with consequent limitation of mobility and long-term health implications, can occur; and soft-tissue injuries may become more common. Hearing impairment is common in osteogenesis imperfecta, as a result of both conductive and sensorineural deficits, and there is an increased incidence of ocular problems. Thus, from the second decade, both audiological screening and regular review by an optician are prudent. As individuals transition to adult services, it is prudent to initiate screening for other complications such as mitral or aortic valve disease (reported incidence of around 5%). It is essential that young people with osteogenesis imperfecta are educated, empowered, and supported. A cornerstone of any approach aiming to achieve these goals is a continuity of coordinated, specialist team care leading into early adult life.

Other causes of primary osteoporosis

The diagnosis of osteogenesis imperfecta is not always straightforward, and the presentation can overlap with those of other diseases affecting connective tissue including Ehlers–Danlos syndrome and Marfan syndrome. A rare but distinct form of primary osteoporosis is osteoporosis–pseudoglioma syndrome, which is caused by homozygous inactivating mutations in *LRP5*, which encodes the low-density lipoprotein receptor-related protein 5 (LRP5). This form of osteoporosis is characterized by fragility fractures, and blindness as a result of aberrant development of the retinal vasculature. Individuals with the condition have also been reported to have learning difficulties, ligamentous laxity, and muscular hypotonia. Idiopathic juvenile osteoporosis is a diagnosis of exclusion but typically presents in a boy or girl during the prepubertal period, with an insidious onset of vertebral fractures and submetaphyseal fragility fractures. Often, there is a history of proximal muscle weakness and chronic pain. Radiology may reveal areas of lucency in the metaphyses. Bone biopsy shows a low rate of bone remodelling. Up to 20% of cases may be due to heterozygous mutations in *LRP5*. There is usually spontaneous remission after puberty but individuals may be left with residual deformities. In both osteoporosis–pseudoglioma syndrome and idiopathic juvenile osteoporosis, intravenous bisphosphonates can be helpful in relieving pain and improving bone density and may prevent vertebral deformity. Mutations in *WNT1*, a key element in activating LRP5-mediated signalling, have been shown to cause early onset primary osteoporosis. Even more recently, mutations in *PLS3* have been found to cause early onset low-turnover osteoporosis inherited in an X-linked manner.

Patient support groups

The following patient support groups may be useful:
- Brittle Bone Society (http://www.brittlebone.org)
- Osteogenesis Imperfecta Foundation (http://www.oif.org)

Future developments

Although bisphosphonates have been successful in improving outcomes in osteogenesis imperfecta and appear to be generally safe and well tolerated, there remain some concerns about their use, particularly in the long term, and they do not offer a cure for osteogenesis imperfecta. Anti-sclerostin antibodies have been used in a number of mouse models of osteogenesis imperfecta, with promising results. Other novel molecular approaches under investigation include mesenchymal stem cell therapy and allele-specific silencing.

Further reading

Cundy T. Recent advances in osteogenesis imperfecta. *Calcif Tissue Int* 2012; 90: 439–49.

Forlino A, Cabral WA, Barnes AM, et al. New perspectives on osteogenesis imperfecta. *Nat Rev Endocrinol* 2011; 7: 540–57.

12.9 Sclerosing bone disorders

Osteopetrosis

Definition and epidemiology

Osteopetrosis describes a genetically and clinically hetero-geneous group of conditions characterized by increased bone density resulting from abnormal osteoclast differentiation or function (Table 12.6). Altogether they are rare: the incidence of autosomal-dominant osteopetrosis is approximately 1 in 20,000 births, whilst that of severe autosomal-recessive osteopetrosis is around 1 in 250,000.

Pathophysiology

Osteoclasts are highly specialized multinucleate cells which enable bone resorption by degrading bone mineral and organic bone matrix. A number of single-gene defects cause osteopetrosis due to their effect on osteoclast differentiation or function. A number of these genes encode for proteins that are key to the acidification of the resorption lacuna that sits between the osteoclast and bone surface, including *CLCN7* (which encodes chloride channel 7), *TCIRG1* (which encodes V-type proton ATPase 116 kDa subunit a isoform 3, a subunit of a vacuolar proton pump), *OSTM1* (which encodes osteopetrosis-associated transmembrane protein 1), and *CA2* (which encodes carbonic anhydrase). Defects in these genes result in normal or elevated numbers of poorly functional osteoclasts, so-called osteoclast-rich osteopetrosis. In contrast, mutations in genes that encode proteins necessary for osteoclast differentiation, such as *RANKL* (which encodes receptor activator of nuclear-kappa B ligand), result in a paucity of mature osteoclasts or

'osteoclast-poor' osteopetrosis. More than half the cases of autosomal-recessive osteopetrosis have a mutation in *TCIRG1*; 10% have one in *CLCN7*. Mutations in *CLCN7* are also the most common cause of the intermediate form of autosomal-recessive osteopetrosis; mutations in *PLEKHM1*, affecting intracellular vesicular transport, are another. Autosomal-dominant osteopetrosis is caused by heterozygous mutations in *CLCN7*.

Clinical features

Osteoclast failure can result in abnormal bone modelling and altered craniofacial morphology and can have an impact on other systems such as bone marrow and the nervous system. The range of severity of osteopetrosis varies greatly. The more severe forms are those with an autosomal-recessive inheritance and tend to present in infancy, whilst autosomal-dominant osteopetrosis is milder, presenting later (even in adulthood) and is generally limited to the skeleton.

Autosomal-dominant osteopetrosis (Albers–Schoenberg disease)

Autosomal-dominant osteopetrosis is typically diagnosed in late childhood or adolescence, often as a chance finding on a radiograph, sometimes following a fracture as a result of the weakness that can paradoxically occur in the condition. A limited skeletal survey will reveal the characteristic radiological features of the condition: diffuse sclerosis; 'rugger jersey spine' (dense areas of sclerosis adjacent to the end plates of the vertebrae; see Figure 12.15); a 'bone-in-bone' appearance due to the persistence of unresorbed primary

Table 12.6 Inheritance and features of sclerosing bone disorders

Disorder	Inheritance (gene)	Clinical and radiological features
Osteopoikilosis	AD (*LEMD3*)	Benign, usually asymptomatic
		Multiple circular/ovoid opacities in ischia, pubic bones, and metaphyses
Melorrheostosis	AD	Can be asymptomatic or painful with deformity
		Cortical hyperostosis resembling dripping candle wax
		Sclerotomal distribution of lesions
Dysosteosclerosis	AR	Manifestation in infancy
		Skin changes and developmental regression
		Platyspondyly, bowed long bones
Osteopathia striata +/ –cranial sclerosis	XLD (*WTX*)	Macrocephaly, cleft palate, hearing loss
		Additional features may include developmental delay, cranial nerve palsies, anal malformations, and cataracts
		Longitudinal striations in the metaphyses
Camurati–Engelman syndrome	AD (*TGFB1*)	Prominent forehead and proptosis
		Presents in childhood with muscular weakness in lower limbs, waddling gait, and limb pain
		Thin limbs, thickened painful bones, and little muscle mass
		Thickening and sclerosis of diaphyses and skull
Van Buchem disease	AR (*SOST*)	Progressive enlargement of jaw in puberty
		Nerve compression
		High bone mass and endosteal hyperostosis
Sclerosteosis	AR (*SOST* or *LRP4*)	High bone mass, gigantism, syndactyly, square jaw, nerve compression

Abbreviations: AD, autosomal dominant; AR, autosomal recessive; XLD, X-linked dominant.

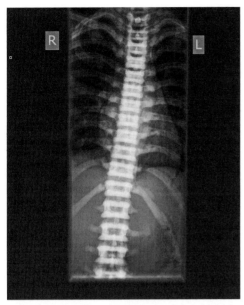

Fig. 12.15 Radiograph showing 'rugger jersey' spine in osteopetrosis.

spongiosa (see Figure 12.16); and undermodelling of the metaphyses of long bones ('Erlenmeyer-flask' deformity). The complications in autosomal-dominant osteopetrosis are largely confined to the skeleton and include fractures, scoliosis, and cranial nerve compression, which can occur in up to 5% of cases. Secondary complications are relatively frequent, such as delayed union or non-union of fractures and osteomyelitis, particularly of the mandible in association with dental disease. Routine dental surveillance and good dental hygiene are an important aspect of management.

In some nosologies, autosomal-dominant osteopetrosis is divided into type 1 and type 2, with Albers–Schoenberg disease being type 2 autosomal-dominant osteopetrosis. Type 1 autosomal-dominant osteopetrosis (or hyperostosis type Worth) is due to gain of function mutations in *LRP5* (see 'Hyperostosis type Worth').

Autosomal-recessive osteopetrosis

Autosomal-recessive osteopetrosis is an altogether more severe disease, usually presenting in the first few months of life, although failure of bone resorption may result in hypocalcaemia and seizures in the neonatal period. Symptoms may be non-specific, including feeding difficulties, poor growth, and anaemia. Infants often present with incipient blindness and may require urgent decompression to preserve vision. There is marked sclerosis of the skeleton with undermodelling of long bones. There is an increased risk of fracture and osteomyelitis. Changes in the skull can

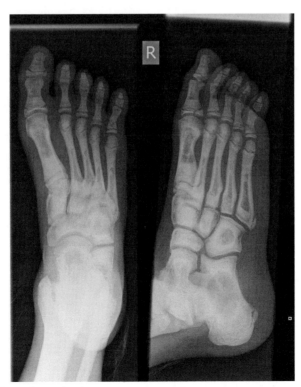

Fig. 12.16 Radiograph showing 'bone-in-bone' appearance in osteopetrosis.

manifest as frontal bossing, macrocephaly, choanal stenosis, and hydrocephalus. There is a high risk of nerve compression resulting in hearing loss or facial palsy as well as blindness. Another serious complication that reduces life expectancy is bone-marrow failure due to the constraint on haematopoiesis resulting from the abnormal expansion of the bone, resulting in pancytopenia and extramedullary haematopoiesis with hepatosplenomegaly.

It is important to distinguish the following rarer variants from classic autosomal-recessive osteopetrosis:

- neuropathic autosomal-recessive osteopetrosis (caused by mutations in CLCN7 and OSTM1):
  - perinatal onset
  - seizures with normocalcaemia
  - developmental delay
  - retinal atrophy
  - delayed myelinization and progressive cortical atrophy on MRI
- autosomal-recessive osteopetrosis with renal tubular acidosis (caused by mutations in CA2):
  - infantile onset with milder course
  - renal tubular acidosis
  - cerebral calcifications
  - developmental delay
  - cranial nerve compression
  - bone-marrow involvement rare
- X-linked osteopetrosis (caused by mutations in IKBKG):
  - infantile onset
  - severe immunodeficiency
  - lymphoedema
  - anhidrotic ectodermal dysplasia

Autosomal-recessive osteopetrosis can also occur in association with other conditions such as common variable immune deficiency and leucocyte adhesion deficiency syndrome.

Individuals with autosomal-recessive osteopetrosis may present later than infancy with a less severe 'intermediate' form of osteopetrosis. They commonly present in the first few years of life with fractures and a predisposition to mandibular osteomyelitis. However, visual impairment can occur in early infancy. These individuals typically have mandibular prognathism, proptosis, anaemia, and hepatosplenomegaly.

Treatment

Division of autosomal-recessive osteopetrosis into 'osteoclast-rich' and 'osteoclast-poor' types, depending on histological characteristics, is helpful in terms of understanding prognosis and the likely effectiveness of any treatment.

For most severe 'osteoclast-rich' forms of autosomal-recessive osteopetrosis, bone-marrow transplantation is justified and presents an opportunity for cure. However, in individuals with neuropathic autosomal-recessive osteopetrosis due to mutations in CLCN7, bone-marrow transplantation does not lead to a regression of the primary encephalopathy and retinopathy. In osteopetrosis due to OSTM1 mutations, bone-marrow transplantation has generally not been considered, given the severity of the neurological problems and bone disease. 'Osteoclast-poor' forms of osteopetrosis are not cured by bone-marrow transplantation but there may be the prospect of treatment with soluble RANKL.

Pycnodysostosis

Pycnodysostosis is a particular form of osteopetrosis due to an inactivating mutation in CTSK, which encodes cathepsin K, a protein secreted by the osteoclast into the resorption lacuna and necessary for the breakdown of type 1 collagen in the bone matrix. Affected individuals have disproportionate and marked short stature with a characteristic head shape and facial features including micrognathia, an increased mandibular angle, dental malocclusion, proptosis, a prominent forehead, and delayed closure of the anterior fontanelle. Total or partial aplasia of the terminal phalanges, with hypoplasia of the fingernails, is characteristic. Similarly, clavicles can be hypoplastic or absent. Treatment is supportive. Complications of the condition include fractures, osteomyelitis of the mandible, upper airway problems, and raised intracranial pressure.

Hyperostosis type Worth

Hyperostosis type Worth used to be known as autosomal-dominant osteopetrosis type 1. However, it is not a disorder of osteoclast activity. Activating mutations in LRP5 result in inhibited binding of the inhibitors sclerostin (encoded by SOST) and Dickkopf-related protein 1 (encoded by DKK1) and, consequently, in excessive bone formation. Individuals may have a large, square jaw and a torus palatinus (a bony lump on the hard palate) and are not prone to fractures. Radiological findings include a marked thickening of the cortices of long bones and the calvarium of the skull.

There are a number of other rare sclerosing bone disorders conditions, many of which have characteristic radiological appearances, emphasizing the importance of judicious but adequate use of plain radiography and access to an experienced radiology opinion. For most of them, there is no effective treatment.

Further reading

Rosen CJ, ed. Primer on Metabolic Bone Diseases and Disorders of Mineral Metabolism (7th edition), 2008. Wiley–Blackwell.

Stark Z and Savarirayan R. Osteopetrosis. Orphanet J Rare Dis 2009; 4: 5.

12.10 Fibrodysplasia ossificans progressiva

Epidemiology and pathophysiology

Fibrodysplasia ossificans progressiva (FOP) is an ultra-rare and extremely disabling condition characterised by progressive ossification of extraskeletal tissues. The incidence of FOP is probably less than 1 in 2 million. Although it is heritable, it has only been multigenerational in a handful of families worldwide. At affected sites, there is lymphocytic infiltration usually followed by a recapitulation of the process of endochondral ossification (i.e. new bone formation). The disease is due to dysregulation of bone morphogenetic protein signalling, with overexpression of bone morphogenetic protein 4. In almost all cases it is due to a specific heterozygous missense activating mutation in a bone morphogenetic protein type 1 receptor gene, *ACVR1*.

Clinical features

The two principal manifestations of FOP are heterotopic ossification of soft tissues such as muscles and tendons, and congenital malformation of the great toe.

Apart from the malformation of the great toes, children appear normal at birth. However, often by 2 years of age, they will develop the earliest lesions as painful swellings of the chest wall. FOP lesions usually develop rapidly over several days. They can regress spontaneously but more commonly progress to permanent ossification. Evolution of the disease is episodic and occurs at a variable rate, even within families. The cumulative effect of increasingly widespread heterotopic ossification determines the level of disability. Specific features include chest-wall constriction, progressive fusion of vertebrae, scoliosis, joint immobility, and contractures, with patients often fixed in unusual positions. Most affected individuals require a wheelchair for mobility by the third decade of life. Many individuals die early as a result of chest-wall disease but, despite the disease, some individuals can live productive lives well beyond middle age.

Routine mineral biochemistry is normal, although serum alkaline phosphatase may be elevated during flare-ups. Radiographic features (other than soft-tissue ossification, abnormality of the hallux, and vertebral fusion) include acetabular dysplasia with large capital femoral epiphyses and wide necks; cervical vertebrae with small bodies and thick pedicles; and shortening of the first metacarpals and middle phalanges of other digits.

Management

There is presently no medical treatment for FOP, and management is therefore supportive. Surgery (e.g. for biopsy or release of contractures) is practically contra-indicated due to the risk of inducing further, potentially catastrophic ossification. Other trauma, such as intra-muscular injections, including vaccinations, should be avoided.

Lesions are induced by trauma and inflammation. Avoidance of these (e.g. falls) is therefore a key element to management. Prior to diagnosis, lesions can sometimes be mistaken for malignancies, and attempts to biopsy or remove lesions can be disastrous, due to the induction of further new bone formation.

In view of the rarity and severity of the condition, once the diagnosis is made, expert opinion should be sought as a matter of urgency.

Patient support groups

The patient support group International Fibrodysplasia Ossificans Progressiva Association (http://www.ifopa.org) may be useful.

Future developments

Although there is currently no treatment available, pharmacological inhibitors of bone morphogenetic protein signalling are undergoing clinical trials for FOP.

Further reading

Pignolo RJ, Shore EM, and Kaplan FS. Fibrodysplasia ossificans progressiva: Clinical and genetic aspects. *Orphanet J Rare Dis* 2011; 6: 80.

Chapter 13

Endocrine oncology and neuroendocrine disorders

Chapter contents

13.1 General introduction

Introduction

Several genetic disorders can be associated with neuro-endocrine tumours. These are summarized in Table 13.1. Several of these genetic disorders will be discussed in separate chapters.

Specific markers

Neuroendocrine tumours may produce specific hypersecretory symptoms and hormones.

The diagnosis of neuroendocrine tumours is based on clinical presentation, hormone assays, radiological and nuclear medicine imaging, and pathology. In patients with clinically functioning neuroendocrine tumours, specific biochemical tests should be requested in blood or 24-hour urine samples obtained with or without provocative testing (see Table 13.2). Levels of circulating markers or urinary excreted products can be monitored and used for tumour follow-up.

Non-specific markers

Chromogranin A

Neurons and neuroendocrine cells contain vesicles with peptide hormones, biogenic amines, and neurotransmitters. These vesicles store and release acidic, soluble secretory proteins known as 'granins'. The three 'classic' granins are chromogranin A, chromogranin B, and secretogranin 2 (sometimes called chromogranin C). Four other members of the granin family are secretogranin 3 (or 1B1075), secretogranin 4 (or HISL-19), secretogranin 5 (or 7B2), and secretogranin 6 (or NESP55).

Chromogranin A has become the most important circulating tumour marker for neuroendocrine tumours, although it cannot differentiate between different subtypes of neuroendocrine neoplasms. It can also have interesting clinical applications in so-called non-functioning neuroendocrine tumours. Chromogranin A levels are increased in most patients with metastatic neuroendocrine tumours of the gastrointestinal tract and pancreas. A significant positive relation between the serum levels of chromogranin A and the tumour mass of most neuroendocrine tumours has been demonstrated, except in gastrinoma. Serum concentrations of chromogranin A are only rarely slightly elevated in subjects with small neuroendocrine tumours such as insulinomas. Increased chromogranin A concentrations can be found in most patients with gastrinoma, even when the tumour burden is limited. It is well known that chronically elevated gastrin levels cause hyperplasia of the neuroendocrine enterochromaffin-like cells of the stomach. As these cells secrete chromogranin A, they might be responsible for the elevated circulating chromogranin A levels. The specificity of elevated levels of chromogranin A in the diagnosis of neuroendocrine tumours is very high (~100%).

Neuron-specific enolase

Serum neuron-specific enolase levels are frequently elevated in patients with several neuroendocrine tumours. Elevated levels are exclusively associated

Table 13.1 Hereditary tumour syndromes associated with neuroendocrine tumours

Syndrome	Neuroendocrine tumour
Von Hippel–Lindau syndrome (OMIM 193300)	Pancreatic neuroendocrine tumours (5%–10%)
	Phaeochromocytomas (10%–20%)
Multiple endocrine neoplasia 1 (OMIM 193300)	Pituitary adenomas (5%–65%)
	Pancreatic neuroendocrine tumours (80%–100%)
	Thymic carcinoids (mostly in men; <10%)
	Bronchial carcinoids (mostly in women; 20%–25%)
	Gastric carcinoids (ZES related) (5%–35%)
Multiple endocrine neoplasia 2A (OMIM 171400)	Medullary thyroid carcinoma
	Phaeochromocytoma (bilateral)
Multiple endocrine neoplasia 2B (OMIM 162300)	Medullary thyroid carcinoma
	Phaeochromocytoma (bilateral)
Familiarly medullary thyroid carcinoma (OMIM 155240)	Medullary thyroid carcinoma
Neurofibromatosis 1 (OMIM 162200)	Periampullary somatostatinomas
	Phaeochromocytomas
Carney complex 1 (OMIM 160980)	Pituitary adenomas
Tuberous sclerosis (OMIM 191100)	Pituitary adenoma
	Pancreatic neuroendocrine tumours (insulinomas)
Multiple endocrine neoplasia 4 (OMIM 610755)	Pituitary adenomas

Abbreviations: OMIM, Online Mendelian Inheritance in Man; ZES, Zollinger–Ellison syndrome.

Table 13.2 Specific neuroendocrine tumour markers in serum or plasma or urine

Tumour/syndrome	Tumour marker(s)	Test result(s)
Foregut carcinoid	24-Hour urinary 5-HIAA	Occasionally elevated
Midgut carcinoid	24-Hour urinary 5-HIAA	Usually elevated
	Tachykinins	Usually elevated
Hindgut carcinoid	24-Hour urinary 5-HIAA	Generally not elevated
Gastrinoma	Basal (fasting) serum gastrin	Generally elevated
Insulinoma	Plasma glucose	<2.2 mmol/L (<40 mg/dL)
	Basal (fasting) serum insulin	Inappropriately elevated
	Basal (fasting) serum proinsulin	Inappropriately elevated
	Basal (fasting) serum C peptide	Inappropriately elevated
	Sulphonylurea screen	Negative
Glucagonoma	Basal (fasting) serum glucagon	Usually elevated
	Basal (fasting) serum pancreatic polypeptide	Generally elevated
VIPoma	Basal (fasting) serum vaso-intestinal polypeptide	Usually elevated
	Basal (fasting) serum peptide histidine-methionine	Usually elevated
PPoma	Basal (fasting) pancreatic polypeptide	Usually elevated
Somatostatinoma	Basal (fasting) somatostatin	Usually elevated
Ectopic acromegaly	Basal growth hormone	Usually elevated
	Basal insulin-like growth factor 1	Usually elevated
	Basal growth hormone-releasing hormone	Usually elevated
Ectopic Cushing's syndrome	Midnight cortisol	Usually elevated
	Basal adrenocorticotrophin	Usually (inappropriately) elevated
Malignant hypercalcaemia	Basal serum calcium	Usually elevated
	Basal parathyroid hormone-related peptide	Usually elevated

Abbreviations: 5-HIAA, 5-hydroxyindoleacetic acid.

with poor tumour differentiation. It is generally not considered to be a good diagnostic marker for neuroendocrine tumours such as chromogranin A but in selected cases can be used as a follow-up marker.

Pancreatic polypeptide
Pancreatic polypeptide is produced by normal pancreas but is found in high concentrations in 80% of patients with pancreatic tumours and in 50% of patients with carcinoid tumours.

13.2 Neuroendocrine imaging

Introduction

Techniques for imaging neuroendocrine tumours can be divided into the following categories:

- anatomical cross-sectional techniques (CT, MRI, and ultrasound)
- nuclear medicine imaging techniques involving radio-nuclide pharmaceuticals
- invasive imaging techniques, including angiography, venous sampling, and endoscopic ultrasound

Functioning neuroendocrine tumours are often small in size at the time of biochemical diagnosis and may arise in many sites throughout the body. This can make tumour localization with anatomical cross-sectional imaging quite challenging. Non-functioning neuroendocrine tumours and malignant neuroendocrine tumours, which are typically larger in size at the time of presentation than functioning neuroendocrine tumours, are usually readily localized, staged, and followed-up using cross-sectional imaging.

Nuclear medicine techniques are based on certain physiological characteristics of the tumour, such as the presence of cell surface receptors or uptake of particular molecules. These techniques are complimentary to cross-sectional imaging in the localization and staging of neuroendocrine tumours. They may be used to predict response to nuclear medicine therapies, and, in some cases, to assess response to treatment.

Invasive imaging techniques are also used in particular circumstances, such as obtaining tissue or venous samples, as well as for angiographic treatments.

The initial choice of imaging modality varies, depending on the suspected site of disease (e.g. the lung, the gastrointestinal tract, or the pancreas), as well as local expertise. There is no consensus as to the single best imaging modality, and combining modalities is standard practice.

Imaging techniques

Anatomical cross-sectional imaging

CT is frequently the initial imaging modality for the detection of suspected gastro-entero-pancreatic and lung neuroendocrine tumours. Multiphase imaging before and after iodinated contrast medium improves detection. In patients with a contraindication to iodinated contrast, a non-contrast study may be helpful (e.g. in cases of lung neuroendocrine tumour) or an alternative imaging technique may be used. CT without specific bowel preparation is of limited use in detecting the primary site of a gastrointestinal neuroendocrine tumour but mesenteric disease, lymphadenopathy, and liver metastases are well demonstrated (see Figure 13.1).

CT enterography and enteroclysis involve distention of the bowel with fluid prior to imaging. These techniques are more sensitive than routine CT in detecting primary gastrointestinal neuroendocrine tumours. The small bowel is distended with fluid, either by oral ingestion (enterography) or by cannulating the jejunum with a nasojejunal tube in order to instil fluid (enteroclysis). Intravenous contrast medium is also used for optimal results.

With regards to MRI, its performance now equals or exceeds that of CT in the detection of gastro-entero-pancreatic neuroendocrine tumours involving the liver,

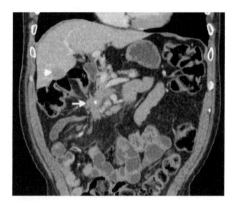

Fig 13.1 Mesenteric disease CT.

the pancreas, and the retroperitoneum (see Figure 13.2). Magnetic resonance enterography is also becoming more widely available and improves detection of the primary lesion. In most cases, intravenous gadolinium contrast will be given to improve the detection of neuroendocrine tumours. MRI is not used in the initial investigation of suspected pulmonary neuroendocrine tumours but may be used in some cases, such as defining the extent of apical tumours.

Ultrasound may be used for the detection and follow-up of liver metastases. In some centres, particularly in cases of slow-growing tumours for which long-term follow-up is anticipated, ultrasound is used alternately with CT in order to reduce radiation dose to the patient. The use of ultrasound contrast media is under investigation in the detection and assessment of response in liver metastases. Ultrasound may also be used to direct biopsy, where clinically indicated.

Nuclear medicine imaging techniques

Somatostatin receptor scintigraphy is the most widely used radiopharmaceutical technique for the localization of neuroendocrine tumours. The radiopharmaceutical used is ^{111}In-pentetreotide, which attaches to somatostatin

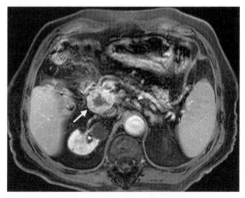

Fig 13.2 MRI of a pancreatic neuroendocrine tumour (arrow). Courtesy of Barts NHS Trust.

receptors on the cell surface of many neuroendocrine tumours. Other radiopharmaceuticals are also available (Table 13.3). Localization of the primary and metastatic tumour sites is then possible by detection of emitted radiation by means of a gamma camera providing whole-body imaging (see Figure 13.3). These techniques complement cross-sectional imaging for complete staging information, and will also identify those tumours with inoperable or metastatic disease but which might be candidates for high-activity targeted therapy, due to their uptake of the radiopharmaceutical.

Where the location of the tumour is not clear from the planar images, the site of the tracer can be plotted in cross-sectional imaging via SPECT and co-localized with CT (see Figure 13.4).

When using scintigraphy for tumour follow-up, care must be taken with interpretation. Some agents, such as interferon, may upregulate somatostatin receptors and so lead to increased tracer uptake without disease progression. In other cases, a tumour that previously expressed somatostatin receptors may dedifferentiate and become 'imaging negative' despite anatomical progression. As such, the clinical context is crucial information for the reporting physician.

Gallium PET/CT uses ^{68}Ga-labelled somatostatin analogues and is reported to be more sensitive than other imaging modalities at detecting most types of neuroendocrine tumour, with the exception of lung and liver metastases. It is currently of limited availability. However, the combination of high detection rate with the gallium tracer and accurate anatomic localization from the integrated CT is likely to lead to this technique being the imaging modality of choice for the detection and staging of neuroendocrine tumours in the future. FDG PET/CT is used is some cases of tumours with highly aggressive behaviour.

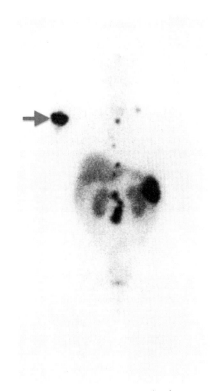

Fig 13.3 Somatostatin receptor scintigraphy of a neuroendocrine tumour (arrow).
Courtesy of Barts NHS Trust.

Table 13.3 Types of radiotracers used in nuclear medicine imaging

Radiotracer	Description	Patient preparation
[111]In-labelled pentetreotide (somatostatin receptor scintigraphy)	An analogue of somatostatin that is more stable in plasma	Octeotide therapy should be discontinued 48 hours prior to imaging
	Binds to cell surface receptors expressed by approximately 80% of enteropancreatic neuroendocrine tumours and some paragangliomas and chromaffin cell tumours	Often best performed at the end of a dosing interval
		A technetium bone scan is necessary to rule out bone metastases
[123]I-labelled metaiodobenzylguanidine	Concentrated by catecholamine producing medullary adrenal tumours, including extra-adrenal paragangliomas, and chromaffin cell tumours	Calcium-channel blockers, labetalol, reserpine, tricyclic antidepressants, antipsychotic drugs, and sympathomimetics such as amphetamines should be discontinued 3 days prior to the study, when possible
[18]-F-labelled glucose analogue (e.g. ^{18}F-FDG)	Concentrated in cells with a rapid glucose metabolism and imaged on PET/CT	Refer to local policy of PET patient preparation
	Well-differentiated NETs may not be FDG avid	The patient must fast prior to FDG administration
	FDG imaging may be useful in cases of aggressive dedifferentiated tumours where conventional scintigraphy is negative[†]	
[68]Ga-labelled somatostatin analogue	Similar to In-labelled somatostatin analogues, but used in PET/CT with greater sensitivity	Octeotide therapy should be discontinued 48 hours prior to imaging
	Not currently widely available	

Abbreviations: CT, computed tomography; FGD, fluorodeoxyglucose; NET, neuroendocrine tumour; PET, positron emission tomography..

† Data from Intenzo CM, Jabbour S, Lin HC, et al. Scintigraphic imaging of body neuroendocrine tumors. *Radiographics*. 2007; 27: 1355–69.

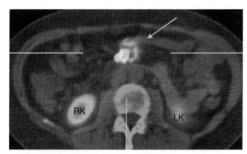

Fig 13.4 Somatostatin receptor scintigraphy with single-photon emission CT; the arrow indicates an octreotide-avid mass at the root of the small bowel mesentery; LK, left kidney; RK, right kidney.
Courtesy of Barts NHS Trust.

^{18}F-DOPA PET/CT and ^{11}C-labelled 5-hydroxytryptophan (5-HTP) PET/CT are promising emerging imaging tools, but neither is routinely available in most centres.

Invasive imaging techniques

Endoscopy with or without endoluminal ultrasound is used for gastroduodenal, pancreatic, and colorectal neuroendocrine tumours. A significant advantage to these techniques is the possibility of obtaining a tissue diagnosis by biopsy or fine-needle aspiration.

Digital subtraction angiography with venous sampling may be used to aid localization in cases where a functioning lesion has not been localized by conventional techniques. Calcium stimulation with venous sampling may be used in patients with multiple endocrine neoplasia type 1 when a functional pancreatic neuroendocrine tumour must be identified among multiple lesions prior to planning surgery.

Angiographic techniques, including transarterial chemoembolization, are used for the treatment of liver metastases.

Technique sensitivity in tumour detection

Each imaging technique has advantages and limitations. The sensitivities for each technique in particular tumour types are given in Table 13.4.

Imaging of specific neuroendocrine tumour types

Commonly used imaging modalities for tumours are listed in Table 13.5.

Gastro-enteric neuroendocrine tumours

Endoscopy is the method of choice for detecting suspected gastric and colonic neuroendocrine tumours. Small-bowel neuroendocrine tumours are typically highly vascular, have a high number of somatostatin receptors, and may be detected using contrast-enhanced CT or magnetic resonance enterography, combined with somatostatin receptor scintigraphy or gallium PET/CT to localize the tumour and to complete staging. Capsule endoscopy has been reported in a few studies to successfully detect small-bowel neuroendocrine tumours when other techniques have failed, but does not precisely localize the position of the tumour within the small bowel. Despite the available imaging

Table 13.4 Reported sensitivities of various imaging modalities for specific neuroendocrine tumours

Location and modality	Sensitivity (%)
Pancreatic NET	
CT	57–94
MRI	74–94
EUS	82–93
Insulinoma SRS	50–60
^{68}Ga-DOTATOC PET/CT	87–96
Gastrointestinal NET	
CT enteroclysis	85
MR enteroclysis	86
SRS	86–95
Gallium PET/CT	87–96
Neuroendocrine liver metastases	
CT	44–82
MR	82–95
Gallium PET/CT	96

Abbreviations: CT, computed tomography; EUS, endoscopic ultrasound; MR, magnetic resonance; MRI, magnetic resonance imaging; NET, neuroendocrine tumour; PET, positron emission tomography; SRS, somatostatin receptor scintigraphy.

Adapted by permission from BMJ Publishing Group Limited. Gut, Ramage JK, Ahmed A, Ardill J et al., Guidelines for the management of gastroenteropancreatic neuroendocrine (including carcinoid) tumours (NETs), 61, Copyright 2012, BMJ Publishing Group Ltd.

techniques, the primary tumour may be difficult to identify on imaging.

Signs of a malignant neuroendocrine tumour on CT include larger tumour size, necrosis, calcification, and invasion of the surrounding structures. In general, gastro-entero-pancreatic neuroendocrine tumours metastasize to lymph nodes and the liver, especially midgut neuroendocrine tumours, of which 40%–80% have metastases at presentation. A mesenteric mass may be seen in midgut neuroendocrine tumours. Metastases to bone and lung may also be seen.

Staging of neuroendocrine tumours is according to the Union for International Cancer Control (UICC) TNM (for tumour, node, metastasis) system. The European Neuroendocrine Tumour Society has also issued a TNM staging system that differs slightly from the UICC system (see Ramage et al., 2012).

Pancreatic neuroendocrine tumours

Pancreatic neuroendocrine tumours may be initially suspected clinically if there is a functioning tumour, such as an insulinoma. Functioning pancreatic neuroendocrine tumours are often very small at the time of initial investigation and can be challenging to identify. Multislice CT with pre-contrast, arterial phase, and portal venous phase imaging with thin slice reformats allow the most sensitive detection, equally that of high-resolution MRI T2, T1 fat-saturated, and dynamic contrast administration. Pancreatic neuroendocrine tumours that are non-functioning or result in non-specific symptoms typically present at a much later stage with a large mass.

Table 13.5 Commonly used imaging modality for tumour types in the assessment of the extent of disease, follow-up, and response to treatment

Tumour type	Commonly used imaging modality	
	Cross-sectional	**Nuclear medicine**
Gastro-entero-pancreatic-NET	Endoscopy + /–EUS	^{111}In-labelled pentetreotide SPECT
	CT or MRI + /–enterography	[68]Ga- labelled PET
Bronchial neuroendocrine tumours	Broncoscopy + /– EUS	[111]In- labelled pentetreotide SPECT
	CT	[68]Ga- labelled PET
Poorly differentiated neuroendocrine tumours	CT and/or MRI	^{18}F-FDG PET/CT
Phaeochromocytoma and paragangliomas	CT and/or MRI	^{111}In-labelled pentetreotide SPECT
		MIBG SPECT

Abbreviations: CT, computed tomography; EUS, endoscopic ultrasound; FGD, fluorodeoxyglucose; MIBG, metaiodobenzylguanidine; MRI, magnetic resonance imaging; NET, neuroendocrine tumour; PET, positron emission tomography; SPECT, single-photon-emission computed tomography; SRS, somatostatin receptor scintigraphy.

Some characteristics of pancreatic neuroendocrine tumours are as follows.

Insulinomas are the most frequent of the pancreatic neuroendocrine tumours, accounting for 50% of cases; 10%–15% are malignant, and more than 99% are found in the pancreas. They are typically small (less than 2 cm in size).

Gastrinomas are the next most common tumours, at 20%–30%. A large proportion are malignant, at 60%–75%, and in addition to be found in the pancreas, they are found in the duodenum and in the lymph nodes. They are of variable size.

Non-functioning tumours and tumours that secrete pancreatic polypeptide make up 15%–20% of pancreatic tumours are frequently malignant, large, and found almost exclusively within the pancreas.

VIPomas make up 3% of these tumours and are malignant in 50%–60%. Most are found in the pancreas (90%), but 10% are adrenal.

Glucagonomas and somatostatinomas are rare and often malignant tumours found most commonly within the pancreas.

Bronchial neuroendocrine tumours

Large-cell neuroendocrine tumours of the lung and small-cell lung cancers, the most aggressive of the lung neuroendocrine tumours, are best detected and staged with CT. The more aggressive tumours show high uptake on ^{18}F-FDG PET/CT (Chong et al., 2006).

Sympathoadrenal tumours

Phaeochromocytomas

CT and MR are highly sensitive but only moderately specific for phaeochromocytoma localization, with some overlap in imaging appearances with other adrenal tumours (see Figure 13.5a).

Nuclear medicine imaging techniques help to confirm the diagnosis as well as localize multifocal and metastatic disease. ^{123}I-MIBG is the preferred nuclear medicine tracer for benign phaeochromocytomas (see Figure 13.5b). Somatostatin receptor scintigraphy and FDG PET/CT are less sensitive than ^{123}I-MIGB for benign phaeochromocytomas but increase in sensitivity for malignant and more poorly differentiated tumours.

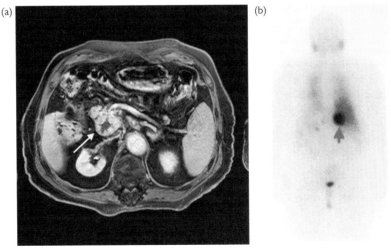

(a)   (b)

Fig 13.5 (a) Adrenal phaeochromocytoma (arrowed). (b) Metaiodobenzylguanidine phaeochromocytoma (arrowed).

For extra-adrenal tumours, paragangliomas, somato-statin receptor scintigraphy is the imaging of choice, as it is more sensitive and specific than MIBG.

Uptake of ^{123}I-MIBG indicates the potential to use high-activity MIBG as treatment in these tumours.

Some case series show promising results for PET-CT using a ^{68}Ga-labelled somatostatin analogue. Sensitivities are likely higher than with MIBG SPECT, but clinical trials are awaited.

Learning points

The choice of imaging modality will depend on local expertise and may involve several complementary techniques, usually including a cross-sectional technique as well as a nuclear medicine imaging technique. Gallium PET/CT is emerging as an important tool in the imaging of gastro-entero-pancreatic neuroendocrine tumours, combining somatostatin receptor imaging with anatomic localization.

Assessment of disease progression is predominantly on CT or MRI. Somatostatin receptor scintigraphy or MIBG scintigraphy may be used in some cases.

Multidisciplinary teams should be consulted for guidance on the choice of imaging at each stage of disease in patients with neuroendocrine tumours.

References and further reading

Ambrosini V, Campana D, Tomassetti P, et al. ^{68}Ga-labelled peptides for diagnosis of gastroenteropancreatic NET. *Eur J Nucl Med Mol Imaging* 2012; 39: S52–60.

Chong S, Lee KS, Chung MJ et al. Neuroendocrine tumors of the lung: Clinical, pathologic, and imaging findings. *Radiographics* 2006; 26: 41–57; discussion 57–8.

Husband J and Reznek RH. *Husband and Reznek's Imaging in Oncology* (3rd edition), 2009. CRC Press.

Intenzo CM, Jabbour S, Lin HC, et al. Scintigraphic imaging of body neuroendocrine tumors. *Radiographics* 2007; 27: 1355–69.

Ramage JK, Ahmed A, Ardill J, et al. Guidelines for the management of gastroenteropancreatic neuroendocrine (including carcinoid) tumours (NETs). *Gut* 2012; 61: 6–32.

Sundin A, Vullierme MP, Kaltsas G, et al. ENETS consensus guidelines for the standards of care in neuroendocrine tumors: Radiological examinations. *Neuroendocrinology* 2009; 90: 167–83.

13.3 Small bowel neuroendocrine tumours ('carcinoids')

Introduction: Epidemiology

The term 'carcinoid' was first adopted by Oberndorfer in 1907, as he wanted to describe a small-bowel tumour that was morphologically distinct and clinically less aggressive than intestinal adenocarcinoma. In the past, pathologists called all gastro-entero-pancreatic neuro-endocrine tumours 'carcinoids', because their histo-pathological features seemed to be quite similar without special immunostaining. Currently, although the term 'carcinoid' is no longer acceptable to pathologists, most clinicians still find it of practical use in describing neuro-endocrine tumours of the gastrointestinal tract, and 'carcinoid syndrome'.

According to the Surveillance, Epidemiology, and End Results Program database from the USA, the small bowel represents the most common primary site of gastrointestinal carcinoids in Caucasian patients, and the second most common one in African-Americans and Asian/Pacific Islanders. For that reason, in this section we will focus on the pathogenesis, diagnosis, and management of small-bowel carcinoids. According to their embryological origin, small-bowel carcinoids are included in the group of 'midgut carcinoids', together with those of appendiceal and proximal colon origin. As with all gastro-entero-pancreatic neuroendocrine tumours, the annual incidence of small-bowel carcinoids has been rising and has recently been estimated as 0.67 in 100,000 per year. Another epidemiological study from USA demonstrated also that small-bowel carcinoids are the most common small-bowel tumours, followed by adenocarcinomas, lymphomas, and stromal tumours. Small-bowel carcinoids seem to be more common in males (incidence 0.80 vs 0.57 in females). Finally, it has been reported that, in approximately 10% of patients with small-bowel carcinoids, particularly males, synchronous or metachronous adenocarcinomas are found. One-third of these carcinomas arise from the gastrointestinal tract, particularly the large bowel.

Pathogenesis: Classification

The aetiology of small-bowel carcinoids is uncertain. Genomic aberrations seem to be less common compared to those detected in pancreatic neuroendocrine tumours, whilst there is no clear correlation between the stage of the disease and the number of aberrations. The most frequent duplications were found on Chromosomes 19 and 17 and at the chromosomal locus 4p14-qter, whilst deletions are usually seen at the chomosomal loci 18p22-qter, 11q22-q23, and 16q21-qter, with Chromosome 18 deletions being the most common. The latter observation, together with the fact that Chromosome 18 deletions are rare in pancreatic neuroendocrine tumours and bronchial carcinoids, may indicate that loss of heterozygosity of Chromosome 18 is involved in the pathogenesis of small-bowel carcinoids.

Small-bowel carcinoids are most commonly located in the distal ileum and, in up to 40% of cases, they are multiple. At the time of diagnosis, they measure >2 cm and have already invaded the muscularis propria. The most common metastatic sites are in the mesentery/peritoneum and the liver. Less commonly, small-bowel carcinoids can metastasize to the lungs and bone; rarely, they can be associated with breast, myocardial, and orbital metastases as well. The metastatic potential of small-bowel carcinoids seems to be associated with the size of the primary lesion.

Small-bowel carcinoids are associated with the abnormal metabolism of tryptophan. In healthy people, about 99% of tryptophan is used to make nicotinic acid, and 1% is made into 5-hydroxytryptamine (serotonin). However, in patients with small-bowel carcinoids, the production of 5-hydroxytryptamine and, subsequently, 5-hydroxyindoleacetic acid predominates, and the latter can be measured in the urine of most patients. A deficiency in nicotinic acid can then develop and the patients may have features of 'pellagra'. Apart from 5-hydroxytryptamine, these tumours may produce several other hormones, such as tachykinins, prostaglandins, substance P, histamine, and so on. In patients mainly with hepatic metastases, these hormonal products, following intestinal drainage into the portal system, circumvent metabolism in the portal vein and are directly secreted into the systemic circulation, causing 'carcinoid syndrome' (see 'Clinical features'). In 5% of patients with retroperitoneal or ovarian metastases, carcinoid syndrome can occur without liver involvement as, in these cases, the hormones directly enter the circulation, bypassing the liver.

Apart from metabolic abnormalities, small-bowel carcinoids may cause pronounced fibrosis locally—in the peritumoral tissues in the mesentery and the retroperitoneal space—and distantly in the heart valves. The consequences of local fibrosis (desmoplasia) include obstruction of bowel loops and occlusion of mesenteric vessels and the ureters. Although previous studies have indicated that desmoplasia is associated with the release of serotonin or tachykinins from these tumours, more recent data suggest a potential role of TGF beta, bone morphogenic protein 4, or connective tissue growth factor. However, the exact cause of mesenteric fibrosis has not been established yet. In contrast, the role of 5-hydroxytryptamine, histamine, and tachykinins released by the malignant cells is clearer in the pathogenesis of heart valve fibrosis, thus causing 'carcinoid heart disease'. The vasoactive tumour products are inactivated in the liver, the lungs, and the brain, but the presence of hepatic metastases may allow large quantities of these substances to reach the right side of the heart, without being inactivated by the liver. Carcinoid heart disease has a preferential right-heart involvement (tricuspid valve, pulmonary valve) that is most likely related to inactivation of vasoactive substances by the lungs (by the monoamine oxidase system; see Figure 13.6). In the 5%–10% of cases with left-sided valvular pathology (affecting mainly the mitral valve), one should suspect extensive liver metastases, a bronchial neuroendocrine tumour, and/or a patent foramen ovale.

Approximately 90% and 80% of small-bowel carcinoids express somatostatin receptors types 2 and 5, respectively, which is important for tumour visualization and treatment.

Small-bowel carcinoids have morphologically the histopathological features of other gastro-entero-pancreatic neuroendocrine tumours and, on immunohistochemistry, they are usually positive for chromogranin A, synaptophysin, and serotonin. According to the WHO 2010 classification, they are divided into well-differentiated neuroendocrine

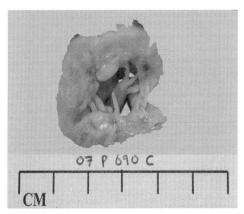

Fig 13.6 Tricuspid valve almost fully replaced by fibrous tissue. Only small areas of normal endocardium can be noted.

tumours (the vast majority of cases) and poorly well-differentiated neuroendocrine carcinomas (rarely). On the basis of the widely accepted grading system (based on the Ki-67 proliferation index), they can be classified into G1 tumours (Ki-67 proliferation index $\leq$ 2%), which represent the majority of small-bowel carcinoids; G2 tumours (Ki-67 proliferation index 3%–20%); and G3 tumours (Ki-67 proliferation index >20%), which are rare. Small-bowel carcinoids can be classified also with the TNM system.

Clinical features
Many small-bowel carcinoids have no specific symptoms and are discovered incidentally at the time of a screening colonoscopy or surgery for other abdominal disorders, and also during investigation in an asymptomatic patient with metastatic disease. Therefore, the presence of these tumours may be undetectable for years without obvious signs or symptoms.

When symptoms occur they are associated with (1) local tumour mass effects, including vague abdominal pain (which often leads to false diagnoses (i.e. irritable bowel syndrome)), nausea, vomiting, or jaundice; (2) complications of mesenteric or retroperitoneal fibrosis, such as intestinal obstruction, mesenteric ischaemia due to occlusion of the superior mesenteric artery or its branches, and ascites or recurrent gastrointestinal bleeding (ectopic varices) due to occlusion of the superior mesenteric vein (SMV) and development of segmental portal hypertension (patients with retroperitoneal fibrosis may also develop hydronephrosis and renal failure secondary to stenosis of the ureters); and (3) the systemic effects of the tumour hormonal products (functional symptoms).

A typical example is the classic carcinoid syndrome. It noted in approximately 20%–30% of patients with hepatic metastases. Carcinoid syndrome consists mainly of (1) paroxysmal flushing (90%) which is dry, is triggered by foods, alcohol, or exercise, and can be noticed in patient's face, neck, and upper trunk; and (2) chronic diarrhoea (70%), which is secretory. However, carcinoid syndrome is not the only cause of diarrhoea in patients with small-bowel carcinoids. The differential diagnosis of diarrhoea in those patients is presented in Box 13.1.

Wheezing (15%) and symptoms associated with carcinoid heart disease (20%–30%), such as bilateral peripheral oedema, fatigue, and shortness of breath, represent less common symptoms of carcinoid syndrome. Rarely, patients may develop pellagra (5%), myopathy (7%), and skin pigmentation (5%). *Carcinoid crisis* is a life-threatening complication of this syndrome, including hypotension (occasionally hypertension), tachycardia predisposing to arrhythmias, bronchial wheezing, flushing, and CNS abnormalities. It can be precipitated by an anaesthetic or interventional procedure in these patients.

Investigations
Apart from the clinical features, which are more evident in patients with functional symptoms, the diagnosis of small-bowel carcinoids is based upon (1) the levels of several peptides and amines, which represent tumour products, in blood and urine (biomarkers); (2) the localization of primary and/or metastatic lesions by imaging studies; and (3) histopathological confirmation (through a biopsy or a surgical specimen), which represents the 'gold standard' and should be obtained whenever possible.

Biomarkers
Chromogranin A belongs to a family of soluble, acidic glycoproteins (chromogranins A, B, and C) and is found throughout the neuroendocrine system. Although chromogranin A is not specific for any particular type of neuroendocrine tumours, it is thought to be the best and most sensitive general marker for the diagnosis and follow-up of gastro-entero-pancreatic neuroendocrine tumours. Levels of chromogranin A may correlate with tumour progression or regression; in addition, changes in the level of chromogranin A may precede radiographic evidence of progression. The highest chromogranin A levels have been found in metastatic small-bowel carcinoids. In these, chromogranin A seems to correlate with tumour burden and biological activity, whilst it may be also an independent prognostic factor. Moreover, in a series of radically resected small-bowel carcinoids, raised chromogranin A was the first sign of recurrence. False-positive increased chromogranin A levels are noted in renal impairment, liver failure, atrophic gastritis, inflammatory bowel disease, and the chronic use of proton-pump inhibitors.

Urinary 5-hydroxyindoleacetic acid, a metabolite of 5-hydroxytryptamine, is a specific marker for small-bowel carcinoids. A 24-hour urine collection is requested, with the patient avoiding certain foods (e.g. bananas, avocados, aubergines, pineapples, plums, and walnuts), drinks (e.g. drinks containing caffeine), and medications (e.g. paracetamol, fluorouracil, methysergide, and naproxen) prior to the test. The test's sensitivity and specificity for metastatic small-bowel carcinoids is 76% and 88%, respectively.

In patients with small-bowel carcinoids, and especially in those with carcinoid syndrome, *N-terminal pro-brain natriuretic peptide* seems to be a very useful biomarker for detection of carcinoid heart disease (at a cut-off level of 260 pg/mL (30.68 pmol/L)) and offers a cost-effective approach to screening. It can identify those patients who will need a cardiac echocardiogram.

Emerging biomarkers include (1) antibodies against paraneoplastic antigen Ma2, which can be helpful for early detection of recurrence following surgery; and (2) circulating neuroendocrine tumours cells, levels of which can be used to monitor tumour growth and response to treatment and may also be of prognostic value. However, more studies are needed before the routine utilization of these novel markers in clinical practice is recommended.

Imaging studies

Radiological and nuclear medicine imaging studies are used for the initial assessment of disease extent and the localization of the primary lesion, especially in preoperative staging.

Transabdominal ultrasound is of limited value in revealing the primary lesion of small-bowel carcinoids, although the use of ultrasound 'microbubble' contrast medium may increase the sensitivity of ultrasound for the detection of liver metastases. Therefore, cross-sectional imaging with CT and MRI is currently the radiological approach of choice in the workup of patients with small-bowel carcinoids.

Multidetector CT is the most widely used cross-sectional imaging study for both assessment of tumour load and follow-up in small-bowel carcinoids. Hepatic metastases in CT demonstrate low attenuation in comparison to liver parenchyma on pre-contrast phase, whilst they strongly enhance post contrast. Small-bowel carcinoids mesenteric metastases associated with fibrosis have commonly a quite typical appearance with radiating strands of soft tissue (see Figure 13.7).

MRI is not the imaging of first choice in patients with small-bowel carcinoids. However, it can be used instead of CT in younger patients, in patients with iodine allergy, and in those with renal impairment, whilst it seems also to be more sensitive than CT for small hepatic metastases.

As approximately 90% of small-bowel carcinoids express somatostatin receptors type 2, the *octreoscan* is recognized as the gold-standard modality for imaging in small-bowel carcinoids, with an overall sensitivity of approximately 90% and 95% for primary tumour and hepatic metastases, respectively. The simultaneous performance of SPECT, using a triple-head camera, increases its sensitivity and specificity. An octreoscan may detect unsuspected lesions not shown by conventional studies, and this is crucial when surgery is planned. Furthermore, it may predict the response to treatment with somatostatin analogues. However, its sensitivity may be lower in small-volume disease and in tumours with a Ki-67 proliferation index of >10%.

Only 40%–50% of small-bowel carcinoids demonstrate uptake with ^{123}I-MIBG scintigraphy. Therefore,

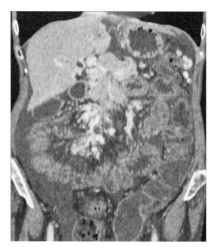

Fig 13.7 Abdominal CT demonstrating extensive mesenteric desmoplasia associated with a metastatic mesenteric mass from a small bowel carcinoid.

the role of this technique in the imaging assessment of small-bowel carcinoids is only complementary; an ^{123}I-MIBG scan is mainly performed to assess whether radio-targeted treatment with ^{131}I-MIBG can be considered.

Whenever conventional CT or an octreoscan fail to reveal the primary lesion, CT or MRI enteroclysis may detect an occult small-bowel carcinoid, with a reported sensitivity and specificity of 85% and 97%, respectively. The detection of the primary lesion can be also facilitated with small-bowel endoscopic studies such as *wireless small-bowel capsule endoscopy* or *double-balloon small-bowel enteroscopy*. However, not many centres have access to these endoscopic modalities, and their role in the diagnostic algorithm has not been fully established. In contrast, if a small-bowel carcinoid is suspected to be present in the terminal ileum, *colonoscopy with terminal ileum intubation*, a technique which is widely available, can be quite useful.

Recently, the labelling of somatostatin analogues with PET isotopes such as ^{68}Ga has led to the development of *[68]Ga-DOTATOC* and *[68]Ga-DOTATATE PET* scans (see Figure 13.8). These new imaging modalities can be completed within a few hours, compared to the 24–48 hours needed for an octreoscan, and also seem to identify additional tumour lesions. Moreover, new tracers, such as 5-HTP labelled with ^{11}C, and L-DOPA labelled with ^{18}F, have led to the development of *[11]C-5-HTP PET* and *[18]F-DOPA PET*, respectively. These types of PET seem to be valuable diagnostic tools, as they can detect small lesions not revealed by other methods. However, they are not widely available yet. Centres that have access to these techniques are utilizing them in patients with small-volume disease and a negative octreoscan and also for detection of an occult primary lesion. The most widely available technique, *[18]F-FDG PET*, is of limited value in most small-bowel carcinoids, as they are slow-growing malignancies and thus, have a largely normal glucose metabolism; it is only helpful in high-grade small-bowel carcinoids (very rare) and when a second malignancy is suspected.

32

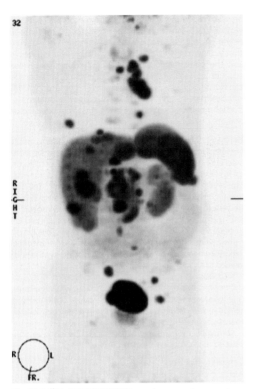

Fig 13.8 ^{68}Ga-DOTATATE PET scan demonstrating extensive mesenteric, hepatic, myocardial, and bone metastases from a patient with small bowel carcinoid.

Additional imaging studies that can be used for specific indications include *cardiac echocardiography*, for the initial assessment and the follow-up of patients with carcinoid heart disease; *cardiac MRI*, for the assessment of cardiac metastases; and *Tc bone scan* and *MRI spine*, when bone metastases, especially in the spine, are suspected.

Other investigations
Although the clinical features of steatorrhoea are quite typical (see 'Clinical features'), it can be confirmed with low levels of *faecal elastase*. Diarrhoea due to small-bowel bacterial overgrowth or bile-salt malabsorption can be confirmed with an *H_2-breath test* and a *nuclear medicine small-bowel malabsorption study*, respectively.

Treatment
The major goals of treatment in patients with small-bowel carcinoids are (1) medical control of patient's symptoms and improvement of their quality of life; (2) resection of the primary tumour and, if possible, metastatic lesions; and (3) control of tumour growth, in cases of advanced disease.

Symptom control
Carcinoid syndrome and carcinoid crisis
Somatostatin analogues may be used for symptom control, as follows. The monthly depot formulations *octreotide LAR* (for long-acting-repeatable) and *lanreotide Autogel* are administered as intramuscular and deep subcutaneous

injections, respectively. The licensed dosage of octreotide LAR is 10, 20, or 30 mg every 4 weeks; for lanreotide Autogel, the recommended doses are 60, 90, or 120 mg every 4 weeks. Long-acting somatostatin analogues provide sustained levels in plasma and also eliminate the need for daily injections. Studies have demonstrated that depot formulations have efficacies comparable to those of short-acting immediate release preparations. The depot formulations are currently considered to comprise the 'standard of care' for symptom control in patients with carcinoid syndrome, as these agents can control flushing and diarrhoea in >80% and >70% of patients, respectively. These agents also seem to reduce the incidence of carcinoid heart disease and delay its progression. There are no randomized studies to date comparing the efficacy of octreotide versus lanreotide in carcinoid syndrome. Loss of response to treatment with somatostatin analogues has been explained by tachyphylaxis, which, according to recent data, appears later than was previously thought. In cases of breakthrough symptoms, it is common practice to increase the dose of octreotide LAR to 30 mg per month, or the dose of lanreotide Autogel to 120 mg every 28 days. If symptoms occur throughout the month, the options are (1) to increase the dose of octreotide LAR up to 60 mg/month (doses >60 mg do not seem to be more efficacious); (2) to administer subcutaneous booster injections as required; or (3) to switch to a continuous subcutaneous octreotide pump. Alternatively, if breakthrough symptoms occur mainly during the week before the next long-acting injection, a reduction of administration intervals from 28 to 21 days can be considered.

In cases of carcinoid crisis, intravenous octreotide is given as a 50–500 μg bolus, and may be continued as an infusion at 50 μg/hour for a further 24–48 hours. Additionally, intravenous antihistamines and hydrocortisone may be of some benefit. For the prevention of carcinoid crisis, prophylactic administration of octreotide is given by constant intravenous infusion at a dose of 50 μg/hour for 12 hours prior to, and at least 48 hours after, an interventional procedure (e.g. an operation, or any other procedure that involves general anaesthesia or transarterial hepatic embolization). For the same reason, patients who have carcinoid syndrome and are, for any reason, on inotropes should be on concomitant intravenous octreotide as well. Somatostatin analogues are well-tolerated medications in the vast majority of patients. However, some adverse effects, such as cholelithiasis (in up to 50% of patients), steatorrhoea, abdominal discomfort, and bloating have been described.

Interferon alfa is a well-established treatment for gastro-entero-pancreatic neuroendocrine tumours and a second-line treatment in patients with carcinoid syndrome. Combining interferon alfa with somatostatin analogues seems to be beneficial in patients with breakthrough symptoms refractory to somatostatin-analogue monotherapy. The recommended dose for interferon alfa in the treatment of gastro-entero-pancreatic neuroendocrine tumours is 3–9 million units, usually three times per week subcutaneously. Symptomatic as well as biochemical responses (e.g. reduction of 5-hydroxyindoleacetic acid levels) have been noted in about 50% of patients. A common problem with interferon treatment is the adverse effects associated with it, and these may influence patients' compliance with treatment. The effects include chronic fatigue syndrome, flu-like symptoms, bone-marrow suppression, depression, thyroid-function disorders, and other autoimmune phenomena.

Transarterial hepatic embolization is an interventional procedure which is performed in patients with predominantly metastatic disease in the liver, and severe carcinoid syndrome that is refractory to the aforementioned treatment options. Symptomatic and biochemical responses have been noted in 40%–80% and 7%–75% of patients, respectively. This treatment requires careful patient selection. Contraindications include hepatic failure, tumour burden exceeding 50% of the hepatic volume, portal vein occlusion, and hyperbilirubinaemia. Relative contraindications are contrast allergy, coagulopathies, severe carcinoid heart disease, extra-hepatic tumour dominance, and poor performance status. Post-embolization syndrome (abdominal pain, fever, and nausea) is the commonest adverse effect. Serious complications may occur in individual patents and include gallbladder necrosis, renal failure, liver abscess, vascular damage, hepatorenal syndrome, and carcinoid crisis.

Peptide receptor therapy is another option in cases of symptomatic progression despite treatment with somatostatin analogues (see 'Control of tumour growth').

Complications of mesenteric fibrosis

There is no established medical treatment to date for the prevention of the development or treatment of mesenteric fibrosis; therefore, at present, we need to focus on the medical treatment of its complications. For mesenteric ischaemia-type pain, oral analgesics are used, and rotating oral antibiotics (ciprofloxacin, metronidazole, rifaximin, etc.) comprise the main treatment for small-bowel bacterial overgrowth. In cases of SMV occlusion, there is limited experience with placement of SMV stents by interventional radiologists.

Other medications

In patient who are on treatment with somatostatin analogues and have developed steatorrhoea, oral pancreatic enzyme supplements can be very helpful. Oral cholestyramine is the treatment of diarrhoea related to bile-salt malabsorption. It is also recommended to commence patients with carcinoid syndrome on oral vitamin B compounds to prevent symptoms of pellagra. Finally, initial medical management of patients with carcinoid heart disease and features of right-heart dysfunction includes oral diuretics.

Resection of primary and metastatic disease

It is preferable that patients who are due to undergo elective surgery for small-bowel carcinoids should be operated in centres with experience in neuroendocrine tumours. Patients with known carcinoid syndrome should receive peri-operative intravenous octreotide for the prevention of a carcinoid crisis (see symptoms control).

Primary tumour

Curative resection should be the aim in all patients with localized disease and should involve, apart from resection of the primary lesion, dissection around the mesentery and clearance of regional lymph nodes. If the tumour is located in the terminal ileum, a concomitant right hemicolectomy is recommended.

Palliative resection should be used in patients with distant metastases who are symptomatic from the primary tumour, to prevent further deterioration of symptoms and increased morbidity. This palliative resection can

be also recommended even in asymptomatic patients in order to prevent complications related to mesenteric desmoplasia. The decision should be made after discussion in a neuroendocrine multidisciplinary team meeting, and the patient's co-morbidities should be taken into account as well. Although the latter recommendation cannot be supported by randomized studies, data from retrospective series have shown that logo-regional resection of the primary tumour is a positive prognostic factor and may influence survival.

Resection of hepatic metastatic disease

Hepatectomy with curative intent should always be considered in patients with advanced small-bowel carcinoids, as it seems that it is associated with increased survival. However, according to the existing guidelines, the following criteria need to be met: (1) the tumours should be histologically G1 or G2, and the predicted morbidity and mortality rates in the individual patient should be acceptable; (2) there should be no unresectable lymph nodes, extra-hepatic distant metastases, or peritoneal carcinomatosis; and (3) there should be no features of severe carcinoid heart disease.

Debulking liver resection can be considered if >90% of the hepatic tumour load can be removed, whilst *palliative resection for symptom control* can only be recommended in selective cases, following discussion in a neuroendocrine multidisciplinary team meeting.

Orthotopic liver transplantation should be only be considered in exceptional circumstances.

Concomitant cholecystectomy

Although prospective data are lacking, it is recommended that patients who are having an elective surgery for small-bowel carcinoids should have a concomitant cholecystectomy as well. These patients may be already on or will be treated in the future with somatostatin analogues, and there is always a risk of cholelithiasis and its complications.

Non-gastrointestinal surgery

Cardiac surgery for heart valve replacement can be considered on individual basis in patients with severe carcinoid heart disease. Cardiac surgery should be only performed in specialist centres, and patients who get referred should have well-controlled carcinoid-syndrome symptoms, stable disease radiologically, good nutritional status, and no significant co-morbidities.

Control of tumour growth
Active surveillance

In asymptomatic patients with low-grade (G1) tumours, low tumour load, and non-progressive disease, no treatment but only active surveillance could be a reasonable management option.

Somatostatin analogues

The use of somatostatin analogues as anti-proliferative agents has only been established recently. Retrospective studies have shown stabilization of tumour growth in ≥50% of patients with progressive disease. The results of a recent randomized Phase III trial (PROMID; for *p*lacebo-controlled, double-blind, prospective, randomized study of the effect of *o*ctreotide LAR in the control of tumour growth in patients with metastatic neuroendocrine *mid*gut tumours) demonstrated that the median time to progression in patients with small-bowel carcinoids treated with octreotide LAR was more than twice as long, compared to that of patients treated with placebo. The most favourable results were seen in patients in whom the primary tumour had been resected, and in those who had a low (<10%) hepatic tumour load. The results of a Phase III study of lanreotide versus a placebo have also demonstrated the effect of this somatostatin analogue to retard neuroendocrine tumour growth, regardless of hepatic load and for a Ki-67 proliferation index <10% (the CLARINET study).

Interferon alpha
The anti-proliferative role of interferon alpha has been assessed in combination with somatostatin analogues in two randomized trials, in which interferon alfa was combined with either lanreotide or octreotide. These studies failed to show that the combination was superior to monotherapy with somatostatin analogues with regards to progression-free survival or overall survival. Not surprisingly, the adverse effect profile was more pronounced in the combination group.

Peptide receptor radiotherapy
According to retrospective, non-randomized trials treatment with radiolabelled peptides, apart from improvement of symptoms and quality of life, the peptides can also provide control of the tumour growth in patients with advanced small-bowel carcinoid. This treatment can target all tumours that show positive uptake on octreoscan or in ^{68}Ga-DOTATOC/DOTATATE PET scans. A large series of patients with several types of advanced neuroendocrine tumours (including small-bowel carcinoids) has shown complete responses and partial responses in 2% and 28%, respectively, of patients who were treated with ^{177}Lu-DOTATATE, and such positive results were confirmed in the recent NETTER-1 study which used a randomized design with a control arm comprising an increased dose of octreotide LAR. Encouraging results have been also demonstrated with ^{90}Y-DOTATATE in patients who progressed despite previous treatments. The main adverse effects of peptide receptor therapy include bone-marrow suppression and renal toxicity.

^{131}I-MIBG
According to data from a large series, in patients with metastatic small-bowel carcinoids, ^{131}I-MIBG is associated with symptomatic response in 60%–65%, hormonal response in 12.5%, and objective tumour response in 0%–15%. However, it is usually considered to be a second-line radio-targeted treatment, as tumour uptake is usually better with radiolabelled peptides, and the hospitalization period is shorter.

Systemic chemotherapy
It is generally not effective in patients with advanced small-bowel carcinoids, and can only be considered in selective cases where all other treatments have failed to control tumour growth. However, it is a first-choice treatment in the rare situation when a small-bowel carcinoid is poorly differentiated (G3).

Loco-regional treatments
They are considered in patients with predominantly metastatic disease in the liver. Transarterial hepatic embolization (see 'Symptom control') is associated with 8%–60% objective responses; however, the mean duration of response is sometimes short, lasting for only 6–8 months.

Radiofrequency ablation of hepatic metastases can be considered when the tumour size in the liver is <3 cm and the number of metastases is small; better results are seen when it is combined with liver surgery.

New molecular targeted treatments
A recent randomized study has shown that *everolimus (an mTOR inhibitor) plus octreotide LAR* may improve progression-free survival in comparison to octreotide LAR alone in patients with advanced small-bowel carcinoids. However, further randomized studies are needed to assess the new molecular targeted treatments in terms of symptomatic and quality of life benefit, as well as overall survival.

Follow-up
According to the existing guidelines, all patients should be followed up every 6–12 months, whilst high-grade small-bowel carcinoids need to be followed up every 3 months. The follow-up should be life long and consist of clinical evaluation, estimation of blood and urine biomarkers, and review of cross-sectional imaging studies. An octreoscan does not need to be performed routinely at follow-up.

Prognosis: Survival
According to the results of a large study from a tertiary referral centre in Uppsala, Sweden, and a multicentre study supported by the United Kingdom and Ireland Neuroendocrine Tumours Society, the median overall survival from date of diagnosis was 8.4 years for all small-bowel carcinoids. In patients who had hepatic metastases, the median survival from the date of diagnosis was 7.69 years, and 5.95 years from date of diagnosis of liver metastases. On the basis of univariate and multivariate analyses, increasing age at diagnosis, increasing levels of chromogranin A and 5-hydroxyindoleacetic acid, a high Ki-67 level, carcinoid heart disease, and peritoneal carcinomatosis were associated with a poorer outcome. In contrast, resection of hepatic metastases, resection of the primary tumour, treatment with somatostatin analogues, and peptide receptor radiotherapy were associated with improved prognosis.

Patient support groups/useful websites
The following patient support groups and websites may be useful:
- http://www.netpatientfoundation.org
- http://www.ukinets.org
- http://www.enets.org

Further reading
Ahmed A, Turner G, King B, et al. Midgut neuroendocrine tumours with liver metastases: Results of the UKINETS study. *Endocr Relat Cancer* 2009; 16: 885–94.

Bhattacharyya S, Davar J, Dreyfus G, et al. Carcinoid heart disease. *Circulation* 2007; 116: 2860–5.

Boudreaux JP, Klimstra DS, Hassan MM, et al. The NANETS consensus guideline for the diagnosis and management of neuroendocrine tumors: Well-differentiated neuroendocrine tumors of the jejunum, ileum, appendix, and cecum. *Pancreas* 2010; 39: 753–66.

Caplin ME, Pavel M, Ćwikła JB, et al. Lanreotide in metastatic enteropancreatic neuroendocrine tumors. *N Engl J Med* 2014; 371: 224–33.

Norlén O, Stålberg P, Öberg K, et al. Long-term results of surgery for small intestinal neuroendocrine tumors at a tertiary referral center. *World J Surg* 2012; 36: 1419–31.

Pape UF, Perren A, Niederle B, et al. ENETS Consensus Guidelines for the management of patients with neuroendocrine neoplasms from the jejuno-ileum and the appendix including goblet cell carcinomas. *Neuroendocrinology* 2012; 95: 135–56.

Pavel M, Baudin E, Couvelard A, et al. ENETS Consensus Guidelines for the management of patients with liver and other distant metastases from neuroendocrine neoplasms of foregut, midgut, hindgut, and unknown primary. *Neuroendocrinology* 2012; 95: 157–76.

Ramage JK, Ahmed A, Ardill J, et al. Guidelines for the management of gastroenteropancreatic neuroendocrine (including carcinoid) tumours (NETs). Gut 2012; 61: 6–32.

Rindi G, Arnold R, Bosman FT, et al. 'Nomenclature and classification of neuroendocrine neoplasms of the digestive system', in Bosman FT, Carneiro F, Hruban RH, et al., eds, *WHO Classification of Tumours in the Digestive System* (4th edition), 2010. IARC, pp. 13–14.

Rinke A, Müller HH, Schade-Brittinger C, et al. Placebo-controlled, double-blind, prospective, randomized study on the effect of Octreotide LAR in the control of tumor growth in patients with metastatic neuroendocrine midgut tumors: A report from the PROMID Study Group. *J Clin Oncol* 2009; 27: 4656–63.

Toumpanakis CG and Caplin ME. Molecular genetics of gastroenteropancreatic neuroendocrine tumors. *Am J Gastroenterol* 2008; 103: 729–32.

13.4 Insulinomas

Definition
Insulinoma is a neuroendocrine tumour arising from the beta cells of the pancreas (the islets of Langerhans) and so is capable of secreting insulin.

Epidemiology
Insulinoma is reported to be the most common cause of hypoglycaemia in patients who are well without systemic illness (including diabetes mellitus), once factitious hypoglycaemia has been excluded. However, it is a rare tumour, with an estimated incidence of 4 per million population per year. Autopsy studies suggest a higher prevalence and therefore tumours may remain undiagnosed in life. The median age of presentation is in the fifth decade of life and there is a female-to-male preponderance.

Pathophysiology
Insulinomas are the commonest type of functional pancreatic neuroendocrine tumours and they are usually benign. The majority are sporadic, although they are also associated with multiple endocrine neoplasia type 1 and, in this setting, they are more likely to be malignant. Prediction of malignancy depends on WHO criteria, which include tumour size, the presence of metastases, local invasiveness, vascular invasion, and mitotic index; however, these criteria are not always reliable.

Clinical features
Insulinoma must appear in the differential diagnosis of fasting hypoglycaemia in a person who is otherwise healthy. Hypoglycaemia may present as unexplained collapse, loss of consciousness, or 'funny turns'. Symptoms may include adrenergic symptoms and neuroglycopenic symptoms. Although the symptoms may be highly suggestive, there are frequently no physical signs. There is often evidence of weight gain due to snacking to prevent or overcome the symptoms, or secondary to the hyperinsulinaemia, and there may be signs from other endocrine tumours if the presentation is in the context of a tumour-prone syndrome. It is important to demonstrate Whipple's triad either at the time of symptoms or with a provocation test (see Chapter 15, Section 15.1).

Investigations
Making the diagnosis
The diagnosis relies upon the demonstration of biochemical hypoglycaemia (see Chapter 15, Section 15.1) in the context of inappropriately elevated serum insulin concentrations. The provocation test is the prolonged supervised fast, which is positive in 94% of cases (either alone or as well as the occurrence of reactive hypoglycaemia). This is run as an inpatient investigation according to a formalized protocol. Up to 6% of patients will have post-prandial hypoglycaemia alone. Historically, this was provoked by an oral glucose load but the number of false positives has encouraged a shift towards a mixed-meal test, which is also a more physiological investigation. Corroborative evidence, such as C-peptide, beta hydroxybutyrate, and a sulfonylurea screen, do not assist with the biochemical diagnosis of hyperinsulinaemic hypoglycaemia, but are important in order to help rule out differential diagnoses, such as self-administration of insulin or oral hypoglycaemic

agents. Inappropriately elevated insulin without elevated C-peptide is suggestive of exogenous insulin administration, whilst classical biochemistry but with concurrent detectable sulfonylurea in the blood implies use of oral hypoglycaemic agents. However, not all oral hypoglycaemic agents (e.g. repaglinide) can be detected in this way (see Chapter 15, Section 15.1).

Over time there has been an increasing economic pressure to demonstrate Whipple's triad (see also Chapter 15, Section 15.1) without resorting to a 3-day admission, and reports from some centres have suggested that up to 83% of patients with subsequent insulinoma diagnoses are hypoglycaemic within the first 22 hours of the fast, enabling the majority of procedures to be carried out under day-case supervision.

The original diagnostic criteria required an insulin level of >6 mU/L in the presence of hypoglycaemia—the specified glucose level at which this should be measured is 2.2 mmol/L (39.6 mg/dL). We have found that the threshold of 3.0 mmol/L (54.1 mg/dL) advised by some groups reduces specificity. This insulin level is applicable when the insulin level is measured by double-antibody radioimmunoassay, with a lower limit of detection of 5 mU/L. The use of polyclonal antibodies leads to as much as 40%–80% cross-reactivity with proinsulin. Monoclonal assays overcame this issue, and their use has enabled lower minimum concentrations of insulin to be detected: this is important where highly specific measures of insulin are required. The cross-reactivity of highly specific insulin assays has been evaluated; whilst they have a place in the diagnosis of insulinoma, as insulin levels are measured 14%–93% lower than those from non-specific assays, it has been suggested that, if they are used, the diagnostic cut-off for hyperinsulinaemia should be revised downwards. A level of 3 mU/L (18 pmol/L; 0.3 mg/dL) has been proposed within recent consensus guidelines. Normative values during prolonged fasting are still needed for newer insulin assays. It is important to exclude alternative diagnoses such as exogenous insulin administration and covert use of oral hypoglycaemic agents, as described previously.

Cases have been described in which insulin levels have been measured below the 6 mU/L critical threshold, and even below the level of 3 mU/L. Several authors have proposed additional measurements to enhance the diagnostic accuracy of the fast. These include measurement of proinsulin and C-peptide. Proinsulin is known to have a hypoglycaemic effect, and tumours that secrete predominantly proinsulin have been documented to cause hypoglycaemia. Under such circumstances, measurement of proinsulin as well as C-peptide has proved helpful. Current guidelines suggest diagnostic thresholds of >200 pmol/L (0.6 ng/mL) for C-peptide and <2.7 mmol/L (28.11 mg/dL) for beta hydroxybutyrate. It is only once the diagnosis of inappropriate endogenous hyperinsulinaemia in the presence of hypoglycaemia is achieved that the next step in investigation will usually be taken: tests to localize the source of excess insulin.

Insulinoma localization
At the time of diagnosis, the vast majority of insulinomas are small, intrapancreatic, and curable by surgery. Preoperative localization improves the chance of cure and reduces the likelihood of complications, but can prove to

be a clinical challenge. Cross-sectional imaging techniques such as abdominal ultrasound and CT scanning have been extensively used but, in general, published data have not shown these to be particularly accurate, with reported sensitivities in the range 17%–50%, although occasional series suggest sensitivities much higher. For example, a CT sensitivity of 94% using multidetector scanning and fine reformats has been demonstrated, whilst MRI performs better, with sensitivities described of 79% for delayed enhanced T1-weighted images or with the use of combined sequences up to 85%. Endoscopic ultrasound is evolving and improving, but this semi-invasive technique is highly dependent on operator experience. However, such a technique may, with the addition of ultrasound-guided biopsy, provide an opportunity for histological diagnosis. Selective intra-arterial injection of the pancreatic arteries with calcium and hepatic venous sampling for insulin, correlates anatomy with function, and in many series appears to be the most sensitive method: a twofold step-up in insulin release suggests that the injected artery supplies the territory feeding the tumour. It allows regionalization (according to the arterial supply territory) rather than localization but this can be corroborated with 2D imaging and this is often sufficient to guide surgical planning (see Figure 13.9).

Results of localization from patients with tumour-prone syndromes are difficult to compare due to the small numbers and the fact that, in general, many such patients present with incidental findings of pancreatic nodules and undergo one or more prior pancreatic resections, making further preoperative localization strategies challenging. For this group of patients, the conclusions regarding sporadic insulinoma localization are unlikely to be suitable for extrapolation.

Management

Symptomatic management
The aim of medical management is to prevent hypoglycaemic episodes during periods of fasting. The initial approach may involve smaller and more frequent meals containing predominantly low-glycaemic-index foods. This may be supplemented by the use of guar gum or acarbose. The most effective drug for controlling hypoglycaemia is diazoxide (starting with as little as 50 mg daily and increasing up to 200 mg three times daily). It suppresses insulin secretion by direct action on the beta cell and by enhancing glycogenolysis. Other useful drugs include glucocorticoids, verapamil, phenytoin, and somatostatin analogues (although these may also paralyse the glucagon-induced hyperglycaemic response to hypoglycaemia and worsen symptoms).

Definitive management
Once the diagnosis and the location of the tumour have been established, the definitive management of insulinoma is surgical. Intraoperative blood glucose monitoring is necessary, together with intravenous glucose infusion. The majority are small and may be managed by enucleation; localization may be aided by intraoperative ultrasound. The most common complication of this operation is pancreatic leak, which may be managed with fibrin glue. More extensive surgery may be required if the tumour is located in particular areas which may be difficult to access, such as the head of the pancreas. In some cases, a partial pancreatectomy or even a Whipple's procedure may prove necessary. Blood sugar may rise shortly after a successful operation and there may even be prolonged rebound hyperglycaemia. Histopathological findings help to determine the optimal follow-up strategy. After a complete resection, a patient may be considered cured but prolonged follow-up is important, especially for patients with suspected malignancy or with tumour-prone syndromes such as multiple endocrine neoplasia type 1.

Management of malignant insulinoma
For patients with persistent or recurrent hypoglycaemia due to local tumour recurrence, reoperation may be appropriate. Where this is not feasible or where there is metastatic spread, systemic treatments must be considered in addition to strategies for medical management of the hypoglycaemia. In pancreatic neuroendocrine tumours, somatostatin analogues may reduce hormonal secretion and have a cytostatic effect. Insulinomas in general appear to have fewer surface somatostatin receptors than other neuroendocrine tumours but these agents may nonetheless be helpful in some cases and small studies now also suggest a benefit from everolimus in the management of malignant insulinoma, both to treat progressive disease but also to treat the hypoglycaemia.

Future developments
For benign insulinomas, improvements in localization and in surgical technique (including intraoperative ultrasound) are enabling a more focused approach to surgery and a greater proportion of patients treated laparoscopically, or by enucleation. For malignant insulinomas, if uptake is present, peptide receptor radiotherapy with radiolabelled octreotide analogues may be helpful. Available chemotherapy regimens are essentially palliative and tailored to the proliferative index.

Further reading
de Herder WW, van Schaik E, Kwekkeboom D, et al. New therapeutic options for metastatic malignant insulinoma. *Clin Endo* 2011; 75: 277–84.

Druce MR, Muthuppalaniappan VM, O'Leary B, et al. Diagnosis and localisation of insulinoma: The value of modern MRI in conjunction with calcium stimulation catheterisation. *Eur J Endo* 2010; 162: 971–8.

Guettier JM, Kam A, Chang R, et al. Localisation of insulinomas to regions of the pancreas by intraarterial calcium stimulation: The NIH experience. *J Clin Endocrinol Metab* 2009; 94: 1074–80.

Plackzowski KA, Vella A, Thompson GB, et al. Secular trends in the presentation and management of functioning insulinoma at the Mayo Clinic 1987-2007. *J Clin Endocrinol Metab* 2009; 94: 1069–73.

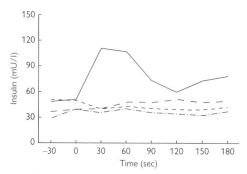

Fig 13.9 Results of a calcium-stimulation catheter, demonstrating insulin excess from the superior mesenteric artery territory which covers the head of the pancreas.

13.5 Gastrinomas

Definitions

- Gastrinomas are neuroendocrine tumours, usually located in the duodenum or pancreas, that secrete gastrin and cause a clinical syndrome known as Zollinger–Ellison syndrome.
- Zollinger–Ellison syndrome is characterized by gastric acid hypersecretion resulting in severe peptic disease (peptic ulcer disease or gastro-oesophageal reflux disease).
- Duodenal tumours now make up 50%–88% of gastrinomas in sporadic Zollinger–Ellison syndrome patients, and 70%–100% of gastrinomas in patients with multiple endocrine neoplasia type 1 together with Zollinger–Ellison syndrome.
- Approximately 25% of patients with Zollinger–Ellison patients have gastrinomas that pursue an aggressive course, and aggressive growth occurs in 40% of patients who presented with liver metastases.
- At diagnosis, 5%–10% of duodenal gastrinomas and 20%–25% of pancreatic gastrinomas are associated with liver metastases.

Incidence

The incidence of gastrinomas is 0.5–3.0 per million population per year.

At the onset of symptoms the mean age of patients with sporadic gastrinomas is 48–55 years; 54%–56% are male, and the mean delay in diagnosis from the onset of symptoms is 5.2 years.

Histopathology

The WHO classifies functioning endocrine tumours of the pancreas into three well-defined categories:

- well-differentiated endocrine tumours, with benign or uncertain behaviour at the time of diagnosis
- well-differentiated endocrine carcinomas with low-grade malignant behaviour
- poorly differentiated endocrine carcinomas, with high-grade malignant behaviour

Clinical presentation

Zollinger–Ellison syndrome should be suspected if there is:

- recurrent, severe, or familial peptic ulcer disease
- peptic ulcer disease without *Helicobacter pylori*
- peptic ulcer disease resistant to treatment or associated with complications (perforation, penetration, bleeding)
- peptic ulcer disease with endocrinopathies or diarrhoea
- peptic ulcer disease with prominent gastric folds on an upper-gastrointestinal series or at endoscopy (92% of Zollinger–Ellison syndrome patients), or with hypocalcaemia or hypergastrinaemia
- abdominal pain (primarily due to peptic ulcer disease or gastro-oesophageal reflux disease; occurs in 75%–98% of cases)
- diarrhoea (occurs in 30%–73% of cases)
- heartburn (occurs in 44%–56% of the cases)
- upper-gastrointestinal bleeding (occurs in 44%–75% of cases)
- nausea/vomiting (occurs in 12%–30% of cases)
- weight loss (occurs in 7%–53% of cases)

Patients with multiple endocrine neoplasia type 1 together with Zollinger–Ellison syndrome (20%–30%) present at an earlier age (mean 32–35 years) than patients with sporadic disease.

Biochemical investigations

Initially fasting serum gastrin levels (FSG) and gastric pH should be determined (off proton-pump inhibitors for at least 1 week, with H2-blocker coverage, *if possible*).

The diagnosis of Zollinger–Ellison syndrome generally requires the demonstration of an inappropriate FSG elevation by demonstrating hypergastrinaemia in the presence of hyperchlorhydria or an acidic pH (preferably ≤2).

At presentation, >98% of patients have an elevated FSG, 87%–90% have marked gastric acid hypersecretion (basal acid output greater than 15 mEq/hour), and 100% have a gastric acid pH ≤2.

If the FSG is <10-fold elevated, and the gastric pH ≤2, then a secretin test and a basal acid output should be done.

Importantly, elevated FSG levels can *also* be caused by hypochlorhydria/achlorhydria (chronic atrophic fundus gastritis, often associated with pernicious anaemia) as well as *H. pylori* infection, gastric outlet obstruction, renal failure, antral G-cell syndromes, short bowel syndrome, and retained antrum.

Of patients with Zollinger–Ellison syndrome and peptic ulcer disease, only 24%–48% have *H. pylori* infection, in contrast to patients with idiopathic peptic disease, of whom >90% have *H. pylori* infection. Therefore, a lack of *H. pylori* infection should lead to a suspicion of Zollinger–Ellison syndrome in a patient with recurrent peptic ulcer disease.

Tumour localization

Sixty to ninety per cent of gastrinomas are malignant, and tumour localization studies are necessary to determine whether surgical resection is indicated, to localize the primary tumour, to determine the extent of the disease and whether metastatic disease to the liver or distant sites is present, and to assess changes in tumour extent with treatment.

Localization studies include conventional imaging studies (CT, MRI, ultrasound), selective angiography, functional localization methods (angiography with secretin stimulation for hepatic venous gastrin gradients, portal venous sampling for gastrin gradients), somatostatin receptor scintigraphy, and endoscopic ultrasound, as well as intraoperative localization methods, including intraoperative ultrasound, intraoperative transillumination of the duodenum, and duodenotomy.

Treatment

Medical treatment

Both H2 blockers and proton-pump inhibitors can control acid hypersecretion in all patients who can take oral medications and are cooperative.

Somatostatin analogues will reduce the hypergastrinaemia.

Surgical treatment

Surgery is the only treatment that can cure gastrinomas. Patients with sporadic Zollinger–Ellison syndrome with resectable disease and without serious contraindications to surgery or with concomitant illnesses limiting life expectancy should undergo routine surgical exploration (laparotomy) for cure by a surgeon experienced in treating these tumours.

Surgery has been shown to decrease the rate of development of liver metastases.

Long-term curative resection without a pancreaticoduodenectomy (Whipple resection) occurs in 20%–45% of patients with sporadic Zollinger–Ellison syndrome when the surgery is performed by a surgeon skilled in the treatment of this disease, but in 0%–1% of patients with multiple endocrine neoplasia type 1 and Zollinger–Ellison syndrome.

Tumours in the pancreatic head area should be enucleated, distal pancreatic resection should be performed for caudally located tumours, and duodenotomy should be performed routinely to detect small duodenal gastrinomas. A lymph node dissection should be performed even if no primary tumour is found, because lymph node primary tumours are reported, although their role is controversial.

The use of routine surgical exploration in patients with multiple endocrine neoplasia type 1 and Zollinger–Ellison syndrome is controversial, since these patients usually have multiple duodenal gastrinomas, which occur frequently with lymph node metastases, the patients are rarely cured, and they have an excellent life expectancy if only small tumours (<2 cm) or no tumours are present on imaging studies.

Advanced disease treatment

Cytoreductive surgery, chemotherapy, biotherapy (somatostatin analogues/interferon), peptide receptor radionuclide therapy, liver transplantation, and hepatic artery embolization or chemo-embolization have all been recommended as being of value in patients with advanced Zollinger–Ellison syndrome.

Prognosis

The 10-year survival without liver metastases is 95%, falling to 80% with liver metastases.

Further reading

Ito T, Igarashi H, and Jensen RT. Zollinger-Ellison syndrome: Recent advances and controversies. *Curr Opin Gastroenterol* 2013; 29: 650–1.

Ito T, Cadiot G, and Jensen RT. Diagnosis of Zollinger-Ellison syndrome: Increasingly difficult. *World J Gastroenterol* 2012; 18: 5495–5503.

13.6 Glucagonomas

Introduction
- Glucagonomas arise from the glucagon-producing alpha cells of the pancreas.
- About 90% of patients already have liver (in 67% of patients) or lymph-node metastases at presentation.
- Approximately 5%–20% of glucagonomas are associated with multiple endocrine neoplasia type 1.

Incidence
The estimated incidence of glucagonomas is 0.01–0.1 per million population per year.

Histopathology
For the histopathology of endocrine tumours of the pancreas, see Section 13.5.

Clinical presentation
The most common presenting features of the glucagonoma syndrome are:
- necrolytic migratory erythema (occurs in more than 70% of patients); this characteristic rash may also involve the mucous membranes, leading to cheilitis, glossitis, and stomatitis
- notable weight loss or cachexia (occurs in more than 60% of patients)
- complaints pointing to the diagnosis of diabetes mellitus (occur in more than 50% of all cases)
- diarrhoea
- psychiatric disturbances, such as depression or psychosis
- enhanced tendency to venous thrombosis (occurs in approximately 11% of patients)

Biochemical investigations
The most common presenting features of glucagonoma are:
- elevated blood glucose levels (occur in more than 50% of all cases)
- normochromic normocytic anaemia (occurs in approximately 33% of cases)
- elevated fasting plasma glucagon levels (occur in all patients)
- elevated levels of pancreatic polypeptide (occur in approximately 50% of patients)

Tumour localization
As for other neuroendocrine pancreatic tumours, tumour localization with transabdominal ultrasonography, CT, MRI, selective abdominal angiography, endoscopic ultrasonography, or somatostatin receptor scintigraphy can be performed.

Treatment
- Diabetic patients may require insulin therapy.
- Aspirin therapy has been used to prevent thrombosis.
- Total surgical removal may be curative only for patients with local, benign disease.
- In patients with more extensive disease, cytoreductive debulking surgery can effectively reduce symptoms, even without necessarily normalizing plasma glucagon levels.
- Liver transplantation has only rarely been performed in glucagonoma patients.
- Single or repeated hepatic artery embolization of metastases initially results in symptomatic symptom relief in the majority (>80%) of patients but, in >50% of patients, symptoms will progress within half a year.
- In both benign and malignant disease, somatostatin analogues are effective in controlling the rash, but less effective in the management of weight loss and diabetes mellitus and ineffective in reducing the incidence of venous thrombosis.
- Palliative combination chemotherapy with dacarbazine, fluorouracil, and streptozotocin seems of only temporary benefit, but is often given in advanced disease.
- Targeted therapy using sunitinib or everolimus has been used for tumour control.
- Peptide receptor radionuclide therapy may also show favourable therapeutic effects.

Further reading
Vinik A, Feliberti E, and Perry RR. Glucagonoma syndrome. Available at http://www.ncbi.nlm.nih.gov/books/NBK279041/ (accessed 13 Jan 2018).

13.7 VIPomas

Introduction

- Tumours that secrete vasoactive intestinal polypeptide, also called VIPomas, account for less than 10% of islet cell tumours.
- VIPomas are mostly solitary tumours, arising from pancreatic cells that secrete vasoactive intestinal polypeptide; these are usually located in the pancreatic tail and body.
- More than 60% of these tumours are malignant and metastasize to lymph nodes, the liver, the kidneys, and bone.
- Rarely, extra-pancreatic tumours appearing as neuroblastomas, ganglioneuroblastomas, or ganglioneuromas have been found.
- VIPomas occur occasionally in patients with multiple endocrine neoplasia (approximately 1%).

Incidence

The estimated incidence of VIPomas is 0.05–0.20 per million per year.

Histopathology

See Section 13.5.

Clinical presentation

A VIPoma, also called Verner–Morrison syndrome or WDHA (for watery diarrhoea, hypokalaemia, and acidosis) syndrome, presents with the following features:

- secretory watery diarrhoea, resulting from stimulation of intestinal fluid secretion by vasoactive intestinal polypeptide; this can lead to hypovolaemia (and hypokalaemia, hypomagnesaemia, hypophosphataemia, and acidosis)
- hypotension resulting from peripheral vasodilatation caused by the direct cardiovascular effects of vasoactive intestinal polypeptide (occurs in some patients)
- signs and symptoms of diabetes mellitus (occurs in 18% of cases)
- flushing (occurs in in approximately 20% of patients)

  Untreated patients usually die within 1 year from diagnosis as a result of severe metabolic disturbances leading to cardiac arrest and renal insufficiency.

Biochemical investigations

The most common presenting features of a VIPoma are:

- hypokalaemia (occurs in virtually all patients)
- hypophosphataemia
- acidosis
- hypomagnesaemia
- hypochlorhydria or achlorhydria (occurs in approximately 75% of patients)

- hypercalcaemia (occurs in 25%–75% of patients)
- glucose intolerance (occurs in 50% of patients) and elevated glucose levels (occur in 18% of cases)
- elevated fasting plasma vasoactive intestinal polypeptide and peptide histidine–methionine concentrations (occur in virtually all patients)
- elevated pancreatic polypeptide levels (occur in 75% of patients) and elevated neurotensin levels (occur in 10% of patients)

Tumour localization

- As for other neuroendocrine pancreatic tumours, tumour localization with transabdominal ultrasonography, CT, MRI, selective abdominal angiography, endoscopic ultrasonography, or somatostatin receptor scintigraphy can be performed.

Treatment

- Severe cases of Verner–Morrison syndrome often require intensive intravenous supplementation of fluid losses (often exceeding 10 L/day) and careful correction of electrolyte and acid–base abnormalities.
- Somatostatin analogues reduce tumoural secretion of vasoactive intestinal polypeptide by more than 50% and inhibit intestinal water and electrolyte secretion. By this mechanism, these drugs control the secretory diarrhoea in more than 50% of patients and, in another 25%, significant clinical improvement is attained.
- Glucocorticoids can also potentially improve diarrhoea, presumably by inhibiting the release of vasoactive intestinal polypeptide and enhancing sodium absorption in the intestines.
- Total surgical removal of the primary tumour may be curative in approximately 40% of patients with either benign VIPomas or non-metastatic malignant tumours.
- In patients with metastatic VIPomas, cytoreductive debulking surgery may result in considerable palliation.
- Palliative combination chemotherapy with streptozotocin and fluorouracil has a limited (approximately 33%) response.
- Interferon alpha has also been used in a small number of patients, with variable success.
- Targeted therapy using sunitinib or everolimus has been used for tumour control.
- Peptide receptor radiotherapy may also show therapeutic effects.

Further reading

Vinik A. Vasoactive intestinal peptide tumor (VIPoma). Available at http://www.ncbi.nlm.nih.gov/books/NBK278960/ (accessed 13 Jan 2018).

13.8 Somatostatinomas

Introduction
- Somatostatinomas are very uncommon islet cell tumours.
- More than 60% are large tumours (mean diameter 5 cm) located in the head and body of the pancreas.
- The remainder occurs in the periampullary region of the duodenum and in the small intestine; these tumours are usually smaller.

Histopathology
See Section 13.5.

Clinical presentation
Pancreatic somatostatinomas usually present with:
- diabetes mellitus
- gallstones
- steatorrhoea

Extra-pancreatic tumours can present in association with von Recklinghausen's disease (OMIM #162240) and phaeochromocytoma. Extra-pancreatic somatostatinomas usually present with:
- obstructive pancreatitis
- obstructive jaundice
- small intestinal haemorrhage
- small intestinal obstruction
- abdominal pain

Biochemical investigations
The most common presenting features of somatostatinomas are:

- elevated blood glucose levels
- elevated fasting plasma somatostatin levels

Tumour localization
Large pancreatic somatostatinomas and metastases can be easily detected with transabdominal ultrasonography and CT. Duodenal tumours are usually found during endoscopy. Most of these tumours are benign, but those larger than 2 cm are considered malignant, and patients harbouring these larger tumours should be screened for metastases.

Treatment
- Because of their large size, pancreatic somatostatinomas can rarely be cured by extensive surgery, and often a Whipple's procedure has to be performed.
- Cytoreductive debulking surgery may result in palliation. The prognosis ranges from weeks to years.
- Duodenal tumours can be cured by surgery alone, although often Whipple's procedure has to be performed.
- Hepatic embolization can be used for palliation of metastatic disease.
- Combination chemotherapy with streptozotocin and fluorouracil can also give temporary relief.
- Peptide receptor radiotherapy may also show therapeutic effects.

Further reading
Vinik A, Pacak, Feliberti E, et al. Somatostatinoma. Available at http://www.ncbi.nlm.nih.gov/books/NBK279034/ (accessed 13 Jan 2018).

13.9 Ectopic hormone production

Introduction

Any neoplasm, whether malignant or benign, may differentiate into diverse cell types, some of which can secrete hormones regardless of whether the cell line of origin of the tumour is endocrine in nature. A syndrome of ectopic hormone production results when these hormones are active and cause a specific clinical picture. There have been many varied case reports of ectopic hormone production by neoplastic lesions, from well-described examples such as vasopressin secretion in small-cell lung cancer to rarer examples such as prolactin production from colonic adenocarcinomas. This section will focus on the more commonly observed syndromes of ectopic hormone production.

Syndrome of inappropriate anti-diuretic hormone secretion

See also Chapter 4, Section 4.3. Syndrome of inappropriate anti-diuretic hormone secretion (commonly abbreviated as SIADH) results from excessive production of vasopressin by a tumour. It is frequently associated with malignancy (although it also has many other precipitants), and is one of the primary causes of hyponatraemia in cancer patients.

Pathophysiology

Vasopressin is usually secreted from the posterior pituitary gland in response to a high serum osmolality or a reduction in circulating volume. One of its primary functions, acting via V2 receptors in the kidney, is to facilitate the retention of water by the epithelial cells of the renal distal convoluted tubule and collecting duct. On binding V2 receptors, vasopressin triggers the upregulation and insertion of aquaporins, which are water channels, into the apical membrane of these renal epithelial cells. They allow water to be reabsorbed down an osmotic gradient, out of the tubular filtrate, and back into the circulation.

Clinical features

In syndrome of inappropriate anti-diuretic hormone secretion, inappropriately high circulating levels of vasopressin cause retention of water in excess of sodium in the kidney. The resulting biochemical abnormality is a euvolaemic hyponatraemia, with decreased serum osmolality and concentrated urine (Table 13.6). The clinical picture is dependent on the level of hyponatraemia achieved. Mild hyponatraemia (125–134 mmol/L) may not cause any symptoms, particularly if the syndrome has developed gradually. Moderate (115–124 mmol/L) or severe (<115 mmol/L) hyponatraemia give an escalating clinical picture of confusion, lethargy, seizures, and coma, and may be life-threatening.

Investigations

Initial investigations of hyponatraemia in a patient with a known tumour should include:

- matched serum and urine osmolalities
- urine sodium

Other investigations should also be carried out, as in any case of hyponatraemia, and include:

- thyroid and renal function
- a 9:00 h cortisol test or a short Synacthen® test
- full medication and fluid intake history
- lipids and glucose

If the patient is not known to have a tumour, and the hyponatraemia remains unexplained, then a neoplasm should be actively sought. It is essential to confirm the diagnosis of syndrome of inappropriate anti-diuretic hormone secretion before starting on the management plan below, to ensure appropriate treatment. One of the commonest errors is to fail to assess the hydration status of the patient with hyponatraemia. Both cerebral salt wasting (a dehydrated, hypovolaemic patient) and psychogenic polydipsia need to be excluded.

Management

If possible, definitive treatment involves removal of the underlying cause.

Initial management is usually via *fluid restriction*. In some cases, it may be necessary to impose severe restrictions of as little as 500 mL fluid intake per day. Careful monitoring of the serum sodium is mandatory, and fluid restriction may be relaxed once sodium begins to normalize.

If hyponatraemia is ongoing or the patient is unable to maintain a fluid restriction, expert help needs to be sought. The treatment options are outlined below. All can potentially be dangerous if patients are not carefully assessed and monitored.

If fluid restriction alone is inadequate, it is possible to treat with *demeclocycline*, a tetracycline antibiotic. This prevents water reabsorption in the kidney, causing an effective diabetes insipidus and helping to correct the hyponatraemia. Demeclocycline is commenced at a dose of 900–1200 mg/day in divided doses [1]; once sodium levels are controlled, the agent is continued at the lowest dose necessary to maintain normal sodium levels. It is contraindicated in renal failure, and hydration status should be carefully monitored, particularly if patients remain on a fluid restriction in combination with demeclocycline, as there is a risk of dehydration.

More recently, a class of drugs which specifically block the V2 receptor in the kidney has been developed. These drugs are known as *V2-receptor antagonists* (often called 'vaptans'). Vasopressin is prevented from initiating the insertion of aquaporins into renal epithelial cells, and reabsorption of water is unable to occur. These drugs may prove useful for the treatment of syndrome of inappropriate anti-diuretic hormone secretion, and tolvaptan (starting at 15 mg daily, up to 60 mg daily) is currently licenced for this use in the UK [1]. However, V2-receptor antagonists are not cost effective at present and have no real advantage over demeclocycline. Hypovolaemic

Table 13.6 Characteristics of syndrome of inappropriate anti-diuretic hormone secretion

Metric	Characteristic
Serum osmolality	↓ (<270 mOsm/kg)
Serum sodium	↓ (<130 mmol/L)
Urine osmolality	↑ (>100 mOsm/kg)
Urine sodium	↑ (>30 mmol/L)
Volume status	Euvolaemia (or mild hypervolaemia)

Table 13.7 Serum biochemical changes in the syndrome of excess parathyroid-hormone-related protein versus primary hyperparathyroidism

Serum markers	PTHrP excess	Primary hyperthyroidism
Calcium	↑↑	↑
Phosphate	↓	↓
Intact PTH	↓	↑
PTHrP	↑	↓

Abbreviations: PTH, parathyroid hormone; PTHrP, parathyroid-hormone-related protein.

hyponatraemia is an absolute contraindication to the use of V2-receptor antagonists, reinforcing the need to carefully assess hydration status. If sodium levels rise too fast (>12 mmol/L in 24 hours) the drug should be discontinued [1].

In severe cases, with a sodium level <115 mmol/L and critical clinical features, it may be necessary to treat with *hypertonic (3%) saline*. This should be done under closely monitored conditions, usually in an intensive care setting. The dose should be carefully calculated to raise sodium by no more than 0.5 mmol/L per hour or 12 mmol/L per 24 hours [2]. Some clinicians advocate an even more cautious increment, with the rise in sodium not exceeding 8 mmol/L per 24 hours [3]. If used, hypertonic saline may be discontinued once serum sodium reaches 120 mmol/L [2]. Over-rapid correction of hyponatraemia, particularly if the onset has been insidious, can lead to the devastating complication of central pontine myelinolysis. Hypertonic saline is rarely necessary in hyponatraemia related to syndrome of inappropriate anti-diuretic hormone secretion as, in this case, the hyponatraemia tends to develop relatively slowly and seldom exhibits the critical features described.

Ectopic secretion of vasopressin has been described in many different types of malignancy, including small-cell and squamous-cell lung carcinomas and carcinoid neoplasms (Table 13.7).

Ectopic PTHrP production

See also Chapter 11, Section 11.3. Humoral hypercalcaemia of malignancy may arise due to an excess of PTHrP produced by a tumour. PTHrP is a peptide that exhibits N-terminal homology to PTH. Ordinarily, it is present at very low levels and has its own distinct physiological role [4].

Pathophysiology
When PTHrP is overproduced by a neoplasm, its homology with native PTH allows it to exert its effect on PTH receptors. This gives a clinical picture not unlike that of primary hyperparathyroidism, with increased bone resorption and a decrease in renal calcium clearance. However, the increased intestinal calcium absorption seen in primary hyperparathyroidism does not appear to be a feature of PTHrP excess.

A list of the biochemical changes caused by PTHrP excess can be seen in Table 13.7. It is possible to measure PTHrP but this is not commonly performed in clinical practice.

Clinical features
The features associated with humeral hypercalcaemia of malignancy are related to the degree of hypercalcaemia.

Patients often have an underlying squamous-cell carcinoma (Table 13.8) and may exhibit:
- polydipsia and polyuria
- nausea, anorexia, and constipation
- weakness and fatigue
- bone pain
- cognitive impairment

In malignancy-associated hypercalcaemia, presentation can be acute, with very high calcium levels—often >3.5 mmol/L (14 mg/dL).

Management
The first-line management of hypercalcaemia of malignancy is *fluid resuscitation*, with patients often requiring large amounts of normal saline, particularly in the first 24 hours (up to 6 L in some cases). Rehydration promotes renal calcium clearance. Previously, loop diuretics were added to inhibit the reabsorption of calcium in the thick ascending limb of the loop of Henle and increase renal calcium excretion. This is no longer in practice in the majority of cases, due to poor evidence of effect, and the risk of further intravascular depletion with electrolyte imbalance. However, loop diuretics can be useful to enable further rehydration once a patient is euvolaemic. Underuse of rehydration is a common error. Rehydration continues to have benefit over several days, and lack of response usually means that the patient needs more fluid replacement rather than any other therapy.

Table 13.8 Common syndromes of ectopic hormone excess and frequently associated tumour types

Syndromes	Tumour types
SIADH	Small-cell lung carcinoma
	Squamous-cell lung carcinoma
	Carcinoid tumours (bronchial/gut/pancreatic)
Ectopic PTHrP production	Mesothelioma
	Adenocarcinoma of the prostate or the pancreas
	Squamous-cell carcinomas of the lung, the skin, the head, the neck, and the oesophagus
	Renal cell carcinoma
	Myeloma
Ectopic ACTH/CRH production	Small-cell carcinoma of the lung
	Carcinoid tumours
	Medullary thyroid carcinoma
	Pancreatic neuroendocrine tumours
	Phaeochromocytoma
Ectopic beta-hCG production	Predominantly from carcinomas such as lung, adrenal, ovary, cervix, prostate, bladder, liver, and breast
	Testicular tumours (seminoma, germinoma, teratoma)
	Choriocarcinoma

Abbreviations: ACTH/CRH, adrenocorticotrophic hormone/corticotrophin-releasing hormone; hCG, human chorionic gonadotrophin; PTHrP, parathyroid hormone-related protein; SIADH, syndrome of inappropriate anti-diuretic secretion.

Bisphosphonates can be used in hypercalcaemia, and are particularly useful in cases of known bone metastases, especially when there is bone pain. An intravenous bisphosphonate, such as pamidronate disodium (15–60 mg) or zoledronic acid (4 mg) may be used *following* adequate fluid replacement, although they are commonly administered prematurely, before rehydration has been given a chance to work. Bisphosphonates act by blocking bone resorption by osteoclasts, with a maximal effect expected 2–4 days after administration, and are often credited with improvement that really is due to continued fluid replacement. Delayed hypocalcaemia often then results as a consequence. Bisphosphonates can cause flu-like symptoms or transient bone pain when administered intravenously. There has been concern over osteonecrosis of the jaw after intravenous bisphosphonate treatment, but this is generally associated with repeated, high-dose, long-term therapy. Bisphosphonates are usually inappropriate when the initial diagnosis is primary hyperparathyroidism, and can make investigation of the cause of hypercalcaemia difficult. They should therefore not be used without the involvement of experts.

In resistant hypercalcaemia, it may be beneficial to use *calcitonin* 100 units every 6–8 hours [1]. This is given either intramuscularly or subcutaneously, and can cause significant nausea and vomiting, as well as abdominal pain. It is not widely used. *Glucocorticoids* can be a valuable adjunctive therapy in hypercalcaemia of malignancy, although they are more useful in haematological malignancies, where the underlying cause is less likely to be syndrome of inappropriate anti-diuretic hormone secretion. Steroids are also effective for granulomatous causes of hypercalcaemia, such as sarcoidosis.

Treatment of the underlying cause is essential if this is feasible, but hypercalcaemia is often a poor prognostic sign in malignancy.

Adrenocorticotrophic hormone

See also Chapter 6, Section 6.8. Ectopic adrenocorticotrophic-hormone production is responsible for approximately 5% of presentations of Cushing's syndrome in adults. The majority of cases of ectopic production of adrenocorticotrophic hormone originate from either small-cell lung carcinomas or neuroendocrine tumours (Table 13.8).

Clinical features

Features of ectopic adrenocorticotrophic-hormone production are essentially those of Cushing's syndrome, although any central weight gain may be less pronounced due to the cachectic effects of the underlying malignancy. Clinical features may also differ depending on the nature of the underlying tumour. For example, carcinoid neoplasms producing adrenocorticotrophic hormone generally give a more classical Cushing's phenotype, whilst small-cell lung carcinomas frequently produce much higher levels of adrenocorticotrophic hormone, resulting in a rapidly progressive syndrome predominantly featuring proximal myopathy, hypokalaemia, hypertension, and glucose intolerance [5]. Some patients also exhibit hyperpigmentation. This is due to an excess of melanocyte-stimulating hormone, a peptide hormone which shares a common precursor molecule, pro-opiomelanocortin, with adrenocorticotrophic hormone.

Investigation

The clinical presentation of Cushing's syndrome prompts a search for the source of hormonal excess. Investigations

include the following [6] (see also Chapter 3, Section 3.4, and Chapter 4, Section 4.5):

- midnight measurement of cortisol, to confirm lack of overnight nadir
- measurement of adrenocorticotrophic hormone
- low-dose DST (0.5 mg dexamethasone 6 hourly for 48 hours)
  - adrenocorticotrophic hormone and cortisol are measured at $T = 0$ and $T = 48$ hours
  - in Cushing's syndrome, there is failure to suppress cortisol to <50 nmol/L (1.8 mg/dL) at $T = 48$ hours
- bilateral simultaneous inferior petrosal sinus sampling:
  - used in cases of high adrenocorticotrophic-hormone production and Cushing's syndrome but no definite pituitary source
  - is the preferred current method for confirming an ectopic source of adrenocorticotrophic-hormone production
- high-dose DST:
  - previously used to distinguish an ectopic versus a pituitary source of adrenocorticotrophic hormone
  - has limited diagnostic accuracy and has therefore mostly been replaced by bilateral simultaneous inferior petrosal sinus sampling where available
- CT scan chest/abdomen/pelvis (with MRI, if CT is equivocal)
- ^{111}In-octreotide scintigraphy: may be useful in identifying a covert source of ectopic adrenocorticotrophic hormone [7]
- ^{68}Ga-DOTATOC or ^{68}Ga-DOTATATE PET/CT:
  - have proven to be advantageous in localizing neuroendocrine tumours, which express somatostatin receptors [8]
  - many of the common tumours giving rise to ectopic secretion of adrenocorticotrophic hormone (Table 13.8) have been demonstrated to express somatostatin receptors [9], making ^{68}Ga-labelled peptides a potentially useful tool

Management

Curative surgical or cytotoxic treatment of the underlying cause should always be considered. This may be practicable if the source of ectopic adrenocorticotrophic hormone is, for example, an isolated neuroendocrine tumour. Unfortunately, a cure is not always achievable. The other therapeutic options for treatment of ectopic adrenocorticotrophic-hormone secretion mainly involve control of hypercortisolism. *Ketoconazole* (initially 200 mg twice daily, doubled to 400 mg twice daily if necessary), which is an antifungal medication, and *metyrapone* (initially 250 mg three times daily, up to 750 mg three times daily as required), which is an inhibitor of 11-beta-hydroxylase, are both inhibitors of steroidogenesis and are commonly used [6]. Liver functions should be monitored on ketoconazole, and cortisol should be measured at least weekly on both medications to ensure the adrenal glands are not over-suppressed.

Mitotane chemotherapy, typically used for adrenocortical carcinoma, also inhibits steroidogenesis and may be useful. This should be initiated only after multidisciplinary team discussion with clinicians experienced in its use. The starting dose is 2–3 g/day in divided doses [1]. Plasma monitoring of mitotane concentrations is necessary, and the dose should be adjusted accordingly [1]. Patients may need concurrent corticosteroid replacement, depending on the degree of adrenal suppression achieved. Although not commonly used, *cabergoline*, a dopamine agonist usually seen in the treatment of prolactinomas rather than for the treatment of adrenocorticotrophic-hormone excess has been employed as medical therapy for ectopic adrenocorticotrophic-hormone secretion. If source tumours are positive for dopamine receptors, then dopamine agonists can be useful as an additional therapy [10]. The somatostatin analogue *octreotide* can also be considered, and may be particularly useful in carcinoid tumours causing adrenocorticotrophic-hormone excess. A trial of a short-acting preparation should be initiated to assess response and side effects prior to the consideration of any longer-acting depot preparation.

In the event that medical therapy fails to control the cortisol excess, *bilateral adrenalectomy* with subsequent glucocorticoid and mineralocorticoid replacement may be necessary.

Emerging treatment options include *peptide receptor radionuclide therapies* such as ^{90}Y-DOTATOC or ^{177}Lu-DOTATATE. These use radionuclides coupled with a somatostatin analogue, which then targets somatostatin receptors expressed by some ectopic adrenocorticotrophic-hormone sources [11].

Many cases of ectopic adrenocorticotrophic-hormone secretion represent a covert source; once hormonal control is achieved, long-term follow-up and review is essential, as lesions may become apparent after months or even years.

Other examples of ectopic hormone secretion

There are many other (albeit rarer) examples of ectopic hormone secretion from tumours. Overproduction of hCG may cause gynaecomastia and feminization in men. Growth hormone or GHRH excess will give a clinical picture of acromegaly, and tumours secreting IGF-2 may cause hypoglycaemia. In cases of hormonal excess with no obvious source, a tumour presenting with ectopic hormone secretion should be sought.

References and further reading

1. Joint Formulary Committee. *British National Formulary* (63rd edition), 2012. Pharmaceutical Press.

2. Thompson C and Crowley R. Hyponatraemia. *J R Coll Physicians Edinb* 2009; 39: 154–7.

3. Adrogue H and Madias N. Hyponatraemia. *New Engl J Med* 2000; 342: 1581–9.

4. Burtis W. Parathyroid hormone-related protein: Structure, function and measurement. *Clin Chem* 1992; 38: 2171–83.

5. DeLellis R and Xia L. Paraneoplastic endocrine syndromes: A review. *Endocr Pathol* 2003; 14: 303–18.

6. Imperial Centre for Encocrinology. Imperial Centre for Encocrinology. Available at http:\\impce.com (accessed 13 Jan 2018).

7. Sookur P, Sahdev A, Rockall A, et al. Imaging in covert ectopic ACTH secretion: A CT pictorial review. *Eur Radiol* 2009; 19: 1069–78.

8. Frilling A, Sotiropoulos G, Radtke A, et al. The impact of 68Ga-DOTATOC positron emission tomography/computed tomography on the multimodal management of patients with neuroendocrine tumours. *Ann Surg* 2010; 252: 850–6.

9. Tsuta K, Wistuba I, and Moran C. Differential expression of somatostatin receptors 1–5 in neuroendocrine carcinoma of the lung. *Pathol Res Pract* 2012; 208: 470–4.

10. Petrossians P, Thonnard A, and Beckers A. A Medical treatment in Cushing's syndrome: Dopamine agonists and cabergoline. *Neuroendocrinology* 2010; 92: 116–19.

11. Davi M, Bodei L, Ferdeghini M, et al. Multidisciplinary approach including receptor radionuclide therapy with 90Y-DOTATOC ([90Y-DOTA0, Tyr3]-octreotide) and 177Lu-DOTATATE ([177Lu-DOTA0, Tyr3]-octreotate) in ectopic Cushing syndrome from a metastatic gastrinoma: A promising proposal. *Endocr Pract* 2008; 14: 213–18.

13.10 Endocrine function following chemotherapy and radiotherapy

Introduction

The last 30 years have seen a dramatic improvement in the medium- and long-term survival of children and adults treated for malignant disease. The development of more effective supportive therapy has allowed oncologists to use more intensive treatments. In children, overall survival is approximately 75%, with rates as high as 80% for acute lymphoblastic leukaemia, and 95% for germ cell tumours. In adults, the use of multiple, sequential treatment regimens has led to longer survival. It has been estimated that approximately 2 million adults are living with a diagnosis of cancer in the UK in 2012, a figure expected to rise to 3 million by 2025.

Cancer treatment is known to impact upon the endocrine system; endocrinopathies are the most common consequence of cancer therapy in adults treated for malignant disease during childhood, affecting up to 40%. Endocrine deficits can develop immediately following treatment or develop over many years. It is likely that many patients have, or are at risk of suffering, an undiagnosed endocrinopathy. An understanding of the impact of cancer treatment on the endocrine system identifies those patients at risk and allows appropriate monitoring to be in place, to provide early treatment to reduce the impact on the patient's life.

Traditionally cancer therapy has been divided into surgery, cytotoxic chemotherapy, and radiotherapy. More recently, cytokines and monocolonal antibodies, which target components of the immune system, have been introduced; these can have significant effects on the endocrine system.

Radiotherapy

General principles

The impact of radiotherapy is determined by a number of factors. The greater the total dose received, the greater the impact on both the diseased tissue and the neighbouring healthy tissue. The total radiation dose is divided into fractions delivered over many days. The fraction size contributes to the overall effect; the larger the fraction, the greater the toxicity. The sensitivity of the tissue to radiation will determine the speed with which complications of radiotherapy develop. Tissue sensitivity is determined by the rate of cell division. Radiation effects are observed promptly in tissues with rapid cell division, such as the germinal epithelium, gut lining, or malignant tissue, but may develop over many years in tissues that turn over slowly, for example neural tissue. The time from treatment is, therefore, an important consideration, especially for tissues that are less sensitive to radiation, such as the hypothalamo-pituitary axis. Diagnoses which may be associated with radiation-induced hypopituitarism are shown in Table 13.9. Different modalities of radiotherapy, such as stereotactic radiotherapy or proton beam therapy, aim to reduce the dose received by healthy tissue. The principles of monitoring pituitary function in patients treated for intracranial lesions remain the same, determined by the dose received to the hypothalamo-pituitary axis.

Table 13.9 Diagnoses, typical radiation doses, and risk of hypothalamo-pituitary dysfunction

Diagnosis	Typical radiation dose (Gy)	Risk of pituitary dysfunction
Total body irradiation	14.4	Moderate (adult)
Acute lymphoblastic leukaemia	24	Moderate (adult)
Nasopharyngeal carcinomas	65	High
Sinonasal adenocarcinomas or squamous-cell carcinomas	60–65	High
Astrocytoma (low grade)	50.4–54.0	Only if in close proximity to the hypothalamo-pituitary axis
Glioblastoma multiforme	55–60	Not clinically relevant for many
Medulloblastoma		
• standard–craniospinal	23.4	Moderate
• posterior fossa boost	30.6	
• metastatic–craniospinal	31–39	High
• posterior fossa boost	Up to 60	
Pineal germinoma		
• craniospinal	24	Moderate
• tumour site	14	
Meningioma Grade 1	50.4	High if close proximity
Meningioma Grades 2, 3	54–60	High if close proximity
Pituitary adenoma	45.0–50.4	High
Craniopharyngioma	50.4	High

The pituitary

Pituitary dysfunction

Pituitary dysfunction is common in patients treated with radiotherapy which encompasses the hypothalamo-pituitary axis. The initial insult is to the hypothalamus: the serum prolactin level rises and the pituitary remains sensitive to hypothalamic-releasing hormones. Eventually, the pituitary becomes atrophic and unresponsive to direct stimulation, and serum prolactin falls.

The anterior pituitary hormones are usually lost in a characteristic order: growth hormone is the most sensitive to radiation, followed by the gonadotrophins, adrenocorticotrophic hormone, and TSH. The presence of hypothalamo-pituitary disease accelerates the rate of development of endocrinopathy (see Figure 13.10).

Growth-hormone deficiency

Growth-hormone deficiency can occur as soon as 6 months following radiation or take many years to develop. Radiation doses as low as 9 Gy delivered in a single fraction or 18 Gy delivered in ten fractions can cause severe growth-hormone deficiency in adults. Doses of 18–24 Gy were used prophylactically in children treated for acute lymphoblastic leukaemia and caused growth-hormone deficiency in 65% of subjects within 5 years. Those who did not develop growth-hormone deficiency during childhood were still at risk of developing severe growth-hormone deficiency in adult life (growth-hormone response <3 µg/L during an ITT). All children treated for intracranial tumours with doses in excess of 30 Gy developed growth-hormone deficiency within 3 years. In adults, the speed with which growth-hormone deficiency develops is determined by the pretreatment growth-hormone level (see Figure 13.11).

Gonadotrophin deficiency

It is not clear what the radiation threshold dose is for developing gonadotrophin deficiency, but it is more common following doses in excess of 35 Gy, occurring in up to 27% of those adults treated for lesions not involving the pituitary. In children, radiotherapy to the hypothalamo-pituitary axis can initially cause precocious puberty. Doses above 24 Gy increase the risk of precocious puberty in both boys and girls, but doses of 18–24 Gy only increase the risk in girls. Paradoxically, children receiving high-dose radiotherapy, who develop precocious puberty, may subsequently develop gonadotrophin deficiency and pubertal arrest.

Adrenocorticotrophic-hormone deficiency

Adrenocorticotrophic-hormone deficiency has been described in 21%–27% of adults treated for non-pituitary tumours with more than 50 Gy, but is much less common at lower doses.

TSH deficiency

TSH deficiency is very rare following low doses of radiation (<24 Gy) but the incidence increases as the dose rises. It is important to recognize that some patients treated with radiotherapy are at significant risk of primary hypothyroidism; those treated with total body irradiation or craniospinal radiation suffer exposure to the thyroid, which is at a high risk of failing (see 'The thyroid').

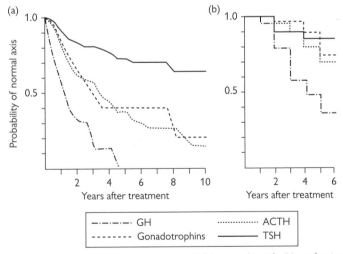

Fig 13.10 The impact of pituitary disease on evolution of hypopituitarism following radiation for (a) non-functioning pituitary adenomas and (b) nasopharyngeal carcinoma; ACTH, adrenocorticotrophic hormone; GH, growth hormone; TSH, thyroid-stimulating hormone.

Panel a: Reproduced with permission from Littley MD, Shalet SM, Beardwell CG et al., Hypopituitarism following external radiotherapy for pituitary tumours in adults, *QJM: An International Journal of Medicine*, Volume 70, Issue 2, pp. 145–160. doi: 10.1093/oxfordjournals.qjmed.a068308. Copyright (1989), by permission of Oxford University Press on behalf of the Association of Physicians of Great Britain and Ireland. Panel b: Reproduced from Lam KSL, Tse VK, Wang C et al., Effects of Cranial Irradiation on Hypothalamic—Pituitary Function—a 5-Year Longitudinal Study in Patients with Nasopharyngeal Carcinoma, *QJM: An International Journal of Medicine*, Volume 78, Issue 2, pp. 165–176. doi:0.1093/oxfordjournals.qjmed.a068535. Copyright (1991), by permission of Oxford University Press on behalf of the Association of Physicians of Great Britain and Ireland.

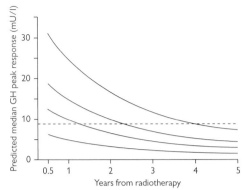

Fig 13.11 The evolution of growth-hormone (GH) deficiency in patients undergoing radiotherapy for non-functioning pituitary adenoma, as determined by the baseline GH status. The lines shown are for pretreatment GH peaks to insulin tolerance tests using 50, 30, 20, and 10 mU/L (3 mU/L = 1 μg/L). Reproduced from Toogood AA, Ryder WDJ, Beardwell CG et al., The evolution of radiation-induced growth hormone deficiency is determined by the baseline growth hormone status, *Clinical Endocrinology*, pp. 97–103, Copyright (1995), with permission from John Wiley and Sons.

Posterior pituitary dysfunction

Posterior pituitary dysfunction, if it occurs, in patients suffering intracranial tumours is caused by the lesion itself or as a complication of surgery. There is no evidence that radiation to the hypothalamo-pituitary axis causes diabetes insipidus.

Monitoring pituitary function

Assessment of pituitary function requires a detailed history, with particular attention to menstrual status in women, and sexual function in men. Basal measurements should be taken of FSH, LH, TSH, and FT4, together with basal measurements of estradiol in women, and testosterone in men. Diagnosis of adrenocorticotrophic-hormone deficiency requires a dynamic function test. The short tetracosactrin test, popular in many endocrine units, should be used with caution in patients treated with cranial radiation, as it appears to under-diagnose adrenocorticotrophic-hormone deficiency, compared with the ITT. Posterior pituitary function should be assessed if there is a history of thirst and polyuria, using paired plasma and urine osmolalities, or a water-deprivation test, if necessary.

It is important to assess pituitary function as soon as an intracranial lesion has been diagnosed, particularly if it is close to or involves the hypothalamo-pituitary axis. Thereafter, pituitary function should be repeated on an annual basis. If the lesion does involve the axis, an additional assessment should be undertaken 6 months following treatment. Annual testing should continue for 10 years; following this, it should be every 5 years or if there is clinical suspicion of a new pituitary hormone deficit. Assessment of the growth-hormone status should be undertaken if growth-hormone replacement is being considered. The ITT is often contraindicated in patients with intracranial lesions due to a history of seizures, so an alternative stimulus such as glucagon or GHRH and arginine should be considered.

Children treated with cranial radiation should undergo regular assessment of height velocity and pubertal status,

to identify evolving growth-hormone deficiency or precocious puberty.

The thyroid and parathyroid

The thyroid is sensitive to radiation, which can result in hypothyroidism, hyperthyroidism, and nodules, a proportion of which will be malignant. The thyroid may be exposed as a result of neck irradiation used to treat lymphoma or head and neck lesions; spinal radiotherapy; or total body irradiation used during conditioning prior to stem cell transplantation.

Hypothyroidism is the most common abnormality, affecting up to 50% of adults treated during childhood. The risk increases as the dose of radiation increases. In the British Childhood Cancer Survivorship Study, 7.7% of subjects (n = 10,091) had been diagnosed with hypothyroidism. Those at greatest risk had been treated for Hodgkin's disease (19.9%), intracranial tumours (15.3%), non-Hodgkin's lymphoma (6.2%), or leukaemia (5.2%). Hypothyroidism can develop up to 25 years following treatment, so monitoring of thyroid function is vital. In patients undergoing total body irradiation, 6.5% had developed hypothyroidism within 30 months of treatment; an additional 3% developed thyroiditis.

Thyrotoxicosis is less common following neck irradiation. In one large study of adults treated for childhood cancer, the relative risk of developing thyrotoxicosis was eightfold that observed in a sibling control group.

Thyroid nodules

The risk of thyroid nodules increases as the dose of radiation increases. Nodules may be benign or malignant. Malignant nodules are papillary carcinomas in approximately two-thirds of cases, and follicular carcinomas in one-third. The young thyroid is very sensitive to radiation; the greatest risk of developing thyroid cancer is seen in patients irradiated before the age of 10. Thyroid nodules can occur many years following treatment. In one cohort of patients treated for Hodgkin's disease, the mean interval between treatment and diagnosis of thyroid cancer was 20.7 years.

Monitoring and management

Patients in whom the thyroid has been exposed to radiation should be monitored on an annual basis. The thyroid should be palpated, and thyroid function checked annually. Hypothyroidism should be treated with levothyroxine promptly. It is recognized that prolonged exposure to excess TSH may increase the risk of thyroid cancer in those already at increased risk, so treatment should be instigated if the TSH exceeds the upper limit of normal on two occasions.

If a thyroid nodule is detected, the patient should undergo an ultrasound of the thyroid, with fine-needle aspiration for cytology. Patients in whom the cytology is suspicious should be referred for total thyroidectomy.

Parathyroid dysfunction

Neck irradiation is associated with an increased risk of hyperparathyroidism that can occur up to 40 years following treatment. Patients at risk should have their calcium monitored annually.

The testis

The germinal epithelium of the testis is exquisitely sensitive to the effects of radiation due to its rapid cell turnover. Doses as low as 1.2 Gy have resulted in permanent azoospermia. Those at greatest risk of azoospermia are men undergoing total body irradiation as conditioning prior to stem cell transplant and those treated for acute lymphoblastic leukaemia, as they receive radiation directed at the testes for testicular disease. In contrast, the Leydig cells are relatively resistant to the effects of radiation, so circulating testosterone levels are often in the normal range. The typical hormone profile in a man who has received testicular radiotherapy shows a markedly raised FSH, mildly raised or normal LH, and normal testosterone. If the radiation dose exceeds 20 Gy and 30 Gy in the prepubertal and adult testis, respectively, then Leydig cell failure is likely resulting in testosterone deficiency.

The ovary
The number of primordial follicles contained in the human ovary peaks shortly after birth, at approximately 2 million, and then declines as a result of atresia or recruitment, with the latter resulting in ovulation. The follicle population can be diminished by insults such as radiation or chemotherapy. Ovarian failure following cancer treatment can be characterized in two ways: as acute ovarian failure that develops during or shortly after treatment is completed, or as a premature menopause which occurs many years following treatment. The effect of radiation on ovarian function is determined by the dose delivered to the ovary, and the age at treatment (see Figure 13.12).

Chemotherapy
The impact of what might be considered traditionally as cytotoxic chemotherapy is primarily limited to the gonads. In men, gonadotoxic agents cause damage to the germinal epithelium, causing oligo- or azoospermia. In women, these agents cause either acute ovarian failure or premature menopause. Cytotoxic agents are frequently delivered in combinations known as regimens. The most gonadotoxic regimens are those used in the past to treat Hodgkin's lymphoma, called ChOP and ChlVPP, which contain the alkylating agent chlorambucil and procarbazine. Other agents known to have gonadotoxic effects are shown in Box 13.2. The impact of chemotherapy in the ovary is similar to that of radiation and is determined by the dose delivered and the age of the woman at the time of treatment. If the ovary is irradiated at the time of treatment with chemotherapy, the risk of

---

Box 13.2 Chemotherapeutic agents that are gonadotoxic in men and women

Alkylating agents
Cyclophosphamide
Ifosfamide
Nitrosoureas
Chlorambucil
Melphalan
Busulfan

Vinca alkaloids
Vinblastine

Antimetabolites
Cytarabine

Platinum agents
Cisplatin

Other agents
Procarbazine

Reproduced from John A.H. Wass, Paul M. Stewart, Stephanie A. Amiel et al., *Oxford Textbook of Endocrinology and Diabetes*, Second Edition, Box 7.4.2, Copyright © 2011 with permission from Oxford University Press.

---

acute ovarian failure is increased; for example, the combination of cyclophosphamide and total body irradiation in women prior to stem cell transplantation invariably results in acute ovarian failure.

New anticancer agents
Modern cancer treatments can manipulate specific components of the immune system. Ipilimumab is a monoclonal antibody which enhances the ability of cytotoxic T-lymphocytes to destroy malignant cells by inhibiting CTLA-4. This effectively causes an autoimmune process not wholly limited to the malignant tissue. Autoimmune hypophysitis, adrenalitis, and thyroiditis have been described. Other agents include can cause hypothyroidism in up to 50% of cases (see Table 13.9). Endocrinopathies can occur during therapy, or several months after treatment has been completed, and appropriate screening should be undertaken by the treating oncologist. Box 13.3 lists agents which are known to cause endocrine dysfunction, most frequently hypothyroidism. It is recommended that the baseline thyroid function be checked before

---

Box 13.3 Newer antineoplastic agents associated with endocrine dysfunction

Tyrosine kinase inhibitors
  Imatinib
  Sunitinib
  Sorafenib
  Motesanib
  Dasatinib
  Nilotinib
  Axitinib
  Cediranib
  Retinoids
Bexarotene
  Immunomodulatory agents
  Ipilimumab and tremelimumab
  Nivolumab
  Pembrolizumab
  Alemtuzumab
  Interferon alfa

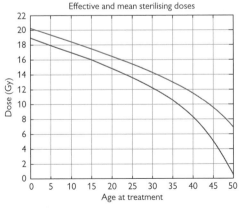

Effective and mean sterilising doses

Fig 13.12 The relationship between radiation dose to the ovary, and age at treatment.
Reprinted from *International Journal of Radiation Oncology, Biology, Physics*, Volume 62, Issue 3, Wallace WH, Thomson AB, Saran F et al., Predicting age of ovarian failure after radiation to a field that includes the ovaries, pp. 738–744, Copyright 2005, with permission from Elsevier.

treatment is started and that thyroid function be monitored every 3 months thereafter.

Adrenal insufficiency

The adrenal glands appear to be resistant to the effects of both chemotherapy and radiotherapy. Primary adrenal failure may occur as the result of disease infiltration or bilateral adrenalectomy. The greatest risk to adrenal function is high-dose glucocorticoid therapy, which may be used to manage the tumour, the effects of the tumour (e.g. the cerebral oedema associated with primary brain tumours), or graft-versus-host disease following allogeneic stem cell transplantation. Patients who become symptomatic when steroids are withdrawn should undergo assessment of adrenal function and be treated with hydrocortisone when appropriate. Adrenal function can be reassessed every 6 months if recovery is expected.

Endocrine replacement therapy

On the whole, hormone deficits should be replaced in line with standard practice. Exceptions are growth hormone, and oestrogen in women with a history of breast cancer or thromboembolic disease.

There is a theoretical concern that growth hormone may influence the natural history of an intracranial lesion. Data from children suggest that growth hormone is safe in this context, with no significant difference in relapse rates between those who did and those who did not receive growth hormone to promote growth. Similar data are not available from adults. As a precaution, it is standard practice to delay growth-hormone replacement in patients with a malignant intracranial lesion for 2 years from the completion of treatment. In adults, it is sensible to seek the agreement of the treating oncologist before embarking upon growth-hormone replacement.

Oestrogen is contraindicated in women who have been treated for breast cancer. In women with ovarian failure resulting from cancer treatment, oestrogen replacement should be used to protect skeletal health and alleviate the symptoms of oestrogen deficiency. There are no data on the safety of oestrogen in this patient cohort, so the lowest dose necessary to be effective should be used, and women should be advised to examine their breasts on a regular basis. If a woman has suffered thromboembolic disease during treatment and there is an identifiable cause, for example a line-associated thrombus, low-dose transcutaneous oestrogen should be used.

Further reading

Absolom K, Eiser C, Turner L, et al. Ovarian failure following cancer treatment: Current management and quality of life. *Hum Reprod* 2008; 23: 2506–12.

Brabant G, Toogood AA, Shalet SM, et al. Hypothyroidism following childhood cancer therapy: An under diagnosed complication. *Int J Cancer* 2011; 130: 1145–50.

Fernandez A, Brada M, Zabuliene L, et al. Radiation-induced hypopituitarism. *Endocr Relat Cancer* 2009; 16: 733–72.

Greenfield DM, Walters SJ, Coleman RE, et al. Prevalence and consequences of androgen deficiency in young male cancer survivors in a controlled cross-sectional study. *J Clin Endocrinol Metab* 2007; 92: 3476–82.

Maddams J, Brewster D, Gavin A, et al. Cancer prevalence in the United Kingdom: Estimates for 2008. *Br J Cancer* 2009; 101: 541–7.

Oeffinger KC, Mertens AC, Sklar CA, et al. Chronic health conditions in adult survivors of childhood cancer. *N Engl J Med* 2006; 355: 1572–82.

Toogood AA. 'Late effects of cancer treatment', in Wass JA and Stewart PM, eds, *Oxford Textbook of Endocrinology and Diabetes*, 2011. Oxford University Press, 1148–59.

Inherited endocrine syndromes and multiple endocrine neoplasia

Chapter contents

14.1 McCune–Albright syndrome

Introduction

McCune–Albright syndrome is a rare disorder characterized by the clinical triad of polyostotic fibrous dysplasia, irregular café-au-lait spots, and precocious puberty.

Characteristic features

At least two of the features must be present to consider the diagnosis. Other endocrinopathies include hyperthyroidism, adrenal nodules with Cushing's syndrome, hyperprolactinaemia, acromegaly, and hyperparathyroidism; hypophosphataemic hyperphosphaturic rickets may also be present. Rarely, severely affected patients may present with hepatic and gastrointestinal dysfunction (e.g. hepatobiliary disease, pancreatitis, gastrointestinal polyposis), cardiac arrhythmias, and aortic root dilatation.

Epidemiology

The estimated prevalence of McCune–Albright syndrome ranges between 1/100,000 and 1/1,000,000. Most commonly, it is found in early childhood but severe cases have also been reported in infancy. Both sexes can be affected, but the syndrome is more common and occurs earlier in girls.

Pathophysiology

The disorder is caused by early somatic mutation in the gene encoding the G-protein alpha subunit that stimulates cAMP formation. This mutation impairs GTPase activity of the alpha-subunit and results in constant stimulation of adenylyl cyclase, and persistently high levels of intracellular cAMP. Increased cAMP levels can mediate mitogenesis and increased cell function. The tissues affected depend on the point in time in embryogenesis at which the mutation occurs. Genetic analysis of GNAS1 is available in some centres.

Clinical features

Typically, the signs and symptoms of either sexual precocity or fibrous dysplasia account for the initial presentation. Precocious puberty is more common in girls than in boys and is heralded by irregular vaginal bleeding due to excess oestrogen production from ovarian follicular cysts. Development of breast tissue without growth of pubic hair may also occur. Increased growth velocity and skeletal maturation are observed, but the rapid epiphyseal development leads to short final stature. The ovaries may display asymmetrical enlargement and regression as a result of a large follicular cyst. Despite the fact that serum estradiol is elevated, the LH response to GnRH is prepubertal. The early oestrogen exposure though, can ultimately result in central precocious puberty. Sexual precocity is also observed in male patients who exhibit testicular (bilateral or unilateral) and penile enlargement, pubic and axillary hair growth, and precocious sexual behaviour.

Fibrous dysplasia ranges from asymptomatic lesions to painful bone involvement, visible bony deformities, or pathologic fractures. The lesions tend to be unilateral, and the sites most commonly involved are the proximal femur and the skull base. They are dysplastic and undermineralized, with poorly organized collagen support, and may lead to fractures or deformities such as the 'shepherd's crook' of the proximal femur. Asymmetry of the jaw, dysmorphism, and difference in limb length may be observed. If the skull is involved, there may be compression of the optic or auditory nerve, leading to blindness, deafness, and vertigo. Rarely, entrapment of spinal nerves may occur as a result of compression following spine fractures. Radionuclide bone scans can detect lesions before they become visible radiographically. Radiographs show multiple areas of cystic lesions and sclerosis, and the typical appearance is that of 'ground glass'. The majority of affected children display bone abnormalities by 8 years of age. The existing lesions may worsen or remain stable; rarely, new lesions may develop. The incidence of fractures is higher during the sixth to the tenth year, but fractures may continue to occur in adulthood.

Café-au-lait spots are the most common clinical sign. They are usually present in infancy and become more prominent with age. Their borders are irregular ('coast of Maine') and their colour ranges from light to dark brown. Pigmented areas usually have a segmented distribution, do not cross the midline, and are located on the side where bone lesions are present.

Cushing's syndrome may be seen in infancy and is related to hyperfunction of bilaterally enlarged and nodular adrenals. It can develop without obvious clinical signs of the syndrome and sometimes regresses during the first years after onset. Cushing's disease is considered to be uncommon.

Growth-hormone excess caused by somatotroph adenomas of the pituitary may be observed, leading to gigantism or acromegaly. In addition, these patients are at increased risk for impaired glucose intolerance, hypertension, and cancer, whilst increased levels of serum growth hormone have adverse effects on craniofacial bone disease. Most growth-hormone secreting tumours may co-secrete growth hormone and prolactin, leading to hypogonadotrophic hypogonadism.

Autonomous hyperfunction may also involve the thyroid. Nodular hyperplasia with thyrotoxicosis or commonly with euthyroid status has been observed. Primary hyperparathyroidism caused by adenoma or hyperplasia is rare and may worsen fibrous dysplasia.

Furthermore, some patients develop hypophosphataemic rickets or osteomalacia. This is attributed to overproduction of a phosphaturic factor, FGF23, by the bone lesions. Severity is directly related to FGF23 levels, as the greater the disease burden, the higher is the secretion of FGF23. Therefore, severe hypophosphataemia is observed in patients with extensive bone disease.

Complications

A few cases of malignant transformation of bone lesions have also been described, especially after high doses of external beam radiation. In addition, there is a greater tendency for malignant transformation in patients who display concomitant growth-hormone hypersecretion. Female patients are at greater risk for breast cancer, whilst thyroid and testicular malignancies have also been observed. A recent study revealed higher incidence of pancreatic and hepatobiliary neoplasms in patients with McCune–Albright syndrome.

Management

McCune–Albright syndrome is a multisystemic disease, and its treatment depends on clinical presentation. Precocious puberty is gonadotrophin independent and does not respond to GnRH agonists. Aromatase inhibitors are the drugs most commonly used, since the main purpose is to block oestrogen effects. Letrozole, a third-generation aromatase inhibitor, has been shown to be effective. The oestrogen-receptor modulator tamoxifen has shown promising results, and a recent study revealed moderate effectiveness of the oestrogen receptor antagonist fulvestrant in girls presenting with the syndrome. Additional treatment options include cyproterone acetate and medroxyprogesterone acetate, whilst male patients are typically treated with a combination of spironalctone and aromatase inhibitors.

There is no established treatment for fibrous dysplasia. Bisphosphonates are frequently used, mostly for pain relief and/or pathologic fracture prevention, but they have no effect on the evolution of bone disease. Surgical intervention is indicated for the treatment of fractures or severe painful malformations. Radiation therapy should be avoided because it is associated with high risk for malignant transformation.

If Cushing's syndrome does not resolve spontaneously, bilateral adrenalectomy is the treatment of choice. Growth-hormone excess is treated with pharmacotherapeutic agents such as long-acting somatostatin analogues or pegvisomant (see Chapter 3, Section 3.6). Dopamine agonists may be necessary if prolactin is also secreted from the tumour.

Further reading

Bercaw-Pratt JL, Moorjani TP, Santos XM, et al. Diagnosis and management of precocious puberty in atypical presentations of McCune-Albright syndrome: A case series review. *J Pediatr Adolesc Gynecol* 2012; 25: e9–13.

Collins MT, Singer FR, and Eugster E. McCune-Albright syndrome and the extraskeletal manifestations of fibrous dysplasia. *Orphanet J Rare Dis* 2012; 7: S4.

Collins MT. Spectrum and natural history of fibrous dysplasia of bone. *J Bone Miner Res* 2006; 21: 99–104.

De Sanctis C, Lala R, Matarazzo P, et al. McCune-Albright syndrome: A longitudinal clinical study of 32 patients. *J Pediatr Endocrinol Metab* 1999; 12: 817–26.

Diaz A, Danon M, and Crawford J. McCune-Albright syndrome and disorders due to activating mutations of GNAS1. *J Pediatr Endocrinol Metab* 2007; 20: 853–80.

Dumitrescu CE and Collins MT. McCune-Albright syndrome. *Orphanet J Rare Dis* 2008; 3: 12.

Eugster EA, Rubin SD, Reiter EO, et al. Tamoxifen treatment for precocious puberty in McCune-Albright syndrome: A multicentre trial. *J Paediatr* 2003; 143: 60–6.

Feuillan P, Calis K, Hill S, et al. Letrozole treatment of precocious puberty in girls with the McCune-Albright Syndrome: A pilot study. *J Clin Endocrinol Metab* 2007; 92: 2100–6.

Gaujoux S, Salenave S, Ronot M, et al. Hepatobiliary and pancreatic neoplasms in patients with McCune-Albright syndrome. *J Clin Endocrinol Metab* 2014; 99: E97–101.

Ippolito E, Bray EW, Corsi A, et al. Natural history and treatment of fibrous dysplasia of bone: A multicenter clinicopathologic study promoted by the European Pediatric Orthopaedic Society. *J Pediatr Orthop B* 2003, 12:155–77.

Sims EK, Garnett S, Guzman F, et al. Fulvestrant treatment of precocious puberty in girls with McCune-Albright syndrome. *Int J Pediatr Endocrinol* 2012; 2012: 26.

14.2 Endocrine tumours in neurofibromatosis type 1

Neurofibromatosis type 1: Definition and epidemiology

Neurofibromatosis type 1 is one of the most common autosomal-dominant inherited disorders, with complete penetrance by adulthood. The incidence ranges from 1/2,600–3,000 births/year. The disease is caused by heterozygous mutations in *NF1*, a large tumour-suppressor gene, which spans over 350 kb of genomic DNA and contains 60 exons. Mutations of the gene are one of the most commonly observed genetic changes in humans (1/7,800–23,000 gametes). Consequently, about 50% of patients with neurofibromatosis type 1 have de novo mutations. Due to these findings and a lack of a distinct genotype–phenotype correlation, mutation screening is rarely performed.

Despite the extremely variable clinical signs and symptoms, even within an individual of the same family and at different times in life, the diagnosis is based on highly specific and sensitive clinical criteria developed by the NIH Consensus Conference in 1987 and updated 1997 (see Box 14.1). Careful evaluation of the medical and family history together with a thorough physical examination and regular follow-up screening are therefore sufficient for the diagnosis of neurofibromatosis type 1, but also necessary to prevent life-threatening complications. The disease can affect multiple organ systems, but its hallmarks are pigmentary abnormalities, such as axillary or inguinal freckling and café-au-lait spots, neurofibromas, and Lisch nodules of the iris. Neurofibromatosis type 1 is also associated with a two- to fourfold increased risk of tumour development, which leads to a reduction of life expectancy by about 15 years. Endocrine tumours in neurofibromatosis type 1 are rare (see Box 14.2).

Phaeochromocytoma in neurofibromatosis type 1

Also see Chapter 6, Section 6.14. Phaeochromocytoma is the most common neuroendocrine tumour associated with neurofibromatosis type 1. Its prevalence is reported to be 0.1%–5.7%. The excessive catecholamine production and secretion from these tumours leads to palpitation, headaches, and sweating but can also cause a severe, life-threatening catecholamine crisis with arrhythmias, heart failure, or stroke. Phaeochromocytoma associated with neurofibromatosis type 1 are seemingly identical to other phaeochromocytomas from the viewpoint of conventional histopathology. They were the first-described hereditary phaeochromocytoma (1904).

Clinical characteristics of phaeochromocytomas associated with neurofibromatosis type 1

The European-American Phaeochromocytoma Registry based in Freiburg comprises now 55 patients with phaeochromocytomas associated with neurofibromatosis type 1, including 29 females and 26 males, who were diagnosed with phaeochromocytoma at age 14–75 (median 43). In 39 of the patients, there was only a single phaeochromocytoma, and it was extra-adrenal in 1 patient. In 16 of the patients, there were multiple phaeochromocytomas; these were extra-adrenal in 2 of the patients, and malignant in 4. None of the patients had thoracic or head and neck paragangliomas.

Clinical diagnosis and treatment of phaeochromocytomas associated with neurofibromatosis type 1

The diagnosis of phaeochromocytoma in patients with neurofibromatosis type 1 is based on elevated plasma levels and/or urinary excretion of adrenaline, noradrenaline, metanephrine, and normetanephrine. Tumours can be detected by CT scan or MRI. Functional imaging methods include [127]I-MIBG or ^{131}I-MIBG and FDG PET. The method of choice for treatment is minimally invasive organ-sparing tumour resection from the adrenal gland and, similarly, endoscopic resection of extra-adrenal

---

Box 14.1 Clinical criteria for the diagnosis of neurofibromatosis type 1, developed by the NIH Consensus Conference in 1987 and updated 1997

These criteria are highly specific and highly sensitive in adults with neurofibromatosis type 1. The diagnosis in children under the age of 8 years can be more problematic because many of these striking features increase in frequency with the age and become more dominant.

The NIH diagnostic criteria are met in an individual who presents two or more of the following features in the absence of another diagnosis:

- six or more café-au-lait macules over 5 mm in greatest diameter in prepubertal individuals, and over 15 mm in greatest diameter in post-pubertal individuals
- two or more neurofibromas of any type or one plexiform neurofibroma
- freckling in the axillary or inguinal region
- optic glioma
- two or more Lisch nodules (iris hamartomas)
- a distinctive osseous lesion such as sphenoid dysplasia or thinning of long bone cortex, with or without pseudarthrosis
- a first-degree relative (parent, sibling, or offspring) with neurofibromatosis type 1 by the above criteria

Neurofibromatosis. NIH Consensus Statement Online 1987 Jul 13–15;6(12):1–19.

Box 14.2 Endocrine tumours observed in neurofibromatosis type 1

Phaeochromocytoma
Parathyroid adenoma
Medullary thyroid carcinoma
Pancreatic islet cell tumour
Gastrointestinal stroma tumour

---

tumours. This includes also patients with large tumours and those with metastases, since reduction of tumour mass is one component of treatment of malignant phaeochromocytoma, in addition to nuclear medical radiation (by MIBG and other tracers) and chemotherapy.

Molecular genetic characteristics

In 25 neurofibromatosis type 1 patients with phaeochromocytomas, germ-line mutations in *NF1* were identified in 23 (92%). These patients were compared to patients with mutations of one of the other susceptibility genes, *RET, VHL, SDHB,* and *SDHD,* as well as to patients without mutations (sporadic phaeochromocytoma); patients with neurofibromatosis type 1 showed clinical characteristics that were closely similar to those of patients with sporadic tumours. Furthermore, molecular genetic analyses of *NF1* do not provide genotype–phenotype correlations and are not indicated for the genetic classification of such patients. The diagnosis of neurofibromatosis type 1 is based on defined clinical criteria.

Other neuroendocrine tumours related to neurofibromatosis type 1

Gastrointestinal stroma tumours have been repeatedly reported in patients with neurofibromatosis type 1. The prevalence of these tumours in neurofibromatosis type 1 patients has been shown to be less than 1%, and minimally invasive surgery is usually indicated. Parathyroid adenoma and subsequent hyperparathyroidism may occur as a single condition or together with other tumours which are very uncommon in patients with neurofibromatosis type 1.

Patient support groups/useful websites

The following patient support website may be useful:

- http://www.inspire.com/groups/neurofibromatosis-network/

Further reading

Anonymous: Neurofibromatosis. Conference statement. National Institutes of Health Consensus Development Conference. *Arch Neurol* 1988; 45: 575–8.

Bausch B, Borozdin W, and Neumann HP: Clinical and genetic characteristics of patients with neurofibromatosis type 1 and phaeochromocytoma. N Engl J Med 2006; 354: 2729–31.

Bausch B, Koschker AC, Fassnacht M, et al. Comprehensive mutation scanning of NF1 in apparently sporadic cases of phaeochromocytoma. *J Clin Endocrinol Metab* 2006; 91: 3478–81.

Mannelli M, Castellano M, Schiavi F, et al. Clinically guided genetic screening in a large cohort of Italian patients with phaeochromocytomas and/or functional or nonfunctional paragangliomas. *J Clin Endocrinol Metab* 2009; 94: 1541–7.

Neumann HP, Bausch B, McWhinney SR, et al. Germ-line mutations in nonsyndromic phaeochromocytoma. *N Engl J Med* 2002; 346: 1459–66.

Riccardi VM. Von Recklinghausen neurofibromatosis. *N Engl J Med* 1981; 305: 1617–27.

Sorensen SA, Mulvihill JJ, and Nielsen A. Long-term follow-up of von Recklinghausen neurofibromatosis. Survival and malignant neoplasms. *N Engl J Med* 1986; 314: 1010–15.

Walker L, Thompson D, Easton D, et al. A prospective study of neurofibromatosis type 1 cancer incidence in the UK. *Br J Cancer* 2006; 95: 233–8.

14.3 Von Hippel–Lindau disease

Introduction

Von Hippel–Lindau disease is a rare autosomal-dominant tumour syndrome affecting 1 in 36,000 people. Approximately 80% of cases are inherited, whilst 20% arise as de novo mutations with no family history.

Clinical presentation is usually in the second or third decade of life, with >90% penetrance by the age of 65 years. There is both inter- and intra-familial phenotypic heterogeneity, suggesting that both genotype effects specific to von Hippel-Lindau disease and genotype effects caused by modifier genes affect clinical features.

Von Hippel–Lindau disease is associated with highly vascular benign and malignant tumours—most frequently, CNS haemangioblastomas, retinal angiomas, clear cell renal cell carcinomas, phaeochromocytomas, pancreatic islet tumours, and endolymphatic sac tumours, in addition to visceral cysts in the kidney, the pancreas, the epididymis, and the broad ligament (see Figure 14.1).

A clinical diagnosis of von Hippel–Lindau disease is made in the presence of two or more tumours associated with von Hippel–Lindau disease, or one tumour occurring in an at-risk individual with a family history of von Hippel–Lindau disease.

Although there is no cure, with better imaging, screening (see Box 14.3) and treatment, the outlook for patients with von Hippel–Lindau disease is improving.

Clinical features

CNS haemangioblastomas typically affect the cerebellum, brain stem, or spinal cord, sparing supratentorial sites. These tumours are best detected by MRI; it is suggested that individuals be screened every 1–3 years from adolescence. Although benign, these tumours may produce symptoms due to mass effect, haemorrhage, or CSF obstruction. Surgery is generally reserved for symptomatic patients, and alternatives include stereotactic radiotherapy.

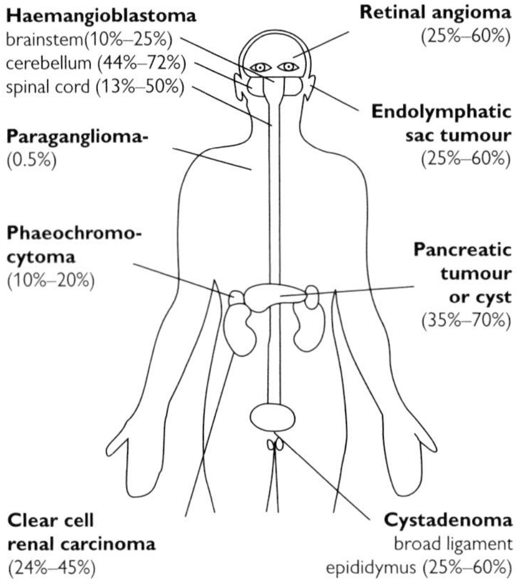

Retinal angiomas are histologically identical to CNS haemangioblastomas and are frequently bilateral. Annual ophthalmic screening is recommended from infancy since complications such as exudation, retinal traction and haemorrhage may threaten sight. Laser photocoagulation or cryotherapy is generally successful, although anti-angiogenic therapies may be used in difficult cases (e.g. optic nerve haemangioblastomas).

Clear cell renal cell carcinoma is the most frequent cause of mortality. Tumours are malignant, multifocal, and bilateral, but when they are <3 cm in diameter, the risk of metastasis is low. The strategy is generally to screen annually by ultrasound or MRI from the age of 16 and to undertake nephron-sparing approaches such as partial nephrectomy or radiofrequency ablation for lesions >3 cm in diameter. Despite this approach, repeated surgery may ultimately lead to loss of renal function, requiring dialysis.

Phaeochromocytoma (see also Chapter 6, Section 6.14) may be the sole manifestation of von Hippel–Lindau disease, and von Hippel–Lindau disease accounts for as many as 50% of familial and 11% of apparently sporadic cases of phaeochromocytomas. Phaeochromocytomas due to von Hippel–Lindau disease are less likely to be malignant (approximately 5%) than sporadic phaeochromocytomas; 98% of phaeochromocytomas secrete norepinephrine, and it is suggested that screening begin in early childhood, by annual measurement of blood pressure and plasma normetanephrine or urinary catecholamine metabolites. Extra-adrenal paragangliomas (mostly carotid body tumours) have also been observed.

Pancreatic neuroendocrine tumours (see Chapter 13) associated with von Hippel–Lindau disease are usually non-functional islet cell tumours. They can be detected by MRI, and are frequently malignant. Surgery is indicated for tumours >3 cm in diameter.

Endolymphatic sac tumours are frequently bilateral and may present with hearing loss, tinnitus or vertigo.

Cystic disease is often seen in the kidney and pancreas, where it is usually clinically silent, as well as in relation to CNS haemangioblastomas.

Cystadenomas of the epididymis and the broad ligament are usually asymptomatic and rarely require treatment.

Haemangioblastoma
brainstem(10%–25%)
cerebellum (44%–72%)
spinal cord (13%–50%)

Retinal angioma
(25%–60%)

Paraganglioma-
(0.5%)

Endolymphatic sac tumour
(25%–60%)

Phaeochromo-cytoma
(10%–20%)

Pancreatic tumour or cyst
(35%–70%)

Clear cell renal carcinoma
(24%–45%)

Cystadenoma
broad ligament
epididymus (25%–60%)

Fig 14.1 Clinical features of von Hippel–Lindau disease.

Box 14.3 Suggested screening guidelines

Birth: neurological, eye, and hearing assessments

Age 1–4: annual ophthalmic, neurological, hearing, and blood pressure assessments

Age 5–15: annual ophthalmic, neurological, and blood pressure assessments; annual plasma/urine normetanephrine and abdominal ultrasound; alternate year audiology assessments

Age 16 and above: annual ophthalmic examination, plasma/urine normetanephrine and abdominal ultrasound; alternate year audiology assessment and contrast enhanced MRI scan of abdomen, brain, and cervical spine

Table 14.1 Von Hippel–Lindau subtypes

Type	Phaeochromocytoma	Haemangioblastoma	Renal cancer	Mutation type	HIF activation
1		✓	✓	Deletion/ nonsense	+++
2B	✓	✓	✓	Missense	++
2A	✓	✓		Missense	+
2C	✓			Missense	−

Abbreviations: HIF, hypoxia-inducible factor.

Molecular genetics

The tumour-suppressor gene *VHL* lies on the short arm of Chromosome 3 (3p25–26) and comprises three exons with two alternate translational start sites that encode for 159 and 213 amino-acid proteins, respectively. Each isoform has tumour-suppressor function and, to date, all of the >900 *VHL* mutations reported affect both forms.

Patients with von Hippel–Lindau disease harbour a germ-line mutation in one *VHL* allele. In accordance with Knudson's 'two-hit' hypothesis, tumours arise following somatic loss or inactivation of the remaining wild-type allele. *VHL* inactivation is also commonly observed in sporadic tumours such as clear cell renal cell carcinomas, following somatic loss or inactivation of both alleles.

The *VHL* gene product pVHL is a multi-purpose protein, the best-studied role of which is as a member of an E3 ubiquitin ligase complex that targets the transcription factor HIF for rapid degradation by the proteasome. Inactivation of pVHL stabilizes HIF, mimicking cellular hypoxia and activating transcriptional pathways involving many hundreds of hypoxia-responsive genes. These include *VEGF* and *PDGFB*, which underlie the highly vascular phenotype of von Hippel–Lindau-associated tumours and provide a rationale for new anti-angiogenic therapies. However, since both pVHL and HIF are ubiquitously expressed, this does not explain the tissue specificity of tumours associated with von Hippel–Lindau disease.

Genotype–phenotype associations seen in von Hippel–Lindau disease appear to associate with effects on the HIF pathway (see Table 14.1). Families with truncating mutations or exon deletions in *VHL*, mutations that have a large effect on HIF dysregulation, have a low frequency of phaeochromocytoma (von Hippel–Lindau disease type 1).

Families with a high incidence of phaeochromocytoma (von Hippel–Lindau disease type 2) generally have germ-line missense mutations and are further classified according to risk of renal cell carcinoma and haemangioblastoma. Mutations associated with phaeochromocytoma only (von Hippel–Lindau disease type 2C) retain their ability to regulate HIF; thus, this pathway may be important in some tumour types but not others.

Finally, some germ-line *VHL* mutations that result in subtle defects in hypoxia pathways may result in an autosomal-recessive familial polycythaemia (Chuvash polycythaemia) and not be associated with tumours at all.

Differential diagnosis

The differential diagnosis of von Hippel–Lindau disease type 2C (phaeochromocytoma only) includes multiple endocrine neoplasia types 2A and 2B, neurofibromatosis type 1, and mutations in subunits of succinate dehydrogenase.

Germ-line mutations in *FH* (which encodes fumarate hydratase, *FLCN* (which encodes folliculin), and the oncogene *MET* may lead to familial forms of renal cancer but generally these are of non-clear cell histology.

Genetic counselling

Genetic testing is highly sensitive and specific and is indicated in all patients with a known or suspected clinical diagnosis of von Hippel–Lindau disease, although in the 20% with de novo mutations, genetic mosaicism can lead to false-negative results.

Where the mutation is known, it can be used to determine the need for surveillance in family members. Since detection of at-risk individuals affects medical management from a young age, genetic testing should be offered as early as possible and may also be employed for prenatal counselling in at-risk pregnancies.

Genetic testing may also be used in patients with a single *VHL*-associated tumour, particularly of early onset. In particular, since phaeochromocytoma is the sole manifestation of von Hippel–Lindau disease type 2C, individuals with multifocal, bilateral, or familial phaeochromocytoma should be offered *VHL* testing.

Patient support groups

Information for patients, families, and physicians is available through the VHL Family Alliance (http://www.vhl.org).

Further reading

Jafri M and Maher ER. The genetics of phaeochromocytoma: Using clinical features to guide genetic testing. *Eur J Endocrinol* 2012; 166: 151–8.

Kaelin WG. Von Hippel-Lindau disease. *Annu Rev Pathol* 2007; 2: 2145–173.

Latif F, Tory K, Gnarra J, et al. Identification of the von Hippel-Lindau disease tumor suppressor gene. *Science* 1993; 260: 1317–20.

Lonser RR, Glenn GM, Walther M, et al. Von Hippel-Lindau disease. *Lancet* 2003; 361: 2059–67.

Maher ER, Neumann HP, and Richard S. Von Hippel-Lindau disease: A clinical and scientific review. *Eur J Hum Genet* 2011; 19: 617–23.

VHL Family Alliance. *The VHL Handbook: What You Need To Know about VHL* (4th edition), 2012. VHL Family Alliance.

Wind JJ and Lonser RR. Management of von Hippel-Lindau disease-associated CNS lesions. *Expert Rev Neurother* 2011; 11: 1433–41.

14.4 Carney complex

Definition and epidemiology

Carney complex is a familial multiple neoplasia and lentiginosis syndrome inherited in an autosomal-dominant manner. The exact prevalence of this rare disease is difficult to establish; approximately 750 cases from many ethnicities have been reported worldwide since 1985.

Diagnosis and clinical manifestations of Carney complex

Carney complex can present with a number of endocrine and non-endocrine manifestations which vary between patients.

Endocrine tumours

Cushing's syndrome and PPNAD

PPNAD, a form of adrenocorticotrophic-hormone-independent Cushing's syndrome, is the most frequent endocrine manifestation of Carney complex and is present in 60%–70% of Carney complex patients. PPNAD is characterized by small-pigmented nodules, most less than 10 mm in their greatest diameter, often surrounded by atrophic cortex (see Figure 14.2; also see Chapter 6, Section 6.8). The disease is bilateral and is more frequent in females and in young adults, with a peak incidence during the second and third decades of life. The administration of dexamethasone in the course of Liddle's test establishes the diagnosis of PPNAD biochemically (Table 14.2). Bilateral adrenalectomy is the most effective treatment.

Pituitary tumours

Pituitary tumours in Carney complex typically develop from somatomammotrophs only and are often associated with gigantism and/or acromegaly; isolated prolactinomas are rare. Acromegaly in Carney complex (see also Chapter 3, Section 3.6) typically has a slow, progressive course. Increased levels of IGF-1 and growth hormone can be present in up to 75% of Carney complex patients, whereas clinical acromegaly may be seen in only 10%–20% of the patients. These biochemical abnormalities before the radiological evidence of a frank pituitary tumour are due to somatomammotrophic hyperplasia that precedes the development of tumours.

Other endocrine tumours

Multiple thyroid nodules are present by ultrasonography in up to 75% of patients. Follicular adenoma is the most common finding; follicular or papillary thyroid cancer develops in less than 10% of patients.

Testicular tumours are a common finding in male patients with Carney complex and can be of three types:
- large-cell calcifying Sertoli cell tumour:
  - is the most common testicular lesion in Carney complex
  - appears in the first decade of life, often before puberty
  - is almost always benign, with the exception of those in a few older patients who developed testicular cancer
  - almost always occurs bilaterally and is multifocal (in more than half of the patients)
  - presents as a calcification in ultrasonography
- testicular adrenal rest tumour:
  - is due to (ectopic) PPNAD
  - can lead to Cushing's syndrome
- Leydig cell tumour:
  - rare in Carney complex

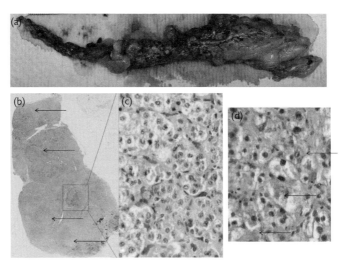

Fig 14.2 (a) Macroscopic appearance of the adrenal gland in primary pigmented nodular adrenocortical disease; the surface shows multiple pigmented micronodules. (b) Haematoxylin and eosin staining (magnification, 5×) of the tissue from Panel a; multiple nodules are indicated by the arrows. (c) Magnification (20×) showing a single nodule. (d) magnification (40×) showing intracellular pigmentation (lipofuscin granules; arrowed).

Table 14.2 Liddle's test for the diagnosis of Cushing's syndrome in pigmented nodular adrenocortical disease

Day	Dexamethasone dose	Steroids measured[†]
−2 (baseline)	—	24-Hour urinary free cortisol and 17-hydroxysteroids
−1(baseline)	—	24-Hour urinary free cortisol and 17-hydroxysteroids
Days 1–4	0.5 mg[‡] × 4 in 24 hours, orally, starting at 06:00 h	24-Hour urinary free cortisol and 17-hydroxysteroids
Days 5–6	2 mg[‡] × 4 in 24 hours, orally, starting at 06:00 h	24-hour urinary free cortisol and 17-hydroxysteroids

Note: Patients with pigmented nodular adrenocortical disease show a 'paradoxical' increase in their 24-hour urinary free cortisol and/or 17-hydroxysteroids; this increase is progressive and reaches its peak on the second day of the high-dose dexamethasone administration.

[†] The 24-hour urinary free cortisol level is expressed in micrograms per square meter of body surface area; 17-hydroxysteroid excretion is expressed in milligrams per grams of creatinine excreted in 24 hours.

[‡] For children, the lowest dexamethasone dose is adjusted to 7.2 μg/kg of body weight, and the highest dose to 28.5 μg/kg.

- can be seen alongside large-cell calcifying Sertoli cell tumours (unlike the latter, Leydig cell tumours are never seen isolated in the context of Carney complex)

Women with Carney complex commonly develop ovarian cysts and other tumours, including serous cystadenomas and teratomas. These tumours may progress occasionally to ovarian carcinoma (mucinus adenocarcinoma or endometrioid carcinoma); reported cases of ovarian cancer occurred in the fifth decade of life.

Cardiac myxomas

Cardiac myxomas are neoplasms found relatively frequently among patients with Carney complex (30%–40% of all Carney complex patients develop at least one cardiac myxoma in their lifetime). Although benign by nature, these tumours cause most of the mortality among patients with Carney complex because of their location. Cardiac myxomas may be within any chamber of the heart, often at multiple sites, and tend to recur frequently. Once they appear, they tend to grow rather fast, sometimes within the course of weeks. Cardiac myxomas can grow in utero, during infancy, and recur even in the elderly; in other words, screening for these tumours should be undertaken at any age, although most tumours are seen in young adults. Early detection of cardiac myxomas by echocardiography and their surgical excision are essential to prevent sudden death or severe morbidity due to embolism, strokes, or cardiac failure.

Skin lesions

Skin lesions are among the major criteria of Carney complex (see Table 14.2). The most common skin lesions are lentigines, epithelioid blue naevi, and cutaneous myxomas.

Lentigines present in 70%–75% of cases. Morphologically, they are flat, poorly circumcised, brown-to-black macules that are less than 0.5 cm in diameter and are located around the lips, the eyelids, the ears, and the genital area (see Figure 14.3a, b, and e). They can be found at birth but usually they acquire their typical distribution at the peripubertal period and tend to fade after the fourth decade of life. They do not substantially change with sun exposure, unlike other pigmented lesions of the skin, and are not associated with a known increased risk for melanoma.

Epithelioid blue naevi are small (usually <5 mm), circular or star-shaped, and dark blue to black in colour. They are variably distributed (face, trunk, limbs; see Figure 14.3c).

Cutaneous myxomas are found in 30%–55% of patients. They present as asymptomatic, small (up to 1 cm), opalescent or dark-pink papules located on the eyelids, the ears, the trunk, and the perineum (see Figure 14.3d, f). Occasionally, they are multiple on one site; rarely, they are associated with local pain due to pressure on a nerve. They are often misdiagnosed as neurofibromas, ganglioneuromas, lipomas, or collagenomas. However, early diagnosis is essential, since it is estimated that almost 80% of patients with Carney complex with a life-threatening cardiac myxoma had presented earlier in life with cutaneous myxoma.

Other skin lesions, such as Spitz naevi, café-au-lait spots, and hypopigmented macules have all been reported but they are rarer than the ones described above.

Breast lesions

Breast tissue lesions in Carney complex include lobular or nodular myxomatosis, myxoid fibroadenomas, or ductal adenomas. Despite extensive involvement of the breast in Carney complex, there does not appear to be increased risk for breast cancer in this condition.

Psammomatous melanotic schwannomas

Psammomatous melanotic schwannomas are present in 8% of Carney complex. These lesion can be found anywhere in the peripheral nervous system, but are most frequently found in the gastrointestinal tract (oesophagus and stomach) and the paraspinal sympathetic chain. Malignancy may be observed in 10% of the cases, with frequent metastasis to the lungs, the liver, the brain, and/or the spinal cord.

Bone lesions

Osteochondromyxoma is a bone tumour found in less than 5% of patients with Carney complex. It occurs early in life, usually before the age of 2, and clinically presents as a painless mass in distal long bones (diaphyseal) and small flat bones (nasal).

Cancers

In addition to thyroid, ovarian, and testicular carcinomas, hepatocellular and rare pancreatic tumours (acinar cell

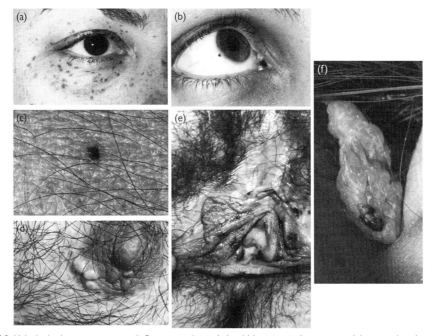

Fig 14.3 Multiple skin lesions in patients with Carney complex, including (a) lentigines in the area around the eye and on the eyelids, (b) inner canthal pigmentation, (c) a blue naevus, (d) multiple myxomas around the nipple, (e) intensely pigmented genital macules, and (f) a complex myxomatous lesion of the external ear.

carcinoma, adenocarcinoma, and intraductal pancreatic mucinous neoplasm) were recently described among Carney complex patients. Metastatic adrenocortical carcinoma has also developed in at least two patients with a background of PPNAD.

Genetics of Carney complex

Genetic linkage analysis identified two independent chromosomal loci for Carney complex: 17p22–4 and 2p16. The gene on 2p16 remains unknown. In most cases, Carney complex is caused by inactivating mutations in *PRKAR1A*, which is located on 17q22–4 and encodes the most widely expressed of the regulatory subunits of protein kinase A, type 1 alpha.

Diagnostic criteria

The diagnosis of Carney complex is made if two or more major manifestations of the syndrome are present (see Box 14.4). The diagnosis may also be made when only one of the major criteria is present and the patient is a carrier of a known inactivating mutation of *PRKAR1A* (see Box 14.4, 'Supplemental criteria').

Screening and follow-up

Paediatric patients

The following is recommended for paediatric patients with Carney complex:

- echocardiographic evaluation should be performed during the first 6 months of life and annually thereafter; if there is a history of an excised myxoma, the evaluation should be performed every 6 months

- other imaging or hormonal screening in prepubertal children is not considered necessary, unless there are clinical issues, such as, for example, growth failure or overgrowth; obesity; or precocious puberty

Post-pubertal children and adult patients

In post-pubertal children and adult patients, the following annual workup is recommended:

- an echocardiogram
- UFC (diurnal cortisol levels and an overnight 1 mg dexamethasone testing may be performed as needed and if clinical symptoms of Cushing's syndrome exist)
- serum IGF-1 levels
- an oral glucose tolerance test, to measure levels of growth hormone
- a testicular ultrasound (if calcification suggesting the presence of a large-cell calcifying Sertoli cell tumour was seen during the initial workup)
- a thyroid ultrasound should be obtained at the initial evaluation and then repeated annually as needed; fine-needle aspiration should be performed if large nodules are present
- an ovarian ultrasound is recommended at the initial evaluation and repeated if an abnormality was detected
- brain and spine MRIs should be obtained during the initial evaluation of any adult patient with Carney complex, but not repeated, unless clinical neurological signs suggest the possibility of a schwannoma (psammomatous melanotic schwannoma)

Box 14.4 Diagnostic criteria for Carney complex

Major diagnostic criteria

1. Spotty skin pigmentation with a typical distribution (lips, conjunctiva and inner or outer canthi, vaginal and penile mucosa)
2. Myxoma (cutaneous and mucosal)
3. Cardiac myxoma
4. Breast myxomatosis or fat-suppressed magnetic resonance imaging findings suggestive of this diagnosis
5. PPNAD or paradoxical positive response of urinary glucocorticosteroids to dexamethasone administration during Liddle's test
6. Acromegaly due to GH-producing adenoma
7. LCCSCT or characteristic calcification on testicular ultrasonography
8. Thyroid carcinoma or multiple, hypoechoic nodules on thyroid ultrasonography, in a young patient
9. Psammomatous melanotic schwannoma
10. Blue nevus, epithelioid blue nevus (multiple)
11. Breast ductal adenoma (multiple)
12. Osteochondromyxoma

Supplemental criteria

1. Affected first-degree relative
2. Inactivating mutation of the *PRKAR1A* gene

Abbreviations: GH, growth hormone; LCCSCT, large-cell calcifying Sertoli cell tumour; PPNAD, pigmented nodular adrenocortical disease.
Reproduced from Horvath A, Stratakis CA, Carney complex and lentiginosis, *Pigment Cell & Melonoma Research*, Volume 22, Issue 5, pp. 580–587, Copyright (2009) with permission from John Wiley and Sons.

Further reading

Anselmo J, Medeiros S, Carneiro V, et al. A large family with Carney complex caused by the S147G PRKAR1A mutation shows a unique spectrum of disease including adrenocortical cancer. *J Clin Endocrinol Metab* 2012; 97: 351–9.

Bertherat J, Horvath A, Groussin L, et al. Mutations in regulatory subunit type 1A of cyclic adenosine 5'-monophosphate-dependent protein kinase (PRKAR1A): Phenotype analysis in 353 patients and 80 different genotypes. *J Clin Endocrinol Metab* 2009; 94: 2085–91.

Briassoulis G, Kuburovic V, Xekouki P, et al. Recurrent left atrial myxomas in Carney Complex: A genetic cause of multiple strokes that can be prevented. *J Stroke Cerebrovasc Dis* 2012; 21: 914.e1–e8.

Carney JA and Toorkey BC. Myxoid fibroadenoma and allied conditions (myxomatosis) of the breast. A heritable disorder with special associations including cardiac and cutaneous myxomas. *Am J Surg Pathol* 1991; 15: 713–21.

Carney JA, Boccon-Gibod L, Jarka DE, et al. Osteochondromyxoma of bone: A congenital tumor associated with lentigines and other unusual disorders. *Am J Surg Pathol* 2001; 25: 164–76.

Chrousos GP and Stratakis CA. Carney complex and the familial lentiginosis syndromes: Link to inherited neoplasias and developmental disorders, and genetic loci. *J Intern Med* 1998; 243: 573–9.

Gaujoux S, Tissier F, Ragazzon B, et al. Pancreatic ductal and acinar cell neoplasms in Carney complex: A possible new association. *J Clin Endocrinol Metab* 2011; 96: E1888–95.

Gennari M, Stratakis CA, Hovarth A, et al. A novel PRKAR1A mutation associated with hepatocellular carcinoma in a young patient and a variable Carney complex phenotype in affected subjects in older generations. *Clin Endocrinol (Oxf)* 2008; 69: 751–5.

Kirschner LS, Carney JA, Pack SD, et al. Mutations of the gene encoding the protein kinase A type I-alpha regulatory subunit in patients with the Carney complex. *Nat Genet* 2000; 26: 89–92.

Morin E, Mete O, Wasserman JD, et al. Carney complex with adrenal cortical carcinoma. *J Clin Endocrinol Metab* 2012; 9: E202–6.

Premkumar A, Stratakis CA, Shawker TH, et al., Testicular ultrasound in Carney complex: Report of three cases. *J Clin Ultrasound* 1997; 25: 211–14.

Pringle DR, Yin Z, Lee AA, et al. Thyroid-specific ablation of the Carney complex gene, PRKAR1A, results in hyperthyroidism and follicular thyroid cancer. *Endocr Relat Cancer* 2012; 19: 435–46.

Rothenbuhler A and Stratakis CA. Clinical and molecular genetics of Carney complex. *Best Pract Res Clin Endocrinol Metab* 2010; 24: 389–99.

Shenoy BV, Carpenter PC, and Carney JA. Bilateral primary pigmented nodular adrenocortical disease. Rare cause of the Cushing syndrome. *Am J Surg Pathol* 1984; 8: 335–44.

Stergiopoulos SG, Abu-Asab MS, Tsokos M, et al. Pituitary pathology in Carney complex patients. *Pituitary* 2004; 7: 73–82.

Stratakis CA, Carney JA, Lin JP, et al. Carney complex, a familial multiple neoplasia and lentiginosis syndrome. Analysis of 11 kindreds and linkage to the short arm of chromosome 2. *J Clin Invest* 1996; 97: 699–705.

Stratakis CA, Papageorgiou T, Premkumar A, et al. Ovarian lesions in Carney complex: Clinical genetics and possible predisposition to malignancy. *J Clin Endocrinol Metab* 2000; 85: 4359–66.

Stratakis CA, Sarlis N, Kirschner LS, et al. Paradoxical response to dexamethasone in the diagnosis of primary pigmented nodular adrenocortical disease. *Ann Intern Med* 1999; 131: 585–91.

Stratakis CA, Kirschner LS, and Carney JA. Clinical and molecular features of the Carney complex: Diagnostic criteria and recommendations for patient evaluation. *J Clin Endocrinol Metab* 2001; 86: 4041–6.

Vezzosi D, Vignaux O, Dupin N, et al., Carney complex: Clinical and genetic 2010 update. *Ann Endocrinol (Paris)* 2010; 71: 486–93.

14.5 Cowden syndrome

Definition and epidemiology

Cowden syndrome is a multiple hamartoma tumour syndrome with a high risk for benign and malignant tumours of the thyroid, breast, endometrium, and kidney. Affected individuals usually have macrocephaly, pathognomonic mucocutaneous skin lesions such as trichilemmomas, and papillomatous papules. Because of the variable and often subtle external manifestations of Cowden syndrome, many individuals remain undiagnosed, so the true prevalence is unknown. The prevalence has been estimated at 1 in 200,000, although this is probably an underestimate. Up to 85% of individuals who meet the diagnostic criteria for Cowden syndrome have a detectable *PTEN* mutation and fall under the category of *PTEN* hamartoma tumour syndrome (PHTS). PHTS includes Cowden syndrome, Bannayan–Riley–Ruvalcaba syndrome (BRRS), and *PTEN*-related Proteus syndrome. BRRS is a congenital disorder characterized by macrocephaly, intestinal hamartomatous polyposis, lipomas, and pigmented macules of the glans penis. *PTEN*-related Proteus syndrome is a complex, highly variable disorder involving congenital malformations and hamartomatous overgrowth of multiple tissues, as well as connective tissue nevi, epidermal nevi, and hyperostoses.

Clinical features

A presumptive diagnosis of PHTS is based on clinical signs; by definition, however, the diagnosis of PHTS is made only when a *PTEN* mutation is identified. Clinical diagnostic criteria for Cowden syndrome have been developed to help clinicians identify patients with Cowden syndrome. Clinical criteria have been divided into three categories: pathognomonic, major, and minor (see Box 14.5).

Molecular genetic testing

Historically, it was suggested that up to 85% of individuals who meet the diagnostic criteria for Cowden syndrome and 65% of individuals with a clinical diagnosis of BRRS have a detectable *PTEN* mutation. More recently, it was found that approximately 25% of individuals who meet the strict diagnostic criteria for Cowden syndrome have a pathogenic *PTEN* mutation, including large deletions. Approximately 10% of individuals with BRRS who do not have a mutation detected in the *PTEN* coding sequence have large deletions within or encompassing *PTEN*.

Investigations

Given the many protean features of Cowden syndrome, the Cleveland Clinic developed a risk calculator for estimating a patient's risk of having a *PTEN* mutation (http://www.lerner.ccf.org/gmi/ccscore).

Optimal *PTEN* testing for individuals suspected of having Cowden syndrome includes sequencing of *PTEN* Exons 1–9 and flanking intronic regions. If no mutation is identified, deletion/duplication analysis should be performed. If still no mutation has been identified, consider research testing, especially in those with Cowden syndrome and Cowden-like syndrome (e.g. *PTEN* promoter, other susceptibility genes).

Complications

Malignant and non-malignant tumour risk

Individuals with Cowden syndrome have a high risk of breast, thyroid, and endometrial cancers. As with other hereditary cancer syndromes, the risk of multifocal and

---

Box 14.5 Operational diagnostic criteria for Cowden syndrome

Criteria

Pathognomonic criteria
  Mucocutaneous lesions:
  • trichilemmomas (facial)
  • Acral keratoses
  • papillomatous papules
  • mucosal lesions

Major criteria
  Breast cancer
  Thyroid cancer (especially follicular)
  Macrocephaly (>97th percentile)
  Endometrial cancer
  Lhermitte–Duclos disease

Minor criteria
  Other thyroid lesions (goitre or nodule)
  Mental retardation
  Hamartomatous intestinal polyps
  Lipomas
  Fibrocystic breast disease
  Uterine fibroids
  Fibromas
  Genitourinary tumours (uterine fibroids, renal cell carcinoma) or malformations

Requirements for diagnosis

Individuals with no family members diagnosed with Cowden syndrome
  Mucocutaneous lesions, if there are one of the following conditions:
• six or more facial papules (of which three or more must be trichilemmomas)
• cutaneous facial papules and oral mucosal papillomatosis
• oral mucosal papillomatosis and acral keratoses
• six or more palmoplantar keratoses
  Two or more major criteria met (one must be macrocephaly or Lhermitte–Duclos disease)
  One major criteria and three minor criteria
  Four minor criteria

Individuals with a family member diagnosed with Cowden syndrome
  A pathognomonic mucocutaneous lesion
  Any one major criteria, with or without minor criteria
  Two minor criteria

Data from *Clinical Cancer Research*, Volume 18, Issue 2, Lifetime Cancer Risks in Individuals with Germline PTEN Mutations, Tan MH, Mester JL, Ngeow J et al., 2012, pp. 400–407.

---

bilateral cancer (in paired organs, such as the breasts) is increased.

Breast disease

Women with Cowden syndrome have as high as a 67% risk for benign breast disease. Prior to gene identification, estimates of lifetime risk to females of developing breast cancer were 25%–50%, with an average age of diagnosis between 38 and 46 years; however, a recent analysis of prospectively accrued and followed probands and family members with a *PTEN* mutation reveal an 85% lifetime risk for female breast cancer, with 50% penetrance by the age of 50 and increased risk overall for second malignant neoplasms.

Thyroid disease

See also Chapter 2, Section 2.8. Benign multinodular goitre of the thyroid as well as adenomatous nodules and follicular adenomas are common, occurring in up to 75% of individuals with Cowden syndrome. The life-time risk for epithelial thyroid cancer is approximately 35%. The median age of onset was 37 years but the disease can present as early as 7. Significantly, follicular thyroid cancer histology is over-represented in adults compared to the general population, in which papillary histology is over-represented and no medullary thyroid carcinoma was observed. Clinicians should be clinically vigilant for other features of Cowden syndrome (e.g. macrocephaly or other benign tumours) in assessing thyroid cancer patients for the possibility of Cowden syndrome.

Endometrial disease

Benign uterine fibroids are common among patients with PHTS. The lifetime risk for endometrial cancer is estimated at 28%, with the starting age at risk in the late thirties to early forties.

Gastrointestinal neoplasias

More than 90% of individuals who had a *PTEN* mutation and underwent at least one upper or lower endoscopy were found to have polyps. Histologic findings varied, ranging from ganglioneuromatous polyps, hamartomatous polyps, and juvenile polyps to adenomatous polyps. The lifetime risk for colorectal cancer is estimated at 9%, with the starting age at risk in the late thirties.

Renal cell carcinoma

In individuals with Cowden syndrome, the lifetime risk for renal cell carcinoma is estimated at 35%, with the starting age at risk in the forties. The predominant hist-ology is papillary renal cell carcinoma.

Other

In individuals with Cowden syndrome, the lifetime risk for cutaneous melanoma is estimated at more than 5%. Brain tumours as well as vascular malformations affecting any organ are occasionally seen in individuals with Cowden syndrome.

Neurodevelopmental sequelae

Lhermitte–Duclos disease

Most, if not all, adult-onset Lhermitte–Duclos disease (dysplastic gangliocytoma of the cerebellum, a hamartomatous overgrowth known to be a feature of Cowden syndrome) can be attributed to mutations in *PTEN*, even in the absence of other clinical signs of Cowden syndrome or BRRS.

Autism/pervasive developmental disorder and macrocephaly

Germ-line *PTEN* mutations were identified in individuals with these findings, especially in the presence of other personal or family history consistent with Cowden syndrome or BRRS. The 10%–20% prevalence of germ-line *PTEN* mutations in autism spectrum disorders with macrocephaly has now been confirmed by several independent groups.

Management

Treatment of manifestations

Treatment for the benign and malignant manifestations of PHTS is the same as for their sporadic counterparts. Cutaneous lesions should be excised only if malignancy is suspected or symptoms (e.g. pain, deformity) are significant.

Surveillance

Screening recommendations that can be used to detect tumours at the earliest, most treatable stages are listed in Table 14.3.

Testing of relatives at risk

PHTS is inherited in an autosomal-dominant manner. The majority of Cowden syndrome cases are simplex. Perhaps 10%–50% of individuals with Cowden syndrome have an affected parent. Each child of an affected individual has a 50% chance of inheriting the mutation and developing PHTS. When a *PTEN* mutation has been identified in a proband, molecular genetic testing of asymptomatic at-risk relatives can identify those who have the family-specific mutation and warrant ongoing surveillance.

Useful websites

The following websites may be useful:
- GeneReviews: http://www.ncbi.nlm.nih.gov/books/NBK1488/
- Cleveland Clinic Risk Calculator for PTEN: http://www.lerner.ccf.org/gmi/ccscore/

Table 14.3 Screening recommendations for patients with *PTEN* hamartoma tumour syndrome

Cancer	General population risk (%)	Lifetime risk with PHTS (%)	Screening
Breast	12.0	~85	Starting at age 30: annual mammogram; consider MRI for patients with dense breasts
Thyroid	1.0	35	Annual ultrasound
Endometrial	2.6	28	Starting at age 30: annual endometrial biopsy or transvaginal ultrasound
Renal cell	1.6	34	Starting at age 40: renal imaging every 2 years
Colon	5.0	9	Starting at age 35: colonoscopy every 2 years
Melanoma	2.0	6	Annual dermatologic examination

Abbreviations: MRI, magnetic resonance imaging; PHTS, *PTEN* hamartoma tumour syndrome.

Data from *Clinical Cancer Research*, Volume 18, Issue 2, Lifetime Cancer Risks in Individuals with Germline PTEN Mutations, Tan MH, Mester JL, Ngeow J et al., 2012, pp. 400–407.

Further reading

Eng C. *PTEN* Hamartoma tumor syndrome. Available at http://www.ncbi.nlm.nih.gov/books/NBK1488/ (accessed 14 Jan 2018).

Ngeow J, Mester J, Rybicki LA, et al. Incidence and clinical characteristics of thyroid cancer in prospective series of individuals with Cowden and Cowden-like syndrome characterized by germline PTEN, SDH, or KLLN alterations. *J Clin Endocrinol Metab* 2011; 96: E2063–71.

Ngeow J, Stanuch K, Mester JL, et al. Second malignant neoplasms in patients with Cowden syndrome with underlying germline PTEN mutations. *J Clin Oncol* 2014; 32: 1818–24.

Mester J, Eng C. Estimate of de novo mutation frequency in probands with PTEN hamartoma tumor syndrome. *Genet Med* 2012; 14: 819–22.

Mester JL, Zhou M, Prescott N, et al. Papillary renal cell carcinoma is associated with PTEN hamartoma tumor syndrome. *Urology* 2012; 79: 1187e1–7.

Tan MH, Mester J, Peterson C, et al. A clinical scoring system for selection of patients for PTEN mutation testing is proposed on the basis of a prospective study of 3042 probands. *Am J Hum Genet* 2011; 88: 42–56.

Tan MH, Mester JL, Ngeow J, et al. Lifetime cancer risks in individuals with germline PTEN mutations. *Clin Cancer Res* 2012; 18: 400–7.

14.6 POEMS syndrome

Introduction
POEMS (for *p*olyneuropathy, *o*rganomegaly, *e*ndocrinopathy, *M*-protein, and *s*kin changes) syndrome is a rare multisystem disorder with monoclonal plasma cell proliferation and overproduction of cytokines such as vascular endothelial growth factor (VEGF). POEMS syndrome has also been called Crow–Fukase syndrome, Takatsuki syndrome, and PEP (for *p*lasma cell dyscrasia, *e*dema, and *p*igmentation) syndrome. The prevalence of POEMS syndrome is unclear, but a national survey conducted in Japan showed a prevalence of approximately 0.3/100,000. The disease was initially thought to be more common in Japan, given that the largest initial reports were from Japan. However, large series have also been reported from France, the United States, China, and India, and the disorder has been increasingly recognized in many areas of the world. Although the majority of patients have osteosclerotic myeloma, these same patients usually have only 5% bone marrow plasma cells or less (almost always monoclonal lambda), and rarely have anaemia, hypercalcaemia, or renal insufficiency. These characteristics and the superior median survival differentiate POEMS syndrome from multiple myeloma.

Pathophysiology
The pathogenesis of POEMS syndrome is not well understood, but overproduction of VEGF and other cytokines (interleukins 6 and 12, TNF alpha), possibly secreted by plasmacytomas, is likely to be responsible for many of the characteristic symptoms. Almost all patients with POEMS syndrome have highly elevated serum VEGF levels, and disease activity appears to correlate with VEGF levels. VEGF is a potent multifunctional cytokine that induces prominent angiogenesis and microvascular hyperpermeability, and therefore could cause many of the symptoms of POEMS syndrome such as oedema/effusion, organomegaly, and skin angiomas. However, mechanisms for the peripheral neuropathy and endocrinopathy are still unclear.

Diagnosis and clinical features
In the advanced stage of the disease, when many systemic manifestations already develop, the diagnosis of POEMS syndrome is not difficult. However, in the early phase, patients show a part of the symptoms or laboratory abnormalities, the disease is often under-diagnosed. Skin changes include angiomas, skin thickening, pigmentation, and hypertrichosis. Important clinical features other than the five cardinal symptoms of 'POEMS' include peripheral oedema, pleural effusion, ascites, sclerotic bone lesions, Castleman disease, papilloedema, polycythaemia, and thrombocytosis (see Figure 14.4). Proposed diagnostic criteria are shown in Box 14.6. Polyneuropathy is present in all patients, and the diagnosis is made by a combination of characteristic symptoms and laboratory findings. Serum VEGF level is a useful diagnostic biomarker.

Endocrinopathy is a central but poorly understood feature of POEMS. Approximately 80% of patients have a

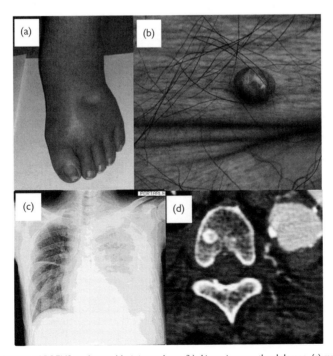

Fig 14.4 Clinical features of POEMS syndrome: (a) pitting oedema, (b) skin angioma on the abdomen, (c) massive pleural effusion, and (d) osteoclastic lesions on bone CT.

Box 14.6 Criteria for the diagnosis of POEMS syndrome

Major criteria
(a) Polyneuropathy (mandatory)*
(b) Monoclonal plasma cell proliferative disorder
(c) Elevation of serum or plasma VEGF levels
Minor criteria
(a) Sclerotic bone lesions
(b) Castleman disease**
(c) Organomegaly (hepato-splenomegaly or lymphadenopathy)
(d) Oedema (oedema, pleural effusion, or ascites)
(e) Endocrinopathy (adrenal, thyroid, pituitary, gonadal, parathyroid, or pancreatic)***
(f) Skin changes (hyperpigmentation, hypertrichosis, plethora, cyanosis, hemangiomata, or white nails)
(g) Papilloedema
(h) Thrombocytosis and/or polycythaemia

(1) Definite POEMS syndrome: Three major criteria and at least one minor criterion.
(2) Probable POEMS syndrome: Two major criteria, with at least one minor criterion.

Abbreviations: VEGF, vascular endothelial growth factor.
* Defined by M-protein, or monoclonal plasma cell proliferation in bone marrow biopsy or biopsy of a plasmacytoma or sclerotic lesion
** There is a Castleman disease variant of POEMS syndrome that occurs without evidence of a clonal plasma cell disorder that is not accounted for in this list. This entity should be considered separately.
*** Because of the high prevalence of diabetes mellitus and thyroid abnormalities, this diagnosis alone is not sufficient to meet this minor criterion.
Adapted from Dispenzieri, A, POEMS syndrome: 2014 Update on diagnosis, risk-stratification, and Management, 2014, *American Journal of Hematology*, Volume 89, Issue 2. Copyright (2014) with permission from John Wiley and Sons.

---

recognized endocrinopathy, with hypogonadism as the most common endocrine abnormality, followed by thyroid abnormalities, glucose metabolism abnormalities, and, lastly, adrenal insufficiency. The majority of patients had evidence of multiple endocrinopathies in the four major endocrine axes (gonadal, thyroid, glucose, and adrenal). For male patients, gynaecomastia is frequently present.

Treatment

POEMS syndrome is a potentially fatal disease, and patients' quality of life deteriorates because of progressive neuropathy, massive peripheral oedema, pleural effusion, or ascites. Serious complications such as multi-organ failure from capillary leak syndrome, restrictive lung disease, pulmonary hypertension, and thromboembolic events may occur, contributing to the poor prognosis.

There are no randomized controlled trials for POEMS syndrome, presumably because of the rarity of the disorder, and therefore no established treatment regimen. Case reports and series report the use of irradiation, resection of plasmacytomas, chemotherapies, corticosteroids, plasmapheresis, and intravenous immunoglobulin infusion for the treatment of POEMS syndrome. Irradiation has usually been proposed for patients with a solitary plasmacytoma. If patients have wide spread osteosclerotic lesions, systemic chemotherapy is necessary. In appropriate candidates, high-dose chemotherapy with autologous peripheral blood stem cell transplantation is recommended. This treatment resulted in obvious improvement in neuropathy as well as other symptoms, with a significant decrease in serum VEGF levels. From

data of published experience, the transplant-related mortality was initially reported to be 7.4%, but a recent update in 2008 suggested a lower transplant-related mortality (3.3%) with better peri-transplant supportive care (Dispenzieri 2008). Indications for this treatment have not yet been established, and long-term prognosis is unclear. Treatments that may be considered in the future include lenalidomide or thalidomide, anti-VEGF monoclonal antibody (bevacizumab), and bortezomib. The first randomized controlled trial with thalidomide has been completed in Japan, and efficacy of this agent has been proved.

References and further reading

Bardwick PA, Zvaifler NJ, Gill GN, et al. Plasma cell dyscrasia with polyneuropathy, organomegaly, endocrinopathy, M-protein, and skin changes: the POEMS syndrome. Report of two cases and a review of the literature. *Medicine* 1980; 59: 311–22.

Dispenzieri A. POEMS syndrome. *Blood Rev* 2007; 21: 285–99.

Dispenzieri A, Kyle RA, Lacy MQ, et al. POEMS syndrome: Definitions and long-term outcome. *Blood* 2003; 101: 2496–506.

Katayama K, Misawa S, Sato Y, S et al. Japanese POEMS Syndrome with Thalidomide (J-POST) Trial: Study protocol for a phase II/III multicentre, randomised, double-blind, placebo-controlled trial. *BMJ Open* 2015; 5: e007330.

Kuwabara S, Dispenzieri A, Arimura K, et al. Treatment for POEMS (polyneuropathy, organomegaly, endocrinopathy, M-protein, and skin changes) syndrome. *Cochrane Database Syst Rev* 2012; 6: CD006828.

Watanabe O, Arimura K, Kitajima I, et al. Greatly raised vascular endothelial growth factor (VEGF) in POEMS syndrome. *Lancet* 1996; 347: 702.

14.7 Multiple endocrine neoplasia type 1

Definition
Multiple endocrine neoplasia type 1 is characterized by the combined occurrence of parathyroid adenomas, pancreatic islet cell tumours, and anterior pituitary tumours. In addition, some patients may develop bronchial, thymic, or gastric neuroendocrine tumours or adrenocortical tumours (Table 14.4). Cutaneous tumours may manifest in patients with multiple endocrine neoplasia type 1 and they may be multifocal.

Epidemiology
The population prevalence of multiple endocrine neoplasia type 1 is 1 in 30,000 individuals. This disease shows a >50% penetrance by the age of 20, and >98% penetrance by the age of 50. Untreated, patients with multiple endocrine neoplasia type 1 have a 50% chance of death by the age of 50.

Diagnosis
A diagnosis of multiple endocrine neoplasia type 1 may be made if:
* two or more primary endocrine tumours of the type associated with multiple endocrine neoplasia type 1 occur in a patient
* one endocrine tumour of the type associated with multiple endocrine neoplasia type 1 is diagnosed in a patient with a first-degree relative with multiple endocrine neoplasia type 1
* a germ-line mutation is identified in an individual, even if they are asymptomatic

Genetics
Multiple endocrine neoplasia type 1 is an autosomal-dominant condition that results from germ-line mutations in a ten-exon gene called *MEN1*, which is located on Chromosome 11q13 and encodes a 610-amino-acid protein named menin. *MEN1* is a tumour-suppressor gene, and the clinical condition arises from the combination of an inherited inactivating germ-line mutation and a subsequent, inactivating, somatic DNA mutation which then drives tumour development within a specific tissue. It is important to note that not every patient with a germline mutation will have a past family history of multiple endocrine neoplasia, as de novo mutations occur in approximately 10% of cases.

In approximately 10% of patients with multiple endocrine neoplasia type 1, germ-line mutations in the coding region of *MEN1* are not found with standard mutational analysis. Additional techniques can be utilized to help to diagnose those cases where large gene deletions are responsible.

Indications for genetic testing for multiple endocrine neoplasia type 1
Genetic counselling should precede genetic testing. Testing should be offered to:
* any patient with a clinical diagnosis of multiple endocrine neoplasia type 1
* all asymptomatic first-degree relatives of a patient with multiple endocrine neoplasia type 1 (ideally in the first decade of life, as manifestations of multiple endocrine neoplasia type 1 have been reported in patients as young as 5)

Consider testing when the following clinical features, which are strongly suspicious of multiple endocrine neoplasia type 1, are present:
* multiple parathyroid tumours before the age of 40
* recurrent hyperparathyroidism
* multiple pancreatic islet tumours
* a diagnosis of gastrinoma

Care recommendations
Multiple endocrine neoplasia type 1 is associated with a decreased life expectancy. The majority of patients with multiple endocrine neoplasia type 1 will die from a cause related to the disease. On the basis of the high disease penetrance and the significant associated morbidity and mortality, lifelong biochemical and radiological screening should be offered to all patients with multiple endocrine neoplasia type 1. This recommendation should be accompanied by the explanation that the detection and treatment of early disease may improve prognosis and life expectancy, although this remains unproven. Patients with multiple endocrine neoplasia type 1 should be cared for by experienced multidisciplinary teams.

Input from patient support groups (e.g. AMEND UK and the NET Patient Foundation) may be invaluable to patients and their families.

Parathyroid tumours
Clinical features
Primary hyperparathyroidism is the most common manifestation of multiple endocrine neoplasia type 1, and multiple glands may be affected.

Screening recommendations
Biochemical screens
Biochemical screens should include annual measurements of calcium and PTH, from the age of 8.

Imaging
No routine imaging is recommended.

Management
The timing of parathyroid surgery remains controversial. Possible indications include deteriorating bone density, the

Table 14.4 Tumour types in multiple endocrine neoplasia type 1, and their estimated penetrance

Tumour type	Estimated penetrance (%)
Parathyroid adenoma	90
Pancreatic islet cell tumour	30–70
Pituitary tumour	30–4
Bronchial NET	2
Thymic NET	2
Gastric NET	10
Adrenocortical tumour	40
Angiofibroma	85
Collagenoma	70
Lipomas	30
Meningiomas	8
Phaeochromocytoma	<1

Abbreviations: NET, neuroendocrine tumour.

presence of a gastrinoma, uncontrolled hypercalcaemia, planning pregnancy, or patient preference. The recommended first procedure is an open bilateral neck exploration, performed by an experienced surgeon, with a total or subtotal (3.5 glands) parathyroidectomy. A simultaneous prophylactic transcervical thymectomy should be considered; however, this measure does not completely eliminate the risk of developing a thymic neuroendocrine tumour. Cinacalcet may be helpful in targeting the hypercalcaemia of primary hyperparathyroidism associated with multiple endocrine neoplasia type 1, but the long-term effect of this agent on proliferating tissues in multiple endocrine neoplasia type 1 remains unknown.

Anterior pituitary tumours

Clinical features

Macroadenomas with invasive features may be more common in patients with multiple endocrine neoplasia type 1 than those with sporadic disease. Notably, though, the frequency of pituitary carcinoma does not appear to be increased. Prolactinomas are the commonest subtype (60%), followed by somatotrophinomas (25%) and non-functioning adenomas; adrenocorticotrophic-hormone-secreting adenomas are rare (<5%). Plurihormonal expression is not uncommon.

Screening recommendations

Biochemical screens
Biochemical screens should include annual measurements of prolactin and IGF-1, from the age of 5.

Imaging
Three-yearly pituitary MRI scans should be performed.

Management
Interventions are similar to those used for the management of sporadic pituitary disease.

Gastropancreatic neuroendocrine tumours

Clinical features
Malignant pancreatic islet cell tumours are the commonest cause of death in patients with multiple endocrine neoplasia type 1. In light of this, surveillance of the pancreas is inevitably a major focus of care. However, pancreatic lesions are extremely common in multiple endocrine neoplasia type 1, and optimal management of much of this diverse spectrum of disease (from benign to malignant and from non-functioning to overt syndromes of hormone excess) remains unclear (Table 14.5).

Screening recommendations

Biochemical screens
Biochemical screens should include annual measurements of fasting glucose, insulin, chromogranin A, glucagon, vasoactive intestinal polypeptide, and pancreatic polypeptide, from the age of 5. In addition, there should be an annual measurement of FSG, from the age of 20.

Imaging
Imaging should include annual pancreatic imaging via MRI, CT, or endoscopic ultrasound.

Management
Gastrinomas are frequently elusive, small, and multiple/metastatic at diagnosis; consequently, aggressive surgery remains a controversial approach. The mainstay of managing Zollinger–Ellison syndrome is with proton-pump inhibitor therapy. In contrast, attempted curative surgery is the treatment of choice for the majority of insulinomas in multiple endocrine neoplasia type 1, as these are typically solitary. Glucagonomas and VIPomas are also best treated surgically, if this is feasible, although metastatic disease at baseline is common. Stabilization of tumour progression and/or control of functional effects may be achieved by a variety of modalities, including somatostatin analogues, chemotherapy, embolization, and radiolabelled or other, newer therapies. Surgery for non-functioning pancreatic neuroendocrine tumours in multiple endocrine neoplasia type 1 is recommended for lesions >2 cm or those of 1–2 cm and with rapid growth. Surveillance appears acceptable for lesions <1 cm (overall risk of synchronous malignancy ~4%).

Other tumours associated with multiple endocrine neoplasia type 1

Bronchial/thymic neuroendocrine tumours
Bronchial/thymic neuroendocrine tumours are rare but aggressive tumours that are associated with an increased risk of death in patients with multiple endocrine neoplasia type 1, especially, it appears, for male cigarette smokers. Imaging with MRI/CT every 1–2 years from the age of 15 is proposed, although the optimal frequency of imaging is unknown, and the rationale for screening must be balanced against cumulative radiation exposure.

Adrenocortical tumours
Most adrenocortical tumours are non-functional benign lesions. Radiological surveillance is achieved via pancreatic imaging. Biochemical evaluation is indicated in symptomatic patients or for lesions >1 cm. A slight increase risk of adrenocortical carcinoma is seen in multiple endocrine neoplasia type 1.

Facial angiofibromas/collagenomas/lipomas
Facial angiofibromas/collagenomas/lipomas are benign, common, and often multifocal lesions that may help raise the clinical suspicion of multiple endocrine neoplasia type 1. Any medical intervention is typically directed by patient preference.

Further reading

Brandi ML, Gagel RF, Angeli A, et al. Guidelines for diagnosis and therapy of MEN1 and MEN2. *J Clin Endocrinol Metab* 2001; 86: 5658–71.

Goudet P, Murat A, Binquet C, et al. Risk factors and causes of death in MEN1 disease. A GTE (Groupe d'Etude des Tumeurs Endocrines) cohort study among 758 patients. *World J Surg* 2010; 34: 249–55.

Thakker RV. Multiple endocrine neoplasia type 1 (MEN1) and type 4 (MEN4). *Mol Cell Endocrinol* 2014; 386: 2–15.

Thakker RV, Newey PJ, Walls GV, et al. Clinical practice guidelines for multiple endocrine neoplasia type 1 (MEN1). *J Clin Endocrinol Metab* 2012; 97: 2990–3011.

Table 14.5 Estimated penetrance of pancreatic islet tumour subtype in multiple endocrine neoplasia type 1

Islet tumour type	Estimated penetrance (%)
Gastrinoma	40
Non-functioning and PPoma	20–55
Insulinoma	10
Glucagonoma	<1
VIPoma	<1

14.8 Multiple endocrine neoplasia types 2 and 4

Introduction

Multiple endocrine neoplasia type 2 is a familial tumour syndrome conferring the risk of medullary thyroid cancer, phaeochromocytoma, and hyperparathyroidism: it occurs in 1 in 30,000 people, and over 1000 families carrying the disease have been identified worldwide. This disease is of particular interest because mutations in the *RET* onco-gene are causative in more than 99% of families, and the identification of carriers of a *RET* mutation enables these people to be offered prophylactic surgery to remove the thyroid gland, which is the most likely site of malignancy. There is now extensive experience in the management of these families and, furthermore, drugs have been developed which can inhibit the actions of the activated onco-gene product, the RET receptor, which has tyrosine kinase activity.

The *RET* proto-oncogene is located at chromosomal position 10q11.2 and encodes a cell-surface receptor with extracellular, transmembrane, and intracellular domains. Activation via a point mutation leads to dimerization of the receptor, phosphorylation of tyrosine residues, and activation of a number of second-messenger pathways. Activated RET, through its signalling cascades, leads to cellular growth, proliferation, and migration. It is these pathways that are targeted by the newer therapeutic agents for medullary thyroid cancer.

Genotype–phenotype correlation

There are three main phenotypes of multiple endocrine neoplasia type 2: 80% of cases have multiple endocrine neoplasia type 2a (also referred to simply as 'multiple endocrine neoplasia type 2'), in which medullary thyroid cancer occurs in over 95% of cases and may be accompanied by phaeochromocytomas in 50% of cases, and parathyroid tumours in 30%; 10% of cases have familial medullary thyroid carcinoma, where medullary thyroid cancer occurs alone; and 5% of cases have multiple endocrine neoplasia type 2b (also called 'multiple endocrine neoplasia type 3') in which medullary thyroid cancer is accompanied by marfanoid habitus, enlarged corneal nerves, mucosal neuromas, especially on the tongue, and generalized ganglioneuromatosis. It should be noted that the medullary thyroid cancer associated with multiple

endocrine neoplasia type 2b is particularly aggressive and can occur in infants.

The *RET* mutations in multiple endocrine neoplasia type 2a are clustered mainly in Exons 10 and 11, with rarer mutations in Exons 13 to 15. Multiple endocrine neoplasia type 2b is usually associated with a mutation in Codon 918 in Exon 16. The location of the resulting mutated amino acid (i.e., whether it is extracellular or intracellular) has implications for the way in which RET signalling is activated, and this affects phenotype (see Figure 14.5).

The genotype–phenotype correlations in multiple endocrine neoplasia type 2 have enabled recommendations to assist in surveillance of people who carry *RET* mutations and to guide timing of prophylactic surgery (see Table 14.6).

Investigation and management of medullary thyroid cancer

Medullary thyroid cancer occurs sporadically in 75% of patients and, in 25%, occurs as part of multiple endocrine neoplasia type 2. All cases of medullary thyroid cancer (even if apparently sporadic) should undergo germ-line *RET* mutation testing to exclude multiple endocrine neoplasia type 2. Studies show that, even with careful elicitation of family history, unrecognized familial cases of medullary thyroid cancer are common (up to 10%).

Analysis of tumour DNA for somatic *RET* mutations is not part of clinical management but for research purposes has provided some prognostic clues. Somatic mutation of Codon 918 is common in sporadic medullary thyroid cancer, occurring in 10%–80% of cases. It is thought to indicate a poorer prognosis with a higher rate of recurrence and distant metastases.

Primary treatment for a tumour confined to the thyroid involves thyroidectomy and removal of lymph nodes in the central compartment of the neck, in the region bounded by the carotids laterally, the sternal notch inferiorly, and the hyoid bone superiorly. Additional lateral nodes are removed if metastases are present. If the tumour has metastasized extensively, then debulking surgery is performed, if appropriate.

Metastatic disease in bone can be irradiated, and metastatic disease in soft tissue can be considered for treatment with one of the new tyrosine kinase inhibitors.

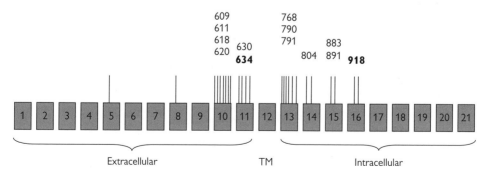

Fig 14.5 Schematic of the *RET* proto-oncogene, showing clustered mutations (e.g. Codon 634 in Exon 11 in multiple endocrine neoplasia type 2A, and Codon 918 in Exon 16 in multiple endocrine neoplasia type 2B); TM, transmembrane.

Table 14.6 Genotype–phenotype correlations for *RET* mutations, and associated recommendations for management and surveillance (based on the American Thyroid Association guidelines)

Feature	Risk category		Moderate	High	Highest
	A		B	C	D†
Location of *RET* mutation (codons)	532, 533, 768, 790, 791, 891, 912, 804, 844, or 912		609, 611, 618, 620, or 630	634	883 or 918
Associated syndrome	FMTC		FMTC	MEN 2A	MEN 2B
	MEN 2A		MEN 2A		
Earliest onset of MTC	Adult		5 years old	<5 years old	<1 year old
Recommended time of thyroidectomy‡	>5 years old, if criteria are met		When criteria are met	<5 years old, if criteria are met	ASAP
Recommended age for initiation of phaeochromocytoma screening§	20 years old		20 years old	8 years old	8 years old
Recommended age for initiation of hyperparathyroidism screening	20 years old		20 years old	8 years old	N/A

Abbreviations: FMTC: familial medullary thyroid carcinoma; MEN 2A, multiple endocrine neoplasia type 2a; MEN 2B, multiple endocrine neoplasia type 2b; MTC, medullary thyroid cancer.

† Category D, which is associated with the mutations that cause MEN 2B, is the highest-risk category. Patients falling into this category must be screened as early as possible, and gene carriers will need prophylactic thyroidectomy in the first 1–2 years of life.

‡ Patients in Category C should have prophylactic surgery in childhood, but those in Categories A and B, the decision should be guided by criteria such as whether the basal calcitonin and neck ultrasound are normal.

§ Patients needing surgery should always have urine catecholamine screening prior to undergoing general anaesthesia.

Data from American Thyroid Association Guidelines Task Force, Kloos RT, Eng C et al, Medullary thyroid cancer: management guidelines of the American Thyroid Association, *Thyroid*, 2009, Volume 19, Issue 6, pp. 565–612.

The follow-up of patients with medullary thyroid cancer involves measurement of the serum calcitonin, initially every 4–6 months. The calcitonin doubling time is a good predictor of survival; doubling every 6–24 months is associated with a 10-year survival of 37%, but doubling less than every 6 months is associated with a 10-year survival of 8%. Once the calcitonin level rises, CT of the neck, chest, and abdomen, combined with PET, is indicated, with the aim being to identify resectable disease, or disease that could be staged in preparation for treatment with a tyrosine kinase inhibitor. MRI scanning is more sensitive than CT for the detection of liver metastases. Management of the psychological stress associated with calcitonin measurement in frequently asymptomatic patients is important, with decreased frequency of measurement once the rate of calcitonin increase is known. There is controversy as to the age and extent of prophylactic surgery for asymptomatic *RET* mutation carriers. Total thyroidectomy is the minimum procedure, combined with prophylactic central node dissection when indicated by either specific *RET* genotype and/or pre-operative calcitonin level (see Table 14.6).

The histological precursor of medullary thyroid cancer, C-cell hyperplasia, may be seen in the thyroids of *RET* mutation carriers, but can also be seen in normal thyroids at autopsy and its histological definition is controversial. Calcitonin stimulation tests using agents such as pentagastrin are rarely required in the genetic era, due to the risks of false positivity and inaccurate reference ranges.

Prognosis of medullary thyroid cancer

The prognosis of medullary thyroid cancer depends on the extent of the disease at the initial diagnosis. Patients who have tumours that are less than 1 cm and confined to the thyroid, and whose basal calcitonin is undetectable after surgery, have a 10-year survival of nearly 100%, whereas patients with cervical metastases at diagnosis have a 75%–85% 10-year survival.

Targeted molecular therapies for medullary thyroid cancer

A number of new agents have been the subject of both Phase 2 and Phase 3 studies. These agents inhibit multiple kinases, including RET itself, and other molecules such as VEGFR. The degree of RET inhibition may differ according to *RET* genotype, with V804L-mutation tumours showing resistance to several tyrosine kinase inhibitors.

Vandetanib, in patients with familial medullary thyroid cancer and, more recently, in those with sporadic medullary thyroid cancer, has shown promising anti-tumour effects. Lenvatinib is the subject of an ongoing Phase 3 study. Tyrosine kinase inhibitors have been demonstrated to prolong disease-free survival and reduce symptoms of flushing and diarrhoea due to elevated calcitonin levels. Vandetanib and cabozantinib are now approved by the US Food and Drug Administration for use in medullary thyroid cancer.

Side effects of tyrosine kinase inhibitors are related to the multiple proteins inhibited and include diarrhoea, fatigue, anorexia, photosensitive skin rashes, hypertension, and prolonged QT syndrome. The long-term prognosis of medullary thyroid cancer patients taking tyrosine kinase inhibitors is not yet known.

Phaeochromocytoma in multiple endocrine neoplasia type 2

Phaeochromocytomas occur in >50% of patients with multiple endocrine neoplasia type 2b and in up to 50% of patients with multiple endocrine neoplasia type 2a, depending on their specific genotype. In 65% of cases, tumours are bilateral at presentation; in the remaining cases, contralateral tumours may develop within a decade. Usually in multiple endocrine neoplasia type 2, phaeochromocytomas are diagnosed 10–25 years after medullary thyroid cancer (or C-cell hyperplasia). In the uncommon circumstance when phaeochromocytoma is the index presentation of multiple endocrine neoplasia type 2, thyroidectomy will still be indicated, since medullary thyroid cancer will nearly always be present.

Phaeochromocytomas associated with multiple endocrine neoplasia type 2 are typically adrenal in location, benign, and associated with mixed production of adrenaline and noradrenaline (and metanephrines). In contrast, Von Hippel–Lindau syndrome is typically associated with noradrenaline-secreting adrenal tumours and, in *SDH* subunit-associated familial paraganglioma syndromes, phaeochromocytomas are more likely to occur in extra-adrenal locations and are (in the case of *SDHB*) at higher risk of malignancy. Patients with multiple endocrine neoplasia type 2 should be screened annually from age 8 (if in the highest-risk category) or 20 (if in the least-high risk category), with measurements of serum or urinary catecholamines and/or metanephrines. Positive tests should trigger adrenal CT or MRI imaging. Functional imaging with ^{123}I-MIBG or DOPA PET may be helpful in some cases.

Treatment of the phaeochromocytoma is surgical. Preoperative preparation includes alpha blockade and then beta-blocker treatment as needed to control tachycardia. Perioperative monitoring and blood pressure control is crucial. Patients with bilateral disease may benefit from cortex-sparing surgery. Although metastatic phaeochromocytoma is rare in multiple endocrine neoplasia type 2, patients who develop it may benefit from treatment with ^{131}I-MIBG.

Hyperparathyroidism in multiple endocrine neoplasia type 2

Hyperparathyroidism occurs mainly in patients with the C634R *RET* mutation and is mild. Treatment is usually total parathyroidectomy and autotransplantation into the forearm. Some patients have a single parathyroid adenoma, in which case it is worthwhile using preoperative imaging with the radionuclide sestamibi to enable single-gland removal. In contrast, the hyperparathyroidism associated with multiple endocrine neoplasia type 1 is usually associated with four-gland hyperplasia, for which open-neck exploration is required and preoperative imaging may be unhelpful.

Multiple endocrine neoplasia type 4

Multiple endocrine neoplasia type 4 is a very rare genetic endocrine tumour syndrome associated with mutations in the cyclin-dependent kinase inhibitor gene *CDKN1B*, which encodes p27. A variety of different endocrine syndromes and tumours associated with this disease have been described, including primary hyperparathyroidism, pituitary adenomas, testicular tumours, neuroendocrine cervical tumours, and, possibly, renal and adrenal tumours.

Further reading

Barbet J, Campion L, Kraber-Bodere L, et al. Prognostic impact of serum calcitonin and carcinoembryonic antigen doubling times in patients with medullary thyroid carcinoma. *J Clin Endocrinol Metab* 2005; 90: 6077–84.

Elisei R, Cosci B, Romei C, et al. Prognostic significance of somatic RET oncogene mutations in sporadic medullary thyroid carcinoma: A 10-year follow-up study. *J Clin Endocrinol Metab* 2008; 93: 682–7.

Hoegerle S, Nitzsche E, Altehoefer C, et al. Pheochromocytomas: Detection with ^{18}F-DOPA whole-body PET: Initial results. *Radiology* 2002; 222: 507–12.

Learoyd DL and Robinson BG. Do all patients with RET mutations associated with multiple endocrine neoplasia type 2 require surgery? *Nat Clin Prac Endocrinol Metab* 2005; 1: 60–1.

Machens A, Brauckhoff M, Holzhausen HJ, et al. Codon-specific development of pheochromocytoma in multiple endocrine neoplasia type 2. *J Clin Endocrinol Metab* 2005; 90: 3999–4003.

Robinson BG, Paz-Ares L, Krebs A, et al. Vandetanib (100 mg) in patients with locally advanced or metastatic hereditary medullary thyroid cancer. *J Clin Endocrinol Metab* 2010; 95: 2664–71.

Wells SA Jr, Asa SL, Dralle H, et al. Revised American Thyroid Association guidelines for the management of medullary thyroid carcinoma. *Thyroid* 2015; 25(6): 567–610.

Wells SA Jr, Robinson BG, Gagel RF, et al. Vandetanib in patients with locally advanced or metastatic medullary thyroid cancer: A randomised, double blind phase III trial. *J Clin Oncol* 2012; 30: 134–41.

Chapter 15

Endocrinology of metabolism

Chapter contents

15.1 Hypoglycaemia

Definition

Hypoglycaemia is defined as a level of plasma or serum glucose concentration low enough to cause symptoms and/or signs, including impairment of brain function. The threshold for symptoms varies between individuals and under different circumstances; for example, there is a lower threshold in patients suffering recurrent episodes. Some utilize a threshold for plasma glucose of <3.0 mmol/L (54 mg/dL) but, when the appropriateness of the insulin response is evaluated, a threshold of 2.2 mmol/L (40 mg/dL) is more frequently applied and is one we recommend. Hypoglycaemia is confirmed by documenting the following criteria comprising Whipple's triad, either during spontaneous symptoms or by provocation testing:

- symptoms and/or signs consistent with hypoglycaemia
- documented low plasma glucose
- resolution of these once the glucose levels have been corrected by the administration of food or glucose

Measurement issues

Blood tests should be obtained after overnight fast to ensure repeatability. Whole blood values are approximately 10% below plasma values, and values from capillary samples can be 1.7–2.2 mmol/L (30–40 mg/dL) lower than plasma values. Low glucose values can, rarely, also be due to errors in sample handling. If the samples are not processed rapidly or collected with glycolytic inhibitors, then glycolysis by blood cells may result in a 0.6–1.1 mmol/L (10–20 mg/dL) drop in blood glucose per hour at room temperature, and more so in samples with excessive cell numbers, such as in polycythaemia or leukaemia. Hypertriglyceridemia may reduce plasma glucose levels as much as 15% below the actual value. Additionally, alterations in the peripheral circulation may cause pseudohypoglycaemia.

Epidemiology

Hypoglycaemia is common in patients with diabetes mellitus, most particularly those taking oral hypoglycaemic medications and insulin. It is increasingly recognized in patients following bariatric surgery. Malignancy and insulin-secreting tumours are rarer but important causes.

Physiology of glucose homeostasis

In normal physiology, the sources of circulating glucose are dietary carbohydrate, gluconeogenesis, and glycogenolysis. During fasting, gluconeogenesis and glycogenolysis, principally in the liver, are sufficient to maintain glucose concentrations within normal limits even without glucose absorption from the gut. By 48 hours of fasting, glycogen stores in the liver are diminishing, and gluconeogenesis in liver and kidneys provides an increasing percentage of circulating glucose. In order to prevent hypoglycaemia, insulin levels are suppressed and counter-regulatory hormones stimulated. Glucagon stimulates glycogenolysis and gluconeogenesis, increasing hepatic glucose release, and its absence (after pancreatectomy or in type 1 diabetes) results in more serious hypoglycaemic episodes. Epinephrine and norepinephrine stimulate hepatic glycogenolysis and renal gluconeogenesis, augment lipolysis, and inhibit insulin

Table 15.1 Hormonal effects on glucose flux

Hormone	Effect on glucose	Mechanism
Insulin	↓	Inhibition of gluconeogenesis
		Stimulation of liver and muscle glycogen synthesis
		Stimulation of cellular glucose uptake
Adrenaline	↑	Stimulation of liver and muscle glycogenolysis
Glucagon	↑	Stimulation of liver glycogen glycogenolysis
		Stimulation of liver gluconeogenesis
Cortisol	↑	Stimulation of liver gluconeogenesis
Growth hormone	↑	Glucose-sparing metabolism by mobilization of triglycerides

release and insulin-stimulated glucose uptake. Growth hormone and cortisol suppress insulin-mediated glucose uptake and augment glucose release (see Table 15.1)

Causes of hypoglycaemia

The causes of hypoglycaemia can be broadly divided into those that cause a decrease in the rate of delivery of glucose into the circulation from the gut or organs, and those that cause an increase in the rate of glucose removal. Removal of glucose from the circulation may be due to excessive substrate utilization, excess insulin, abnormal insulin counter-regulatory responses, and abnormal target tissue responses. Frequently, for example in sepsis, several factors contribute. Classification of hypoglycaemia according to symptomatology (postprandial vs fasting) or in terms of likely diagnosis (such is in an ill patient vs a well patient) may sometimes be helpful. The differential diagnosis also differs in neonates and children compared to adults (see Tables 15.2 and 15.3).

Table 15.2 Causes of hypoglycaemia in adults

Well-seeming adult	Unwell adult
Drug-induced	Drug-induced sepsis
Factitious hypoglycaemia	Trauma and burns
Malnutrition	Cardiac failure
Tumours:	Renal disease
• islet cell	Liver disease
• non-islet cell	Hormone deficiencies (growth hormone, cortisol)
• nesidioblastosis	Insulin/food or parenteral intake mismatch
Autoimmune (anti-insulin antibodies) reactive hypoglycaemia	
Exercise	
Post-bariatric surgery	
Other	

Table 15.3 Symptoms of hypoglycaemia

Adrenergic	Neuroglycopenic
Sweating	Visual changes
Hunger	Confusion
Tingling	Unusual behaviour
Tremulousness	Weakness
Palpitations	Warmth
Anxiety	Lethargy
	Dizziness
	Seizures
	Coma

Drug-induced hypoglycaemia

In evaluating the hypoglycaemic diabetic patient, one should recognize all the possible precipitating factors, including dietary habits, dosage errors, other medications, age, physical activity, and co-morbidities. Even in non-diabetic patients, medication evaluation is crucial. Hypoglycaemia may be a direct effect of drugs (intentional or accidental insulin overdose, sulfonylureas, etc.) or an effect on the body's regulatory mechanisms (e.g. drug-induced hepatic dysfunction resulting in impaired glycogenolysis). Other well-known agents include salicylates (for which the mechanism is not clear but may involve inhibition of hepatic release of glucose and stimulation of insulin secretion), sulfonamides (which may act similarly to sulfonylureas in this context), and pentamidine, which is pancreatoxic.

Post-bariatric surgery hypoglycaemia

In patients who have undergone gastric surgery such as pyloroplasty or bariatric procedures, hypoglycaemia 90–150 minutes after eating is not uncommon. Rapid transit of glucose into the small intestine results in a vigorous insulin release and leads to hypoglycaemia as the circulation. The post-surgical hormonal changes have been postulated to drive beta-cell hyperplasia and even the development of nesidioblastosis or insulinoma.

Counter-regulatory hormonal deficits

Although, in theory, hypoglycaemia may be caused by deficiencies in any hormones that normally maintain euglycaemia, it is seen mainly in the setting of diabetes mellitus. Glucagon deficiency can occur with long-standing diabetes, after pancreatectomy, and with chronic pancreatitis. Bilateral adrenalectomy or removal of a phaeochromocytoma may contribute to hypoglycaemia.

Non-islet cell tumours and insulinoma

Large, indolent, and malignant tumours of mesenchymal origin have been linked with hypoglycaemia. In some cases, this may be due to increased glucose utilization but, in most instances, it is caused by excessive production of IGF-like molecules by the tumour, which thus suppresses glucose production and reduces the level of counter-regulatory hormones. An insulinoma, in contrast, is a tumour which arises from the beta cells of the pancreas and causes hypoglycaemia by the direct action of excess insulin secretion (see also Chapter 13, Section 13.4).

Catabolic states and organ failure

Hypoglycaemia may also occur in patients who are critically unwell with sepsis or following burns or trauma. It may be a feature of cardiac, renal, or hepatic failure.

Box 15.1 Causes of hypoglycaemia in children

Hyperinsulinism/glucose-sensing abnormalities
Persistent hyperinsulinaemic hypoglycaemia of infancy (nesidioblastosis)
  Mutations in SUR1 (encoded by *ABCC8*), Kir6.2 (encoded by *KCNJ11*)
  Activating mutations in *GCK* (which encodes glucokinase)
    Other rare genetic defects (e.g. *GLUD1*)
    Insulin-producing tumour
    Insulin administration

Glucose underproduction or overutilization
Krebs cycle defects
Defects in alternative-fuel production
Glycogen-storage disorders
Galactosaemia
Fructose intolerance
Hyperthyroidism
Sepsis
Deficiency of cortisol or growth hormone

Drugs and toxins
As for adults, especially ethanol, salicylates, propranolol

Reactive hypoglycaemia

Some would regard an excreted glucose fall postprandially as a pathological state, but this remains controversial, and most would not now recognize the term 'reactive hypoglycaemia' as a useful diagnosis.

Clinical features

Hypoglycaemia should form part of the differential diagnosis in patients with unexplained collapse, loss of consciousness, or a 'funny turn'. Symptoms may include adrenergic symptoms such as pallor, sweating, tremor, and tachycardia. They may also include neuroglycopenic symptoms such as poor concentration, irritability, blurred or double vision, confusion, behavioural changes, focal neurological deficits, seizure, and coma (see Box 15.1).

Plasma glucose levels vary over a relatively narrow range (3.0–9.1 mmol/L (55–165 mg/dL)), despite wide fluctuations in supply and consumption. The brain cannot store or produce glucose and is reliant on plasma levels to function, except in prolonged fasting, during which time the brain utilizes ketone bodies. As plasma glucose levels fall, there is a typical progression of physiologic responses and symptoms. As levels fall to approximately 4.0 mmol/L (72 mg/dL), brain glucose uptake falls, insulin secretion is suppressed, and release of counter-regulatory hormones is initiated. This typically restores normoglycaemia. Adrenergic symptoms, which appear at levels of 3.3 mmol/L (60 mg/dL), tend to motivate eating, although recurrent episodes can blunt these symptoms and lead to 'hypoglycaemia unawareness'. With glucose levels <3.0 mmol/L (55 mg/dL), neuroglycopenic signs and symptoms and EEG changes can be seen. Levels <2.2 mmol/L (40 mg/dL) produce somnolence and behavioural abnormalities, and prolonged levels below 1.7 mmol/L (30 mg/dL) lead to coma, seizures, permanent neurologic deficits, and death. Severe hypoglycemia can also trigger arrhythmia, myocardial infarction, and stroke in patients with who have pre-existing cardiovascular disease.

Box 15.2 Risk factors for hypoglycaemia in diabetes mellitus

Conventional risk factors (relative or absolute insulin excess)
Insulin or tablet doses are excessive, badly timed, or incorrect
Missed meals
Exercise
    Alcohol inhibiting glycogenolysis
    Enhanced insulin sensitivity (weight loss)
    Reduced insulin clearance (renal failure)

Risk factors for hypoglycaemia unawareness
Total endogenous insulin deficiency
Previous severe or recurrent hypoglycaemia
Tight glycaemic control targets

Complete recovery of function with correction of glucose is usual but, if the hypoglycaemia is severe or prolonged, persistent neurological deficit may be present. The clinical features are enhanced if cerebral blood flow is impaired, whilst they may be attenuated in patients taking beta-blocking drugs.

Diagnosis and investigation

In evaluating the hypoglycaemic diabetic patient, one should recognize all the factors that may have precipitated the event, including dietary habits, dosage errors, other medications, age, physical activity, and co-morbid conditions (see Box 15.2).

In non-diabetic patients, first confirm the low blood glucose, either at a time of spontaneous occurrence of symptoms or by provocation using a prolonged supervised fast or a mixed meal test. Clues to the cause may be available from the history, including whether the hypoglycaemia occurs in the context of fasting or postprandially ('reactive hypoglycaemia'), together with an evaluation of possible risk factors, including a careful drug history. Evaluation of a number of factors concurrent with the hypoglycaemia can help to further elucidate the cause. This can be divided into hypoglycaemia with appropriately suppressed insulin, and hypoglycaemia with a detectable insulin level (see Table 15.4).

Management

Acute management

If the patient is conscious, correction of hypoglycaemia should be with oral glucose followed by long-acting carbohydrates. This should then prompt a search for the cause of the hypoglycaemia. If the patient is disoriented or confused, but conscious, treat with intravenous 10% glucose at a rate of 100 mL per hour.

If the patient is unconscious, treat with intravenous 20% glucose at a rate of 75–80 mL over 10–15 minutes. Follow with a saline flush to prevent venous irritation. If intravenous access is impossible, 1 mg of glucagon intramuscularly will increase hepatic glucose efflux. The effect is short-lived but the temporary improvement in glucose level may improve the patient's level of consciousness, to enable oral glucose intake. This will not be effective if the hypoglycaemia is due to hepatic dysfunction.

Management of recurrent hypoglycaemia

Hypoglycaemia due to diabetes mellitus requires amendments to diet or drug therapy (as well as evaluation for cortisol deficiency in type 1 diabetes mellitus). Long-term management depends on a detailed evaluation of the cause of the symptoms. Insulinoma is usually managed surgically (see Chapter 13, Section 13.4). Numerous medical therapies that can raise blood glucose, including diazoxide, prednisolone, venlafaxine, and phenytoin, are discussed elsewhere.

Complications and prognosis

Hypoglycaemia is a potentially serious condition. Its symptoms usually resolve rapidly with administration of glucose. If prolonged or severe, it may result in persistent neurological deficit. Patients with recurrent hypoglycaemia may develop blunted adrenergic symptoms which may make early recognition and correction more difficult.

Future developments

Tight glycaemic control in long-term diabetes management is associated with an increase in hypoglycaemia frequency. The increase in numbers of bariatric procedures mandates better understanding and management of post-surgical hypoglycaemia.

Table 15.4. Differential diagnosis of hypoglycaemia

Symptom	Insulin (μU/mL)	C-peptide (nmol/L)[†]	beta-HB (mmol/L)[‡]	OHA	Diagnosis
No	<3	<0.2	>2.7	No	Normal
Yes	≫3	<0.2	≤2.7	No	Exogenous insulin
Yes	≥3	≥0.2	≤2.7	No	Insulinoma
Yes	≥3	≥0.2	≤2.7	Yes	OHA
Yes	≫3	≫0.2	≤2.7	No	Insulin autoimmune
Yes	<3	<0.2	≤2.7	No	IGF
Yes	<3	<0.2	>2.7	No	Not insulin or IGF

Abbreviations: beta-HB, beta-hydroxybutyrate; IGF, insulin-like growth factor; OHA, oral hypoglycaemic agent.

[†] For C-peptide, 0.2 nmol/L is equal to 0.6 ng/L.

[‡] For beta-HB, 2.7 mmol/L is equal to 28.1 mg/L.

Further reading

Cryer PE, Axelrod L, Grossman AB, et al. Evaluation and management of adult hypoglycemic disorders: An Endocrine Society Clinical Practice Guideline. *J Clin Endocrinol Metab* 2009; 94: 709–28.

Dhatariya K, Levy N, Kilvert A, et al. NHS Diabetes guideline for the perioperative management of the adult patient with diabetes. *Diabet Med* 2012; 29: 420–33.

15.2 Obesity

Definition

Obesity is defined as an excess of body fat sufficient to adversely affect health. A BMI (expressed in kilograms per square metre; weight/height $\times$ height) $\geq$30 defines obesity, and a BMI $\geq$25 defines overweight. Lower cut-off values for BMI and waist circumference may be applicable to non-Caucasian ethnic groups (Table 15.5)

BMI imprecisely estimates adiposity, and does not account for fat distribution, which may better determine metabolic and cardiovascular risk at lower BMI values. Central obesity reflects increased visceral (intra-abdominal fat) stores and/or 'ectopic' fat (fat stored in the liver, the muscles, the pancreas, and the epicardium) more directly linked to pathology such as insulin resistance. Waist circumference is a proxy measure of visceral/abdominal fat distribution. BMI and waist circumference criteria are shown in Table 15.5.

Clinical staging, for example using the Edmonton Obesity Staging System, is increasingly being used to define obesity 'severity'.

Pathophysiology and genetics

Obesity results from a positive chronic energy imbalance: an approximate 7000 kcal or 29.3 MJ energy surplus will result in a 1 kg weight gain. Physiological control of energy balance resides in the hypothalamus, which integrates signals from fat stores (e.g. leptin), reward pathways (e.g. nucleus accumbens), the gastrointestinal tract (from the vagal nerve, via the nucleus of tractus solitarius), and gut hormones (e.g. orexigenic ghrelin and satiating glucagon-like peptide 1, peptide YY, and oxyntomodulin). Bile acids and gut microbiota also have important roles.

Obesity is strongly heritable; >300 loci (in particular, the gene *FTO*) are associated with adult and childhood obesity but explain <5% of the variance in BMI values; almost all of the loci impact on energy intake rather than expenditure. Single-gene mutations causing leptin loss of function are rare but are associated with severe early onset obesity and hyperphagia; more common, with a less severe obesity phenotype, are mutations affecting the hypothalamic melanocortin signalling pathway.

Syndromic obesity (Prader–Willi syndrome, Bardet–Biedl syndrome) presents at birth, before the onset of obesity.

The disease consequences of obesity are largely driven by the increased secretion of adipose tissue products, including hormones, cytokines (adipocytokines), and growth factors, resulting in a state of chronic, low-grade, systemic inflammation.

Few organ systems are spared the consequences of obesity (see Box 15.3).

Obesity epidemiology

Between 1980 and 2013, the worldwide prevalence of overweight and obesity increased to 27.5% for adults, and 47% for children. The number of overweight and obese individuals increased from 857 million, in 1980, to 2.1 billion, in 2013: 20%–25% of the adult population in developed countries is now obese. Obesity onset is occurring earlier in life and, in 2012, >40 million children under age 5 were overweight or obese.

Table 15.5 Anthropometric criteria for diagnosis and risk classification of overweight and obesity

	Body mass index (kg·m⁻²)	Obesity class	Disease risk (relative to normal weight and waist circumference)	
Caucasian				
Waist circumference (cm)			Men <102	Men ≥102
			Women <88	Women ≥88
Underweight	<18.5			
Normal	18.5–24.9			
Overweight	25.0–29.9		Increased	High
Obesity	30.0–34.9	I	High	Very high
	35.0–39.9	II	Very high	Very high
Extreme obesity	≥40.0	III	Extremely high	Extremely high
International Diabetes Federation Criteria for South Asian, Chinese				
Waist circumference (cm)			Men <90	Men ≥102
			Women <80	Women ≥88
Underweight	<18.5			
Normal	18.5–22.9			
Overweight	23.0–24.9		Increased	High
Obesity	25.0–29.9	I	High	Very high
	35.0–39.9	II	Very high	Very high
Extreme obesity	≥30	III	Extremely high	Extremely high

Reproduced from Clinical Guidelines on the Identification, Evaluation, and Treatment of Overweight and Obesity in Adults—The Evidence Report. National Institutes of Health, *Obesity Research*, 1998, Volume 6, pp. 51s–209s. Copyright (2012) with permission from John Wiley and Sons. Data from Alberti KGMM, Zimmet P and Shaw, International Diabetes Federation: a consensus on Type 2 diabetes prevention, *Diabetic Medicine*, 2007, Volume 24, pp. 451–463.

Box 15.3 Clinical consequences and associations with obesity

Pulmonary
Hypoventilation
Obstructive sleep apnoea
Asthma

Musculoskeletal
Osteoarthritis
Gout

Gastrointestinal
Gallstones
Non-alcoholic fatty liver
Colon cancer
Reflux oesophagitis
Oesophageal cancer
Periodontal disease

Gynaecological/obstetric
Oligomenorrhoea
Infertility
Cancer of uterus, breast, cervix
Pregnancy morbidity

Dermatological
Hirsutism
Sweating
Psoriasis

Metabolic
Diabetes
Dyslipidaemia
Hyperinsulinaemia

Andrology related
Hypogonadism
Prostate cancer

CNS related
Intracranial hypertension
Stroke
Dementia
Migraine severity

Psychological
Depression

Cardiovascular
Hypertension
Ischaemic heart disease
Heart failure
Thromboembolism

Obesity development in an individual is gradual (over many years); sudden 'explosive' onset suggests other pathology (e.g. drug-induced obesity (via steroids, antipsychotic drugs, or anti-epileptic drugs), hypothalamic disease, or tumour).

Clinical features

Symptoms relate to mechanical effects (e.g. exertional dyspnoea, joint pain, sweating, gastro-oesophageal reflux, lymphoedema, impaired activities of daily living), associated endocrine changes (e.g. oligomenorrhoea, subfertility, hypogonadism), or associated complications (e.g. obstructive sleep apnoea, type 2 diabetes, cardiovascular disease). Low mood, depression, and psychosocial distress are common, as is a history of childhood trauma or sexual abuse, especially in those with associated disordered eating (e.g. binge-eating

disorder). Clinical assessment of the abdomen, heart, and lungs is often impaired in severe obesity. A large cuff is needed to assess blood pressure. Acanthosis nigricans is common and suggests hyperinsulinaemia/insulin resistance; intertrigo and hidradenitis are also common.

Investigations

Exclusion of secondary obesity
- Children with severe obesity before age 5, or with apparent syndromic obesity (e.g. associated with learning disability, dysmorphism, retinal pigmentation), should be offered genetic screening.
- Tests to exclude hypothyroidism or Cushing's syndrome (rare causes of obesity) should be performed.

Assessment of cardiometabolic consequences
The following cardiometabolic assessments should be performed:
- fasting glucose and haemoglobin A1c: to detect diabetes or prediabetes
- liver function: to detect non-alcoholic liver disease or non-alcoholic steatohepatitis
- haemoglobin: to detect iron deficiency, anaemia due to menorrhagia (women), gastro-oesophageal reflux disease, or colon cancer
- testosterone and SHBG: to assess gonadal status

Assessment of nutritional status
Levels of the following nutrients should be measured, to assess the nutritional status of the patient:
- vitamin D (up to 80% of patients presenting for bariatric surgery have a severe vitamin D deficiency)
- folate, iron, and vitamin B_{12} (often the patient's diet provides inadequate levels of these nutrients)

Imaging (where indicated by symptoms or signs)
The following imaging investigations should be performed:
- electrocardiogram, echocardiogram: to detect ischaemic heart disease, and heart failure
- liver ultrasound: to detect non-alcoholic liver disease or non-alcoholic steatohepatitis
- overnight oximetry, sleep studies: to detect sleep apnoea
- MRI brain (if a hypothalamic cause is suspected): to exclude intracranial hypertension

Management

Advice on lifestyle modification
- Advice on lifestyle modification is appropriate for all degrees of obesity. Low-fat, high-protein, low-energy-dense and low-glycaemic diets (typically, a Mediterranean diet) are preferred.
- Recommend energy restriction: assess or estimate energy intake/needs and advise a 500 kcal/day/2.1 MJ reduction. This will predict an initial 0.5 kg/week weight loss.
- Recommend increased activity:
- 45–60 minutes daily of moderate activity is recommended for people who want to avoid gaining any more weight
- 60–90 minutes daily of moderate activity is recommended for people who want to actively lose weight or maintain loss
- Behavioural therapy components address self-monitoring, stimulus control, goal setting, reward contracting, and social support. A cognitive component may be indicated, especially if an eating disorder or prominent psychosocial issues are present.

Table 15.6 Summary of drugs available or submitted for registration for the treatment of overweight and obesity

Drug	Max daily dose (mg)	Placebo-subtracted weight loss	Per cent with >5% loss (vs placebo)	Mode of action	Frequent side effects	Uncommon side effects
Orlistat[a,b]	360	−2.9 kg	—	Lipase inhibitor causing 30% malabsorption of ingested triglycerides	Steatorrhea	Faecal incontinence
Lorcaserin[b]	20	−3.2 kg	45 (20)	Highly selective serotonergic 5-HT2C receptor agonist Causes appetite suppression	Dry mouth Fatigue Dizziness Headache.	Nausea Urinary tract infection Constipation/diarrhoea Hypoglycaemia (in patients with type 2 diabetes)
Phentermine/topiramate extended release[b]	15/92	9.4%	67 (17)	Noradrenergic + GABA-receptor activator Kainite/AMPA glutamate receptor inhibitor Causes appetite suppression	Paraesthesia Dry mouth Constipation Headache Dysgeusia Insomnia Dizziness	Palpitations Disturbances in attention Alopecia Diarrhoea Anxiety Irritability Depression Fatigue Blurred vision Glaucoma
Liraglutide[a,b]	3.0	5.4%	64 (27)	GLP-1 agonist Produces satiety and incretin-mediated insulin release	Nausea Vomiting Constipation Diarrhoea	Gallstones
Naltrexone/bupropion extended release[a,b]	32/360	−5.1	17 (51)	Stimulates hypothalamic POMC neurons Blocks opioid-receptor-mediated POMC auto-inhibition Inhibits DA and NA reuptake	Nausea Constipation Headache Restlessness Abdominal pain Joint pain Dizziness	—

Abbreviations: DA, dopaminergic; GABA, gamma-aminobutyric acid; GLP-1, glucagon-like peptide 1; NA, noradrenergic; POMC, pro-opiomelanocortin.

[a] Approved in Europe.

[b] Approved in the USA.

Pharmacotherapy

- Several options for pharmacotherapy are available; these approximately double weight loss over lifestyle treatment alone, and increase the number of patients achieving 5%, 10%, and 15% losses by two- to three-fold (see Table 15.6).
- Drug-induced weight loss may diminish cardiometabolic risk factors but long-term outcomes have not been established.

- Pharmacotherapy will need to be maintained in the long term; withdrawal of the drug will result in weight regain.

Bariatric surgery

Traditionally, bariatric surgery was classified as restrictive (e.g. adjustable gastric band; sleeve gastrectomy) or malabsorptive (e.g. biliopancreatic diversion; Roux-en-Y gastric bypass; see Figure 15.1), but current evidence

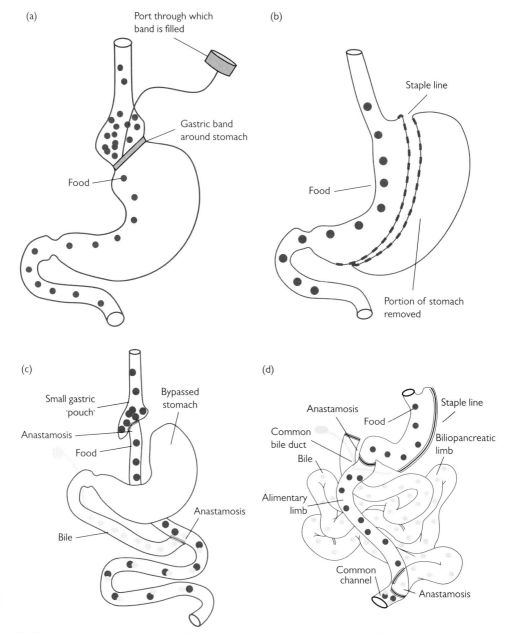

Fig 15.1 Four main types of bariatric surgery: (a) adjustable gastric band, (b) sleeve gastrectomy, (c) Roux-en-Y gastric bypass, and (d) biliopancreatic diversion with duodenal switch.

points to effects on satiety induced by changes in gut-hormone responses to ingested food, bile acid metabolism, and gut flora. Guidelines suggest surgery be offered to patients with a BMI >30 kg/m² with type 2 diabetes, >35 kg/m² with an obesity-related co-morbidity, or >40 kg/m². Weight loss after the adjustable gastric band, Roux-en-Y gastric bypass, and biliopancreatic diversion surgical procedures averages 15%, 30%, and 50%, respectively. About 40%–60% of patients with type 2 diabetes of <5 years duration are able to achieve normoglycaemia without medication. Weight loss associated with bariatric surgery reduces all-cause mortality, cancer mortality, and cardiovascular mortality. Unwanted effects include excessive weight loss, loose skin, nutritional deficiencies, 'reactive' hypoglycaemia, renal stones, and depression and increased suicide.

Future developments

- Preventative strategies are needed but require social/political interventions to encourage healthy lifestyles. These may include taxation on sugar and/or fat, and restrictions of 'unhealthy food' availability, especially in the workplace or schools.
- Endoscopic devices to mimic surgical intervention are being developed.
- Pharmacotherapy research is currently looking for new central brain and peripheral targets and combinations.

Patient support groups/useful websites

- World Obesity Federation: http://www.worldobesity.org/
- Weight Concern: http://www.weightconcern.org.uk
- WLSinfo (Weight Loss Surgery Information and Support): http://www.wlsinfo.org.uk
- The Obesity Society (North America): http://www.obesity.org/resources-for/consumer.htm

Further reading

Centre for Public Health Excellence at NICE and National Collaborating Centre for Primary Care (UK). Obesity: The prevention, identification, assessment and management of overweight and obesity in adults and children. Available at http://www.ncbi.nlm.nih.gov/books/NBK63696/ (accessed 15 Jan 2018).

Kuk JL, Ardern CI, Church TS, et al. Edmonton Obesity Staging System: Association with weight history and mortality risk. Appl Physiol Nutr Metab 2011; 36: 570–6.

le Roux CW, Astrup A, Fujioka K, et al. 3 years of liraglutide versus placebo for type 2 diabetes risk reduction and weight management in individuals with prediabetes: A randomised, double-blind trial. Lancet 2017;389: 1399–409.

Li JV, Ashrafian H, Bueter M, et al. (2011). Metabolic surgery profoundly influences gut microbial-host metabolic cross-talk. Gut 2011; 60: 1–11.

Manning S, Pucci A, and Finer N. Pharmacotherapy for obesity: Novel agents and paradigms. Ther Adv Chronic Dis 2014; 5: 135–48.

National Institute for Health and Care Excellence. Obesity: Identification, assessment and management. Available at http://www.nice.org.uk/guidance/cg189 (accessed 15 Jan 2018).

National Institute for Health and Care Excellence. Preventing excess weight gain. Available at http://www.nice.org.uk/guidance/ng7 (accessed 15 Jan 2018).

Ng M, Fleming T, Robinson M, et al. Global, regional, and national prevalence of overweight and obesity in children and adults during 1980–2013: A systematic analysis for the Global Burden of Disease Study 2013. Lancet 2014; 384: 766–81.

Peng S, Zhu Y, Xu F, et al. FTO gene polymorphisms and obesity risk: A meta-analysis. BMC Med 9: 71.

Pournaras DJ, Aasheim ET, Søvik TT, et al. Effect of the definition of type II diabetes remission in the evaluation of bariatric surgery for metabolic disorders. Br J Surg 2012; 99: 100–3.

Smith R, Batterham R, and Finer N. (2013). Prevalence of vitamin D insufficiency in severely obese patients seeking bariatric surgery. Endo Abst 2013; 31:216.

WHO. Obesity and overweight, 2017. Available at http://www.who.int/mediacentre/factsheets/fs311/en/ (accessed 15 Jan 2018).

WHO/IASO/IOTF. The Asia-Pacific Perspective: Redefining Obesity and Its Treatment, 2000. Health Communications Australia Pty.

Wing RR. 'Behavioural approaches to the treatment of obesity', in Bray GA and Bouchard C, eds, Handbook of Obesity, Clinical Applications, 2004. Marcel Dekker, pp. 147–62.

Yanovski SZ and Yanovski JA. Long-term drug treatment for obesity: A systematic and clinical review. JAMA 2014; 311: 74–86.

15.3 Eating disorders and starvation

Introduction

Anorexia nervosa is a psychiatric disorder characterized by distorted body image, pathological fear of becoming fat, and severe restriction of food intake despite low weight. Anorexia nervosa predominantly affects females (the focus of this section), although males can also develop this disorder. The lifetime prevalence of anorexia nervosa in women is up to 4%, more than ten times the rate in men, with the highest prevalence in the teenage years. Anorexia nervosa is associated with significant medical complications and the highest mortality of any psychiatric disease. Endocrine abnormalities include hypothalamic-pituitary dysfunction, dysregulation of hormones involved in appetite, and profound bone loss (see Box 15.4). Whilst some hormonal alterations are due to chronic starvation, others persist after weight recovery, suggesting that they may be involved in disease pathogenesis.

Hypothalamo-pituitary dysfunction: Anterior pituitary

Reproductive hormones

Females with anorexia nervosa may develop pre-pubertal patterns of GnRH secretion, leading to hypogonadotrophic hypogonadism and infertility. Oestrogen deficiency and low testosterone levels contribute to bone loss. With weight recovery, reproductive function generally returns to normal.

Adrenal axis

Increased hypothalamo-pituitary–adrenal activation may lead to hypercortisolemia in anorexia nervosa. Although this is likely related to the stress of chronic starvation, subtle abnormalities in hypothalamo-pituitary–adrenal signalling may remain after weight restoration, suggesting that cortisol dysregulation could play a role in the pathogenesis of anorexia nervosa. Hypothalamo-pituitary–adrenal abnormalities have been linked to symptoms of anxiety and depression, as well as severity of bone loss in anorexia nervosa.

Growth hormone

Growth-hormone secretion is increased and levels of the downstream hormone IGF-1 are low in anorexia nervosa, consistent with growth-hormone resistance, which is likely due to chronic starvation. IGF-1 is anabolic to bone, and decreased systemic levels likely contribute to the bone loss induced by anorexia nervosa. IGF-1 improves bone mineral density in adult women with anorexia nervosa and concomitantly receiving oestrogen replacement. However, IGF-1 is not FDA-approved for this indication, and additional research is needed to confirm the efficacy and safety of IGF-1 treatment in anorexia nervosa.

Thyroid

Chronic undernutrition in anorexia nervosa results in a 'sick-euthyroid' pattern of TFTs. Typically, T3 levels are low, and rT3 levels are high. TSH and T4 levels may be normal or low. Alterations in the thyroid axis in anorexia nervosa likely represent a mechanism to reduce the metabolic rate and conserve energy in the setting of chronic starvation. Thyroid function normalizes with weight recovery. Given the risk of cardiac arrhythmias and increased mortality in anorexia nervosa, TFT abnormalities in these patients are not treated with thyroid hormone replacement in the absence of overt hypothyroidism.

Hypothalamo-pituitary dysfunction: Posterior pituitary

There is evidence of abnormal release of posterior pituitary hormones vasopressin and oxytocin in anorexia nervosa. Vasopressin release can be erratic, and serum sodium levels high, normal, or low in anorexia nervosa. Clinically, these patients are at risk for hyponatraemia, which can be compounded by excessive water intake and commonly prescribed psychotrophic medications. Regulation of vasopressin normalizes with weight recovery. Secretion of oxytocin, a peptide that has been implicated in regulation of appetite, is also dysregulated in anorexia nervosa. The clinical significance of this is not yet clear.

Appetite-regulating peptides

Levels of leptin, a fat-derived anorexigenic hormone, are low in anorexia nervosa, signalling a chronic energy deficit. Leptin levels normalize after weight recovery. Levels of ghrelin, an orexigenic hormone secreted by the stomach in response to food intake, are high in anorexia nervosa, as expected in the undernourished state. Secretion of peptide YY, a gut hormone that signals satiety, is also increased in anorexia nervosa, and does not appear to normalize with weight restoration. This raises the question of whether abnormal peptide YY dynamics could contribute to the development and maintenance of anorexia nervosa.

Osteopenia

Background

Anorexia nervosa is associated with profound bone loss. It has been reported that more than 90% of women with anorexia nervosa have osteopenia, and nearly 40% meet WHO criteria for osteoporosis. There is a two- to seven-fold increase in the risk of fractures. In adults with anorexia nervosa, markers of bone turnover are uncoupled, with low markers of formation and high markers of

---

Box 15.4 Endocrine abnormalities in anorexia nervosa

Hypothalamo-pituitary dysfunction

Anterior
  Low gonadotrophins, estradiol, and testosterone
  High cortisol
  High growth hormone, low IGF-1
  Low T3, high rT3, and high T4:T3 ratio

Posterior
  High or low vasopressin
  Low oxytocin
  Low leptin, high ghrelin, high peptide YY
  Bone loss

Abbreviations: rT3, reverse triiodothyronine; T3, triiodothyronine; T4, thyroxine.

resorption. During adolescence, a time when bone turnover is typically high, girls with anorexia nervosa have reduced bone formation and resorption markers.

Pathogenesis
The severity of bone loss associated with anorexia nervosa is greater than that seen in normal-weight hypothalamic amenorrhea, indicating that factors in addition to oestrogen deficiency play a role. These include nutritional deficiencies and endocrine dysfunction, including low levels of IGF-1 and testosterone and hypercortisolemia. Abnormalities in secretion of appetite-regulating hormones, including leptin, peptide YY, and oxytocin, may also contribute, although the evidence is less clear.

*Management of bone loss in
anorexia nervosa*
Approaches for the management of bone loss in anorexia nervosa are shown in Box 15.5. A DXA test is indicated at baseline to evaluate for bone loss in females with anorexia nervosa. In those with persistent low weight, bone mineral density should be followed over time. Patients should be encouraged to gain weight and recover menstrual cycles, as both have been shown to improve bone mineral density. Lifestyle modifications, such as appropriate calcium and vitamin D intake and avoidance of smoking and excessive alcohol intake, should be addressed. Exercise programmes must be individualized, as weight-bearing exercise may be beneficial to bone, whereas excessive exercise may promote weight loss, amenorrhea, and fracture risk. In adolescents with anorexia nervosa, transdermal estradiol with cyclic oral progestin may be considered. Bisphosphonates or teriparatide may also be considered

---

Box 15.5 Management of bone loss in anorexia nervosa

Serial dual-energy X-ray absorptiometry testing
Encourage weight gain, restoration of menstrual cycles
Lifestyle modifications
   Adequate calcium/vitamin D intake
   Avoid smoking, excessive alcohol
   Avoid excessive exercise
Consider transdermal estradiol with cyclic oral progestin in adolescents
Consider bisphosphonate or teriparatide on an individual basis (e.g., postmenopause)

---

on an individual basis (e.g. in a postmenopausal woman with anorexia nervosa).

Further reading

American Psychiatric Association. *Diagnostic and statistical manual of mental disorders* (5th edition), 2013. Arlington, VA: American Psychiatric Publishing.

Baskaran C, Misra M, and Klibanski A. Effects of anorexia nervosa on the endocrine system. *Pediatr Endocrinol Rev* 2017; 14(3): 302–11.

Lawson EA and Miller KK. 'Anorexia nervosa: Endocrine complications and their management', in Martin KA, ed, *UpToDate*, 2017. https://www.uptodate.com/contents/anorexia-nervosa-endocrine-complications-and-their-management (accessed 28 Feb 2018).

Schorr M and Miller KK (2017). The endocrine manifestations of anorexia nervosa: mechanisms and management. *Nat Rev Endocrinol* 2017; 13(3): 174–86.

15.4 Sports and endocrinology

Introduction

Since ancient times, unethical athletes have attempted to gain an unfair competitive advantage through the use of doping substances. Hormones are among the most widely abused agents in sports by virtue of their properties as chemical messengers that are carried in the blood and modulate the function of tissues and organs elsewhere in the body. The field of endocrinology has been at the forefront of abuse in sports in the last half-century, a phenomenon brought about by advances in steroid and peptide chemistry. In the last decades, recombinant DNA technology has revolutionized peptide synthesis, so that synthetic peptides are now available in unprecedented quantities.

The pressure to perform in sport is immense. In a frequently cited survey conducted in 1997 by Bamberger in *Sports Illustrated*, over 50% of elite athletes said they would take a performance-enhancing substance that would guarantee they won every competition for the next 5 years and would not get caught, even if they would die from its adverse effects.

Doping

Performance-enhancing substances are widely used to gain a competitive advantage by optimizing body composition, increasing strength, power, and endurance, and accelerating recovery from injury; the use of such substances is called 'doping'. Some of the beneficial effects of doping are believed to be due to central mechanisms that enhance mental effort, whilst others are thought to be due to reducing anti-inflammatory responses and thus improving tolerance to pain. In some cases, these beliefs are well founded; for others, the scientific evidence is scant. This section will focus on three major types of doping: androgenic anabolic steroids, growth hormone, and blood doping.

Androgenic anabolic steroids

Of all the performance-enhancing substances, androgenic anabolic steroids are the most widely abused. Systematic doping at a national level was uncovered in the former German Democratic Republic after the fall of the Communist government in 1990. The use of androgenic anabolic steroids, previously exclusive to strength-intensive sports, spread gradually to other sports. Androgenic anabolic steroids are used in two regimens: cycling and stacking. Cycling refers to intermittent but regular use in an on–off regimen, whereas stacking involves use in escalating doses over weeks. Testosterone stimulates skeletal muscle mass, strength, and power in a dose-dependent manner, the upper limit for which has not yet been defined [1]. Because of these effects on strength and power, abuse of androgenic anabolic steroids is seen among weightlifters and among athletes involved in power sports, such as sprinting. Androgenic anabolic steroids induce a range of adverse effects, including high haematocrit levels, hepatotoxicity, myocardial dysfunction, and aggressive behaviour.

Growth hormone

The increasing popularity of growth hormone among athletes stems from its anabolic and lipolytic properties and the difficulty of its detection. There appears to be no evidence that growth hormone enhances muscle strength, power, or aerobic capacity in trained adult athletes [2]. However, growth hormone does increase anaerobic exercise capacity when administered alone, and to a greater extent when combined with testosterone. Thus, growth hormone appears to benefit sporting events that are powered by the anaerobic energy system, such as sprinting and those requiring intermittent bursts of intensive physical activity. Nonetheless, despite the wide abuse of growth hormone by athletes, there is little support of performance benefit except for a selective effect on anaerobic exercise capacity.

Blood doping

Blood doping is the misuse of certain techniques to increase red blood cell mass or introduce synthetic oxygen carriers, to allow the body to transport more oxygen to muscles and therefore increase endurance-based performance (the VO2 max is increased by 5%–10% when haemoglobin is raised by 10%) [3]. There are three methods for blood doping: using erythropoietin, using synthetic oxygen carriers, and using blood transfusions. Erythropoietin stimulates the production of red blood cells. Synthetic oxygen carriers, such as haemoglobin-based oxygen carriers or perfluorocarbons, are purified proteins or chemicals that have the ability to carry oxygen. There are two types of transfusions: (i) autologous, which is transfusion of one's own blood after a period of storage, and (ii) homologous, which is transfusion of blood from a group-compatible donor.

Doping control

One of the most significant achievements in the fight against doping in sport to date has been the drafting, acceptance, and implementation of a harmonized set of anti-doping rules, the World Anti-Doping Code.

A list of doping substances and methods banned in sports is published yearly by the World Anti-Doping Agency (WADA). A substance or method is included in the list if it fulfils at least two of the following criteria: it enhances sports performance, it represents a risk to the athlete's health, or it violates the spirit of sports. The major categories of prohibited substances for 2016 are summarized in Table 15.7. The list is constantly updated to reflect new developments in the pharmaceutical

Table 15.7 Categories of substances prohibited by the World Anti-Doping Agency

S1	Anabolic agents
S2	Peptide hormones, growth factors and related substances
S3	Beta-2 adrenoceptor agonists
S4	Hormone and metabolic modulators
S5	Diuretics and other masking agents
S6	Stimulants
S7	Narcotics
S8	Cannabinoids
S9	Glucocorticosteroids

Data from World Anti-Doping Code, Prohibited List, January 2017, published September 29, 2016. https://www.wada-ama.org/en/resources/science-medicine/prohibited-list-documents.

Table 15.8 Adverse analytical findings and atypical findings reported in 2015 by accredited laboratories in the Anti-Doping Administration and Management System

Substance group	Occurrences (out of 4500 total)	% of all ADAMS reported findings
S1 Anabolic agents	2279	50.60
S6 Stimulants	679	15.50
S8 Cannabinoids	406	9.00
S9 Glucocorticosteroids	365	8.10
S5 Diuretics and other masking agents	322	7.20
S2 Peptide hormones, growth factors and related substances	181	4.00
S3 Beta-2 adrenoceptor agonists	131	2.90
S4 Hormone metabolic modulators	74	1.60
S7 Narcotics	26	0.60
P2 Beta blockers	13	0.30
P1 Alcohol	5	0.10
M1 Enhancement of oxygen transfer	0	0.00
M2 Chemical and physical Manipulation	1	0.02

Abbreviations: ADAMS, Anti-Doping Administration and Management System.

2015 Anti-Doping Testing Figures, World Anti-Doping Agency, pp. 1–274. https://www.wada-ama.org/en/anti-doping-statistics.

industry as well as doping trends and enumerates the drug types and methods prohibited in and out of competition (see http://www.wada-ama.org/en/resources/science-medicine/prohibited-list-documents).

WADA has exercised an effective governance system for the control of doping through a system of in-competition and out-of-competition testing. In tests conducted in 2015, androgenic anabolic steroids were the most frequently identified performance-enhancing substances, being present in over 50% of all positive tests (Table 15.8; also see http://www.wada-ama.org/en/anti-doping-statistics).

Therapeutic use exemptions

Athletes, like all others, may have illnesses or conditions that require them to take particular medications. If the medication required to treat an endocrine deficiency happens to fall under the prohibited list, a therapeutic use exemption may give that athlete the authorization to use it. The criteria for issuing therapeutic use exemptions are shown in Box 15.6. Under the World Anti-Doping Code, WADA has issued an international standard for therapeutic use exemptions. The standard states that all international federations and national anti-doping organizations must have a process in place whereby athletes with documented medical conditions can request a therapeutic use exemption, and have such a request appropriately dealt with by a therapeutic use exemption committee consisting of a panel of independent physicians (see Box 15.6 and http://

Box 15.6 Criteria for a therapeutic use exemption

The following criteria should be used to determine whether a therapeutic use exemption should be provided:
1. The athlete would experience significant health problems without taking the prohibited substance or method.
2. The therapeutic use of the substance would not produce significant enhancement of performance.
3. There is no reasonable therapeutic alternative to the use of the otherwise prohibited substance or method.
4. The necessity for use cannot be a consequence of prior non-therapeutic use of the prohibited substance.

Data from *Therapeutic Use Exemptions Guidelines*, version 8, 2016, World Anti-Doping Agency.

---

www.wada-ama.org/en/resources/science-medicine/guidelines-therapeutic-use-exemptions-tue).

Methods for the detection of doping

Methods for detecting androgenic anabolic steroids

Androgenic anabolic steroids include testosterone and a large and ever increasing number of synthetic androgens. The methods for the detection of these vary.

Methods for detecting testosterone

The detection of exogenous testosterone abuse is based on the quantification of the concentration of testosterone to its metabolite epimer, epitestosterone in urine. The population mode of testosterone-to-epitestosterone ratios is about 1:1; ratios above 4:1 are indicative of testosterone doping. Often, hCG or LH is used to stimulate endogenous testosterone production, as a way of avoiding exogenous testosterone administration, but the principle underlying the testosterone-to-epitestosterone test applies equally well to the detection of stimulated endogenous testosterone production. However, genetic variations in the function of the UGT2B17 enzyme, which converts testosterone to epitestosterone, can confound the accuracy and interpretation of this doping test. Establishing different cut-offs from genotyping of this enzyme will improve the accuracy of detecting testosterone abuse.

The advent of the carbon isotope ratio test was a major advance for detecting testosterone abuse, even in those who pass the testosterone-to-epitestosterone ratio test. This test is able to differentiate between natural and synthetic testosterone by examining the carbon make-up of testosterone in the urine, as follows. Humans make testosterone from dietary sources which have a higher content of a naturally occurring carbon isotope, C^{13}, than the reagents used to make synthetic testosterone; thus, natural testosterone contains more C^{13} than synthetic testosterone does. Thus, the test is able to detect the use of synthetic testosterone by determining the ratio of C^{13} to C^{12} in testosterone from the urine sample.

Methods for detecting other androgenic anabolic steroids

The method used for the detection of synthetic anabolic steroids is based on differences in molecular weights between native and synthetic androgens. This is achieved by the high-precision, sensitive technique of mass spectrometry. The method usually involves liquid chromatography, which separates the molecules of interest before the masses are measured. In this way, synthetic androgens as varied as methytestosterone, stanozolol, nandrolone, mesterelone, and tetrahydrogestrinone can be detected with accuracy.

Methods for detecting growth hormone

Two methods have been developed for detecting growth hormone abuse. The first is based on the measurement of different pituitary isoforms of growth hormone in serum by using specific immunoassays [4]. Growth hormone is produced and secreted not as a single peptide but as a family of isoforms formed from alternate splicing and post-translational modification. The 22 kDa form of growth hormone predominates in the circulation. The administration of recombinant 22 kDa growth hormone inhibits the production of the other isoforms; thus, the ratio of these forms to the 22 kDa form changes. A method involving the detection of such changes was implemented by WADA during the Athens Olympics in 2004. Because growth hormone is usually taken by doping athletes in the off season, this test is expected to be more effective when implemented in a no-advance-notice, out-of-competition setting. The second approach is based on the measurement of growth hormone-responsive markers in blood, such as components of the IGF axis and collagen turnover (procollagen 3) [5]. At the 2012 London Olympics, WADA introduced a test involving the simultaneous measurement of IGF-1 and procollagen 3; during the Paralympic events, two tests were positive.

Methods for detecting blood doping

Measurement of the haematocrit level is widely employed as a screening test for blood doping. A haematocrit level of 49% in men and 45% in women is the threshold for suspicion of blood doping. In June 2003, the WADA endorsed a urine test as a scientifically valid method for detecting erythropoietin doping. The test is based on the differences between the electrophoretic mobility of recombinant erythropoietin and that of endogenous human erythropoietin, reflecting differences in the glycosylation patterns and isoelectric points of the two proteins [3].

In 2004, WADA introduced a test for homologous transfusion during the Athens Olympics. This test is based on fluorescence-activated cell sorting, using antisera that detect minor differences in blood group antigens. The technique can detect small populations (<5% of the total population) of cells that are antigenically distinct from an individual's own red blood cells. A test for autologous transfusion is not yet available.

The Athlete Biological Passport

Recently, WADA implemented an alternative anti-doping approach: the Athlete Biological Passport (ABP). The fundamental idea behind the ABP is that, rather than directly detect the doping substance itself, it would be better to monitor selected biological parameters over time, as changes in these would, indirectly, reveal the effects of doping. The guidelines for the ABP were approved by WADA's Executive Committee and first took effect on 1 December 2009. The ABP statistical software system is based on personalized monitoring of biomarkers indicative of doping, and is hence not a direct test programme for a given substance. The approach can be used for a variety of doping practices. The effectiveness of the ABP is under active evaluation.

Future challenges

The field is also facing the spectre of the use of genomic technology in sports, that is, gene doping—the technique of modifying or enhancing organ function by gene transfer. WADA has appointed an expert group to address this issue and held workshops on the topic since 2002, with the most recent one held in 2013.

Effective deterrence of sports doping requires novel, increasingly sophisticated detection options calibrated to defeat these challenges, without which fairness in sport is tarnished and the social and health idealization of sporting champions devalued.

References and further reading

1. Basaria S. Androgen abuse in athletes: Detection and consequences. *J Clin Endocrinol Metab* 2010; 95: 1533–43.
2. Birzniece V, Nelson AE, and Ho KK. Growth hormone and physical performance. *Trends Endocrinol Metab* 2011; 22: 171–8.
3. Lundby C, Robach P, and Saltin B. The evolving science of detection of 'blood doping'. *Br J Pharmacol* 2012; 165: 1306–15.
4. Bidlingmaier M and Strasburger CJ. Detecting growth hormone abuse in athletes. *Nat Clin Pract Endocrinol Metab* 2007; 3: 769–777.
5. Powrie JK, Bassett EE, Rosen T, et al. Detection of growth hormone abuse in sport. *Growth Horm IGF Res* 2007; 17: 220–6.

15.5 Possible endocrine syndromes

Excessive flushing

Introduction

Clinically significant flushing, in need of further characterization, would consist of episodes of heat and redness affecting mostly the face, the neck, the upper chest, and, occasionally, the abdomen. Flushing can be constant, transient, or episodic, depending on the aetiology. Although the list of differential diagnoses can be broad (Table 15.9), there are distinct diagnostic features that can be utilized in reaching the correct diagnosis. The key in deciphering the aetiology of these symptoms is careful history taking, in the first instance. Further endocrine characterization is outlined below.

Indicative features of an endocrine cause on history and examination

Intermittent episodes of flushing (or more commonly pallor), headaches, and sweating, as well as possible abdominal pain and hypertension (usually requiring more than three agents to treat), give clues to the possible diagnosis of phaeochromocytoma (see Chapter 5, Section 5.10). A family history of this condition should stimulate further investigation.

Table 15.9 Differential diagnosis and treatment of clinically significant 'flushing syndrome'

Diagnosis	Clues to diagnosis	Possible investigations	Treatments to consider
Endocrine causes			
Neuroendocrine tumours	Episodic diarrhoea	24-Hour urine collection for 5-HIAA	Surgical resection if possible
	Sweating generally not a feature	Liver CT/MRI	Somatostatin analogue therapy
Hypogonadism	Loss of secondary sexual characteristics	09:00 h testosterone/estradiol	Hormone replacement therapy
	Reduced libido	LH	
	Amenorrhoea (women)	FSH	
	Erectile Dysfunction (men)	Prolactin	
	'Youthful' appearance		
Medullary thyroid cancer	Thyroid mass	Calcitonin levels	Surgical resection: total thyroidectomy
	Flushing	Thyroid ultrasound ± biopsy	
	Diarrhoea		
Phaeochromocytoma/ paraganglioma	Hypertension	Plasma and 24-hour urinary metanephrines and catecholamines	Symptom control with alpha blockade
	Sweating		Surgical resection
	Headaches	CT/MRI of the adrenals and the abdomen	
	Pallor (much more common than flushing)		
Pancreatic cancer: VIPoma	Facial flushing, watery diarrhoea, and abdominal cramping may be present	Plasma VIP levels	Somatostatin analogue therapy
		Abdominal imaging: CT	Correction of electrolyte imbalance
			Surgical resection, if possible
			Systemic chemotherapy
Cushing's syndrome	Hypertension	24-Hour urinary free cortisol	Surgical removal of lesion
	Cushingoid body habitus	Overnight (1 mg) dexamethasone suppression test	Medications aimed at lowering endogenous steroid levels, such as metyrapone and fluconazole
	Proximal muscle weakness	Midnight cortisol measurement	
	Skin atrophy		
	Easy bruising		
	Striae: large, purple/dark		
	Supraclavicular fat pad		
	Dorsocervical fat pad		
Common non-endocrine causes			
Systemic mastocytosis	Generally, hypotensive during episodes	Serum tryptase levels	H2 and H1 blockade
	Major and minor criteria described by WHO†	Skin biopsy	
		Bone marrow biopsy	

(continued)

Table 15.9 Continued

Diagnosis	Clues to diagnosis	Possible investigations	Treatments to consider
Panic attack	Situational symptoms	None may be needed	Supportive therapy
		If the history is not clear, may require investigations to out rule other diagnoses	
Neurological/ autonomic dysfunction	Many neurological syndromes can lead to autonomic dysfunction	Investigations should be guided by history but may include brain imaging and autonomic function testing	Treatment is aimed at the underlying cause
	Gustatory sweating		
	Headache		
	Parkinsonian features		
	Hemifacial sweating may indicate cluster headaches		
Drugs	Many, including nicotinic acid, LHRH-agonist therapy, and anti-oestrogen therapy	Discontinuation of possible offending agents	Discontinuation of offending agent, if possible
Alcohol use	Temporal relation of alcohol use with flushing episodes	Alcohol dehydrogenase levels	Alcohol avoidance
Benign cutaneous flushing	Temporal relation to exercise, food intake, and emotion	—	Often, none required
			Non-selective beta blockade
Rarer non-endocrine causes			
Panayiotopolous syndrome	Rare childhood seizure disorder with hypertension, tachycardia, and flushing preceding seizures	—	—
Eosinophilic gastrointestinal disorders	Depends on the layers of mucosa involved	Stool culture	Empiric (based on symptoms)
		Serum IgE levels	
	Can present with abdominal pain, vomiting, diarrhoea, weight loss, and fatigue		
Idiopathic	—	—	—

Abbreviations: 5-HIAA, 5-hydroxyindoleacetic acid; CT, computed tomography; FSH, follicle-stimulating hormone; MRI, magnetic resonance imaging; LH, luteinizing hormone; LHRH, luteinizing hormone releasing hormone; VIP, vasoactive intestinal polypeptide.

† Major criteria are as follows: multifocal flushing, and 15 or more aggregates of mast cells on bone marrow biopsy, confirmed with tryptase staining. Minor criteria are as follows: serum tryptase levels persistently >20 ng/mL; in a biopsy section, more than 25% of mast cells in infiltrates have an abnormal morphology or of all the mast cells in the aspirate are immature or atypical; co-expression of CD117 with CD2 and/or CD25; and detection of a *KIT* point mutation at Codon 816 in bone marrow, blood, or other extracutaneous tissues. Three minor criteria or one major and one minor criteria are needed for the diagnosis to be made (Valent P, Horny HP, Escribano L, et al. Diagnostic criteria and classification of mastocytosis: A consensus proposal. *Leuk Res* 2001; 25: 603–25).

Neuroendocrine tumours (see Chapter 13, Section 13.1)—previously referred to as carcinoid tumours—can have a similar presentation to that outlined above. However, sweating is not frequently seen with these tumours. In the case of gut and bronchial neuroendocrine tumours, symptoms are rarely seen in the absence of liver metastasis. Episodic flushing is seen in up to 85% of patients presenting with this condition, although some patients with this condition have a fixed violaceous discolouration. Diarrhoea is also a common feature of this condition and is due to rapid intestinal transit time. Dyspnoea and bronchospasm, particularly during the episodes of flushing, may point to the presence of bronchial neuroendocrine tumours.

Medullary thyroid cancer (see Chapter 2, Section 2.8) may be identified incidentally or the patient may be symptomatic with flushing and diarrhoea. A thyroid nodule may be palpable, and telangiectasia may be visible on examination.

Hypogonadal aetiology for the symptoms may be evident from the history. Fatigue, loss of secondary sexual characteristics, low libido, and erectile dysfunction in men, or amenorrhoea in women, may be present. If the symptoms have been long-standing, a youthful appearance may be evident, with a lack of temporal hair recession. Gynaecomastia and/or low testicular volumes may be evident.

Flushing may be a feature of Cushing's syndrome (see Chapter 3 and Chapter 6, Section 6.87), although it is unusual as a presenting feature. This can also be seen secondary to glucocorticoid therapy (see Chapter 6, Section 6.12).

Investigations and treatment

Investigations to be undertaken in deciphering the aetiology of flushing are largely guided by the history of the symptoms and have been included in Table 15.9. Full examination to include thyroid examination is useful in deciphering the possible aetiology of symptoms.

Treatment is aimed at the underlying pathology. Antihistamines can be useful in the setting of mastocytosis, allergy, or histamine-producing neuroendocrine tumours. Non-selective beta blockade can also be useful in the treatment of benign cutaneous flushing. An overview of the treatment of the specific conditions has been included in Table 15.9.

Sweating

Introduction

Excessive sweating or hyperhidrosis refers to sweating not appropriate for the level of environmental temperature or thermoregulatory need. Primary hyperhidrosis (no obvious cause identifiable, although it may be related to sympathetic overdrive) and secondary hyperhidrosis (related to medications or medical disorders) are described. There are several endocrine disorders that are known to have hyperhidrosis as a presenting feature (summarized in Table 15.10). There is considerable overlap with the endocrine disorders that may present with flushing (see Table 15.9).

Investigations to consider and treatments

The investigations to consider in the workup of a patient with sweating are outlined in Table 15.10. The priority of tests chosen is largely dependent on the history provided. Treatment is aimed at the correction of the underlying disorder. Other treatments that are aimed at either refractory or primary hyperhidrosis would include antiperspirant topical therapy; botulinum toxin A injection into the local area; local excision of sweat glands; sympathetic denervation; and clonidine therapy (may cause somnolence, so night-time dosing is recommended). Again, the treatment option would largely be dependent on patient preference and physician assessment of risk and potential benefit.

Fatigue

Introduction

The sensation of tiredness or fatigue can be quite debilitating for the patient and a diagnostic quandary for the clinician. Careful targeted history is of vital importance, and the duration and setting of symptoms should be clarified. It is particularly important to decipher whether the patient has true fatigue or weakness (muscular). There is a long list of differential diagnosis. However, the potential causes and the investigations to consider have been summarized in Table 15.11. It can be helpful to consider the potential causes as those possibly related to endocrine disorders, those related to general medical problems (with or without endocrine features), and those related to psycho-neurological causes.

Table 15.10 Endocrine causes of hyperhidrosis, and the diagnostic tests for each condition that should be considered

Endocrine disorder	Diagnostic test to consider
Thyrotoxicosis	Thyroid function tests
Hypogonadism	LH
	FSH
	Testosterone (male)
	Estradiol (female)
Hypocortisolaemia	09:00 h cortisol, short Synacthen® test, or insulin-stimulation test (or glucagon-stimulation test, if the insulin-stimulation test is contraindicated) if a pituitary cause suspected
Phaeochromocytoma/ paraganglioma	Plasma and 24-hour urinary metanephrines and catecholamines
	CT/MRI of the adrenals and the abdomen
Acromegaly	IGF-1 and oral glucose-tolerance test with GH measurements (a failure to suppress GH is in keeping with the diagnosis)
Diabetes mellitus	Plasma glucose
	HbA1c
	Oral glucose-tolerance test
Hypoglycaemia	Plasma glucose levels
Gustatory sweating (autonomic dysfunction)	Autonomic function tests
Hypothalamic disorder (temperature dysregulation)	MRI brain

Abbreviations: FSH, follicle-stimulating hormone; GH, growth hormone; HbA1c, haemoglobin A1c; IGF-1, insulin-like growth factor 1; LH, luteinizing hormone.

Investigations and treatments to consider

A full examination should be undertaken. Baseline investigations should include a full blood count, liver function tests, TFTs, and measurement of electrolytes. Other investigations are guided by the history and clinical findings and have been outlined in Table 15.11.

Treatment is aimed at the underlying pathology (Table 15.11). From an endocrine perspective, correction of underlying hormonal abnormality may lead to rapid improvement of symptoms in certain cases (such as cortisol deficiency); in others, the response to treatment can be more gradual.

Table 15.11 Possible diagnoses, investigations, and treatments to consider when evaluating a patient with fatigue

Diagnosis	Investigations to consider	Treatment
Endocrine disorders		
Hypo- or hyperthyroidism	Thyroid function tests	Aimed at the underling aetiology
Cortisol deficiency/ Addison's disease	09:00 h cortisol	Glucocorticoid and mineralocorticoid replacement
	Short Synacthen® test	
	ACTH levels	
Growth-hormone deficiency	Pituitary function tests, including LH, FSH, estradiol/testosterone, prolactin, IGF-1	Growth-hormone replacement
	Consider dynamic testing, such as the insulin-stimulation test	
Hypogonadism	LH	Hormone replacement therapy
	FSH	
	Testosterone/estradiol	
	Prolactin	
Hypopituitarism	Can present with hypothyroidism, cortisol deficiency, growth-hormone deficiency, or hypogonadism Investigations as above	Hormone replacement therapy
Diabetes mellitus	Blood glucose	Dietetic input as well as treatment aimed at improved insulin sensitivity, insulin secretagogue therapy, or insulin, depending on the underlying diagnosis and the patient's needs
	Oral glucose-tolerance test	
Recurrent hypoglycaemia	Prolonged oral glucose-tolerance test if reactive hypoglycaemia suspected	—
	Short Synacthen® test if hypocortisolaemia suspected	
	Prolonged fast (72 hour) if insulinoma/insulin excess suspected with paired glucose, C-peptide, insulin, and possibly sulfonylurea levels	
Obesity	Investigations aimed at out ruling other causes	Weight-reduction strategies
General medical causes		
Anaemia	Full blood count	Treat underlying cause
	Iron, vitamin B_{12}, ferritin, and folate levels	
Malignancy	Guided by history	Treat underlying cause
	Consider imaging studies	
Obstructive sleep apnoea	Epworth score	Possible CPAP therapy
	Overnight oximetry	
Vitamin B_{12} deficiency	Vitamin B_{12} levels	Vitamin B_{12} replacements
Vitamin D deficiency	Vitamin D and calcium levels	Vitamin D replacement-
	PTH	
Toxins	Plasma levels	Directed against the toxin present
Psycho-neurological causes		
Neurological disorders (e.g. myasthenia gravis; more weakness rather than fatigue)	Aimed at underlying aetiology, in the case of myasthenia gravis	Anticholinesterase agents
		Immunosuppressive agents
	Acetylcholine receptor antibodies	Immunomodulating treatments
	Antibodies to the muscle specific receptor tyrosine kinase	Thymectomy
	Thymic imaging	
Chronic fatigue syndrome	Severe fatigue of >6 months duration	Cognitive behavioural therapy
	Other medical conditions excluded	Psychological support

(continued)

Table 15.11 Continued

Diagnosis	Investigations to consider	Treatment
Fibromyalgia	Based on history	Exercise
		Psychological support
		Selective serotonin and norepinephrine reuptake inhibitors
		Tricyclic antidepressant treatment
Depression	Based on history	Exercise
		Psychological support
		Selective serotonin and norepinephrine reuptake inhibitors
		Tricyclic antidepressant treatment

Abbreviations: ACTH, adrenocorticotrophic hormone; CFAP, continuous positive airway pressure; FSH, follicle-stimulating hormone; PTH, parathyroid hormone.

Further reading

Benson RA, Palin R, Holt PJE, et al. Diagnosis and management of hyperhidrosis. *BMJ* 2013; 347: 6800.

National Institute for Health and Care Excellence. Chronic fatigue syndrome and investigation. Available at http://www.nice.org.uk/Guidance/CG53 (accessed 16 Jan 2018).

Valent P, Horny HP, Escribano L, et al. Diagnostic criteria and classification of mastocytosis: A consensus proposal. *Leuk Res* 2001; 25: 603–25.

Chapter 16

Hormone resistance syndromes

Chapter contents

16.1 Resistance to thyroid hormone

Introduction

Thyroid hormone action in target tissues is dependent on a series of tightly regulated extra- and intracellular processes (see Figure 16.1). Following secretion from the thyroid gland, in response to hypothalamic TRH and pituitary TSH, T4 and T3 are transported to target tissues, bound (>99.5%) to TBG, albumin, and transthyretin (see Figure 16.1a). Cellular uptake of thyroid hormone, especially in the CNS, is mediated by specific transporters (e.g. MCT8; see (Figure 16.1b). An important additional tier of intracellular regulation is provided by a family of deiodinases (deiodinases 1–3), which mediate the conversion of T4 to bioactive T3 (and of T4 and T3 to the inactive metabolites rT3 and T2, respectively). The principal effects of T3 are mediated through a nuclear thyroid receptor, which is a member of the steroid/nuclear receptor superfamily and modulates target gene expression (Figure 16.1b). In humans, two highly homologous thyroid hormone receptors, denoted thyroid hormone receptor alpha (TR-alpha) and thyroid hormone receptor beta (TR-beta), are encoded by separate genes on Chromosomes 17 (*THRA*) and 3 (*THRB*), respectively, with alternate splicing generating three major isoforms (TR-alpha 1, TR-beta 1, and TR-beta 2) which are widely expressed but with differing tissue distributions: TR-alpha 1 is ubiquitously expressed, with particular abundance in the CNS, the myocardium, the gastrointestinal tract, the skeletal muscles, and the bones; TR-beta 1, which is also widely expressed, is the predominant isoform in the liver and the kidneys; and TR-beta 2 is most highly expressed in the pituitary and hypothalamus, but is also found in the inner ear and retina. A fourth splice variant, TR-alpha 2, which lacks the ability to bind thyroid hormone, is expressed in a variety of tissues (e.g. brain, testis), and may act as a functional antagonist of thyroid-hormone-receptor signalling.

Genetic disorders affecting each of the steps in the pathway of thyroid hormone transport, metabolism, and action are increasingly recognized, and give rise to differing syndromes with a common denominator of reduced sensitivity to thyroid hormone (see Table 16.1).

TR-beta resistance to thyroid hormone

Pathophysiology
Most individuals affected by TR-beta resistance to thyroid hormone (TR-beta RTH) harbour heterozygous mutations in the hormone-binding domain of TR-beta.

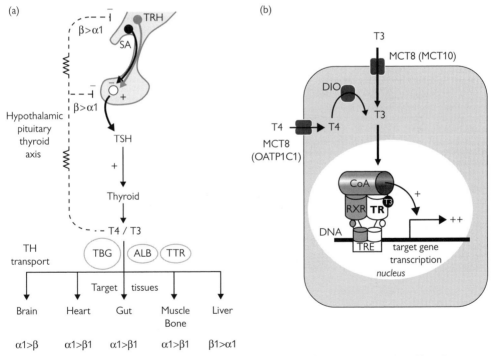

Fig 16.1 Schematic representation of the pathways governing thyroid hormone (a) secretion and transport, and (b) uptake, metabolism, and action. Three deiodinases are involved in the activation or inactivation of thyroxine and triiodothyronine, but only the conversion of thyroxine to bioactive triiodothyronine is shown, for simplicity; α, thyroid receptor alpha; β, thyroid receptor beta; ALB, albumin; CoA, transcriptional coactivator family; DIO, deiodinase; DNA, deoxyribonucleic acid; MCT8/10, monocarboxylate transporters 8 and 10; OATP1C1, organic anion-transporting polypeptide 1C1; RXR, retinoid X receptor; SA, somatostatin; T3, triiodothyronine; T4, thyroxine; TBG, thyroxine-binding globulin; TR, thyroid receptor; TRE, thyroid hormone response element; TRH, thyrotrophin-releasing hormone; TSH, thyrotrophin; TTR, transthyretin.

Table 16.1 Clinical and biochemical features in resistance to thyroid hormone, and other disorders of thyroid-hormone transport and metabolism

		TR-alpha RTH	TR-beta RTH	Allan–Herndon–Dudley syndrome[1]	Selenoprotein deficiency disorder[2]
Gene		THRA	THRB	SLC16A2 (MCT8)	SECISBP2
Laboratory findings (serum)	TSH	Normal	Normal or mildly ↑	High normal or mildly ↑	Normal or mildly ↑
	FT4	Low normal or mildly ↓	↑ (or ↑↑)	Low normal or mildly ↓	↑ (or ↑↑)
	FT3	High normal or mildly ↑	↑	↑ (or ↑↑)	Low normal or ↓
	rT3	↓	↑	Low normal or ↓	↑
	SHBG	Normal or ↑	Normal	↑ (or ↑↑)	Normal
	Se	—	—	—	↓
	IGF-1	↓ or low normal	—	—	—
Clinical features		Hypothyroid skeleton (delayed fusion of cranial sutures; macrocephaly; 'wormian bones'; delayed dentition; abnormal hip ossification) with growth retardation (predominantly lower segment) Variable/selective impairment of cognitive and motor function Constipation and abdominal distension ↓ BMR Low BP and resting HR Macrocytosis; ↓ red cell mass ? Skin tags	Adult: <ul><li>goitre</li><li>tremor</li><li>palpitations (sinus tachycardia; AF)</li><li>dyslipidaemia</li><li>↓ BMD</li><li>↑ BMR in some subjects</li></ul> Childhood: <ul><li>failure to thrive; low BMI; ↑ BMR and ↑ REE ± hyperphagia</li><li>short stature</li><li>hyperkinetic behaviour</li><li>ADHD and/or ↓ IQ in some subjects</li><li>ear, nose, and throat infections (± hearing loss)</li></ul>	Typically, severe cognitive impairment (IQ < 40) Psychomotor retardation (limb hypotonia, spastic quadriplegia, poor head control) Difficulty swallowing (with low body weight) A small number of patients with a milder phenotype have been described and may harbour less deleterious loss-of-function mutations Seizures in some subjects	Growth retardation Mild mental and motor impairment Skeletal myopathy Hearing loss Hypoglycaemia (in childhood) Male infertility Photosensitivity

Abbreviations: ADHD, attention-deficit hyperactivity disorder; AF, atrial fibrillation; BMD, bone mineral density; BMI, body mass index; BMR, basal metabolic rate; BP, blood pressure; HR, heart rate; FT3, triiodothyronine; free FT4, free thyroxine; IGF-1, insulin-like growth factor 1; rT3, reverse triiodothyronine; REE, resting energy expenditure; RTH, resistance to thyroid hormone; Se, selenium; SHBG, sex hormone-binding globulin; T3, triiodothyronine; T4, thyroxine; TR, thyroid receptor; TSH, thyrotrophin.

[1] X-linked disorder.

[2] Selenocysteine is a crucial component of the catalytic subunits of deiodinases 1–3; impaired function of the selenocysteine insertion sequence (SECIS)-binding protein 2 (SECISBP2) results in defective selenoprotein synthesis and a syndrome with wide-ranging features, including impaired deiodination of thyroid hormone.

Mutant receptors have impaired transcriptional function but, importantly, are able to inhibit normal (wild-type) receptor action in a dominant-negative manner. A small number of cases of homozygous TR-beta RTH have been described, and have a particularly severe phenotype. Resistance to thyroid hormone action centrally (due to abnormal TR-beta signalling in the hypothalamus and pituitary) gives rise to the biochemical hallmark of this disorder, with pituitary TSH secretion driving T4 and T3 production to establish a new equilibrium/set point, with high serum levels of thyroid hormone together with a non-suppressed TSH.

Epidemiology
The estimated incidence of TR-beta RTH is approximately 1 in 40,000–50,000 live births, and over 1000 individuals (in >350 families) with the disorder have been described to date.

Clinical features
TR-beta RTH is dominantly inherited and associated with variable clinical features (see Table 16.1). Many patients are either asymptomatic or have non-specific symptoms—in these individuals, with so-called generalized resistance, the high thyroid hormone levels are thought to compensate for ubiquitous tissue resistance, resulting in a euthyroid state. In contrast, a subset of individuals exhibit thyrotoxic features. When the latter clinical entity was first described, patients were thought to have 'selective' or predominantly pituitary resistance to thyroid hormone action, with preservation of normal hormonal responses in peripheral tissues. However, a careful comparison of the clinical and biochemical characteristics of individuals classified clinically with either generalized or predominantly pituitary resistance indicates that there is significant overlap between these entities.

Investigations and interpretation
When TR-beta RTH is suspected, the following investigations should be performed:
- TFTs: to detect hyperthyroxinaemia with non-suppressed TSH (in the absence of confounding

medication usage and/or intercurrent illness, and following exclusion of assay interference)

- genetic analysis: 85%–90% of patients with TR-beta RTH harbour a loss-of-function mutation in *THRB*

Distinguishing TR-beta RTH from the presence of a TSH-secreting pituitary adenoma can be challenging and may require measurement of TFTs in relatives; a TRH test; an L-T3 suppression test; measurement of SHBG and its alpha subunit; a pituitary MRI; and a trial of depot somatostatin analogue.

Management

Traditionally, no specific management has been deemed necessary for TR-beta RTH (other than advice to avoid inappropriate thyroid ablation). However, emerging evidence suggests that individuals with this disorder may be at risk of accelerated bone loss and metabolic dysfunction (e.g. dyslipidaemia). In addition, a group of patients develop cardiotoxicity, requiring beta blockade. The T3 analogue TRIAC (triiodothyroacetic acid), which preferentially binds to TR-beta, has been used to lower TSH and thyroid hormone levels in some patients; other thyroid-hormone-selective modulators are currently in development.

TR-alpha resistance to thyroid hormone

Pathophysiology

In TR-alpha resistance to thyroid hormone (TR-alpha RTH), as in TR-beta RTH, heterozygous mutations (in *THRA*, in this case) yield non-functional mutant receptors that are capable of inhibiting receptor action in a dominant-negative manner.

Epidemiology

To date, only a small number of individuals harbouring TR-alpha mutations have been reported, but dominant transmission has been observed, suggesting that TR-alpha RTH may be more common than previously suspected.

Clinical features

Unlike TR-beta RTH, TR-alpha RTH presents with features of hypothyroidism in a number of different tissues (e.g. the CNS, the gastrointestinal tract, the myocardium, skeletal muscle, bone) but is not associated with a markedly dysregulated pituitary–thyroid axis (see Table 16.1).

Investigations and interpretation

Low-normal T4 and high-normal T3 levels result in a low T4-to-T3 ratio, which, together with a subnormal rT3 level, signifies a more subtle biochemical signature. Serum TSH is normal.

Management

Current, albeit limited, experience suggests that T4 therapy may be of some benefit in TR-alpha RTH, although the development of hyperthyroidism in tissues that express TR-beta may preclude high-dose treatment. Alternative future therapeutic strategies could involve the development of TR-alpha-selective hormone analogues or inhibition of histone deacetylase activity within the transcriptional repression complex recruited by mutant receptors.

Further reading

Bochukova E, Schoenmakers N, Agostini M, et al. A mutation in the thyroid hormone receptor alpha gene. *New Engl J Med* 2012; 366: 243–9.

Gurnell M, Visser T, Beck-Peccoz P, et al. 'Resistance to thyroid hormone', in Jameson JL and De Groot LJ, eds, *Endocrinology* (7th edition), 2015. Saunders, pp. 1649–65.

Moran C, Agostini M, Visser WE, et al. Resistance to thyroid hormone caused by a mutation in thyroid hormone receptor (TR)α1 and TRα2: Clinical, biochemical, and genetic analyses of three related patients. *Lancet Diabetes Endocrinol* 2014; 2: 619–26.

van Mullem A, Chrysis D, Visser E, et al. Clinical phenotype and mutant TRα1. *New Engl J Med* 2012; 366: 1451–3.

16.2 Androgen insensitivity syndrome

Introduction

See also Chapter 9, Section 9.1. Androgen action is essential for male sex differentiation in embryogenesis, the development of puberty, and subsequent fertility. The Y chromosome initiates the first part of male sex development, which occurs in utero, leading the bipotential gonad to become a testis (sex determination). Hormone action dominates the next part, as androgens secreted by Leydig cells develop the internal and external genitalia (sex differentiation), and anti-Müllerian hormone from Sertoli cells regress the Müllerian ducts. Insl3, another product of Leydig cells, is involved in the transabdominal phase of testis descent.

Androgen insensitivity syndrome is characterized by resistance to testosterone and dihydrotestosterone and is the commonest cause of the 46, XY disorders of sex development. Complete androgen insensitivity syndrome results in a female phenotype, whereas partial androgen insensitivity syndrome is characterized by variable degrees of under-masculinization. The version of the syndrome with the mildest defect of androgen action, mild androgen insensitivity syndrome, may present as infertility in an otherwise normal male. The androgen receptor gene AR is located on the X chromosome (Xq11.2–q12); thus, AR mutations are transmitted in an X-linked recessive manner. Mutations are identified in over 90% of patients clinically diagnosed as having complete androgen insensitivity syndrome. Detection rates are much lower for partial androgen insensitivity syndrome, probably as result of the non-specific phenotype.

Complete androgen insensitivity syndrome

See also Chapter 8, Sections 8.2 and 8.3. The typical presentation for complete androgen insensitivity syndrome is either primary amenorrhoea in adolescence, or an inguinal/labial swelling in an infant with normal female external genitalia. At puberty, breasts and female adiposity develop naturally with a normal growth spurt due to aromatization of androgens, which are expressed at increased levels, to oestrogens. Axillary and pubic hair is sparse or absent. The vagina is short and blind-ending, and the uterus is absent, from the effects of testicular anti-Müllerian hormone.

Finding a testis in a female infant during an inguinal hernia repair should prompt investigation. In addition, while bilateral inguinal herniae are rare in female infants, the incidence of complete androgen insensitivity syndrome in such patients is 1%–2%; thus, if bilateral inguinal herniae are found in a female infant, a karyotype or a gonadal biopsy should be undertaken. In such cases, there is often a history of an older affected sister being missed for diagnosis when having an inguinal repair in infancy. Increasingly, another indication is when prenatal tests, which are done more and more for a myriad of reasons, indicate that the foetus is male but the infant is born as a female. The estimated prevalence of complete androgen insensitivity syndrome is about 1:20,000–64,000 male births.

The endocrine profile is typical for hormone resistance. LH concentrations are elevated in the face of increased male levels of testosterone whilst FSH and inhibin are generally normal. Elevated serum anti-Müllerian hormone is a useful distinction from complete gonadal dysgenesis. Oestrogen levels are between the male and female ranges. There is a postnatal testosterone surge in normal males during the first few months of life. This surge does not occur spontaneously in infants with complete androgen insensitivity syndrome, but there is a testosterone response to hCG stimulation. In contrast, infants with partial androgen insensitivity syndrome usually have this testosterone surge.

Partial androgen insensitivity syndrome

Partial androgen insensitivity syndrome presents a wide spectrum of undervirilized external genitalia ranging from female to male. The typical phenotype is perineoscrotal hypospadias with micropenis, with a bifid scrotum which may or not contain descended testes. Such a phenotype can result from other causes of disorders of sex development, such as 45, X/46, XY gonadal dysgenesis, partial XY gonadal dysgenesis, and androgen biosynthetic defects. Appropriate investigations should include a karyotype, measurement of androgen concentrations in response to hCG stimulation, and a urinary steroid profile. The definitive test is often mutation analysis of the cognate gene. The majority of patients with partial androgen insensitivity syndrome are raised male and may enter puberty spontaneously. Gynaecomastia is a frequent accompaniment. The hormone profile is consistent with androgen resistance.

Mild androgen insensitivity syndrome

Mild androgen insensitivity syndrome is characterized by infertility with normal male development; some reported cases present with normal spermatogenesis with genital sub-virilization. Clinical features suggesting mild androgen resistance include gynaecomastia, sparse body hair, a small penis, and sexual dysfunction. Serum LH is increased even although androgen levels are normal or elevated.

Kennedy's syndrome, or spinal and bulbar muscular atrophy, is a rare X-linked neurodegenerative disease which is caused by an expanded glutamine repeat in AR. It is characterized by slowly progressive muscle weakness in the limb and bulbar regions, and affected males have features of mild androgen insensitivity.

Molecular pathogenesis of androgen insensitivity syndrome

More than 400 AR mutations related to androgen insensitivity syndrome are recorded on an international database (http://androgendb.mcgill.ca/). The most frequent AR defects are single-base-pair changes, causing an amino-acid substitution (missense mutation) or premature stop codon (nonsense mutation). Within the eight-exon gene, the vast majority of missense mutations are located in exons encoding the ligand-binding or DNA-binding domains. These domains are conserved among the steroid receptor family, and their structures have been characterized by three-dimensional analysis. About 30% of AR mutations arise de novo. There are also examples of somatic mutations caused by de novo mutations occurring at the post-zygotic stage.

It is important to assess the pathogenicity of novel mutations identified in patients with androgen insensitivity syndrome, particularly in those with partial androgen insensitivity syndrome. Transcriptional assays have been widely used to determine the residual activity of mutant androgen receptors. Model-based functional analysis can be used as an alternative to labour-intensive in vitro assays, but their use is limited to identifying mutations in the ligand-binding or DNA-binding domains.

Management of androgen insensitivity syndrome

A multidisciplinary approach is essential to the management of androgen insensitivity syndrome and it needs to be adapted according to the androgen insensitivity syndrome subtype and the age and development of the patient. Follow-up is long term, lasting from infancy to adulthood and involving a core team of health professionals. This should include paediatric and adult endocrinologists, a urologist, a gynaecologist, and, above all, a clinical psychologist skilled in providing counselling appropriate for the child's cognitive development and, in adulthood, addressing the range of quality-of-life issues appertaining to disorders of sex development. Additional input from clinical geneticists, social services, and ethicists may be required periodically.

A major backup for families with disorders of sex development can be provided by patient advocacy groups such as the Androgen Insensitivity Support Group (http://www.aissg.org/) and DSD Families (http://www.dsdfamilies.org/).

Management of complete androgen insensitivity syndrome
Gender assignment and sex of rearing is female in complete androgen insensitivity syndrome. There is an increased risk of gonadal tumours in disorders of sex development generally. However, the risk is very low during childhood and adolescence in CAIS. It is now recommended that the gonads should be retained *in situ* until spontaneous puberty is fully achieved. The girl can now be fully informed of her condition and take part in discussions about the timing of gonadectomy. After gonadectomy, hormone replacement therapy is necessary to maintain secondary sexual characteristics, psychosocial well-being and bone health. Several oestrogen preparations are available, including transdermal delivery options. In the absence of a uterus, the treatment can be with continuous, unopposed oestrogen. However, some women also take progestogens and, indeed, androgen supplements. The latter are reported by some women with complete androgen insensitivity syndrome to improve libido and general quality of life. How this effect works is unexplained, based on the molecular mode of androgen action via a single, ubiquitously expressed androgen receptor. Nevertheless, there is evidence for androgens acting in non-genomic fashion.

The child with complete androgen insensitivity syndrome needs an assessment of vaginal anatomy under general anaesthesia during the peripubertal period. This provides an indication for later treatment with vaginal dilators at the time of sexual activity. Rarely, vaginoplasty procedures are required.

Gonadal tumours in androgen insensitivity syndrome are germ cell in origin, comprising gonadoblastoma and dysgerminoma. A premalignant stage of the germ cell tumour is known as carcinoma in situ of the testis, also referred to as intratubular germ cell neoplasia unclassified, or testicular intra-epithelial neoplasia. Carcinoma

in situ of the testis arises from gonocytes (primordial germ cells) and is thought to be the result of a developmental arrest of fetal germ cells. The histology shows clusters of large germ cells occupying the seminiferous tubules and, on immunohistochemistry, the cells are positive for tumour markers such as PLAP, c-KIT, and Oct 3/4. The risk of germ cell tumour in complete androgen insensitivity syndrome is low (0.8%–2%) before puberty, but increases with age, with estimates of 3.6% and 33% at 25 and 50 years, respectively. Consequently, it is recommended that gonadectomy be performed in early adulthood. Nevertheless, some women with complete androgen insensitivity syndrome choose not to have gonadectomy. It is currently recommended that screening for a gonadal tumour with MRI is undertaken at 2-yearly intervals. The aforementioned tumour markers are not present in the circulation. However, detection of microRNA signatures of germ cell tumours in blood shows promise as a method for early screening. Other non-germ cell tumours described in association with androgen insensitivity syndrome include Sertoli cell and Leydig cell tumours, hamartomas, and leiomyomas.

Management of partial androgen insensitivity syndrome
Sex assignment is a complex process for an infant born with ambiguous genitalia, and particularly so for infants with XY disorders of sex development. The decision-making process should be multifactorial, taking account of the appearance of the genitalia, the results of endocrine and genetic tests, the options for successful surgical correction, and, not least, the wishes of the parents. The latter may be strongly influenced by cultural factors and respected by members of the professional team following these patients. A short course of testosterone (25 mg intramuscularly monthly for 3 months) or topical dihydrotestosterone gel can be useful to determine androgen responsiveness.

Infants who have partial androgen insensitivity syndrome and are raised as male require hypospadias repair, often in two or three stages, and orchidopexy for undescended testes. Gynaecomastia arising in adolescence can sometimes be managed with an aromatase inhibitor such as letrozole or an oestrogen antagonist such as tamoxifen. However, affected boys often opt for reduction mammoplasty to achieve a more rapid resolution. Infants who have partial androgen insensitivity syndrome and are assigned as female will need feminizing genitoplasty and early gonadectomy to avoid virilization at puberty. Oestrogen replacement therapy at puberty, and assessment of the vaginal anatomy are required.

Psychosocial management of androgen sensitivity syndrome
As far as is practicable, the clinical psychologist needs to be involved early in supportive management at the time of diagnosis and with discussions on sex assignment, plans for surgery, and concerns relating to outcome at puberty, sexual relationships, and predictions for fertility. A key component of psychosocial management is disclosure, with issues about the implication of an XY karyotype, the gonads being testes, the absence of a uterus, and infertility all being brought to the fore. Planned transition from a paediatric- to an adult-based service for disorders of sex development is often best orchestrated by the clinical psychologist. The need for multidisciplinary specialized services to be provided for disorders of sex development dictates that only tertiary centres operating in a

hub-and-spoke fashion should be caring for patients with complex disorders of sex development, including all the subcategories of androgen insensitivity syndrome.

Further reading

Hughes IA, Davies JD, MacDougall J, et al. Androgen insensitivity syndrome. *Lancet* 2012; 380: 1419–28.

Jääskeläinen J. Molecular biology of androgen insensitivity. *Mol Cell Endocrinol* 2012; 352: 4–12.

Lucas-Herald A, Bertelloni S, Ahmed SF, et al. The long-term outcome of boys with partial androgen insensitivity syndrome and a mutation in the androgen receptor gene. *J Clin Endocrinol Metab* 2016; 101(11): 3959–67.

Cools M, Wolffenbuttel KP, Looijenga LHJ, et al. Malignant testicular germ cell tumors in postpubertal individuals with androgen insensitivity: Prevalence, pathology and relevance of single nucleotide polymorphism-based susceptibility profiling. *Hum Reprod* 2017; 32(12): 2561–73.

Kolesinska Z, Ahmed SF, Niedziela M, et al. Changes over time in sex assignment for disorders of sex development. *Pediatrics* 2014; 134; e710–15.

Mongan NP, Tadokoro-Cuccaro R, Bunch T, Hughes IA. Androgen insensitivity syndrome. *Best Pract Res Clin Endocrinol Metab* 2015; 29(4): 569–80.

Nakhal RS, Hall-Craggs M, Freeman A et al. Evaluation of retained testes in adolescent girls and women with complete androgen insensitivity síndrome. *Radiology*. 2013, 268: 153–60.

Chaudhry S, Tadokoro-Cuccaro R, Hannema SE, et al. Frequency of gonadal tumours in complete androgen insensitivity syndrome (CAIS): A retrospective case-series analysis. *J Pediatr Urol* 2017; 13(5): 498.e1–6.

16.3 Primary generalized glucocorticoid resistance, or Chrousos syndrome

Introduction

In humans, glucocorticoids regulate a broad spectrum of physiologic functions and play a pivotal role in critical biologic processes such as growth, reproduction, intermediary metabolism, and immune and inflammatory reactions, as well as CNS and cardiovascular functions. At the cellular level, the actions of glucocorticoids are mediated by an intracellular receptor protein, the glucocorticoid receptor. It belongs to the steroid/thyroid/retinoic acid superfamily of nuclear receptors and functions as a ligand-dependent transcription factor that regulates the expression of glucocorticoid-responsive genes, both positively and negatively. Alternative splicing in exon 9 of the human glucocorticoid receptor (hGR) mRNA transcript generates two highly homologous receptor isoforms: hGR alpha and hGR beta; hGR alpha represents the classic glucocorticoid receptor, which functions as a ligand-dependent transcription factor and mediates the actions of glucocorticoids, whilst hGR beta does not bind glucocorticoid agonists and exerts a dominant-negative effect upon the transcriptional activity of hGR alpha.

In the absence of ligand, hGR alpha resides mostly in the cytoplasm of cells as part of a hetero-oligomeric complex which contains chaperon heat-shock proteins 90 and 70, as well as other proteins. Following binding to the ligand, the activated hGR alpha dissociates from this multiprotein complex and translocates into the nucleus, where it binds as a homodimer to glucocorticoid response elements in the promoter regions of target genes and regulates their expression positively or negatively. Activated hGR alpha can also modulate gene expression independently of DNA binding, by interacting, possibly as a monomer, with other transcription factors, such as nuclear factor kappa B, activator protein-1, p53, and STAT proteins.

Alterations in the molecular mechanisms of hGR alpha action may lead to alterations in tissue sensitivity to glucocorticoids, such as glucocorticoid resistance or glucocorticoid hypersensitivity. In this section, we summarize the pathophysiology and molecular mechanisms underlying primary generalized glucocorticoid resistance, or Chrousos syndrome.

Clinical manifestations

Chrousos syndrome is a rare familial or sporadic condition initially described and elucidated by Chrousos et al. This condition is characterized by generalized, mostly partial, target-tissue insensitivity to glucocorticoids, leading to compensatory activation of the hypothalamo-pituitary–adrenal axis, increased secretion of adrenocorticotrophic hormone, adrenocortical hyperplasia, increased cortisol secretion as a compensation for the reduced action of glucocorticoids at target tissues, and increased production of adrenal steroids with mineralocorticoid (cortisol, deoxycorticosterone, and corticosterone) and/or androgenic (DHEA and DHEAS) activity.

The clinical manifestations of Chrousos syndrome reflect these pathophysiologic alterations. Clinical manifestations of glucocorticoid deficiency are rare and have only been reported in a young child with hypoglycaemic, generalized, tonic–clonic seizures during the course of a febrile illness; in a newborn baby with severe hypoglycaemia, excessive fatigability with feeding, increased susceptibility to infections, and concurrent growth hormone deficiency; and in several adult patients with chronic fatigue. Clinical manifestations of mineralocorticoid excess include hypertension and hypokalaemic alkalosis. Clinical manifestations of androgen excess include ambiguous genitalia in a karyotypic female at birth; gonadotrophin-independent precocious puberty in children of either gender; acne, hirsutism, and impaired fertility in both sexes; male pattern hair loss, menstrual irregularities, and oligo-anovulation in females; and oligospermia in males. The clinical spectrum of the condition is broad, ranging from extremely severe to mild forms, whilst a number of patients may be asymptomatic, displaying biochemical alterations only.

Molecular mechanisms

The molecular basis of Chrousos syndrome has been ascribed primarily to mutations in NR3C1, which encodes hGR; the mutations impair the molecular mechanisms of hGR alpha action and thus decrease tissue sensitivity to glucocorticoids (see Figure 16.2). We have identified most of the NR3C1 mutations associated with Chrousos syndrome and have systematically investigated the molecular mechanisms through which these mutations affect glucocorticoid signal transduction in almost all reported cases with the condition.

Compared with the wild-type receptor, all mutant receptors demonstrated variable reduction in their ability to transactivate glucocorticoid-responsive genes in response to dexamethasone. The mutant receptors hGR alpha I559N, hGR alpha F737L, hGR alpha I747M, and hGR alpha L773P exerted a dominant-negative effect upon the wild-type receptor; this effect may contribute to the manifestation of the disease in the heterozygous state. All mutant receptors in which the mutations were located in the ligand-binding domain of the receptor showed a variable reduction in their affinity for the ligand. The only mutant receptor that demonstrated normal affinity for the ligand was hGR alpha R477H, in which the mutation was located in the DNA-binding domain. In the absence of ligand, most pathologic mutant receptors were observed primarily in the cytoplasm of cells, except hGR alpha V729I and hGR alpha F737L, which were found in both the cytoplasm and the nucleus. Exposure to dexamethasone induced a slow translocation of the mutant receptors into the nucleus, over a time span which ranged from 20 minutes to 180 minutes; in contrast, the wild-type hGR alpha required only 12 minutes for complete translocation. All mutant receptors in which the mutations were located in the ligand-binding domain preserved their ability to bind to DNA but displayed an abnormal interaction with the GRIP1 coactivator in vitro. The only mutant receptor that failed to bind to DNA but displayed a normal interaction with GRIP1 was hGR alpha R477H, in which the mutation was located in the C-terminal zinc finger of the DNA-binding domain.

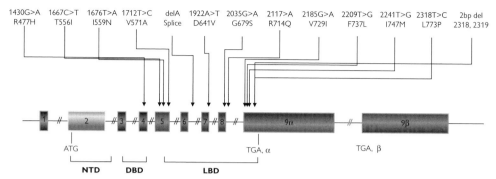

Fig 16.2 Location of the known mutations of the *hGR* gene causing Chrousos syndrome; DBD: DNA-binding domain; LBD: ligand-binding domain; NTD: amino-terminal domain.

Clinical evaluation

In evaluating a patient with suspected alterations in tissue sensitivity to glucocorticoids, it is important to obtain a complete personal and family history, with particular attention to evidence suggesting alterations in the activity of the hypothalamo-pituitary–adrenal axis. Any evidence suggesting possible CNS dysfunction should be noted. In female subjects, the regularity of menstrual cycles should be documented. In children and adolescents, growth and sexual maturation should be evaluated carefully. The physical examination should include an assessment for signs of hyperandrogenism, virilization, and mineralocorticoid excess, as well as a complete neurologic examination. Arterial blood pressure should be recorded and preferably monitored over a 24-hour period.

Endocrinological evaluation

The concentrations of plasma adrenocorticotrophic hormone, plasma renin activity, and aldosterone, as well as those of serum cortisol, testosterone, androstenedione, DHEA, DHEAS, total cholesterol, HDL, LDL, triglycerides, and fasting glucose and insulin, should be recorded in the morning. Determination of the 24-hour UFC excretion on two or three consecutive days is central to the diagnosis, given that patients with Chrousos syndrome demonstrate increased 24-hour UFC excretion in the absence of clinical manifestations suggestive of hypercortisolism. In affected subjects, the rise in serum cortisol and androgen concentrations, as well as the 24-hour UFC excretion, varies considerably depending on the severity of impairment of glucocorticoid signal transduction. Plasma adrenocorticotrophic hormone concentrations may be normal or high.

The responsiveness of the hypothalamo-pituitary–adrenal axis to exogenous glucocorticoids should also be tested with dexamethasone. Increasing doses of dexamethasone should be given orally at midnight every other day, and a serum sample should be drawn at 08:00 h the following morning for determination of serum cortisol and dexamethasone concentrations. Affected subjects demonstrate resistance of the hypothalamo-pituitary–adrenal axis to dexamethasone suppression, which varies depending on the severity of the condition.

Biological and molecular studies

Thymidine-incorporation and dexamethasone-binding assays on peripheral blood mononuclear cells, together with sequencing of *NR3C1*, are necessary to confirm the diagnosis. The thymidine-incorporation assays reveal resistance to dexamethasone-induced suppression of phytohaemagglutinin-stimulated thymidine incorporation, whilst the dexamethasone-binding assays often show decreased affinity of the ligand for hGR, or low hGR concentrations compared to those in control subjects. Sequencing of the coding region of *NR3C1*, including the intron/exon junctions, will reveal mutations or deletions in most, but not all, cases with the condition.

Management

The aim of treatment is to suppress the excess secretion of adrenocorticotrophic hormone and, therefore, the increased production of adrenal steroids with mineralocorticoid and androgenic activity. Treatment involves administration of high doses of mineralocorticoid-sparing synthetic glucocorticoids, such as dexamethasone, which activate mutant and/or wild-type hGR alpha, and suppress the endogenous secretion of adrenocorticotrophic hormone in affected subjects. Adequate suppression of the hypothalamo-pituitary–adrenal axis is of particular importance in order to prevent the development of an adrenocorticotrophic-hormone-secreting adenoma in the pituitary gland and an adrenocortical adenoma in the adrenal glands. Long-term dexamethasone treatment should be carefully titrated according to the clinical manifestations and biochemical profile of the affected subjects.

Further reading

Charmandari E, Kino T, Ichijo T, et al. Generalized glucocorticoid resistance: Clinical aspects, molecular mechanisms, and implications of a rare genetic disorder. *J Clin Endocrinol Metab* 2008; 93: 1563–72.

Charmandari E and Kino T. Chrousos syndrome: A seminal report, a phylogenetic enigma and the clinical implications of glucocorticoid signalling changes. *Eur J Clin Invest* 2010; 40: 932–42.

Charmandari E. Primary generalized glucocorticoid resistance and hypersensitivity. *Horm Res Paediatr* 2011; 76: 145–55.

Chrousos GP, Detera-Wadleigh SD, and Karl M. Syndromes of glucocorticoid resistance. *Ann Intern Med* 1993; 119: 1113–24.

Chrousos GP, and Kino T. Glucocorticoid signaling in the cell: expanding clinical implications to complex human behavioral and somatic disorders. *Proc NY Acad Sci* 2009; 1179: 153–66.

Chrousos GP and Kino T. Intracellular glucocorticoid signaling: A formerly simple system turns stochastic. *Sci STKE* 2005; 304: pe48.

Chrousos GP, Vingerhoeds A, Brandon D, et al. Primary cortisol resistance in man. A glucocorticoid receptor-mediated disease. *J Clin Invest* 1982; 69: 1261–9.

Nicolaides NC, Galata Z, Kino T, et al. The human glucocorticoid receptor: Molecular basis of biologic function. *Steroids* 2010; 75: 1–2.

16.4 Adrenocorticotrophic-hormone resistance syndromes

Introduction

Adrenocorticotrophic-hormone (ACTH) resistance syndromes are a rare group of hereditary disorders resulting in adrenal unresponsiveness to adrenocorticotrophic hormone and include familial glucocorticoid deficiency (FGD) and triple A syndrome.

FGD is an autosomal recessive form of adrenal failure characterized by adrenocorticotrophic-hormone-resistant isolated glucocorticoid deficiency with preserved mineralocorticoid secretion. Affected children develop hypocortisolaemia and compensatory elevated adrenocorticotrophic hormone. Patients with FGD usually present in early childhood with symptoms relating to cortisol deficiency including hypoglycaemia, jaundice, recurrent infection, and failure to thrive. Patients are hyperpigmented, due to grossly elevated levels of adrenocorticotrophic hormone. Renin and aldosterone are typically normal. Unlike Addison's disease, FGD is a genetic disorder resulting from mutations either in genes encoding essential proteins involved in the early response to adrenocorticotrophic hormone or in genes involved in the replicative or oxidative stress pathways.

Triple A syndrome consists of a triad of alacrima (deficient tear production), achalasia (swallowing problems), and adrenal failure. Isolated glucocorticoid deficiency is seen in approximately 80% of patients, with additional mineralocorticoid deficiency present in a further 15%. A wide range of progressive neurological defects have also been associated with triple A syndrome, including motor, sensory, and autonomic neuropathies.

Pathophysiology

Secretion of the adrenocorticotrophic hormone by the anterior pituitary is the most important mechanism controlling cortisol synthesis and secretion from the zona fasciculata in the adrenal gland. The secretion of adrenocorticotrophic hormone is stimulated by corticotrophin-releasing hormone (CRH) from the hypothalamus and follows a circadian pattern. However, adrenocorticotrophic hormone is also released during periods of stress such as trauma, hypoglycaemia, infection, fever, surgery, or anxiety. In addition, cortisol secretion is an example of one of the classical endocrine feedback loops; it is under negative feedback control from the hypothalamo-pituitary–adrenal axis.

Adrenocorticotrophic hormone acts by binding to its specific cell-surface receptor, MC2R (also known as the adrenocorticotrophic-hormone receptor) to induce adrenal steroidogenesis (see Figure 16.3). MC2R is a seven-transmembrane domain G protein-coupled receptor and is part of the melanocortin receptor family, which includes melanocortin receptor types 1–5. The melanocortin receptors are involved in diverse functions including pigmentation and adrenal steroidogenesis, as well as weight and energy homeostasis. The sole ligand for MC2R is adrenocorticotrophic hormone, in contrast to the other melanocortin receptors, which show varying affinities to adrenocorticotrophic hormone and the alpha, beta, and gamma forms of melanocyte-stimulating hormone.

Binding of adrenocorticotrophic hormone to MC2R stimulates intracellular production of cAMP, which in turn

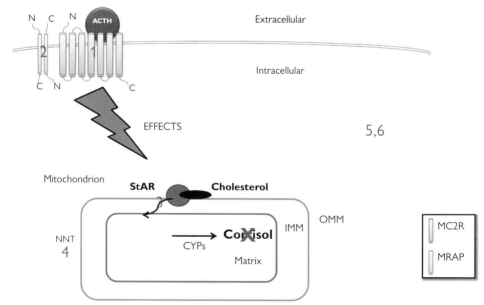

Fig 16.3 Schematic diagram illustrating the location of gene defects causing familial glucocorticoid deficiency: (1) *MC2R* mutations lead to defective MC2R trafficking to the cell surface; (2) *MRAP* mutations lead to defective MC2R trafficking and signalling; (3) *StAR* mutations disrupt cholesterol transport to the inner mitochondrial membrane; (4) *NNT* mutations lead to increased mitochondrial oxidative stress and decreased steroid output; and (5, 6) *MCM4* and *AAAS* mutations lead to early cellular death from increased replicative and oxidative stress.

stimulates cAMP-dependent protein kinase. As a result, cholesterol ester is imported into the cell via the scavenger receptor B1 and hydrolysed by hormone-sensitive lipase. Cholesterol is then introduced into the mitochondria by a complex which includes the steroidogenic acute regulatory protein StAR. Subsequent steroidogenesis requires the concerted action of a number of different steroidogenic enzymes, including cytochrome P450 enzymes and hydroxysteroid dehydrogenase enzymes. Adrenocorticotrophic hormone stimulates increased steroidogenic enzyme expression via a number of mechanisms and ultimately results in an increased rate of cortisol synthesis.

FGD type 1

The gene encoding MC2R, *MC2R*, was first cloned in 1992, enabling researchers to identify point mutations in this gene in patients with FGD (Clark et al., 1993). To date, more than 30 mutations distributed throughout the coding region in *MC2R* have been reported and together account for 25% of cases of FGD. Interestingly, the majority of these are missense mutations. Nonsense mutations are uncommon and usually occur with a missense mutation on the other allele.

FGD type 2

Genetic studies in families with FGD without *MC2R* mutations have linked the gene *MRAP*, which encodes melanocortin-2 receptor accessory protein (MRAP), to the disease. MRAP is a small, single-transmembrane-domain protein. Functional analysis of MRAP revealed that it was essential for normal MC2R function. MRAP forms a unique antiparallel homodimer which directly interacts with the MC2R at the endoplasmic reticulum and is required for correct folding or trafficking of the receptor to the cell surface. Current evidence suggests that MRAP is also required at the plasma membrane for adrenocorticotrophic-hormone binding and signal transduction. Mutations in *MRAP* are found in approximately 20% of cases of FGD.

FGD type 3 (non-classical congenital lipoid adrenal hyperplasia)

StAR is a mitochondrial phosphoprotein that mediates the acute response to steroidogenic stimuli by increasing cholesterol transport from the outer to the inner mitochondrial membrane. Defects in StAR usually result in congenital lipoid adrenal hyperplasia, a severe form of congenital adrenal hyperplasia. However, a small percentage of patients presenting with classical FGD were found to have mutations in *STAR*, the gene that encodes StAR. A review of the history, examination, and biochemical data in the individuals diagnosed with FGD confirmed they had isolated glucocorticoid deficiency with normal or near-normal renin and aldosterone levels. However, some patients did have mild reproductive anomalies, including hypospadias and cryptorchidism, which had not previously been connected to their adrenal failure. The mutations found in *STAR* in FGD appear to lead to only partial impairment of the cholesterol-uptake function of this protein. Thus, classical congenital lipoid adrenal hyperplasia is caused by mutations that completely abolish any functioning StAR, whilst mutations that allow the protein to retain some function are associated with non-classical congenital lipoid adrenal hyperplasia or FGD.

Novel mechanisms of adrenal failure leading to adrenocorticotrophic-hormone resistance

Defects in the DNA replication pathway

Exome sequencing has been utilized in patients with FGD to identify novel genes and pathways involved in adrenal disease. This technique identified a mutation in a gene which encodes one component of the minichromosome maintenance (MCM) protein complex, *MCM4*, in a cohort of Irish patients (Hughes et al., 2012). These patients presented with a unique variant of FGD associated with increased chromosomal fragility, short stature, and natural-killer-cell deficiency. The MCM complex acts as a replicative helicase and is essential for normal DNA replication and genome stability in all eukaryotes. This was the first association between adrenal failure and a gene involved in DNA replication. Depletion of MCM proteins has been proposed to lead to stem cell defects in mice. The relatively specific impingement of the *MCM4* mutation on adrenal function may be a consequence of its effect on the growth of adrenal stem or progenitor cells and their differentiation into steroidogenic cells. This suggests that the protein encoded by *MCM4* has additional functionality beyond DNA replication in adrenal development. This mutation has only been identified in Irish patients and therefore remains a rare cause of FGD.

Defects in antioxidant pathways

Targeted exome sequencing in additional families identified mutations in *NNT*, which encodes nicotinamide nucleotide transhydrogenase, as another cause of isolated glucocorticoid deficiency. These mutations were spread throughout the gene and included deletion of the initiating methionine, splice mutations, and many missense and nonsense mutations. *NNT* is a highly conserved gene that encodes an integral protein of the inner mitochondrial membrane. Under most physiological conditions, this enzyme uses energy from the mitochondrial proton gradient to produce high concentrations of NADPH. In mitochondria, the detoxification of reactive oxygen species by glutathione peroxidases depends on NADPH for regeneration of reduced glutathione from oxidized glutathione. The finding of *NNT* mutations in FGD suggests that, at least in humans, *NNT* is of primary importance for the detoxification of reactive oxygen species in adrenocortical cells, highlighting the susceptibility of the adrenal cortex to this type of pathological damage.

Triple A syndrome

Oxidative stress has also been implicated in the pathogenesis of the closely related triple A syndrome. In this condition, mutations in *AAAS* lead to a deficiency in or mislocalization of the nuclear-pore protein aladin, resulting in impairment of the nuclear import of DNA repair and antioxidant proteins, thus making the patients' cells more susceptible to oxidative stress.

Clinical features

Patients with FGD (Table 16.2) usually present during the neonatal period or in early childhood with symptoms related to cortisol deficiency and adrenocorticotrophic-hormone excess. The most common presenting features are those secondary to hypoglycaemia, including jitteriness, tremors, hypotonia, lethargy, apnoea, poor feeding, and hypoglycaemic seizures. In a small number of patients, undiagnosed hypoglycaemia in infancy may have been sufficiently severe to cause serious long-term neurological sequelae. Neonates may also present with

Table 16.2 Distinguishing clinical features associated with different gene defects causing familial glucocorticoid deficiency

Gene affected	Clinical features in addition to glucocorticoid deficiency
MC2R	Tall stature
MRAP	Early presentation; often in the neonatal period
STAR	Occasionally mild reproductive anomalies in males (e.g. hypospadias and cryptorchidism) when associated with isolated glucocorticoid deficiency only (in contrast to congenital lipoid adrenal hyperplasia)
MCM4	Short stature
	Deficiency in natural killer cells, leading to increased susceptibility to infection
	Delayed puberty in boys
NNT	Infrequent reports of mineralocorticoid deficiency
AAAS	Alacrima
	Achalasia
	Progressive neurological defects
	Twenty per cent of patients have mineralocorticoid deficiency

jaundice, failure to thrive, collapse, and, very rarely, transient neonatal hepatitis.

Hyperpigmentation will usually develop by a few months of age, due to over-stimulation of the type 1 melanocortin receptor by high levels of circulating adrenocorticotrophic hormone, although there are exceptions to this. Older children may present with a variety of features, including increased pigmentation, recurrent infections, hypoglycaemia, lethargy, and shock. As this is an autosomal-recessive disorder, there is frequently a history of consanguinity and there may also be a history of unexplained neonatal or childhood deaths in FGD families.

A feature that has been observed in patients with FGD type 1 is tall stature. The underlying mechanism is not clear but hydrocortisone replacement appears to stop this excessive growth. This suggests that either the high levels of adrenocorticotrophic hormone or the cortisol deficiency itself may have a causative role. It has been proposed that adrenocorticotrophic hormone at high concentrations may activate melanocortin receptors in bone and in the growth plate and thus stimulate growth. Alternatively, it has been reported that cortisol inhibits the synthesis of IGF-binding protein 5 in osteoblasts, suggesting that perhaps cortisol deficiency could result in a lack of inhibition and, hence, increase growth. Tall stature is not a recognized feature of FGD type 2, which tends to present at an earlier age than FGD type 1, meaning patients are treated earlier and do not have chronic exposure to high levels of adrenocorticotrophic hormone or low levels of cortisol.

Adrenocorticotrophic hormone also stimulates adrenal androgen synthesis from the zona reticularis and is required for normal adrenarche in children. In children with FGD adrenarche may not occur, or it may occur with delayed or absent pubic hair development. However, normal pubertal development controlled by the hypothalamo-pituitary–gonadal axis is unaffected, and fertility is normal.

Investigation

The characteristic biochemical feature of FGD is low or undetectable cortisol paired with high levels of adrenocorticotrophic hormone and normal levels of electrolytes, renin, and aldosterone. The levels of adrenocorticotrophic hormone are can be extremely high; often, they are >220 pmol/L (1000 pg/mL; normal range, <18 pmol/L (80 pg/mL)). A standard adrenocorticotrophic-hormone stimulation test will confirm an impaired cortisol response and verify adrenal insufficiency.

The most important feature for distinguishing FGD from other causes of adrenal insufficiency is the absence of mineralocorticoid deficiency. However, FGD patients frequently present with minor abnormalities of the renin–aldosterone axis for various reasons. One reason is that, at presentation, children with FGD are usually stressed and may be hypovolaemic or pyrexial. Alternatively, they may be relatively water overloaded as a result of intravenous fluid replacement and the reduced free-water clearance associated with glucocorticoid deficiency. Usually, after introduction of appropriate hydrocortisone replacement, any minor derangements in renin and aldosterone levels normalize and fludrocortisone replacement will not be required.

Management

The treatment for adrenocorticotrophic-hormone resistance is with physiological glucocorticoid replacement. This is usually given in the form of oral hydrocortisone: 8–10 mg/m^2 per day in children, and 20 mg per day in adults. The total daily dose is given in three to four divided doses throughout the day. Prednisolone and, rarely, dexamethasone can also be used in certain circumstances. In individuals with adequate replacement therapy, levels of adrenocorticotrophic hormone often remain elevated and therefore cutaneous pigmentation can persist. Attempts to suppress levels of adrenocorticotrophic hormone must be avoided, as they will lead to overtreatment, potentially iatrogenic Cushing's syndrome, and poor growth in children.

Hydrocortisone dosing must be increased during times of stress to two to three times the maintenance dose. It is important to ensure the patient and their family have adequate education and understand when and how to increase hydrocortisone doses and emergency management with intramuscular hydrocortisone or hydrocortisone suppositories.

Future developments

It is likely that emerging genetic techniques will identify further novel genes associated with FGD, since approximately 40% of cases have no known cause. This will provide further insights into the action of adrenocorticotrophic hormone and the molecular basis of adrenal development and function.

References and further reading

Achermann JC, Meeks JJ, Jeffs B, et al., Molecular and structural analysis of two novel StAR mutations in patients with lipoid congenital adrenal hyperplasia. *Mol Genet Metab* 2001; 73: 354–7.

Clark, AJ, McLoughlin L, and Grossman, A. Familial glucocorticoid deficiency associated with point mutation in the adrenocorticotropin receptor. *Lancet* 1993; 341: 461–2.

Elias LL, Huebner A, Metherell LA, et al. Tall stature in familial glucocorticoid deficiency. *Clin Endocrinol* (Oxf) 2000; 53: 423–30.

Evans JF, Shen CL, Pollack S, et al. Adrenocorticotropin evokes transient elevations in intracellular free calcium ([Ca2 +]i) and increases basal [Ca2+]i in resting chondrocytes through a phospholipase C-dependent mechanism. *Endocrinology* 2005; 146: 3123–32.

Gabbitas B, Pash JM, Delany AM, et al. Cortisol inhibits the synthesis of insulin-like growth factor-binding protein-5 in bone cell cultures by transcriptional mechanisms. *J Biol Chem* 1996; 271: 9033–8.

Hughes CR, Guasti L, Meimaridou E,. MCM4 mutation causes adrenal failure, short stature, and natural killer cell deficiency in humans. *J Clin Invest* 2012; 122: 814–20.

Lacy DE, Nathavitharana KA, and Tarlow MJ. Neonatal hepatitis and congenital insensitivity to adrenocorticotropin (ACTH). *J Pediatr Gastroenterol Nutr* 1993; 17: 438–40.

Meimaridou E, Kowalczyk J, Guasti L, et al. Mutations in *NNT* encoding nicotinamide nucleotide transhydrogenase cause familial glucocorticoid deficiency. *Nat Genet* 2012; 44: 740–2.

Metherell LA, Chapple JP, Cooray S, et al. Mutations in MRAP, encoding a new interacting partner of the ACTH receptor, cause familial glucocorticoid deficiency type 2. *Nat Genet* 2005; 37: 166–70.

Metherell LA, Naville D, Halaby G, et al. Nonclassic lipoid congenital adrenal hyperplasia masquerading as familial glucocorticoid deficiency. *J Clin Endocrinol Metab* 2009; 94: 3865–71.

Raffin-Sanson ML, de Keyzer Y, and Bertagna X. Proopiomelanocortin, a polypeptide precursor with multiple functions: From physiology to pathological conditions. *Eur J Endocrinol* 2003; 149: 79–90.

Shepard TH, Landing BH, and Mason DG. Familial Addison's disease; case reports of two sisters with corticoid deficiency unassociated with hypoaldosteronism. AMA J Dis Child 1959; 97: 154–62.

Storr HL, Kind B, Parfitt DA, et al. Deficiency of ferritin heavy-chain nuclear import in triple a syndrome implies nuclear oxidative damage as the primary disease mechanism. *Mol Endocrinol* 2009; 23: 2086–94.

Turan S, Hughes C, Atay Z, et al. An atypical case of familial glucocorticoid deficiency without pigmentation caused by coexistent homozygous mutations in *MC2R* (T152K) and *MC1R* (R160W). *J Clin Endocrinol Metab* 2012; 97: 771–4.

16.5 Aldosterone resistance

Aldosterone is secreted in response to sodium deficiency or potassium loading via changes in plasma potassium levels, and to volume depletion in response to angiotensin 2. Its physiological role is to promote reabsorption of sodium ions and, with them, water, in mineralocorticoid-sensitive target tissues such as the kidneys, the distal colon, the sweat glands, and the salivary glands. In the early neonatal period—and more so in prematurity—renal regulation of fluid and electrolyte status is suboptimal, reflecting tubular immaturity and leading to partial and relative resistance to aldosterone in the first week(s) of life; this can be exacerbated by infection. In addition, transient aldosterone resistance can occur in adults in response to surgical procedures or drugs (see 'Differential diagnosis of renal PHA1'). Transient aldosterone resistance is termed 'secondary pseudohypoaldosteronism'.

In contrast with this transient state of relative aldosterone resistance is a rare genetic disease called pseudohypoaldosteronism type 1 (PHA1). In fact, this disease actually comprises three distinct genetic conditions which are caused by mutations in two key molecules in the epithelial response to aldosterone: the mineralocorticoid receptor and ENaC.

PHA1: Classification, diagnosis, aetiology, and treatment

The first report of the syndrome we now know as PHA1 was made by Cheek and Perry, physicians at the Royal Children's Hospital in Melbourne, in 1958; they described a male infant with severe salt wasting and failure to thrive in the absence of overt adrenal or renal disease. They suggested 'that the defect may be due to a refractory state on the part of the tubules to endogenous salt-active steroids or mineralocorticoids'. Today, three different congenital forms of PHA1 have been distinguished. The first is a mild form caused by a dominant mutation in the mineralocorticoid receptor; at the clinical level, the disorder appears confined to the kidney and is thus called renal PHA1. A second, more severe form of PHA1, caused by heterologous mutant mineralocorticoid receptors, has been recently reported; a third form, which is also severe and is more common than the second form, is caused by homozygous recessive mutations in ENaC.

Renal PHA1

Renal PHA1 commonly presents in neonates as salt wasting with excessive weight loss, and, on occasion, vomiting and/or dehydration. Laboratory findings include high levels of urinary potassium, plus high levels of plasma renin and aldosterone. Treatment is by rehydration and supplementary sodium, with the symptoms usually declining over early childhood as the renal tubules mature, with patients upregulating aldosterone secretion. High plasma aldosterone levels persist in the adults, despite plasma renin concentrations falling into the normal range. Treatment—which may involve using ion-exchange resins to lower plasma potassium concentrations—can usually be gradually discontinued from 18 to 36 months of age, providing the infants are on a normal (Western) sodium intake.

Differential diagnosis of renal PHA1

The conditions to be considered in the differential diagnosis for renal PHA1 fall into two categories: conditions which in some way may be mistaken for renal PHA1, and conditions associated with secondary pseudohypoaldosteronism. Among the latter are urinary tract infections or malformations, for which the predisposing factors (other than tubular immaturity, particularly in the premature) are not yet understood. Such secondary conditions in the neonate can be distinguished from the congenital form of PHA1 by urine culture and ultrasound imaging. In adults, a secondary form of pseudohypoaldosteronism may follow massive bowel resection (ileum and colon), reflecting gut loss of sodium. In patients treated with tacrolimus or cyclosporin, secondary pseudohypoaldosteronism probably reflects impaired intracellular signalling downstream of the mineralocorticoid receptor.

Conditions which may be mistaken for renal PHA1 are (most commonly) congenital adrenal hyperplasia, followed by aldosterone synthase deficiency and loss-of-function mutations in ROMK (Bartter's syndrome type 2; see also Chapter 6, Section 6.7). Congenital adrenal hyperplasia (see also Chapter 7, Section 7.5) due to a deficiency in 21-hydroxylase or 3-beta-hydroxysteroid dehydrogenase can be rapidly excluded on clinical and biochemical findings. A similar presentation—dehydration, hyponatraemia, hypokalaemia—may (very rarely) represent aldosterone synthase deficiency, with dehydration often more marked, consistent with animal-knockout data and distinguished by measurement of plasma aldosterone/urinary aldosterone levels. Finally, patients with neonatal Bartter's syndrome type 2 not uncommonly present with hyperkalaemia and elevated levels of plasma renin and aldosterone; these findings revert by the end of the first week of life (in term babies) to the more classic picture of hypokalaemia and metabolic acidosis.

Generalized PHA1

Generalized PHA1 presents as a far more serious and long-lasting phenotype than renal PHA1 does. In a recently described form due to recessive mutations in the gene encoding the mineralocorticoid receptor, a compound-heterozygote infant with two different mutant mineralocorticoid receptors presented with severe dehydration and hyperkalaemia, requiring high levels of administered sodium chloride, as for the more common form of generalized PHA1, which is caused by recessive mutations in the alpha, beta, or gamma subunit of ENaC. Despite the severity of the renal disorder, no obvious effects on the skin or lungs were noted, in contrast with the more common (ENaC-based) form. ENaC is not only the ultimate actor in the epithelial actions of aldosterone, but is also a major contributor to salt and water homeostasis in other organs. In addition to presenting with severe salt wasting via the kidneys, the colon, and sweat glands, patients may have evidence of rhinorrhoea, as the ENaC defect reduces their capacity to clear liquid from their nose; similarly, they may show a variety of pulmonary symptoms, again reflecting difficulty in clearing liquid from the airway.

Vigorous resuscitation and high-dose sodium supplementation (20–50 mEq/kg per day), often by tube, are required in infants, and constant attention to sodium supplementation and, if warranted, the use ion-exchange resins for hyperkalaemia is required in childhood. Early diagnosis is critical for survival, and constant vigilance is required during both childhood and adult life, with the administration of possibly reduced but still very high sodium intake (8–20 mg/kg per day) and the use of ion-exchange resins.

On a final, non-clinical note, the exaggerated dehydration in infants with aldosterone synthase deficiency highlights the difference between mineralocorticoid-receptor-knockout and aldosterone-synthase-knockout mice. The former die in the second week of extrauterine life through uncompensated sodium loss; however, the latter survive if given free access to drinking water, but lose ~1 g of body weight per day and die if allowed to drink only as much as heterozygous littermates.

Finally, for excellent, fully referenced reviews in this area, the author recommends the recent papers by Maria-Christina Zennaro and her colleagues and by Keiko Arai and George Chrousos.

Further reading

Arai K and Chrousos G. Aldosterone deficiency and resistance. Available at http://www.ncbi.nlm.nih.gov/books/NBK279079/ (accessed 17 Jan 2018).

Cheek PB and Perry JW. A salt-wasting syndrome in infancy. *Arch Dis Child* 1958; 33: 252–6.

Funder JW. (2006) Aldosterone and mineralocorticoid receptors: lessons from gene deletion. *Hypertension* 2006; 48: 1018–19.

Hubert EL, Teissier R, Fernandes-Rosa FL, et al. Mineralocorticoid receptor mutations and a severe recessive pseudohypoaldosteronism type 1. *J Am Soc Nephrol* 2001; 22: 1997–2003.

Zennaro M-C, Hubert EL, and Fernandes-Rosa FL. Aldosterone resistance: Structural and functional considerations, and new perspectives. *Mol Cell Endocrinol* 2012; 350: 206–15.

Chapter 17

Endocrinology of different age groups

Chapter contents

17.1 Adolescents in endocrinology

Endocrine care for adolescents

Young people access endocrine care with a range of concerns; some have presentations that are similar to those seen in older adults but some are unique to this age group. Differentiating what is normal physiology from pathology is important to prevent over-investigation, for example, in young people with delayed puberty, menstrual irregularity, or gynaecomastia. Engaging the young person presenting for the first time with signs and symptoms of PCOS, or the growing number of young people with long-term endocrine conditions, could influence outcomes in adult life.

Care and services should be designed to meet the needs of young people, with a focus on making services accessible, emphasizing confidentiality, improving the environment and staff training, offering joined-up working and advice on health issues, and involving young people in designing and evaluating the service. A developmental approach is essential. Different aspects of development can be affected by having an endocrine condition, which may lead to difficulty in having peer relationships, and social isolation; failing to achieve financial independence; and an increase in risky health behaviours and mental-health problems. These should be addressed as part of routine care.

Transition

Transition is just part of healthcare for this age group. Transition is a multifaceted active process that attends to the medical, psychosocial, and educational/vocational needs of adolescents as they move from child into adult care. Transfer to adult services is a single event within this process. This process should begin in early adolescence (11–13 years of age) and continue into young adulthood (23–25 years of age). This broad age range allows for a structured transition programme, adopting a flexible developmental approach with individuals progressing at their own speed. The process should actively encourage the young person to become independent in managing their condition and navigating their own healthcare. The challenge for paediatric and adult endocrine services is to provide continuity of staff, management, and information. Good links between the two services are essential, with an agreed transition policy and mechanisms to reduce the number of young people getting lost during the transfer. Components of care that have shown positive benefit in transition include patient education and skills training, transition care coordinators, joint and young adult clinics, and enhanced follow-up and out-of-hours support.

Consultation skills for adolescents

Healthcare professionals should adapt their consultation style screening for psychosocial issues and health behaviours. If appropriate, young people should be encouraged to be seen for part or all of the consultation without their parents, whilst recognizing and encouraging the parents' important role in supporting the young person. The HEEADDSS screening tool is useful at identifying issues that require attention (see Box 17.1). The tool should ideally be used if the young person is on their own, and going through the meaning and limitation of confidentiality is important.

Common clinical presentations of young people during adolescence

Delayed puberty or interrupted puberty

Puberty represents the biological change seen during adolescence and heralds the development of secondary sexual characteristics, the growth spurt, and, eventually,

---

Box 17.1 HEEADDSS: A psychosocial interview

H Home—Where do you live and who lives there with you? How do you get along with each member? Who could you go to if you needed help with a problem?

E Education & employment—What do you like about school/work? What are you good and not good at? How do you get along with teachers and other students/work colleagues? Inquire about bullying. What are your future plans?

E Exercise & eating incl body image—Are you happy with your weight? If you were going to lose weight how would you do it?

A Activities & peers—What sort of things do you do in your spare time? Are most of your friends from school/work? Do you have one best friend, a few friends or lots of friends?

D Drugs incl smoking & alcohol—Many young people at your age are starting to experiment with cigarettes or alcohol. Have you or your friends tried these or other drugs? How do you pay for them? Do any members of your family smoke or drink?

D Depression incl suicide -What sort of things do you do if you are feeling sad/angry/hurt? Some people who feel really down often feel like hurting themselves or even killing themselves. Have you ever felt this way? Have you ever tried to hurt yourself?

S Sexuality & sexual health- Some young people are getting involved in sexual relationships. Have you had a sexual experience with a boy or girl or both? Inquire about contraception and avoidance of sexually transmitted infections.

S Sleep—Inquire about sleep. Adolescents who are depressed and anxious have difficulty falling asleep.

S Safety—Inquire about driving and internet safety.

fertility. Puberty normally starts between the ages of 8 and 13 in girls, with breast development, advancing to menarche by the age of 16. In boys, puberty starts between 9 and 15 with testicular enlargement (≥4 mL; see Figure 17.1).

Delayed or interrupted puberty is defined as follows:

- females: no signs of breast development by the age of 13, or no periods by the age of 15
- males: no signs of testicular enlargement (<4 mL) by the age of 14

Delayed puberty is more frequently seen in males. The minority will have evidence of hypergonadotrophic hypogonadism, the prevalence of which is estimated to be at 13%. The remainder have impaired secretion and/or action of hypothalamic GnRH. The majority of these patients will have constitutional delay. History and examination need to look for indications of the following causes of hypogonadotrophic hypogonadism:

- functional causes (chronic illness, medication, excessive exercise, malnutrition, or stress)
- pathology-related causes (hypothalamic and pituitary tumours, especially craniopharyngiomas)

- genetic causes (congenital abnormalities (indicated by midline defects, microphallus, cryptorchidism, cleft lip/palate, scoliosis), anosmia (Kalmann's syndrome))

A positive family history is relevant in constitutional delay and congenital GnRH deficiency, which has a significant genetic basis, often with an autosomal-dominant inheritance pattern.

Investigation depends on history and examination and should be tailored accordingly. Imaging of the hypothalamic pituitary axis is only required if history, examination, and investigations suggest a central lesion or if other symptoms/signs such as anosmia need further exploration. Distinguishing constitutional delay from hypogonadotrophic hypogonadism and its causes is challenging, particularly as 10%–15% of adolescents with well-documented isolated hypogonadotrophic hypogonadism undergo spontaneous reversal. A trial of low-dose testosterone (50 mg) monthly for 3–6 months with reassessment of testicular volumes is a pragmatic approach. The psychological and social impact of having delayed puberty, particularly in boys, needs to be recognized and addressed.

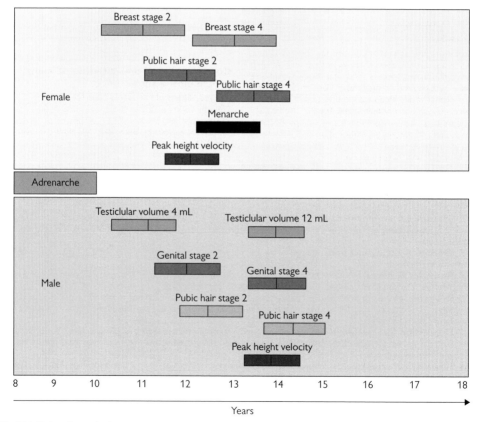

Fig 17.1 Timing of normal puberty.
Reprinted from *The Lancet*, Volume 369, Patton G. C., Viner, R., Pubertal transitions in health, pp. 1130–1139, Copyright (2007), with permission from Elsevier.

Abnormal uterine bleeding in adolescence

During the first 2 years after menarche, there is considerable cycle variability due to anovulatory cycles. In the first year, 50% of cycles are anovulatory, with 80% of cycles occurring within 21–45 days and last 2–7 days. Abnormal uterine bleeding is therefore defined in adolescence as:

- a period of bleeding with a duration >7 days
- a period of bleeding with a flow greater than 80 mL/cycle (more than six pads/tampons a day)
- periods of bleeding that occur more frequently than every 21 days (19 days if first year after menarche) or less frequently than every 45 days (or 90/60 days if first/second year after menarche)
- intermenstrual bleeding or post-coital bleeding

If abnormal uterine bleeding is identified, history, examination, and appropriate investigations should be performed. Excluding pregnancy and enquiring about sexual history and counselling about sexual health are essential. When alternative diagnoses have been excluded, diagnosis of abnormal uterine bleeding due to anovulatory cycles can be made and managed appropriately.

PCOS in adolescence

Symptoms and signs of PCOS frequently begin in adolescence; however, the anovulatory cycles following menarche are just one reason why diagnosing PCOS in adolescence is challenging. Experts have cautioned against over-diagnosing the condition in this age group and a recent collaboration have suggested that the following two criteria should be present before considering a diagnosis of PCOS:

- abnormal uterine bleeding as in periods of bleeding that occur more frequently than every 21 days (19 days if first year after menarche) or less frequently than every 45 days (or 90/60 days if first/second year after menarche) or primary or secondary amenorrhoea
- moderate-severe hirsutism or acne *or* evidence of biochemical hyperandrogenaemia on measuring serum testosterone and SHBG, with calculation of free androgen index, androstenedione, and DHEAS

The psychological and social impact of having PCOS needs to be recognized and addressed. The approach to young people with PCOS depends on presentation and concerns and includes identifying opportunities to discuss lifestyle in young people who are normal weight as well as those who are overweight or obese, to ameliorate the long-term consequences associated with the condition of reduced fertility and type 2 diabetes; recognizing the burden of hirsutism and offering options for management; discussing the importance of contraception whilst on anti-androgens; and reassuring young people about future fertility options.

Gynaecomastia in adolescence

Gynaecomastia is common in adolescence (40%–69%) due to an imbalance of estradiol and testosterone production during puberty. Pubertal gynaecomastia is usually most obvious between 13 and 14 years of age and resolves by the age of 17, although in some instances may persist. Persistent pubertal gynaecomastia accounts for 25% of gynaecomastia presenting in adulthood. Reassurance is often all that is required.

Management of young people with long-term endocrine conditions during adolescence

The completion of puberty and end of linear growth is an important time for young people with a long-term endocrine condition. By this time, young people, if able, should be close to achieving the following:

- being confident in their knowledge about their condition, medication, and issues in adult life
- looking after their own medication and organizing and collecting prescriptions
- being confident enough to be seen on their own in clinic and to contact the clinic independently
- knowing about resources that can offer support and provide information about generic health issues
- having a plan for further education and/or employment
- knowing the plan for their endocrinology care as an adult

This is also the time to reassess the young person and their condition with a focus on health issues relevant to adulthood (reproductive, cardiovascular, and bone health). Medication changes can be considered to those more frequently used in adulthood but may be seen as more desirable to the young person. For information about young people with congenital adrenal hyperplasia and Turner syndrome, see Chapter 7, Section 7.5 and 7.8.

Management of young people with hypopituitarism and growth-hormone deficiency

Young people with childhood-onset growth-hormone deficiency that is persistent have a deficit in muscle and bone mass. Growth-hormone replacement reduces this deficit and, in addition, for some young people, improves energy levels/quality of life, one of the primary indications for growth-hormone replacement in adult life. Young people treated with growth-hormone replacement for growth-hormone deficiency during childhood require reassessment when growth rate fall to <2 cm/year. This is necessary, as a high percentage of young people with idiopathic growth-hormone replacement will retest as normal and could be discharged. Some patient groups who are at risk of evolving pituitary dysfunction,

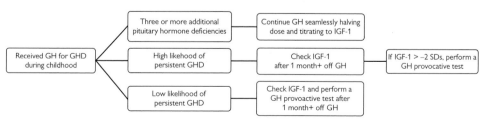

Fig 17.2 Reassessment of growth-hormone status in adolescence; GH, growth hormone; GHD, growth-hormone deficiency; SD, standard deviation.

for example those who have undergone radiation treatment, those with structural abnormalities affecting the pituitary gland, and those with other pituitary hormone deficiencies, should not be discharged, even if found to be normal at reassessment.

Reassessment of growth-hormone status
Reassessment strategies (see Figure 17.2) are based on whether the young person has three or more additional pituitary hormone deficiencies or whether they have a high or low likelihood of growth-hormone deficiency. Peak growth-hormone level during provocative testing in childhood should also be considered.

High likelihood of persistent growth-hormone deficiency
Signs that there is a high likelihood of persistent growth-hormone deficiency are as follows:
- for congenital/idiopathic growth-hormone deficiency:
  - a defined genetic mutation
  - septo-optic dysplasia and other midline defects
  - structural abnormalities that are located in the hypothalamo-pituitary axis and affect positioning of the posterior pituitary gland or the pituitary stalk or are associated with three or more pituitary hormone deficits
- for acquired growth-hormone deficiency:
  - a destructive lesion affecting the hypothalamo-pituitary axis
  - cranial irradiation (high dose)

Low likelihood of persistent growth-hormone deficiency
Signs that there is a low likelihood of persistent growth-hormone deficiency are as follows:
- for idiopathic growth-hormone deficiency: isolated growth-hormone deficiency or growth-hormone deficiency with two or less pituitary hormone deficits in the absence of structural abnormalities located in the hypothalamo-pituitary axis and affecting positioning of the posterior pituitary gland or the pituitary stalk
- for acquired growth-hormone deficiency: cranial irradiation (low dose)

Reinitiation of growth-hormone replacement
In those with persistent growth-hormone deficiency (IGF-1 < −2 standard deviations, and/or peak growth hormone <6 μg/L (for ITT)), growth-hormone replacement should be offered to the young person and restarted at the lower dose of 0.2–0.3 mg, with titration to IGF-1 levels.

Summary
- Care for adolescents in endocrinology should include a developmental approach focusing on psychosocial and educational and vocational outcomes as well as medical; transition is part of this.
- Transition should begin in early adolescence and, to be successful, requires close working between paediatric and adult endocrine teams.
- Knowledge of normal physiology in adolescence relating to puberty and the menstrual cycle allows tailoring of investigations and appropriate management.
- Young people with long-term endocrine conditions require a change of focus in their care in late adolescence and start screening for issues relevant in adult life.

Further reading
Clayton PE, Cuneo RC, Juul A, et al. Consensus statement on the management of the GH-treated adolescent in the transition to adult care. *Eur J Endocrinol* 2005; 152: 165–70.

Crowley R, Wolfe I, Lock K, et al. Improving the transition between paediatric and adult healthcare: A systematic review. *Arch Dis Child* 2011; 96: 548–53.

Derbyshire Children and Young People's Health Promotion Programme. You're Welcome Quality Criteria: Young people friendly health services. Available at http://www.youngpeopleshealth.org.uk/yourewelcome/ (accessed 17 Jan 2018).

Goldenring JM and Rosen DS. Getting into adolescent heads: An essential update. *Contemp Pediatr* 2004; 21: 64–90.

Peacock A, Alvi NS, and Mushtaq T. Period problems: Disorders of menstruation in adolescents. *Arch Dis Child* 2012; 97: 554–60.

Rosenfield RL. The diagnosis of polycystic ovary syndrome in adolescents. *Pediatrics [Internet]* 2015; 136(6): 1154–65. Available from: http://www.ncbi.nlm.nih.gov/pubmed/26598450%5Cnhttp://pediatrics.aappublications.org/cgi/doi/10.1542/peds.2015-1430.

Wales JK. Disorders pubertal development. *Arch Dis Child Educ Pract Ed* 2012; 97: 9–16.

17.2 Endocrinology and ageing

Introduction

As individuals age, endocrine changes result in a decline in endocrine function, involving the responsiveness of tissues as well as reduced hormone secretion from peripheral glands. This is coupled with modifications in the central mechanisms controlling the temporal organization of hormone release, with a dampening of circadian hormonal and non-hormonal rhythms. In evaluating the changes that occur in endocrine function, it is important to distinguish the real effects of ageing on endocrine mechanisms from any confounding factors due to the higher prevalence of age-related illness.

Growth hormone–IGF-1 axis

With ageing, numerous studies have shown that growth-hormone secretion and serum growth-hormone concentrations fall, both basally and in response to stimuli, and this is paralleled by a decline in IGF-1. Growth-hormone production and IGF-1 concentrations decline by more than 50% in healthy older adults. The progressive decline in growth-hormone secretion has been termed the 'somatopause'. In older subjects, the decrease in growth-hormone secretion is known to cause a reduction of protein synthesis, a decrease in lean body and bone mass, and a decline in immune function.

The neuroendocrine mechanisms of the somatopause are uncertain. Early studies suggesting senescent changes in the pituitary have not been supported by the observations that there is no decrease in the number of pituitary somatotroph cells or that exogenous GHRH or GHRH peptide analogues are able to rejuvenate growth-hormone output and plasma IGF-1 levels in older individuals. Consequently, attention has shifted to potential alterations of the hypothalamic regulation of growth-hormone secretion, with data suggesting that an age-dependent decrease in endogenous hypothalamic GHRH output contributes to the age-associated decline in levels of growth hormone.

Low physical fitness and higher adiposity in older individuals also contributes to decreased secretion of growth hormone, although the mechanisms underlying these observations are not clear. Low IGF-1 levels reflect decreased growth-hormone secretion rather than a loss of hepatic responsiveness to growth hormone, as circulating IGF-1 levels increase similarly in young and old men after exogenous administration of either growth hormone or GHRH.

In younger adults who are deficient in growth hormone, alterations in body composition, including physical performance, psychological well-being, and substrate metabolism, resemble those seen in the ageing phenotype. These features are improved by long-term hormone replacement with recombinant human growth hormone. This led to the suggestion that the elderly have genuine growth-hormone deficiency and, by implication, would benefit from growth-hormone treatment.

There are many unanswered questions about the use of growth hormone in older individuals and the effects on lean body mass, adipose tissue, muscle strength, exercise endurance, or quality of life. The initial enthusiasm for the potential benefits of growth-hormone replacement in aged individuals has been severely dampened by its known adverse side effects, including arthralgia, carpal tunnel syndrome, oedema, and hyperglycaemia. There are also particular concerns over the links between the growth hormone–IGF-1 axis and the development of cancer in the normal population.

Currently, there is no 'magic pill' that reverses the process of ageing, and growth-hormone therapy for 'anti-ageing' has currently not been proved to be effective.

Menopause

By the age of 40, ovulation frequency decreases, and reproductive ovarian function ceases within the next 15 years (see also Chapter 7, Section 7.9). Ovarian follicles function less well during this period, with serum estradiol concentrations being lower and FSH concentrations higher than in younger women. Levels of LH are unchanged. Eventually, follicular activity ceases, oestrogen concentrations fall to postmenopausal values, and LH and FSH levels rise above premenopausal concentrations. The changes in these serum concentrations result in a series of further changes, including an increased risk of cardiovascular events, rapid loss of skeletal mass, vasomotor instability, psychological symptoms, and atrophy of oestrogen-responsive tissue.

The risk of cardiovascular disease in premenopausal women is lower than in men but, during the postmenopausal period, the risk increases and is equal to that seen in males of equivalent age and risk-factor profile. Prior to this increase in risk, serum concentrations of atherogenic lipids deteriorate. The decrease in cardioprotective HDL is thought to be one of the causes of increased coronary heart disease, myocardial infarction, and stroke in postmenopausal women.

At the time of menopause, there is rapid loss of bone, due to oestrogen withdrawal. This takes place within the background of age-related bone loss that begins in the fourth decade of life. In the perimenopausal period, women lose 5%–15% of their bone mass, with 80% of this loss being trabecular bone, which is more metabolically active than cortical bone. There is a modest rise in serum calcium without any change in PTH, indicating a possible change in the PTH set point; this change is reversed by hormone action. There is also a fall in the oestrogen-dependent components of intestinal calcium absorption and renal tubular reabsorption of calcium. The associated high bone resorption with normal PTH also suggests an increased sensitivity of bone to PTH. There is no change in the levels of serum 1,25-vitamin D.

During the immediate menopausal period, when the rate of bone loss is greatest, oestrogen replacement maintains bone mass and reduces fracture risk.

Andropause

For many years, there was much debate as to whether serum total testosterone levels were truly lower in healthy older men, or whether this decline was attributable to the ageing process, with the observed decline occurring as a result of confounding effects due to chronic illness and medications. However, from cross-sectional and longitudinal studies, there is now agreement that in healthy men there is a gradual but progressive age-dependent decline in testosterone levels, termed 'andropause'. This is more marked for free testosterone than for total testosterone, due to an age-associated increase of SHBG levels.

The age-related decline in testosterone level does not start at any specific point in older subjects and it varies from modest to severe, which is different from the sharp reduction of oestrogen production in females at the menopause. The decline in serum testosterone concentrations is mainly due to decreased production rates in older men and this is a result of abnormalities at all levels of the hypothalamo-pituitary–testicular axis. In longitudinal studies, serum LH and FSH levels show an age-related increase. However, serum LH concentrations often do not reciprocate the decline in testosterone with age. The testosterone response to LH and hCG decreases with ageing, and the circadian rhythm of plasma testosterone secretion, with higher levels in the morning than in the evening, is generally lost in older men.

The clinical features associated with reduced testosterone levels in ageing men include increased fat mass, loss of muscle and bone mass, fatigue, depression, anaemia, poor libido, erectile deficiency, insulin resistance, and higher cardiovascular risk.

As there is a certain proportion of middle-aged and older men with serum total testosterone levels below the reference range for young adult males, there is a suggestion that supplementing testosterone in older men with low testosterone levels into a range that is mid-normal for healthy, young men may prevent or reverse the effects of ageing. Several clinical studies have been undertaken to determine whether testosterone supplementation in ageing is beneficial. Despite trials examining various parameters, including body composition, muscle strength, bone density, metabolism, and lipid profile, there is still no consensus as to whether androgen treatment is beneficial to men over the age of 50. Much of the uncertainty is due to the brief duration of many of the protocols, such that the effects of prolonged testosterone replacement are not clear.

The recently reported testosterone trials aimed to determine whether testosterone is effective in older with lower testosterone men to improve parameters including sexual function (significantly improved), physical function (improved), and vitality (reduced depressive symptoms). However, adverse effects, including increased haematocrit and PSA, must be carefully monitored.

DHEA

There has been much debate on the anti-ageing properties of DHEA and its potential as a 'hormone of youth'. Unlike the relatively unaffected cortisol biosynthesis, the major age-related change in the human adrenal cortex is a striking decrease in the biosynthesis of DHEA(S). The blood level of DHEA, most of which is present in the sulphated form DHEAS, peaks at approximately 20 years of age and declines rapidly and markedly after the age of 25.

By the age of 80, patients have DHEA levels 10%–20% of those of younger counterparts. The physiological consequences of a decline in DHEA with age are not fully understood. Many have speculated that administration of DHEA may reverse ageing effects, and there is widespread commercial availability of DHEA outside the regular pharmaceutical networks, without adequate scientific evidence. A number of randomized trials assessing the effect of oral DHEA in otherwise healthy older subjects have not shown any clear clinical benefits.

Fluid and electrolyte homeostasis

Hyponatraemia is common (appearing by the age of 75 in the healthy ageing population), due to lower renin and aldosterone levels, reduced renal sensitivity to aldosterone, increased vasopressin secretion in response to an osmotic stimulus, and the concomitant effect of medication.

Adrenal function

Cortisol secretion in ageing individuals is similar to that found in younger persons.

Thyroid function

In ageing individuals, TSH and T4 levels are unchanged; however, there is an increased prevalence of thyroid autoantibodies, and hypo-/hyperthyroidism may present atypically. Sick euthyroid syndrome is more common. Anaplastic thyroid cancer sarcoma and primary lymphoma are more common in the elderly.

Conclusion

Complex changes occurring with ageing are seen in many endocrine systems and occur independently of factors associated with the higher prevalence of age-related illnesses. Endocrine deficiencies in older individuals include a decrease in the peripheral levels of oestrogen and testosterone, with an increase in LH, FSH, and SHBG. In addition, there is a decline in serum concentrations of growth hormone, IGF-1, and DHEA(S). The clinical significance of these deficiencies with age is variable and is still being evaluated.

For each endocrine system, there have been many studies trying to reverse the effects of ageing by restoring the serum hormonal levels of older individuals back into 'younger ranges'. However, it is currently unclear whether treatment of many of these age-related changes is ultimately beneficial. So far, research has not found the 'magic pill' to reverse the process of ageing, and the quest for a 'hormone of youth' still carries on.

Further reading

Araujo AB and Wittert GA. Endocrinology of the aging male. *Best Pract Res Clin Endocrinol Metab* 2011; 25: 303–19.

Chahal HS and Drake WM. The endocrine system and ageing. *J Pathol* 2007; 211: 173–80.

Di Somma C, Brunelli V, Savanelli MC, et al. Somatopause: State of the art. *Minerva Endocrinol* 2011; 36: 243–55.

Snyderr PJ. Effects of testosterone treatment in older men. *New Engl J Med* 2016; 374: 611–24.

Endocrine investigation, nursing, and dietetics

Chapter contents

18.1 Laboratory investigations in endocrine disorders

Introduction

The diagnosis and monitoring of endocrine disorders depend largely on measurements of circulating hormones and growth factors (see also Chapter 1, Sections 1.2–1.4). Although measuring plasma hormone concentrations at a single time point is often adequate, dynamic function tests are needed when the hormone under investigation is secreted episodically. Dynamic tests usually consist of trying to suppress hormones when excess secretion is suspected, or stimulating secretion when hormone deficiency is suspected. It is essential that blood and/or urine specimens are collected appropriately, and the method used for collection will depend on the particular assay being performed (see Tables 18.1 and 18.2).

Methods of investigation

The most popular method for measuring hormones is the immunoassay, but other techniques, such as mass spectrometry interfaced with liquid or gas chromatography, are becoming more common. Most immunoassays use either competitive binding or the immunometric principle. In competitive-binding assays, the molecule of interest (the analyte) in the specimen and a small amount of labelled analyte compete for a limited amount of binder (usually an antibody). Immunometric assays use excess antibody to capture the analyte on a solid surface, and then quantify the amount of bound analyte, usually by a labelled second antibody to a different epitope of the analyte.

Immunological methods are prone to interference, and results should be interpreted taking this into

Table 18.1 Blood tests

Analyte	Tube(s)	Stability	Patient preparation	Special remarks
ACTH	Iced EDTA (plastic)	Unstable	No special requirements	Only useful in delineating the aetiology of hyper-/ hypocortisolism
TSH	Serum, or lithium heparin	Stable	No special requirements	—
Gonadotrophins (LH, FSH)	Serum	Stable	No special requirements	—
Growth hormone	Serum, or lithium heparin	Stable	As required by dynamic test protocols	Only useful as part of a dynamic test
Prolactin	Serum	Stable	Collect 3–4 hours after patient has awakened	—
Copeptin	Serum or plasma	Stable	Use in dynamic function tests	Useful in dynamic tests to diagnose diabetes insipidus
Cortisol	Serum	Stable	Collected at 08:00–09:00 h or as required by dynamic test protocols	Many synthetic corticosteroids cross-react (apart from dexamethasone)
				Oestrogens can give falsely high values because of increase in cortisol-binding globulin
				Single measurement of little value
Free thyroxine and free tri-iodothyronine	Serum	Stable	No special requirements	—
Estradiol	Serum	Stable	No special requirements	Time of sampling with reference to the menstrual cycle is important for interpretation
Progesterone	Serum	Stable	No special requirements	—
Total testosterone	Serum	Stable	No special requirements	Sample at 09:00 h
IGF-1	Serum, or lithium heparin	Stable	No special requirements	Reference interval is highly age and sex dependent
Parathyroid hormone	EDTA	Stable	No special requirements	—
Aldosterone	Serum, lithium heparin, or EDTA	Stable	Patient should be upright for at least 2 hours prior to an ambulatory specimen	—
			Biological interference by many drugs, including diuretics, beta blockers, angiotensin receptor blockers, and ACE inhibitors	
Renin (mass or activity assay)	EDTA, or lithium heparin	Unstable	Patient should be upright for at least 2 hours prior to an ambulatory specimen	Should be separated immediately and frozen
			Biological interferences occur with many drugs, including diuretics, beta blockers, angiotensin receptor blockers, and ACE inhibitors	

(continued)

Table 18.1 Continued

Analyte	Tube(s)	Stability	Patient preparation	Special remarks
DHEAS	Serum or EDTA	Stable	No special requirements	—
Androstenedione	Serum	Stable	No special requirements	—
Sex hormone-binding globulin	Serum	Stable	No special requirements	—
Insulin	Serum, or lithium heparin	Stable	Fasting	Need simultaneous specimen for glucose to demonstrate hypoglycaemia
C-peptide	Serum, or lithium heparin	Stable	Fasting	Need simultaneous specimen for glucose to demonstrate hypoglycaemia
Calcitonin	Serum, or lithium heparin	Unstable	—	Needs to separated and frozen within 30 minutes
17-Hydroxyprogesterone	Serum	Stable	Early morning specimens preferred	—
P1NP	Serum, or lithium heparin	Stable	No special requirements	Need to be separated immediately and frozen
Collagen carboxy-terminal peptide	Plasma (EDTA)	Stable	No special requirements	—
Collagen telopeptides and pyridinium crosslinks	Serum	Stable	—	Freeze separated serum
Osteocalcin	Serum	Stable	No special requirements	Collect on ice, separate within 1 hour, and freeze
25-Hydroxyvitamin D	Serum	Stable	No special requirements	Protect from light
1,25-Hydroxyvitamin D	Serum	Stable	No special requirements	Protect from light
Gut hormone profile	EDTA	Unstable	Fasting Abstain from H2-receptor blockers for 3 days and proton-pump inhibitors for 2 weeks	Needs to be separated immediately and frozen
Catecholamines	EDTA, or lithium heparin	Stable	Discontinue drugs that may cause catecholamine release, for 3–7 days Plasma catecholamine levels can be increased by MAO inhibitors, L-DOPA, methyldopa, and propranolol and decreased by clonidine Avoid tobacco and caffeinated drinks for at least 4 hours before collection	Chill specimens immediately in iced water, and separate within 30 minutes; store frozen
Metanephrines	EDTA	Stable	Fasting for at least 4 hours	Discontinue interfering drugs for at least 1 week (tricyclic antidepressants, phenoxybenzamine, MOA inhibitors)
Serotonin	EDTA (whole blood)	Unstable	—	Appropriate when normal or borderline increases in 5-HIAA are found in patients with clinical evidence of carcinoid syndrome
Chromogranin A	EDTA	Stable	Discontinue proton-pump inhibitors for 2 weeks	—
BNP	EDTA	Stable	No special requirements	—
Lipid profile	Serum, or lithium heparin	Stable	Fasting ≥12 hours	Heparin may cause an artefactual reduction in triglycerides by activating lipases
Haemoglobin A1c	EDTA whole blood	Stable	No special requirements	Haemoglobinopathies can cause false elevations or reductions Affected by red-cell lifetime: reduced in haemolytic anaemia, and elevated in iron-deficiency anaemia

Abbreviations: 5-HIAA, 5-hydroxyindoleacetic acid; ACE, angiotensin-converting enzyme; ACTH, adrenocorticotrophic hormone; BNP, brain natriuretic peptide; DHEAS, dehydroepiandrosterone sulphate; EDTA, ethylenediamine tetra-acetic acid; FSH, follicle-stimulating hormone; IGF-1, insulin-like growth factor 1; LH, luteinizing hormone; MAO, monoamine oxidase; P1NP; procollagen type 1 N-terminal propeptide; TSH, thyroid-stimulating hormone.

Table 18.2 Urine investigations

Analyte	Bottle	Stability	Patient preparation	Special remarks
Free cortisol	Plain	Stable	24-Hour collection preferred	—
			Discontinue all steroid-containing drugs at least 1 week before testing	
Catecholamines	Acid	—	24-Hour collection preferred	Interferences from many antihypertensive drugs
			Discontinue all interfering drugs at least 1 week before testing	
Metanephrines	Plain	Stable	Spot or 24-Hour collection	—
5-HIAA	Acid	—	Spot Random or 24-hour collection	Specimen must be protected from light and stored frozen prior to analysis
			Abstain from drugs and dietary sources for 72 hours	

Abbreviations: 5-HIAA, 5-hydroxyindoleacetic acid.

account. Interference may lead to falsely low or high values. Autoantibodies, such as rheumatoid factors, can cause non-specific interference. Human anti-mouse antibodies (HAMAs) can be problematic when monoclonal antibodies are used in the assay. Heterophile antibodies are antibodies to exogenous antigens and may cross-react with endogenous antigens. Information on clinical conditions that can give rise to these antibodies (e.g. the presence of autoimmune disease; exposure to animal antibodies (in animal workers); monoclonal antibody therapy) is important when interpreting results. These effects can be counteracted by precipitating immunoglobulins using polyethylene glycol, by adsorbing interfering antibodies onto the surface of a reaction tube, or by assaying the specimen after dilution. Assays that are particularly affected included prolactin and thyroid hormones (TSH, FT4).

Cross-reacting substances may cause unreliable results due to their structural similarity to the analyte being measured (e.g. prednisolone in a cortisol assay).

When two antibodies to different parts of a molecule are used in an assay, the assay may give a falsely low result if the molecule is present at a very high concentration, because some molecules are bound by only one of the antibodies. This is called the 'high-dose hook effect'. This can be seen when measuring analytes such as ferritin, alpha-fetoprotein, and hCG, all of which can occur at very high concentrations in certain pathological conditions. This type of interference can be countered by assaying the specimen after dilution.

Assays for free hormones often use so-called analogues to stop the assay from measuring bound hormone. The only true method for measuring free hormones is by equilibrium dialysis, where the free hormone diffuses across a membrane and is measured in the dialysate.

Mass spectrometric methods use a separation step to remove interfering molecules and then ionize the molecule and guide it onto a detector, so that the number of such molecules can be quantified by using a magnetic field. The ratio of mass to charge is characteristic of the molecule. The detector can be tuned to detect particles with a range of mass-to-charge ratios. Potentially, this method offers improved analytical sensitivity, accuracy, and speed, compared to other methods, and can also determine the concentration of multiple hormones or multiple species of a given hormone at the same time.

Interpreting the results of measurements using this technique may be difficult. For instance, some peptide hormones are subject to post-translational processing, such as the removal of small parts of the hormone, or the addition of carbohydrates such as glucose. When measured by antibody methods, the antibodies employed in the assay may bind all of these molecules more or less equally. Mass spectrometry may give separate peaks for all the different species of the molecule of interest, and this may lead to confusing results. For example, immunoassays for UFC frequently measure several different molecules, whereas mass spectrometry methods are much more specific, and will, in general, give lower results. Another example is measurement of 25-hydroxyvitamin D: many immunoassays for 25-hydroxyvitamin D are not equally sensitive for the D3 and the D2 isomers, whereas, with mass spectrometry, it is possible to quantify both of these hormones.

The most important advice is to question results that do not fit with the patient's clinical condition!

18.2 The role of the endocrine specialist nurse

Introduction

The role of the adult endocrine nurse is highly specialized and has changed over recent years in response to local needs. It is recognized that some nurses focus on one specific disease area, whereas others care for patients with a whole range of endocrine disorders. The Society for Endocrinology has a dedicated nurse committee. The committee is made up of highly experienced endocrine nurses who provide advice and support for nurses in order that they may develop their roles within a dynamic and rapidly advancing area of medicine. The committee has written a competency framework for adult endocrine nursing, to help individual nurses, who are new to the specialty, to develop competencies relevant to their area of work.

The committee organizes dedicated sessions for nurses at the society's annual British Endocrine meeting and also organizes an annual endocrine nurse update.

Details of these meetings can be found on the society's website, http://www.endocrinology.org.

Dynamic tests

Named diagnostic investigations can be found in Chapter 3, Section 3.4.

General preparation of patients prior to dynamic tests should include the following:

- before any patient undergoes dynamic testing, it is imperative that he or she is properly prepared, to ensure the test can be performed safely and reliably
- the patient must fully understand the reason for a specific test or tests and what the test involves in order to provide informed consent; the patient may need to stop certain medication which would interfere with the test (e.g. oral oestrogen therapy must be stopped if cortisol levels are to be assessed)

When booking an appointment for a patient to attend for testing, it is important to check the following:

- the medication he or she is taking does not interfere with the test
- he or she fulfils the testing criteria
- if a test requires specific baseline blood tests or ECG to ensure patient safety, he or she should be taken within 3 months of the test (with the exception of potassium levels in the assessment of Conn's syndrome, where a potassium level ≥ 3 mEq/L must be proved biochemically as near to the test date as possible)

It is good practice to send an information sheet outlining the test and the preparation required together with the appointment date.

The day of the test

- On the day of the test, the patient must have the test fully explained by the endocrine specialist nurse, who must outline risks and contraindications, ensuring the patient is able to make a fully informed consent.
- Consent must be obtained before any patient proceeds to testing.
- Each test has a precise protocol which must be adhered to, but it is worth mentioning that, before patients are discharged, there are certain discharge criteria which must not be overlooked (e.g. in Oxford, following an ITT, it is our practice for the patient to stay for 2 hours

on completion of the test; this ensures the patient has lunch, which will promote a normal serum glucose, and is rested following the stress of the procedure).

To ensure patient safety and a reliable interpretation of the results, the endocrine specialist nurse must be familiar with not only the test protocol but also the preparation and discharge criteria and any potential complications or common side effects (e.g. flushing, nausea).

Drug treatment: The role of the endocrine specialist nurse in the education of the patient, the general practitioner, and the practice nurse

Somatostatin-analogue treatment

Patients requiring treatment with a somatostatin analogue are referred by the endocrine doctor to one of the endocrine specialist nurses, who will manage the care pathway, supporting the patient and their family or carers, to ensure a smooth transition onto treatment. The patient will attend the unit for a growth-hormone day curve followed by administration of the first injection (supplied free of charge by the drug company). All subsequent injections are administered at the GP surgery by the practice nurse or by a nurse from the pharmaceutical company.

The endocrine specialist nurse will monitor the patient closely until the patient is stabilized on treatment, after which the care will be managed by doctors in the outpatient setting.

The two pharmaceutical companies that make somatostatin-analogue medication offer a homecare service, whose staff attend the GP surgery to support the practice nurse. This service is essential when the patient lives a long way from the specialist centre.

Treatment for growth-hormone deficiency

Patients who are diagnosed with growth-hormone deficiency are managed and supported in the same way as patients requiring treatment with somatostatin analogues. The endocrine specialist nurse will manage their care pathway until stabilization is reached.

As growth hormone is self-administered the patient will be supported to ensure they are confident and competent to self-inject.

Travel advice is very important for patients receiving growth hormone, as the injection needs to be stored at 2–8 °C. It may be necessary to request pre-filled syringes to cover a holiday period, to avoid the need for cold storage. An up-to-date cover letter from the hospital will ensure patients' ease of passage through customs when they are carrying medication, syringes, and needles.

Patient education and support

The Pituitary Foundation provides expert, up-to-date information on all aspects of pituitary conditions, such as:

- the pituitary gland
- pituitary surgery and radiotherapy
- acromegaly
- Cushing's syndrome

They have an extensive website which provides many educational publications.

*Patients requiring long-term steroid replacement therapy
(e.g. for Addison's disease)*
Education is essential for successful steroid management.
Patients should be given the opportunity to attend steroid
replacement study sessions covering the following:
- why steroids are required
- how steroids work
- what to do if patients become ill
- the emergency steroid pack, and how to administer the
  emergency steroid injection

The emergency steroid pack
The contents of an emergency steroid pack are as follows:
- a 100 mg vial hydrocortisone
- a 2 mL syringe
- a blue needle (23 gauge)
- cotton wool
- a plaster

NB: always check the expiry date of the hydrocortisone.
   The procedure for the administration of the emergency steroid injection is as follows:
1. Place the blue needle on the end of the syringe.
2. Snap off the top of the vial and draw up the hydrocortisone liquid into the syringe.
3. Use the upper outer quadrant of a buttock. (Patients
   or their friends or relatives, following instruction, are
   advised to administer the injection in the leg.)
4. Insert the needle at 90° to the skin.
5. Inject the solution.
6. Remove the needle; press the site of injection with
   cotton wool and then cover it with a plaster.

   As with growth hormone, patients carrying an emergency pack will need an up-to-date cover letter from the
hospital when they are travelling abroad. In addition, patients should be advised to carry an up-to-date steroid
card and wear a medical identification emblem (e.g. a
necklace, bracelet, or watch).

   Some centres in the UK have links with all the area ambulance services covering the UK and offer patients the
opportunity to register their details with their local ambulance service. Patients, if agreeable, are requested to
fill in the paperwork for their specific ambulance service
and to sign and date their entry, together with their endocrine doctor and endocrine specialist nurse. The information is then sent to the appropriate ambulance service
and uploaded into the ambulance service's database. This
gives the paramedic the information and authority to administer the injection of hydrocortisone when attending
the patient, instead of the patient having to wait until
they are admitted to hospital. This avoids any delay in
hydrocortisone administration and helps to promote the
immediate recovery of a patient having an adrenal crisis.

Society for Endocrinology
Nurses are encouraged to become members of the
Society for Endocrinology.
   The Endocrine Nurse Committee within the society
organizes a 2-day educational opportunity for endocrine
specialist nurses annually in September. This is an invaluable way of establishing local and national links. It enables
delegates to form professional relationships which will
support the adult endocrine nurse to further develop
their expertise.
   The Society for Endocrinology has links to patient support groups available on their website.

The Pituitary Foundation local support group
Members of the endocrine nurse team should aim to
support the meetings of the Pituitary Foundation local
support group as often as possible, either as a speaker
or by offering advice and support to the members of
the group.

Multidisciplinary team meetings
A member of the endocrine nurse team should be present at all multidisciplinary team meetings.

18.3 Endocrine dietetics

Dietetic assessment

Appropriate dietetic assessment methods will vary according to patient, condition, and the current aims of medical treatment.

Anthropometric measurements

BMI is a widely used indicator of over- and underweight (see Table 18.3). It is a convenient measure to use in a clinical setting and can be helpful in informing dietetic treatment goals. Weight restoration is often appropriate in underweight individuals with amenorrhoea, and weight loss may be a treatment target for overweight and obese individuals with insulin-resistance-related conditions.

Where BMI is used as an indicator of increased type 2 diabetes and cardiovascular disease risk, the WHO recommends that cut-off points take into account ethnic differences. Those from South Asian, Chinese, and Japanese populations should be considered overweight at a BMI of 23 kg/m^2, and obese at BMI of >27.5 kg/m^2.

As BMI is not a direct measure of body fat, it must be used with care in muscular individuals, the elderly, and conditions that cause muscle atrophy or alter body-fat distribution. For some individuals, alternative measures of body composition, such as waist circumference and bioelectrical impedance analysis, can provide more meaningful feedback regarding nutritional status.

A waist circumference of ≥80 cm in women, and ≥94 cm in men, is associated with increased cardiovascular risk. Waist circumference does not provide any helpful additional measure of risk over and above that already provided by BMI classification in individuals with a BMI >35 kg/m^2.

Eating patterns

Meal frequency and timing can be an important factor in reactive hypoglycaemia, weight restoration in underweight individuals, and weight management. An exploration of meal timing can also highlight unhelpful or disordered eating behaviours such as fasting, grazing, binge eating, and purging. These may, in turn, be exacerbating symptoms or hampering weight-management efforts.

Dietary assessment

All patients will benefit from having a nutritionally adequate diet. Macronutrient intake is a key consideration in managing reactive hypoglycaemia effectively. Carbohydrate quality, soluble fibre, fruit and vegetable intake, and fatty-acid intake will all guide dietary advice

Table 18.3 WHO classification of weight

BMI (kg/m^2)	Weight Classification
Below 18.5	Underweight
18.5–24.9	Healthy
25–29.9	Overweight
30–34.9	Obesity I
35–39.9	Obesity II
40 or above	Obesity III

Reprinted from Obesity: preventing and managing the global epidemic: Report of a WHO Consultation, WHO Technical Report Series 894, World Health Organization, page 9, Copyright (2000).

in the treatment of suboptimal blood lipid levels and cardiovascular risk. Adequate calcium intake is particularly relevant for maintaining and restoring bone density.

Biochemistry

General markers of dietary inadequacy or biochemical imbalances should be considered in all patients but particularly underweight individuals. Of particular importance in endocrine dietetic assessment are:

- 25-hydroxyvitamin D: this is the most clinically relevant measure of Vitamin D insufficiency and deficiency
- total cholesterol, HDL cholesterol, and triglycerides: all provide an indication of cardiovascular risk; each can be targeted individually through specific dietary and lifestyle advice in addition to general cardioprotective dietary advice
- markers of hyperglycaemia: these are relevant in all conditions with an associated risk of type 2 diabetes
- capillary blood glucose monitoring: results collected by the patient can be helpful in severe reactive hypoglycaemia; readings should be accompanied by supporting information regarding food intake, to aid interpretation

See the condition-specific sections in 'Specific advice' for additional factors to consider.

Specific advice

PCOS

Weight management remains one of the most important strategies in treating PCOS. Modest weight losses of 5%–15% in overweight and obese women with the condition are associated with improvements in lipid profiles, serum testosterone levels, SHBG levels, glucose tolerance, ovulation regularity, menstrual cycle regularity, and fasting insulin levels. Weight reduction may also improve levels of depression and self-esteem; however, it should be noted that research findings are mixed as to the ability of weight reduction to improve hirsutism.

The benefits of weight loss are clear and can be helpful to discuss these with individuals whilst also being empathetic to the difficulties of losing weight in PCOS. Weight loss is generally more difficult to achieve than for women who do not have PCOS, and many women report patterns of slow weight loss followed by weight regain. The reasons for this are not fully understood, but postprandial thermogenesis has been shown to be significantly lower in PCOS subjects, particularly in those who are also obese. Whilst the difference is small on a meal-by-meal basis, it can equate to a difference of 17,000 kcal per year, or a 19 kg weight gain over 10 years. In view of this, lean-weight individuals with the condition may benefit from advice aimed at avoiding weight gain.

The optimal diet for weight loss in PCOS has long been a subject of debate, largely due to speculation around the relevance of insulin sensitivity and carbohydrate metabolism. Studies comparing isocaloric reduced-calorie diets with differing macronutrient compositions found high-protein and high-carbohydrate diets to have similar weight-reducing effects. Low-glycaemic-index diets have not shown any consistent greater efficacy over other approaches. Many different diets have been shown to promote similar amounts of weight loss in PCOS, each bringing other additional measurable beneficial clinical outcomes. Dropout rates are high in weight-reducing research studies in this patient group. In view of the lifelong nature of the disorder and the lack of convincing evidence regarding an optimal diet, women should be encouraged to manage their weight using a nutritionally balanced plan that fits with their lifestyle, food preferences, and cooking skills, and which also encompasses activity and behavioural strategies. Referral to a dietitian with particular expertise in weight management is recommended.

The focus of treatment for PCOS may change during a patient's lifetime, encompassing concerns such as body image, fertility, and management of cardiovascular risk. Dietetic advice should be clearly tailored to each individual's current risks, concerns, and treatment goals.

Women with PCOS show a greater incidence of impaired glucose tolerance and type 2 diabetes than those in the general population and frequently have more risk factors for coronary heart disease, including obesity, insulin resistance, hypertension, and dyslipidaemia. It is not yet clear that this is reflected in an increased cardiovascular mortality rate. Dietetic assessment and advice can monitor and address these risk factors where possible.

Current evidence does not support the theory that disordered eating and bulimia nervosa are more common in PCOS, and no causal relationship has been shown. However, where disordered eating habits are present, these are likely to be a significant barrier to successful lifestyle treatment if left unaddressed.

Physical activity has benefits independent of weight loss and can reduce waist circumference and increase insulin sensitivity. Regular activity may also offer weight-independent protection from the development of type 2 diabetes. Exercise levels in line with the guidelines advised for the population at large are usually a suitable starting point for advice. Body image concerns, excess body hair, and significant obesity can all pose barriers to where and how women may be willing to exercise. Advice to be more physically active should include support and information on how to increase activity levels in an acceptable way.

Vitamin D deficiency is common in PCOS (67%–85% of women) and there is cautious evidence of benefits to menstrual dysfunction and insulin resistance from supplementation. Supplementation to correct deficiencies should be considered, whilst dietary and lifestyle changes can play a modest role in maintaining corrected levels.

Amenorrhoea

Nutrition support advice can help to restore body weight to a healthy BMI where this is contributing factor to menstrual irregularity. In most cases, a 'food first' approach is recommended, concentrating on:

- a steady weight gain of 0.5 kg/week
- increased consumption of nutrient- and energy-dense foods, particularly good sources of protein
- a regular pattern of sufficient meals and snacks
- an overall healthy dietary balance
- food-fortification strategies

Energy-dense foods with low nutrient density (e.g. cakes, crisps, and chocolate) may be helpful as an addition to more nutritious options. Self-monitoring strategies such as food diaries can increase meal and snack frequency.

The role of body-fat percentage in amenorrhoea is controversial, but athletic individuals may also need to gain body fat in addition to increasing total body mass. Strenuous exercise may impair efforts to increase in body-fat percentage, and advice should cover both the duration and the intensity of activity. Modest exercise will benefit bone mineral density.

Menstrual irregularity is associated with an increased risk of fractures and reduced bone mineral density and it is important to optimize dietary calcium intake.

A specialist multidisciplinary team should treat when low BMI is accompanied by behaviours suggestive of an eating disorder.

Where amenorrhoea is part of chronic anovulation in PCOS, please see the advice given in 'PCOS'.

Hypoglycaemia

Postprandial (reactive) hypoglycaemia responds well to dietary treatments known to slow glucose absorption and reduce insulin response. Key advice is as follows:

- ensure an adequate frequency of small meals and snacks (4 hourly), avoiding overly large carbohydrate loads
- accompany carbohydrates with protein and/or fibre
- modify intake to reduce the consumption of high-glycaemic-index carbohydrates, replacing them with low-glycaemic-index choices
- reduce the consumption of highly sugar-based foods, such as fizzy drinks
- become educated regarding alcohol and its effects on hepatic gluconeogenesis
- engage in regular physical activity

The aim of treatment is to reduce symptoms to a manageable level, with an emphasis on continuing with dietary changes in order to maintain improvements to the quality of life. A confirmed medical diagnosis is important before giving dietary advice, as hypoglycaemic symptoms are not always accompanied by biochemical hypoglycaemia.

Body shape may have a role in reactive hypoglycaemia, with lean individuals, individuals with moderate lower body overweight, and those who have recently lost very large amounts of weight particularly affected. Reactive hypoglycaemia often coexists with insulin resistance or PCOS; in these cases, dietetic advice should be modified to consider all relevant aims of treatment.

Weight management

Weight management has a significant role to play in symptom reduction, the prevention of secondary complications, and improving quality of life. Appropriate weight-management goals may include:

- weight loss, typically in 5%–10% stages
- weight maintenance following successful weight loss
- primary prevention of weight gain

Before advising on changes

When weight loss is being considered as part of a treatment plan, it is valuable to discuss with individuals their current willingness and motivation to make changes and to ask them to identify any relevant barriers they can foresee to making lifestyle changes. Advice can then be tailored to their readiness and capacity to make changes.

Unsuccessful weight-loss attempts can be demoralizing and, at worst, discourage patients from future engagement with healthcare professionals around this issue. Patients should be referred only when ready to fully engage with a weight-loss intervention, and weight-management services should be delivered by staff with appropriate experience and qualifications.

Where patients have a considerable history of weight cycling (repeated intentional weight loss followed by subsequent unintended weight regain), it is advisable to discuss their concerns and confidence in their ability to lose weight and to encourage a sustainable approach to making changes, if this has not been their approach to weight loss in the past.

Healthcare professionals should be aware of the possibility of binge-eating disorder in patients who have difficulty losing weight and maintaining weight loss. The incidence of binge-eating disorder is around 3% in the general population but may be as high as 30% among those looking to obtain weight-management advice.

Recommendations for weight-loss interventions
The most successful weight-management interventions include physical activity, dietary changes, and behavioural components. This combined approach has been shown to be more effective than diet or diet and exercise alone. Box 18.1 gives some recommendations for evaluating the content and approach of weight-management programmes and resources, adapted from the Scottish Intercollegiate Guidelines Network Management of Obesity clinical guideline. These recommendations should be considered before patients are referred on for weight-management support.

Despite many years of research, there is still no consensus as to the optimal dietary approach for weight loss and, in clinical practice, it is clear that a one-size-fits-all approach does not work. A daily energy deficit of 500–600 kcal per day is adequate to promote weight loss in the region of 0.5 kg per week in most individuals. This can be achieved in a number of different ways, and no particular macronutrient composition provides superior results. The mode by which the calorie deficit is achieved can therefore be readily tailored to suit the individual.

There is insufficient evidence to recommend glycaemic index or glycaemic load as a sole dietary strategy for weight loss, but the satiating effects of low glycaemic carbohydrates can provide a helpful appetite control. There is no particular evidence to recommend very-low-calorie diets (<800 kcal per day) for patients with endocrine conditions, and these diets should only be used with close medical and dietetic supervision.

Box 18.1 Recommended criteria for weight-management programmes and resources

Recommended criteria for weight-management programmes and resources are as follows:
- realistic weight reduction targets, such as 5%–10% of starting weight
- modest weekly weight-loss targets of 0.5–1.0 kg
- a focus on sustainable, long-term changes
- a multi-component approach, addressing diet, activity, and behaviour
- dietary advice that advocates a balanced, healthy diet
- physical activity, encouraged in a practical and regular way
- behavioural strategies such as self-monitoring and how to deal with lapses and difficult situations
- provide or recommend ongoing support

Weight-loss interventions are more effective when regular support can be provided, preferably at 2-week intervals (or, at least, initially), and weight-management services should be designed around a model of offering regular support.

Behavioural strategies and weight management
The following range of behavioural strategies can be advised for individuals aiming to lose weight or maintain a weight loss:
- self-monitoring of food intake and eating behaviours
- cognitive restructuring strategies
- understanding emotional and environmental stimuli to overeat
- setting realistic goals
- using problem-solving skills
- preparing for, and managing, relapses into old behaviours

Physical activity and weight management
Activity alone is a poor strategy for weight reduction, as it is difficult for most individuals to meet the duration and intensity of exercise required on a daily basis. However, increasing activity levels will contribute to weight loss and provides additional metabolic benefits.

Current physical activity guidelines for the population at large are a suitable starting point for most individuals (5×30 minutes of moderate intensity activity per week, or 150 minutes in total). Those who meet or exceed these guidelines can be advised on increasing the duration or intensity of their current activities. Strategies that decrease the amount of time spent being sedentary are appropriate for all, but particularly for those with reduced mobility.

Bone health
Osteoporosis risk increases in a number of endocrine disorders, including hyperthyroidism, hyperparathyroidism, hyperprolactinaemia, Cushing's disease, and persistent amenorrhoea. Individuals who do not have osteoporosis but who are at an increased risk of developing the condition will benefit from adequate calcium and vitamin D, moderation in alcohol consumption, and regular weight-bearing exercise, such as walking.

For those diagnosed with osteoporosis, a regular calcium intake of 1200 mg and vitamin D doses of at least 800 IU are associated with a slower rate of bone loss and a decrease in fracture risk. Intakes substantially above this are unlikely to provide any significant additional benefit. Calcium supplements can be used to make up any shortfall where it is not possible to achieve an adequate intake via food-based sources. Calcium citrate and calcium carbonate supplements are similarly bioavailable.

Where the overall calcium intake is adequate, fracture risk is similar across meat eaters, vegetarians, and vegans.

Moderate alcohol intake is not detrimental to bone mineral density and, in some cases, has been shown to have a moderate protective effect (particularly in postmenopausal women). Long-term chronic alcohol consumption inhibits osteoblast proliferation and has been linked to lower bone mineral density and increased fracture risk; excessive intake should be avoided.

Vitamin B_{12} is known to stimulate osteoblast activity and bone formation, and fracture risk is higher in those with pernicious anaemia. Older adults are particularly at risk of an inadequate vitamin B_{12} status and may require supplements or an increased intake of fortified foods.

The role of carbonated fizzy drinks in bone health remains controversial, with a number of studies indicating an increase in fracture risk with increased carbonated drink consumption, and a negative impact on bone modelling and remodelling in children and adolescents. No clear mechanism has been found and it may be that these beverages are a marker for poor diet quality, as well as sometimes being consumed as a replacement for foods high in calcium.

Further reading

Appleby P, Roddam A, Allen N, et al. Comparative fracture risk in vegetarians and nonvegetarians in EPIC-Oxford. *Eur J Clin Nutr* 2007; 61: 1400–6.

Brun JF, Fédou C, and Mercier J. Postprandial reactive hypoglycemia. *Diabetes Metab* 2000; 26: 337–51.

Moran LJ, Ko H, Misso M, et al. Dietary composition in the treatment of polycystic ovary syndrome: A systematic review to inform evidence-based guidelines. *J Acad Nutr Diet* 2013; 113: 520–45.

Scottish Intercollegiate Guidelines Network. Management of obesity: A national clinical guideline. Available at http://www.sign.ac.uk/sign-115-management-of-obesity.html (accessed 18 Jan 2018).

Tang BM, Eslick GD, Nowson C, et al. Use of calcium or calcium in combination with vitamin D supplementation to prevent fractures and bone loss in people aged 50 years and older: A meta-analysis. *Lancet* 2007; 370: 657–66.

Patient advice and reference

Chapter contents

19.1 Diagrams for explanation to patients

Figures 19.1–19.5 show simplified figures and diagrams to help explain common hormonal conditions to patients in clinic.

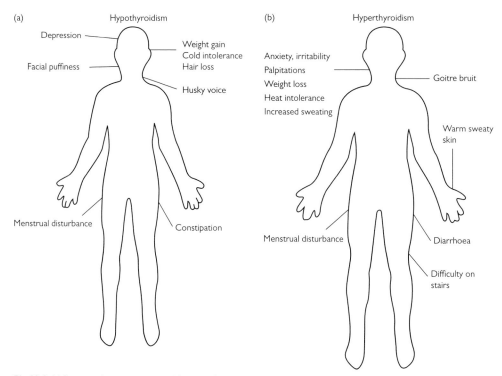

Fig 19.1 (a) Diagram showing some typical features of a patient with hypothyroidism. (b) Diagram showing some typical features in a patient with hyperthyroidism. (c) Diagram showing normal and abnormal thyroid hormone secretion.
Panels a, b: Adapted from Patrick Davey, *Medicine at a Glance, Fourth Edition*, copyright (2014) with permission from John Wiley and Sons.

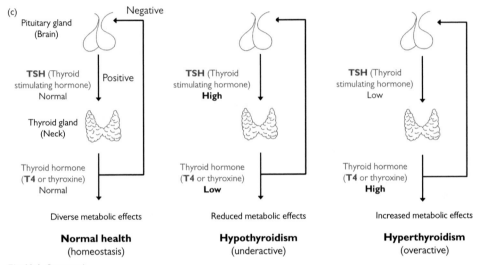

(c)

Negative

Pituitary gland
(Brain)

TSH (Thyroid
stimulating hormone)
Normal

Positive

Thyroid gland
(Neck)

Thyroid hormone
(**T4** or thyroxine)
Normal

Diverse metabolic effects

Normal health
(homeostasis)

TSH (Thyroid
stimulating hormone)
High

Thyroid hormone
(**T4** or thyroxine)
Low

Reduced metabolic effects

Hypothyroidism
(underactive)

TSH (Thyroid
stimulating hormone)
Low

Thyroid hormone
(**T4** or thyroxine)
High

Increased metabolic effects

Hyperthyroidism
(overactive)

Fig 19.1 Continued

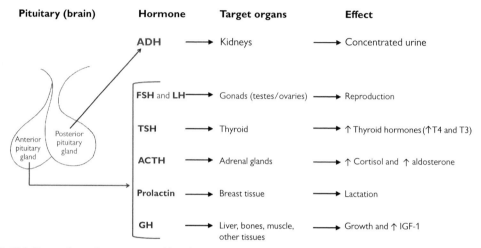

Fig 19.2 Diagram showing hormones secreted from the pituitary gland; ACTH, adrenocorticotrophic hormone; ADH, antidiuretic hormone; FSH, follicle-stimulating hormone; GH, growth hormone; LH, luteinizing hormone; T3, triiodothyronine; T4, thyroxine; TSH, thyroid-stimulating hormone.

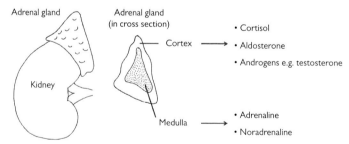

Fig 19.3 Diagram showing hormones secreted from the adrenal gland.

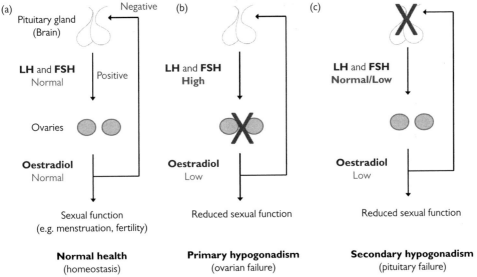

Fig 19.4 Diagram showing female hormonal secretion; FSH, follicle-stimulating hormone; LH, luteinizing hormone.

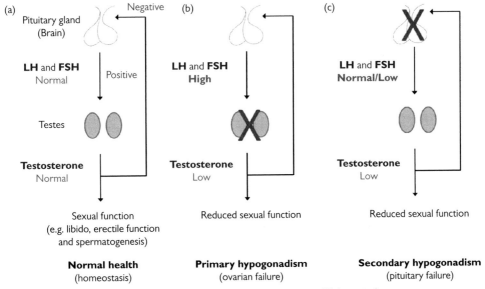

Fig 19.5 Diagram showing male hormonal secretion; FSH, follicle-stimulating hormone; LH, luteinizing hormone.

19.2 Bone and mineral metabolism

The National Osteoporosis Society in the UK (NOS; see http://www.nos.org.uk) is a very useful source of information and support for patients. Their website provides information under the following headings:

- What is osteoporosis?
- Looking for drug treatments?
- Advice for living with osteoporosis
- Can I get involved?
- Healthy bones and risks

- Find a support group
- The latest news about osteoporosis

The website also provides access to leaflets and books about osteoporosis.

The NOS also provides a helpline to deal with individual questions; this can be reached on 0845 450 0230. The NOS can point you towards local services and support groups.

19.3 Clinical genetics

Clinical genetics services in the UK

UK clinical genetics services are regionally based, usually in teaching hospitals. There are only 25 regional genetics services, each covering a wide area (usually about 3 million population]). Most services undertake peripheral clinics in district general hospitals, as well as the main clinics at the teaching hospital.

Genetic counsellors are autonomous health professionals with specialist skills and training. Genetic counsellors generally work as part of a team with consultant clinical geneticists, usually within a regional genetics centre, to deliver genetic counselling to individuals and families who have, or are at risk of having, genetic conditions.

Genetic counselling is defined as 'a communications process which deals with human problems associated with the occurrence, or the risk of occurrence, of a genetic disorder in a family'.

The aims of genetic counselling are to help the individual or family to:

- understand the information about the genetic condition
- appreciate the inheritance pattern and risk of recurrence
- understand the options available
- make decisions appropriate to their personal and family situation
- make the best possible adjustment to the disorder or risk

Genetic counsellors, therefore, use their specialist counselling skills to provide information, support, and advocacy to enable patients to adjust to a genetic diagnosis and reach decisions about intervention and healthcare.

Genetic testing in the UK is undertaken in NHS molecular genetics laboratories. These are all CPA accredited, which means that they have been inspected for the quality of their testing, and also the turnround times for testing. Individual laboratories will offer different genetic tests, and this is regulated by the UK Genetic Testing Network, which administers this on the basis of clinical utility and cost.

Samples submitted for testing will be dealt with via the regional genetics centre laboratory, who will undertake DNA extraction and storage, and then an aliquot of the sample will be distributed appropriately to other laboratories for analysis if required.

Clinical genetics services outside the UK

In most of Western Europe, the USA, Canada, and Australasia, clinical genetics services function in much the same way as they do in the UK. Many countries outside these regions, however, do not have clinical genetics services, and genetic testing is unavailable to huge numbers of people in their own countries. It is therefore becoming increasingly frequent, given the wide level of dispersal of populations in the twenty-first century, for family members in countries where this service does not exist to request testing in the UK on a private basis. This can be facilitated by clinical genetics consultants in the private sector, if required. Private consultations and genetic testing are not usually funded by UK health insurance companies, and hence the UK clinical genetics consultants

do not usually appear on 'approved lists' from these companies, but this is irrelevant when patients are coming from abroad and, since the cost of clinical genetics consultations and testing is not prohibitive, this is increasingly something that UK patients who may not be eligible for genetic testing via the NHS may wishing to pursue.

Role of the clinical geneticist

The British Society for Human Genetics has defined the roles of a clinical geneticist, and the relevant ones for this publication are as follows:

- provide diagnosis of genetic disorders affecting all ages and body systems, birth defects, and developmental disorders
- provide investigation and genetic risk assessment
- provide genetic counselling
- provide predictive testing for late-onset disorders, using agreed protocols
- provide follow-up and support, as well as co-ordination of health surveillance for specific genetic conditions
- offer genetic services to extended families
- maintain genetic family register services
- liaise with genetic laboratories
- provide education and training of genetic professionals and other healthcare professionals
- be a resource of expertise and information for other specialists, primary care doctors, and other health professionals
- develop service guidelines and standards, advise commissioners of service, and advise those establishing screening programmes

Surveillance

Providing follow-up and support and co-ordinating surveillance for specific genetic conditions are felt by many clinical geneticists to be central to their role. An example of such a condition would be Cowden syndrome, for which there are no UK guidelines regarding surveillance.

Family responsibility

Clinical geneticists are unique among health professionals, because their remit is responsibility for the extended family. We have files containing the notes for the whole family, not just the one patient being seen in the clinic appointment that day, and part of the clinical genetics consultation entails an assessment of which other family members may be at risk of a particular condition, and working out a plan with the patient for informing those family members about their risk.

Non-disclosure within families is a relatively common problem, and this can generate ethical dilemmas, particularly when the information regarding the whereabouts of a family member who has not been informed about their risk becomes available to the clinical genetics team. According to rules about patient confidentiality, that patient should not be informed directly. However, in the case of a serious condition such as multiple endocrine neoplasia type 2, many clinicians would feel that the patients' best interests would be served by informing them, regardless of these rules.

Disclosure of information to children is also sometimes difficult. Many individuals affected with genetic conditions do not wish to pass the information onto their children. It seems that they feel that they are paradoxically protecting their children in some way by not informing them, whereas they could be endangering them by withholding access to surveillance and possible treatment. It is therefore the role of a clinical geneticist to liaise with the family and work with them to facilitate the resolution of these types of issue. If there is a danger that a child's best interests are being ignored, and that child may be at serious risk, for example where there is a family history of Von Hippel–Lindau disease, then it is appropriate to involve child protection services, but usually, such drastic measures can be avoided by working with the family for a short time. This has the added advantage of facilitating the continuing engagement of the family with the health services, as this may otherwise be problematic if intervention by child protection services had been invoked. It is really important to emphasize, in this context, that these are roles that do take an amount of time that usually is not possible in a busy endocrinology clinic, and the involvement of clinical geneticists in a multidisciplinary context is not only appropriate but also essential for these types of cases.

Education

The educational role of clinical geneticists is also important. Many endocrinologists may only occasionally have patients with rare genetic conditions, whereas, for a clinical geneticist with a special interest, such patients are relatively common. The clinical geneticist will therefore have the incentive and time to be up to date with recent literature and evidence-based guidelines regarding the surveillance of such patients, and requests for education sessions are therefore appropriate.

It is important to emphasize, however, that it is not the clinical geneticist's role to undertake the management of the problems associated with these conditions. Abnormalities seen during surveillance should be referred on to the appropriate specialist for further investigation and management, and it is important that the clinical geneticists restrict themselves to the 'co-ordination of surveillance and support roles'.

Multidisciplinary clinics

Ideally, in line with the government White Paper 'Integrating Clinical Genetics into Mainstream Services', clinical genetics and endocrinology should see patients together in the context of the multidisciplinary clinic. Increasingly, however, there have been financial and bureaucratic difficulties with these clinics.

The multidisciplinary clinic can work in one of two main ways. Patients can be seen by the geneticist and the endocrinologist together, or (possibly more efficiently) they can be seen sequentially by these specialists. This enables the clinics to run more smoothly, and means that endocrinologists do not have to spend time listening to what may, sometimes, be extended appointments where predictive testing or implications for extended family members are discussed by geneticists.

Genetic testing

Genetic tests are done for a variety of clinical genetic purposes, including the diagnosis of genetic disease in children and adults, the identification of future disease risks, the prediction of response to drugs, and the assessment of risks of disease to future children. These tests currently involve the use of molecular genetic techniques

such as PCR and DNA sequencing, and are likely to involve newer techniques such as next-generation sequencing and whole-exome sequencing in the near future. There are, however, other ways to diagnose genetic disease. Haemoglobin electrophoresis does not involve molecular genetic techniques but would enable a diagnosis of sickle-cell anaemia to be made categorically.

Limitations of genetic testing

It is generally believed that a genetic test is usually done for a patient to fully establish a diagnosis. However, this is complicated by the fact that there are some patients who fulfil the clinical criteria for a particular condition, but in whom genetic testing yields normal results. A good example of this would be multiple endocrine neoplasia type 1, where mutations in *MEN1* are found in only 65% of individuals fulfilling clinical diagnostic criteria (in simplex cases) but in 80%–90% of familial cases. Another example is Cowden syndrome, where the situation is worse in that only 25% of individuals fulfilling clinical diagnostic criteria are found to have mutations in *PTEN*. There are several possible reasons for this. First, it is possible that other genes, as yet undiscovered, may cause Cowden syndrome or multiple endocrine neoplasia type 1. Second, although genetic technology has advanced considerably in recent years, it is possible that not all mutations are detected in the known genes for these conditions, using current techniques. Finally, there always remains the possibility that mutations in regulatory elements of the genes or epigenetic mutations could account for the undiscovered mutations. These would not be detected using current techniques.

A genetic test, therefore, must always be interpreted in the context of the patient. If an individual has extreme macrocephaly, follicular thyroid cancer, several lipomas, and breast cancer, then they should be treated as though they have Cowden syndrome, even if *PTEN* mutation testing yields normal results.

Diagnostic genetic testing

There are circumstances, for example when planning parathyroid surgery in patients with suspected multiple endocrine neoplasia type 1, when, if clinical genetics input is unavailable in a reasonable time frame, it is reasonable for endocrinologists to arrange the genetic testing, but the follow-up (once results are available) should involve the clinical genetics team, for reasons already outlined.

Predictive genetic testing

Once a mutation is known within a family, predictive genetic testing can be undertaken for unaffected family members. This, as its name suggests, predicts the chance that an individual will become affected by the familial condition. Predictive genetic testing should always be undertaken in the context of a clinical genetics appointment. Patients are given the opportunity to receive information about the condition, and to explore the pros and cons of undergoing genetic testing. They are given information about surveillance, and also about risk-reducing surgery options, where appropriate. The psychological implications of the predictive test are also discussed, and it is common for these appointments to take up to 45 minutes, with many patients requiring a second appointment before finally coming to a decision as to whether they would like to go ahead with testing. Clearly, this is not something that would be feasible to undertake in a busy endocrinology clinic, and so the ideal situation would be a multidisciplinary clinic, with clinical geneticists available to see patients independently as required. If a multidisciplinary clinic is not possible, referral to regional genetics services is recommended for the purpose of predictive testing.

Genetic testing and insurance

Under a moratorium which is in place until 2017, but is likely to be renewed, the Department of Health and the Association of British Insurers (2005, p. 4) have agreed to the following:

> Customers will not be required to disclose the results of predictive genetic tests for policies up to £500,000 of life insurance, or £300,000 for critical illness insurance, or paying annual benefits of £30,000 for income protection insurance (the 'financial limits'). More than 97% of policies issued in 2004 were below these limits in each category.

This moratorium was put in place because it was feared that individuals were not undergoing predictive genetic testing because of worries that they would not, in the future, be able to get life insurance or income protection if they undertook a predictive test. It is important to realize that insurance companies are, however, allowed to ask about family history, and can weight premiums accordingly. If an individual has had three relatives who died at young ages from medullary thyroid cancer, the insurance premiums are likely to be weighted according to the high likelihood of multiple endocrine neoplasia type 2 being the condition that has caused these cancers in the family. This weighting would occur completely independently of any genetic testing having occurred.

Although individuals are not required to disclose the results of predictive genetic testing to insurance companies, if a predictive genetic test shows that individual not to have inherited multiple endocrine neoplasia type 2 (using the example above), then it would be in the best interests of that individual to disclose that information to the insurance company, as they would be forced to reduce the premiums accordingly, because it had just been shown that the family history of that individual does not apply to them.

Diagnostic genetic testing results, in an individual who has already experienced features of a condition, should be made available to an insurance company on request.

Genetic testing in children

Since genetic testing is often associated with the prediction of future risk of disease, even when a diagnostic test is being done, careful consideration has been given to the special difficulties associated with the genetic testing of children.

In 2010, the British Society for Human Genetics published guidance regarding this; their conclusions are summarized as follows:

- in circumstances where genetic testing will affect the clinical management of a child, for example the initiation or cessation of treatment or surveillance, genetic testing is appropriate during childhood; the longer-term consequences for that child should, where possible, be discussed with the child prior to testing
- where genetic testing is predictive of disease in the future, and there is no recognized surveillance or treatment available for the condition during childhood, the recommendations are that 'in such circumstances

testing should normally be delayed until the young person can decide for him/herself when, or whether, to be tested. The rationale for this recommendation is that testing in childhood removes the opportunity of the future young person to make their own choices about such decisions, and that opportunity should not be denied to them without good reason'

Although this guidance is not absolute, it does recommend that very careful consideration should be given to circumstances where parents are requesting testing in young children when the child will receive no immediate medical benefit from the testing. The default here should be not to test; however, these cases should always be managed by clinical genetics teams.

Mechanisms of inheritance

Explanation of mechanisms of inheritance is the remit of the clinical geneticist. Table 19.1 summarizes the way in which the conditions detailed in this book are inherited.

Conditions can be inherited in several different ways. However, as a rule of thumb, metabolic conditions tend to be inherited in an autosomal or an X-linked recessive way, whereas conditions predisposing to the development of tumours tend to be inherited in an autosomal-dominant way.

Autosomal-dominant inheritance

In autosomal-dominant inheritance, an affected individual has two copies of the relevant gene: one with a mutation, and the other being normal. 'Dominant' refers to the fact that only one mutated gene is required for the individual to be affected with the condition. The mutated gene therefore 'dominates' over the normal copy.

Table 19.1 Mechanisms of inheritance for common endocrine genetic conditions

Condition	Mechanism of inheritance
Multiple endocrine neoplasia type 1	Autosomal dominant
Multiple endocrine neoplasia type 2	Autosomal dominant
Cowden syndrome	Autosomal dominant
Carney complex	Autosomal dominant
Von Hippel–Lindau disease	Autosomal dominant
Neurofibromatosis type 1	Autosomal dominant
McCune–Albright syndrome	Mosaic disorder (mutations present in not all cells), usually not inherited
Osteogenesis imperfecta	Autosomal dominant, autosomal recessive (depends on type)
Congenital adrenal hyperplasia	Autosomal recessive
X-linked hypophosphataemic osteomalacia	X-linked dominant
Liddle syndrome	Autosomal dominant
Bartter syndrome	Autosomal recessive
Gitelman syndrome	Autosomal recessive
Androgen insensitivity syndrome	X-linked recessive

Each time an affected individual has a child, they will only pass on one copy of the relevant gene. The child therefore has a 50% chance of inheriting the mutated copy, and a 50% chance of inheriting the normal copy. If they inherit the normal copy, they are usually at no more risk of developing the condition than other people in the general population. A caveat to this is the well-documented presence of phenocopies in families with cancer-predisposing conditions (individuals in a family with no mutation who still develop the condition). The reason for the presence of phenocopies is not yet clear. If a child, however, inherits the mutated copy of the relevant gene from an affected parent, then they are at significantly increased risk of developing the condition. This, however, is subject to penetrance.

Penetrance

Penetrance can be simply defined as the chance of an individual developing a condition when they have inherited a relevant mutated gene. This varies between conditions, and can also be variable within one condition. It can also vary by age. Clinical geneticists will be able to explain this to patients during the clinical genetics consultation, and will aim to give the patient and their extended family a personal risk assessment for them of developing particular types of tumour.

Autosomal-recessive inheritance

In autosomal-recessive inheritance, the affected individual will have two mutated copies of the relevant gene. This has occurred because they have received one mutated copy from each parent. Both parents are likely to be unaffected carriers, with one normal copy of the gene, and one mutated copy. In this situation, the gene is said to be 'recessive' because it is necessary for both copies to be mutated before an individual is affected, in contrast to the dominant condition described above. It is possible that one parent is affected with the condition, with two mutated copies of the gene, and the other parent is a carrier, but this does depend on the effect of the condition on reproductive fitness. In a situation, therefore, where both parents are unaffected carriers, these parents have a one-in-four chance of having an affected child.

X-linked recessive inheritance

In X-linked recessive inheritance, the mutated gene is on the X chromosome. Females have two X chromosomes, whereas males have one. The condition is recessive, as in the autosomal-recessive condition, so two mutations are required for an individual to have the condition. Females are therefore usually unaffected carriers, because they have one mutated gene and another (normal) copy of the gene on the other X chromosome. Males, however, who inherit the mutated gene from their mother, will be affected because they only have one X chromosome, and therefore cannot be carriers. For daughters of carrier females, therefore, there is a 50% risk of them being carriers. For sons, there is a 50% risk of them being affected.

X-linked dominant inheritance

In X-linked dominant inheritance, again, the mutated gene is on the X chromosome. The difference here, however, is that the mutation is dominant, so only one mutated gene is required for an individual to be affected with the condition. Females, therefore, can be affected as well as males. There are many conditions which are fatal in males and which are inherited in this way. This is because of the process of X inactivation in females.

X inactivation

Females do not need to have two X chromosomes, as can be seen from the fact that males exist perfectly normally with only one copy of most of the genes present on this chromosome. A process occurs in females, therefore, where one X chromosome is inactivated in all cells of the female. Usually, this process is random, and so a female will inactivate the paternal copy of the X chromosome in 50% of her cells, and the maternal copy of the X chromosome in the other 50%. It is known, however, that if a mutation has occurred on an X chromosome, then that X chromosome will be preferentially inactivated. The mechanism by which this occurs is not entirely understood. This is important when considering X-linked condition, because it means that, in X-linked recessive conditions, female carriers are unaffected because they will preferentially inactivate the mutated X and, in X-linked dominant conditions, females are likely to be less severely affected than males, who do not have this inactivation facility.

Surveillance for inherited genetic conditions

Genetic testing, whether diagnostic or predictive, informs the need for surveillance in individuals with genetic conditions. A confirmed diagnosis of multiple endocrine neoplasia type 2a, for example, in an individual with an apparently isolated phaeochromocytoma, will prompt completely different surveillance from a confirmed diagnosis of Von Hippel–Lindau disease in the same individual.

The surveillance recommendations for the conditions in this book are detailed in the relevant chapters. It is important to realize, however, that, whilst some conditions are common and therefore have well-documented surveillance recommendations, for rare conditions, there may be little or no evidence in this regard, and planning surveillance for these individuals is therefore more difficult. For this reason, clinical geneticists tend to try to group individuals with rare conditions into the multidisciplinary clinics which they attend, and this enables close monitoring of the patients and their families, and also ongoing evaluation of the surveillance that is being offered. The establishment of evidence-based surveillance protocols for these conditions is fraught with difficulty. Historically, clinicians simply recommended what was recognized to be sensible, and then modified it when it seemed to be appropriate but, in the era of evidence-based medicine, this is no longer possible. The difficulty with the establishment of these surveillance protocols is the lack of evidence for the rare conditions. If a condition is extremely rare, there will be not enough individuals with the condition who have undergone follow-up for sufficient time to enable an accurate estimation of what may be appropriate in terms of surveillance.

A good example of this is the relatively recent evidence concerning mutations in SDHB and SDHD. These mutations were only discovered to be a cause of familial phaeochromocytoma and paraganglioma in 2001. At the time, the only individuals who were known to have these mutations were those in whom a young-onset diagnosis of one of these tumours had been made. As more families were discovered with these mutations, however, it was found that there are a relatively high number of unaffected individuals in previous generations who were also mutation carriers but had never developed any tumours. This meant that information regarding the penetrance of the mutations was modified, and centres around the UK and others worldwide began to collaborate to try to establish the true penetrance. This, clearly, affected the surveillance protocols. Further evidence suggested that *SDHB*-mutation carriers could have the features of Cowden syndrome, and this then raised the possibility that additional surveillance might be appropriate for these individuals. Full resolution of this question is not yet available.

Another important issue regarding surveillance is the responsibility for follow-up. It is important to ask the following: 'Who is responsible for requesting this surveillance, and who will feed the results back to the patient, and act upon them appropriately?'

This is one of the strengths of the surveillance which can be arranged via clinical geneticists, particularly as part of a multidisciplinary clinic. Clinical geneticists can take responsibility for arranging the surveillance, some of which (particularly in conditions such as Von Hippel–Lindau disease and Cowden syndrome) does not involve endocrinology. They can then arrange review of the results as the appropriate time.

Reproductive choice: Prenatal testing and preimplantation genetic diagnosis

There are two main options available to individuals who are affected with a genetic disorder and who do not wish to pass this disorder on to their children. Both these options are only possible, however, if the mutation causing the disorder is known.

Prenatal testing: Amniocentesis and chorionic villus sampling
In amniocentesis and chorionic villus sampling, testing occurs during the pregnancy. Amniocentesis occurs at 16–18 weeks of pregnancy, and involves taking a sample of amniotic fluid under ultrasound guidance. Chorionic villus sampling occurs between 10 and 12 weeks of pregnancy, and involves taking a sample of placenta, again under ultrasound guidance. Following culture of either of these types of sample, genetic analysis is performed, and it is therefore possible to determine if the foetus carries the disease-causing mutation. Both these techniques carry an attendant risk of miscarriage; this is slightly higher for chorionic villus sampling than for amniocentesis. These tests are usually arranged by the clinical genetics department, involving liaison with prenatal services, and results of the testing are given by the clinical genetics department. It is common for termination of pregnancy to be requested if the foetus is shown to carry the disease-causing mutation, and this is arranged.

Preimplantation genetic diagnosis
Preimplantation genetic diagnosis is a relatively new technique, involving IVF technology. A series of embryos are created using this technology, and then one cell is removed from each embryo for analysis at the eight-cell stage. Only embryos that do not carry the disease-causing gene alteration are then considered for implantation. Preimplantation genetic diagnosis is regulated by the Human Fertilisation and Embryology Authority, who grant specific licences to centres in order that couples with particular diseases can be helped by this technique. This is particularly relevant in endocrine disease because, although some of these conditions are common (e.g. multiple endocrine neoplasia type 2a), so a licence will already have been granted for them, in the case of very rare diseases such as Carney complex, it is likely that a request for preimplantation genetic diagnosis will not yet have been received, and therefore the whole process will take much longer. This technique can be done at various centres around the UK; however, NHS funding is not definite, and depends on geography. Referral is usually via the clinical genetics service.

References and further reading

Astuti D, Latif F, Dallol A, et al. Gene mutations in the succinate dehydrogenase subunit SDHB cause susceptibility to familial pheochromocytoma and to familial paraganglioma. *Am J Hum Genet* 2001; 69: 49–54.

Brandi ML, Gagel RF, Angeli A, et al. Guidelines for diagnosis and therapy of MEN type 1 and type 2. *J Clin Endocrinol Metab* 2001; 86: 5658–71.

British Society for Human Genetics. Report on the genetic testing of children 2010. Available at http://www.bsgm.org.uk/media/678741/gtoc_booklet_final_new.pdf (accessed 18 Jan 2018).

Department of Health. Our inheritance, our future: Realising the potential of genetics in the NHS. Available at http://webarchive.nationalarchives.gov.uk/+/www.dh.gov.uk/en/Publicationsandstatistics/Publications/PublicationsPolicyAndGuidance/DH_4006538 (accessed 18 Jan 2018).

Department of Health and the Association of British Insurers. Concordat and moratorium on genetics and insurance, 2005. Available at http://webarchive.nationalarchives.gov.uk/20130123204306/http://www.dh.gov.uk/en/Publicationsandstatistics/Publications/PublicationsPolicyAndGuidance/DH_4105905 (accessed 18 Jan 2018).

Department of Health and the Association of British Insurers. Concordat and moratorium on genetics and insurance, 2011. Available at http://www.gov.uk/government/uploads/system/uploads/attachment_data/file/216821/Concordat-and-Moratorium-on-Genetics-and-Insurance-20111.pdf (accessed 18 Jan 2018).

Firth H and Hurst J. *Oxford Desk Reference: Clinical Genetics* (2nd edition), 2017. Oxford University Press.

Guo SS and Sawicki MP. Molecular and genetic mechanisms of tumorigenesis in multiple endocrine neoplasia type-1. *Mol Endocrinol* 2001; 15: 1653–64.

Ni Y, Zbuk KM, Sadler T, et al. Germline mutations and variants in the succinate dehydrogenase genes in Cowden and Cowden-like syndromes. *Am J Hum Genet* 2008; 83: 261–8.

Srirangalingam U, Walker L, Khoo B, et al. Clinical manifestations of familial paraganglioma and phaeochromocytomas in succinate dehydrogenase B (SDH-B) gene mutation carriers. *Clin Endocrinol (Oxf)* 2008; 69: 587–96.

Tan MH, Mester J, Peterson C, et al. A clinical scoring system for selection of patients for *PTEN* mutation testing is proposed on the basis of a prospective study of 3042 probands. *Am J Hum Genet* 2011; 88: 42–56.

19.4 Patient support and information resource

Patient support organizations offer practical and emotional support to those patients who are newly diagnosed, or have been diagnosed for some time, with an endocrine condition. Support can also be provided to families and carers of the patient.

Practical support can include information about their condition, treatment, lifestyle, and well-being issues, plus the opportunity to talk to or meet other patients.

Endocrine conditions can be lifelong; patients can feel alone and bewildered at any stage of their journey. Their diagnosis, tests, and subsequent treatment can be a shock. Patient support can help to alleviate their fears and isolation and empower them physically and emotionally to cope and feel more positive.

Travel advice for patients

It's a good idea to keep a written record of any medical conditions affecting you, and a list of all the medications you are taking (including both proper and trade names). Most importantly, ask your GP or consultant to write a letter describing your condition and the treatments you are taking. You might also find it useful to carry a repeat prescription script with you. If you want to take any sort of medicine with you—either prescribed or bought from a pharmacist—find out if there are any restrictions on taking it in and out of the UK or the country you are visiting. This is particularly important for patients on growth hormone. Ask the relevant embassy or high commission or telephone the Home Office for advice (0207 035 4848).

Always carry medicines in a correctly labelled container, as issued by the pharmacist. The letter from your doctor, the repeat prescription script, and a personal health-record card giving details of the drug prescribed will help you in case you need it to get you through customs.

If you have medications that need to be refrigerated, the following are suggestions on how to keep medications cool during travel.

- Purchase or borrow a small cool bag with two freezer blocks.
- Before you travel, call your accommodation (hotel, motel, bed and breakfast, etc.) and ask if they have refrigerators in the rooms or, if not, if one can be hired for your room.
- If they do not have refrigerators, ask if they have a freezer where they can place your freezer blocks on a rota in order that you can keep your cool bag cool.
- During travel, place your medication into cool bag with both frozen blocks—the blocks should keep cool for around 12 hours.
- If you need to use the hotel's freezer, on arrival, give them one block labelled with your name. Twelve hours later, swap the blocks to ensure you continually have a frozen block to use both day and night in the cool bag.
- In a dire emergency, for example when there is no freezer or refrigerator available, wrap the medication in a cold, wet flannel and keep in the shade. This option is not recommended for the long term.
- If you ask at your local chemist, they may loan you a 24-hour freeze box, free of charge. Be aware, they may

expect you to return it. A 24-hour freeze box is very bulky and you will need to carry it with you.
- Cabin crews may also refrigerate your medications for you on the aircraft (again, they can refuse this request). Be sure it is properly labelled and be certain to retrieve your medications before leaving the plane!
- There are growth hormone products that are available that do not need refrigeration—just kept cool—very useful for holidays!

It is recommended that you find out *before* you travel what options are available to you.

If you frequently travel by car, you may wish to invest in one of the very small refrigerators that are now widely available and are reasonably priced.

Insurance and pensions

Each case will need to be assessed individually. You may find that the insurance company charges extra premiums. If your condition has only recently been diagnosed or treatment started, they may want to postpone a decision for a while. Of course, each insurance company will have its own practices. You need to persevere if the first response is disappointing.

Driving

You have a legal obligation to notify the DVLA of a condition that lasts longer than 3 months and may affect your fitness to drive. Conditions such as pituitary tumour should be notified. More information about driving and medical conditions can be found on the Directgov website (http://direct.gov.uk; see also Chapter 21, Section 21.2)

Many patients with endocrine conditions will find there is no restriction, but you should check with your GP. The only conditions likely to affect you are problems with your eyesight or hypoglycaemia. Having transsphenoidal surgery, for example, does not in itself limit your ability to drive. Your specialist or GP will give you full advice.

For drivers' medical enquiries, contact the DVLA on 0300 790 6806 or email at drivers.dvla@gtnet.gov.uk.

Benefits

More recently, the government has introduced Employment and Support Allowance (usually shortened to ESA) for people unable to work because of a health problem. For this, you do not necessarily need to be up to date with National Insurance contributions. All new claimants go onto ESA, and people currently claiming incapacity benefits are gradually being moved onto ESA. Once again, you have to undertake a medical and have to gain sufficient points for physical and psychological difficulties in order to continue to qualify for ESA.

Official information on ESA can be found on the direct.gov website: http://www.direct.gov.uk/en/MoneyTaxAndBenefits/BenefitsTaxCreditsAndOtherSupport/Illorinjured/DG_171894.

Disability Rights UK also produce a factsheet, F31, about ESA. This includes the scoring system used, located in Appendix 1. It can be found on their website, https://www.gov.uk/employment-support-allowance.

Patient support groups

The Pituitary Foundation

The Pituitary Foundation (http://www.pituitary.org.uk) supports those who have acromegaly, Cushing's syndrome, craniopharyngioma, diabetes insipidus, empty sella syndrome, hypopituitarism, prolactinoma, and Sheehan's syndrome, as well as other, rarer pituitary conditions. Their support services include:

- a national helpline for general pituitary support (0117 370 1320; open Monday–Friday, 10:00–16:00 h)
- a helpline email contact to a support team (helpline@pituitary.org.uk)
- an endocrine specialist nurse helpline (0117 370 1317)
- *Pituitary Life* magazine, three times a year (for members)
- an informative and helpful website and booklet library, plus emergency patient care cards for hydrocortisone and diabetes insipidus
- a forum section of the website, plus Facebook and Twitter
- local support groups around the country, to meet others face to face
- 'Telephone Buddies' with similar conditions, to call or email
- national pituitary conferences

Patient quotations

The quotations are from patients who have joined the Pituitary Foundation:

- 'Just received and read Pit Life; been a patient for 30 years and can't believe the things you cover in the magazine. Delighted with the coverage of HC issues, as had several problems in past with hospitals not understanding HC crisis. So delighted with Pit Life, it is unbelievable; so pleased and happy with it.'
- **'**When I was diagnosed and had my surgery, there was no Foundation; I felt a freak, alone and worried about my future. They have made a huge difference to me and I cannot thank them enough.'

Other endocrine patient support groups

Other endocrine patient support groups are as follows:

- Addison's disease: http://www.addisons.org.uk
- Association for Multiple Endocrine Neoplasia: http://www.amend.co.uk
- British Thyroid Foundation: http://www.btf-thyroid.org
- Hypopara UK (for hypoparathyroidism): http://www.hpth.org.uk
- Thyroid Eye Disease Charitable Trust: http://www.tedct.co.uk
- Turners Syndrome Support Society: http://www.tss.org.uk

Chapter 20

Speedy reference

Chapter contents

20.1 Indications for treatment of subclinical hyperthyroidism

Diagnosis

Subclinical hyperthyroidism is defined biochemically by a TSH persistently below the lower limit of the reference range, with normal levels of FT3 and FT4. Around 3% of the population have subclinical hyperthyroidism; this figure includes healthy individuals whose TSH lies outside the statistically defined reference range. Subclinical hyperthyroidism is more common in women, the elderly, and in areas of low iodine intake (due to the increase in autonomous thyroid nodules).

The commonest cause is inadequately monitored levothyroxine replacement for hypothyroidism or TSH-suppressive levothyroxine treatment for thyroid cancer. Endogenous causes are (i) Graves' disease, (ii) multinodular goitre, (iii) autonomous thyroid nodules, and (iv) thyroiditis.

Progression to overt thyrotoxicosis occurs in 5%–8% of these cases per year, with the highest risk in nodular thyroid disease. Progression is only 1% per year in the elderly with incompletely suppressed TSH levels (0.1–0.4 mU/L). Exposure to excess iodine, from dietary iodine supplements, amiodarone, radiocontrast media, or topical iodine preparations, may precipitate overt hyperthyroidism in subclinical hyperthyroidism.

Other causes of a low TSH must be excluded before diagnosing subclinical hyperthyroidism. These include (i) non-thyroidal illness, (ii) current or recent treatment for overt hyperthyroidism, (iii) pregnancy, (iv) hypopituitarism (in which case, FT4 is usually low), and (v) dopamine or glucocorticoid treatment.

Effects of subclinical hyperthyroidism

Symptoms

Population-based cohort studies have shown no increase in symptoms, including mood and cognition, compared to healthy controls. Individual patients may complain of thyrotoxic symptoms, especially those who are younger. Conflicting data exist on an association between subclinical hyperthyroidism and dementia.

Cardiovascular effects

Left ventricular hypertrophy, impaired diastolic function, and impaired exercise tolerance have been reported inconsistently in subclinical hyperthyroidism. The risk of atrial fibrillation is increased around threefold in subclinical hyperthyroidism and is similar in those whose TSH is undetectable and those in whom the TSH level is 0.1–0.4 mU/L. Most studies of atrial fibrillation have only examined individuals aged 60 or over. Prospective cohort studies have found no increase in cardiovascular mortality but the most comprehensive meta-analysis to date has shown a 41% increase in overall mortality in subclinical hyperthyroidism.

Skeletal effects

Subclinical hyperthyroidism is associated with a decrease in bone mineral density in postmenopausal women but not in premenopausal women or men. Regarding the risk of fracture, there appears to be no effect of subclinical hyperthyroidism if the TSH is 0.1–0.4 mU/L, but an increase in hip and vertebral fracture rate has been observed in individuals over 65 years old with subclinical hyperthyroidism, especially in women with undetectable TSH levels. Alendronate treatment is less effective in patients with iatrogenic subclinical hyperthyroidism.

Recommendations for treatment

Despite its prevalence, there are few good trials of treatment in subclinical hyperthyroidism. Restoring euthyroidism decreases heart rate and left ventricular mass and increases diastolic dysfunction. Atrial fibrillation may revert to sinus rhythm or respond more successfully to cardioversion if subclinical hyperthyroidism is treated, and further loss of bone mineral density is prevented by treatment.

The most comprehensive guidelines for treatment of subclinical hyperthyroidism have been produced jointly by the American Thyroid Association, the American Association of Clinical Endocrinologists, and the Endocrine Society. The following is a summary of these recommendations:

- for iatrogenic subclinical hyperthyroidism (TSH 0.1–0.4 mU/L):
  - review the indication for treatment
  - lower the levothyroxine dosage to return the TSH to within the reference range, except in those patients in whom TSH suppression is deliberate (typically those with thyroid cancer)
- for iatrogenic subclinical hyperthyroidism (TSH < 0.1 mU/L):
  - review the indication for treatment
  - in patients with lower-risk thyroid cancer, it may be adequate to keep the TSH level between 0.1 and 0.4 mU/L
  - in all other non-cancer cases, lower the levothyroxine dosage to return the TSH to within the reference range
- for endogenous subclinical hyperthyroidism (TSH 0.1–0.4 mU/L):
  - routine treatment is not indicated
  - treatment might be considered in elderly patients at risk of cardiovascular disease
- for endogenous subclinical hyperthyroidism (TSH <0.1 mU/L):
  - await resolution if the cause is thyroiditis
  - consider treatment for those aged over 60, those at increased risk of cardiovascular disease or osteoporosis, or those with symptoms suggestive of thyrotoxicosis

It should be noted that these recommendations are based on, at best, fair evidence for a benefit of treatment (and then only with regard to effects on bone density). The choice of treatment, when given, is determined by aetiology and patient preference. Anti-thyroid drugs are reasonable first-line treatment for Graves' disease, given by titration or the block–replace regimen. Radioiodine is required for toxic adenoma (^{131}I, 500 MBq) and for multinodular goitre (^{131}I, 500 MBq for a small goitre, 600 MBq for a moderate or large goitre). Thyroidectomy is rarely indicated in subclinical hyperthyroidism, but may be necessary if there are compressive symptoms from a large multinodular goitre.

When treatment is not given, patients should be offered regular follow-up to detect progression to overt hyperthyroidism. Until the natural history of the condition in the individual patient is established, repeat measurement of the TSH and FT3 is required every 3 months, and more frequently if there are thyrotoxic symptoms or cardiac complications. If the TSH and FT3 do not alter over 6–12 months, annual testing is acceptable, with instructions to the individual to have interim testing if new symptoms develop. In postmenopausal women with subclinical hyperthyroidism, measurement of bone mineral density is useful in determining whether there is any osteopenia or osteoporosis which might require treatment with a bisphosphonate or other agent. This information may also be useful in determining which patients might benefit from thyroid treatment.

Further reading

Blum MR, Bauer DC, Collet TH, et al. Subclinical thyroid dysfunction and fracture risk: A meta-analysis. *JAMA* 2015; 313: 2055–65

Cooper DS and Biondi B. Subclinical thyroid disease. *Lancet* 2012; 379: 1142–54.

Haentjens P, Van Meerhaeghe A, Poppe K, et al. Subclinical thyroid dysfunction and mortality: An estimate of relative and absolute excess all-cause mortality based on time-to-event data from cohort studies. *Eur J Endocrinol* 2008; 159: 329–41.

Ross DS, Burch HB, Cooper DS, et al. 2016 American Thyroid Association guidelines for diagnosis and management of hyperthyroidism and other causes of thyrotoxicosis. *Thyroid* 2016; 26: 1343–21.

Royal College of Physicans. Radioiodine in the management of benign thyroid disease: Clinical guidelines. Available at https://www.bnms.org.uk/images/stories/downloads/documents/2007radioiodine_in_the_management_of_benign_thyroid_disease.pdf (accessed 18 Jan 2018).

Surks MI, Ortiz E, Daniels GH, et al. Subclinical thyroid disease: Scientific review and guidelines for diagnosis and management. *JAMA* 2004; 291: 228–38.

Turner MR, Camacho X, Fischer HD, et al. Levothyroxine dose and risk of fractures in older adults: Nested case-control study. *BMJ* 2011; 342: d2238.

20.2 Differentiated thyroid cancer follow-up

Overview

The prognosis for differentiated thyroid cancer is good, and most patients will be cured of their disease; however, 10%–15% of patients will develop local or distant recurrence. Late recurrences are not uncommon and are usually treatable; therefore, long-term follow-up of this patient group is recommended.

This section provides an overview of how to follow up the patient after primary treatment, which will usually have consisted of surgery (total thyroidectomy ± neck dissection) and radioiodine remnant ablation (RRA).

The purpose of regular, routine follow-up of patients with differentiated thyroid cancer is to:

- detect recurrent disease
- detect and manage toxicities caused by treatment
- ensure patients are on doses of levothyroxine to maintain an appropriate level of TSH suppression
- manage other associated problems, including hypoparathyroidism with subsequent hypocalcaemia
- monitor the impact of thyroid hormone manipulation on bone density and the risk of skeletal events

Disease surveillance

Clinical follow-up

Patients should have their first follow-up appointment within 2–3 months of RRA. The purpose of this visit is to:

- discuss the results of the post-ablation whole-body scan
- assess and manage any radioiodine-induced toxicities
- ensure the dose of levothyroxine is appropriate
- review hypoparathyroidism and consequent requirements for calcium and/or vitamin D replacement

At each review, patients should have:

- a relevant history taken, focusing on:
  - symptoms relating to local disease recurrence, specifically dysphagia, dysphonia, discomfort, or fullness in the neck
  - in high-risk patients, symptoms relating to distant disease, such as persistent cough or pain
  - symptoms relating to thyroid hormone status and hypocalcaemia
- an examination of the thyroid bed and central and lateral compartments of the neck; further physical examination should be directed according to symptoms

Biochemical follow-up

Thyroglobulin

- Serum thyroglobulin should be measured at each clinic visit together with anti-thyroglobulin antibodies which if present may reduce the reliability of thyroglobulin as a tumour marker.
- Following total thyroidectomy and RRA, serum thyroglobulin should fall to become undetectable over approximately 6–12 months.
- Any subsequent rise in serum thyroglobulin is suggestive of recurrent disease.
- Patients should be reassessed at 9–12 months post RRA.
- If the thyroglobulin is undetectable, a stimulated thyroglobulin is recommended for additional sensitivity. A stimulated thyroglobulin requires either withdrawal

from thyroid hormone to cause a rise in TSH or recombinant human TSH given on Days 1 and 2, followed on Day 5 by serum thyroglobulin.

- An ultrasound scan of the thyroid bed and neck is also recommended at this time.
- A stimulated thyroglobulin <0.5 ng/mL has between 98.0% and 99.5% likelihood of identifying patients who are completely free of tumour [1, 2]. Therefore, if a stimulated thyroglobulin is negative at 9–12 months post RRA, the risk of recurrence of disease is extremely low, and follow-up intervals can be increased.
- A raised stimulated thyroglobulin is suggestive of persistent disease or a residual thyroid remnant.
- Surgically resectable disease should first be excluded, usually with ultrasound, CT (without contrast), or MRI.
- If there is no resectable disease, a therapy dose of radioiodine should be considered.

TSH suppression

TSH acts as a growth factor for thyroid cancer cells; therefore T4 should be titrated to keep TSH levels suppressed. To minimize the adverse effects of long-term TSH suppression, notably reduced bone density, atrial fibrillation, and exacerbation of ischaemic heart disease, TSH suppression is tailored to the individual risk of recurrence.

Radiological follow-up

Ultrasound

All patients should have an ultrasound scan of thyroid bed and neck in conjunction with a stimulated thyroglobulin at 9–12 months post treatment. If this is negative for disease, future imaging is based on clinical or biochemical suspicion of relapse.

Whole-body ^{131}I scan

- A whole-body ^{131}I scan is carried out after RRA or radioiodine therapy. This reveals the sites of radioiodine uptake. Correlation with anatomical imaging is useful to clarify the site of residual disease.
- If serum thyroglobulin is rising, a whole-body ^{131}I scan may be considered, to identify sites of disease.

FDG PET/CT

FDG PET/CT can be useful in identifying thyroid cancer when the disease becomes less differentiated and therefore less iodine avid. Preparation for the scan with TSH stimulation either with thyroid-hormone withdrawal or recombinant human TSH can increase the sensitivity [3].

Monitoring of hormone replacement and treatment-induced toxicity

Following surgery and RRA, there is a responsibility to monitor for treatment-related morbidity and biochemical abnormalities. Therefore, alongside assessment of disease status, the following should be reviewed:

- history:
  - symptoms that may suggest under- or over-replacement of T4
  - symptoms of hypocalcaemia
  - symptoms arising from treatment-related morbidity
- examination: thyroid status
- biochemical tests:

- serum phosphate (if on vitamin D)
- serum calcium
- PTH
- wean off of calcium supplements if PTH and calcium levels permit
- radiological: bone density scanning should be considered in postmenopausal women or a family history of osteoporosis

Risk stratification

The risk of recurrence of differentiated thyroid cancer can be stratified into low, intermediate, and high (see Figure 20.1) [4]. Designation into one of these risk groups will guide the intensity of follow-up and level of TSH suppression. This is a dynamic process, and the level of risk may change with time as more information

about an individual's disease and response to treatment becomes available.

Ongoing TSH suppression can be adjusted to the risk level and status of disease at the 9–12 month post-ablation assessment (Table 20.1) [4].

For low- and intermediate-risk patients, frequency of follow-up is 3–6 monthly for the first 2 years, 6–12 monthly for Years 3–5, and annually thereafter. Follow-up of high-risk patients is individualized.

Very-low-risk patients can be followed up less frequently and may be discharged from specialist care to community-based follow-up, if appropriate.

Medullary thyroid cancer

- Patients diagnosed with medullary thyroid cancer require lifelong follow-up in a specialist multidisciplinary clinic.

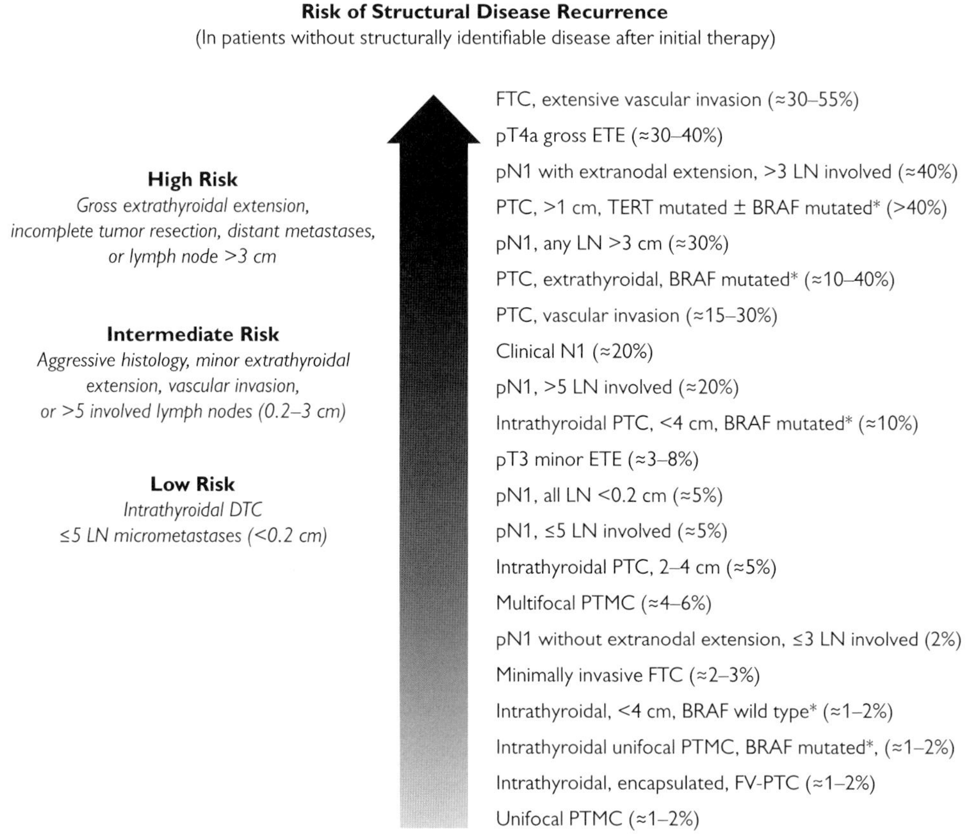

Risk of Structural Disease Recurrence
(In patients without structurally identifiable disease after initial therapy)

High Risk
Gross extrathyroidal extension, incomplete tumor resection, distant metastases, or lymph node >3 cm

Intermediate Risk
Aggressive histology, minor extrathyroidal extension, vascular invasion, or >5 involved lymph nodes (0.2–3 cm)

Low Risk
Intrathyroidal DTC ≤5 LN micrometastases (<0.2 cm)

FTC, extensive vascular invasion (≈30–55%)

pT4a gross ETE (≈30–40%)

pN1 with extranodal extension, >3 LN involved (≈40%)

PTC, >1 cm, TERT mutated ± BRAF mutated* (>40%)

pN1, any LN >3 cm (≈30%)

PTC, extrathyroidal, BRAF mutated* (≈10–40%)

PTC, vascular invasion (≈15–30%)

Clinical N1 (≈20%)

pN1, >5 LN involved (≈20%)

Intrathyroidal PTC, <4 cm, BRAF mutated* (≈10%)

pT3 minor ETE (≈3–8%)

pN1, all LN <0.2 cm (≈5%)

pN1, ≤5 LN involved (≈5%)

Intrathyroidal PTC, 2–4 cm (≈5%)

Multifocal PTMC (≈4–6%)

pN1 without extranodal extension, ≤3 LN involved (2%)

Minimally invasive FTC (≈2–3%)

Intrathyroidal, <4 cm, BRAF wild type* (≈1–2%)

Intrathyroidal unifocal PTMC, BRAF mutated*, (≈1–2%)

Intrathyroidal, encapsulated, FV-PTC (≈1–2%)

Unifocal PTMC (≈1–2%)

Fig 20.1 The 2015 American Thyroid Association risk stratification, showing the risk of structural disease recurrence in patients without structurally identifiable disease after initial therapy. The risk of structural disease recurrence associated with selected clinico-pathological features is shown as a continuum of risk, with percentages (ranges, approximate values) presented to reflect our best estimates based on the published literature reviewed in the text. In the left-hand column, the three-tiered risk system proposed as the 'Modified Initial Risk Stratification System' is also presented, to demonstrate how the continuum of risk estimates informed our modifications of the 2009 American Thyroid Association Initial Risk System; whilst analysis of *BRAF* and/or *TERT* status is not routinely recommended for initial risk stratification, we have included these findings (marked with an asterisk) to assist clinicians in proper risk stratification in cases where this information is available; ETE, extrathyroidal extension; FTC, follicular thyroid cancer; FV, follicular variant; LN, lymph node; PTC, papillary thyroid cancer; PTMC, papillary thyroid microcarcinoma.
Reproduced from table 4, Thyroid, Volume 26, 2015 American Thyroid Association Management Guidelines for Adult Patients with Thyroid Nodules and Differentiated Thyroid Cancer: The American Thyroid Association Guidelines Task Force on Thyroid Nodules and Differentiated Thyroid Cancer, Haugen BR, Alexander EK, Bible KC et al., 2016, pp. 1–133. Copyright © 2016, Mary Ann Liebert, Inc.

Table 20.1 Target TSH levels according to clinical risk of recurrence

TSH <0.1	TSH 0.1–0.5	TSH 0.5–2.0
Initial period post treatment		
High-risk patients	Intermediate-risk patients	Low-risk patients who have undergone remnant ablation and have undetectable serum Tg levels
	Low-risk patients who have undergone remnant ablation and have low-level serum Tg levels	Low-risk patients who have not undergone remnant ablation and have undetectable serum Tg levels
	Low-risk patients who have not undergone remnant ablation and have low-level, stable, detectable Tg	
Following response to treatment assessment at 9–12 months		
Patients with a structural incomplete response to therapy	Patients with a biochemical incomplete response to therapy, taking into account the initial risk classification, Tg level, Tg trend over time, and risk of TSH suppression	Patients with an excellent (clinically and biochemically free of disease) or indeterminate response to therapy
	Patients who presented with high-risk disease but have an excellent (clinically and biochemically free of disease) or indeterminate response to therapy for up to 5 years, after which the degree of TSH suppression can be reduced with continued surveillance	Patients who have not undergone remnant ablation or adjuvant therapy and who demonstrate an excellent or indeterminate response to therapy with a normal neck US, and low or undetectable suppressed serum Tg or anti-Tg antibodies that are not rising

Abbreviations: Tg, thyroglobulin; US, ultrasound.

Data from *Thyroid*, Volume 26, 2015 American Thyroid Association Management Guidelines for Adult Patients with Thyroid Nodules and Differentiated Thyroid Cancer: The American Thyroid Association Guidelines Task Force on Thyroid Nodules and Differentiated Thyroid Cancer, Haugen BR, Alexander EK, Bible KC et al., 2016, pp. 1–133.

- T4 should be replaced but there is no benefit to suppressing TSH.
- Following initial surgery, calcitonin should be measured as a post-operative baseline. An undetectable level at this point is a strong indicator of complete remission.
- Each review should comprise taking a history, performing a clinical examination, and measuring levels of thyroid function, calcitonin, and carcinoembryonic antigen and should take place at 6–12 monthly intervals.
- A rising calcitonin should be investigated with an ultrasound or CT of the neck, CT of the chest and abdomen, and a bone scan. Distant metastatic disease is often not evident until calcitonin levels > 44.9 pmol/L (150 pg/mL); levels below this suggest that the disease remains local to the neck.
- Patients with a diagnosis of multiple endocrine neoplasia 2 should have regular screening for phaeochromocytoma and hyperparathyroidism.

Anaplastic thyroid cancer

Anaplastic thyroid cancer is the most aggressive form of thyroid cancer and responds poorly to surgery and systemic therapies. It is rapidly progressive, with around half of patients presenting with metastatic disease; thus, follow-up should be tailored to the individual needs of the patient.

There are no useful tumour markers for this pathological subtype; however, progressive disease is usually clinically apparent and easily seen on cross-sectional imaging.

It is important that the local palliative care team are involved early in the patient pathway, as symptoms are often difficult to manage, and median survival is short, at around 5 months

References and further reading

1. Kloos RT and Mazzaferri EL. A single recombinant human thyrotropin-stimulated serum thyroglobulin measurement predicts differentiated thyroid carcinoma metastases three to five years later. *J Clin Endocrinol Metab* 2005; 90: 5047–5057.
2. Castagna MG1, Brilli L, Pilli T, et al. Limited value of repeat recombinant human thyrotropin (rhTSH)-stimulated thyroglobulin testing in differentiated thyroid carcinoma patients with previous negative rhTSH-stimulated thyroglobulin and undetectable basal serum thyroglobulin levels. *J Clin Endocrinol Metab* 2008; 93: 76–81.
3. Leboulleux S, Schroeder PR, Busaidy NL, et al. Assessment of the incremental value of recombinant thyrotropin stimulation before 2-[18F]-fluoro-2-deoxy-D-glucose positron emission tomography/computed tomography imaging to localize residual differentiated thyroid cancer. *J Clin Endocrinol Metab* 2009; 94: 1310–16.
4. Cooper DS, Doherty GM, Haugen BR, et al. Revised American Thyroid Association management guidelines for patients with thyroid nodules and differentiated thyroid cancer. *Thyroid* 2009; 19: 1167–214.
5. Haugen BR, Alexander EK, Bible KC, et al. 2015 American Thyroid Association management guidelines for adult patients with thyroid nodules and differentiated thyroid cancer. *Thyroid* 2016; 26: 1–133.

20.3 Indications for growth-hormone treatment

Introduction

Growth-hormone therapy is a substitution treatment to be offered in severe growth-hormone deficiency. The goal of this treatment is to correct metabolic, functional, and psychological abnormalities related to adult growth-hormone deficiency. In principle, any patient with severe growth-hormone deficiency is eligible for replacement treatment; however, there are requirements which vary in different countries.

Definition of severe growth-hormone deficiency

Severe growth-hormone deficiency is defined biochemically in the adult within an appropriate clinical context (i.e. with evidence of hypothalamo-pituitary disease, after cranial irradiation, or after traumatic brain injury). It is associated with an abnormal body composition, as well as psychological and physical features (see Box 20.1).

Biochemical diagnosis requires the demonstration of inadequate growth-hormone stimulation, with a validated test such as the ITT, which should always be performed with medical supervision and is contraindicated in older patients or those with a history of ischaemic heart disease or epilepsy, or a glucagon test. The combined administration of arginine and GHRH is nowadays complicated, since GHRH is not readily available any more, although the situation may change.

If three or four additional pituitary hormone deficiencies are present and IGF-1 is below reference values, no stimulation test is required, since growth-hormone deficiency has been shown to be present in over 97% of these patients.

Isolated idiopathic growth-hormone deficiency occurring de novo is not a recognized entity in the adult; however, there is a trend to treat less severe cases of adult growth-hormone deficiency nowadays, after initial approval.

The threshold for defining severe growth-hormone deficiency is a growth-hormone peak <3 ng/mL (or <5 ng/mL in the United States) after an ITT or glucagon test; for GHRH + arginine, the threshold is 11 ng/mL with a normal BMI, and <4 ng/mL in obese patients (BMI > 30).

Additionally, in the UK, the NICE recommendations require that only patients with impaired health-related quality of life (HRQoL) assessed with the disease-generated questionnaire AGHDA (for *assessment of growth-hormone deficiency in adults*) be offered growth-hormone replacement.

Unauthorized use of recombinant human growth hormone (rhGH) for the prevention of ageing or to increase sport performance is illegal and may be dangerous in someone without growth-hormone deficiency.

Treatment regimens

- rhGH should be administered subcutaneously once daily, preferably in the evening.
- The initial dose should be low: 0.1 mg/day in older individuals, 0.2 mg/day in young males, and 0.3 mg/day in young females.
- Dose escalations should be gradual, considering the biochemical response of IGF-1 (an indicator of hepatic growth-hormone action) as well as clinical features. These include evaluation of waist circumference (an indication of increased abdominal fat present in untreated growth-hormone deficiency), blood pressure, total and LDL cholesterol (which tend to fall after initiating rhGH), and HRQoL, especially energy, vitality, partner satisfaction, mood, sleep quality, and days off work, all of which improve after replacing rhGH.
- Many countries require HRQoL to be evaluated with questionnaires, preferably with disease-specific ones like AGHDA or QLS (for *questions on life satisfaction*). IGF-1 concentrations should be maintained within the age- and gender-related normal reference concentrations. Once established, annual clinical and biochemical control are usually enough to maintain adequate treatment.

Response to rhGH therapy

Reduction of abdominal obesity and an increase in energy levels occur early after starting rhGH therapy, although initial joint stiffness and muscle pain may present concomitantly; however, these problems are usually self-limited, either spontaneously or after a reduction in dose. Explaining this to the patients, so he/she knows what to expect, is useful, so they don't lose confidence in the treatment early on.

On the whole, sustained improvements towards normative scores in HRQoL take place within a few weeks of beginning replacement therapy and are maintained over the years. The more symptomatic the growth-hormone deficiency patients are at baseline, the greater the magnitude of response tends to be after starting substitution therapy with rhGH. Problems with memory and tiredness, the most serious burden for untreated patients, are also the ones that take longer to improve, whilst tenseness, self-confidence, and problems with socializing improve earlier and may even become normal. This lasting improvement and similar pattern of response in the majority of patients, independently of the level of HRQoL impairment at baseline, together with the requirement of daily self-injections, firmly support the evidence that rhGH replacement corrects these patients' psychological and physical problems.

Box 20.1 Common complaints and features found in untreated adult patients with growth-hormone deficiency and which improve after starting therapy with recombinant human growth hormone

- Abdominal adiposity with increased waist/hip ratio
- Reduced muscle strength, exercise performance, and energy
- Thin, dry skin and hair, and defective sweating
- Emotionally lability, depressive mood, and tendency towards social isolation
- Reduced sleep quality
- Lack of concentration and self-confidence
- Low bone density
- Unfavourable lipid profile (low HDL cholesterol; high total and LDL cholesterol and triglycerides)

Interaction of rhGH with concomitant hormone-substitution therapy

- Adult growth-hormone deficiency is most often associated with other pituitary hormone deficiencies, which require concomitant replacement. Interactions between these different therapies occur, which should be recalled if necessary.
- Initiation of rhGH may unmask secondary adrenal insufficiency or mandate an increase in the dose of hydrocortisone substitution.
- Oral oestrogens impair growth-hormone action and increase the required rhGH dose; this does not occur with the transdermal route, which is therefore recommended and should be associated with progestogens unless a hysterectomy has been performed.
- This does not apply to androgen substitution therapy.
- Growth hormone increases the peripheral conversion of T3 to T4, so that adjustments in doses of T4 are often necessary after the initiation of rhGH therapy; it may also unmask pre-existing central hypothyroidism, indicated by a subnormal circulating FT4 concentration, so FT4 should be measured when IGF-1 is monitored to adjust the rhGH dose.

Risks of rhGH

There is no evidence that replacement therapy with rhGH increases type 1 or type 2 diabetes mellitus; hypothalamic or pituitary tumour recurrence; or the risk of malignancy. However, any active malignancy requires stopping rhGH until control of the underlying condition is achieved.

If pituitary tumour rests are known to exist, imaging should be performed regularly to ascertain any progression, although it is not necessary to always halt rhGH if progression is found.

Side effects mainly related to water retention at treatment initiation (i.e. oedema, arthralgia, myalgia, paraesthesiae, joint stiffness, and pain related to carpal tunnel syndrome) are much less frequent nowadays, in parallel with lower-dose adjustments.

Worsening of glucose tolerance and increase in insulin resistance may occur and deserve monitoring, especially in older individuals, obese patients, and those with a strong family history of diabetes. rhGH therapy is not contraindicated in type 1 or type 2 diabetes, so a diabetic patient with growth-hormone deficiency should be treated similarly to any other one with diabetes. However, rhGH therapy is contraindicated in the presence of florid diabetic retinopathy.

Further reading

Attanasio AF, Jung H, Mo D, et al. Prevalence and incidence of diabetes mellitus in adult patients on growth hormone replacement for growth hormone deficiency: A surveillance database analysis. *J Clin Endocrinol Metab* 2011; 96: 2255–61.

Ho KK. Consensus guidelines for the diagnosis and treatment of adults with GH deficiency II: A statement of the GH Research Society in association with the European Society for Pediatric Endocrinology, Lawson Wilkins Society, European Society of Endocrinology, Japan Endocrine Society, and Endocrine Society of Australia. *Eur J Endocrinol* 2007; 157: 695–700.

Koltowska-Haggstrom M, Mattsson AF, Monson JP, et al. Does long-term GH replacement therapy in hypopituitary adults with GH deficiency normalise quality of life? *Eur J Endocrinol* 2006; 155: 109–19

Molitch ME, Clemmons DR, Malozowski S, et al. Evaluation and treatment of adult growth hormone deficiency: An Endocrine Society clinical practice guideline. *J Clin Endocrinol Metab* 2011; 96: 1587–609.

Webb SM, Strasburger CJ, Mo D, et al. Changing patterns of the adult growth hormone deficiency diagnosis documented in a decade-long global surveillance database. *J Clin Endocrinol Metab* 2009; 94: 392–9.

20.4 Follow-up of pituitary tumours

Acromegaly

For a flowchart on the management of acromegaly, see Figure 20.2.

Prolactinomas

For a flowchart on the management of microprolactinomas, see Figure 20.3. For a flowchart on the management of macroprolactinomas, see Figure 20.4.

Corticotroph adenomas

- After pituitary surgery:
  - cure: monitor 09:00 serum cortisol after omitting the previous evening's dose and the morning dose of hydrocortisone, at 6-monthly intervals (or earlier, if there is clinical concern); if serum cortisol >100 nmol/L (3.6 μg/dL), consider checking for relapse of Cushing's syndrome (by overnight DST) or for recovery of the hypothalamo-pituitary adrenal axis (by the short Synacthen® test or ITT)
  - no cure: consider repeat surgery; bilateral adrenalectomy; radiotherapy; or medical treatment
- After radiotherapy or medical treatment:
  - monitor by clinical picture and cortisol day curve (if radiotherapy, monitor for adrenal insufficiency and further pituitary hormone deficits)

- After bilateral adrenalectomy:
  - monitor for Nelson's syndrome

Non-functioning pituitary adenomas

- Non-operated:
  - micros: rescan at 1 and at 5 years
  - macros: rescan yearly for the first 5 years and 2 yearly for the next 5–6 years; monitor visual fields at yearly intervals if the tumour is close to the optic chiasm
- Operated:
  - no post-operative radiotherapy: scan yearly for the first 5 years and 2-yearly for the next 5–6 years
  - post-operative radiotherapy: annual assessment of the pituitary function, if previously intact, and annual formal visual fields

Craniopharyngiomas

- In all cases, perform annual pituitary imaging, annual visual fields assessment (if abnormal), and annual assessment of the pituitary hormone reserve (if radiotherapy). See Figure 20.5.

Rathke's cleft cysts

For a flowchart on Rathke's cleft cysts, see Figure 20.6.

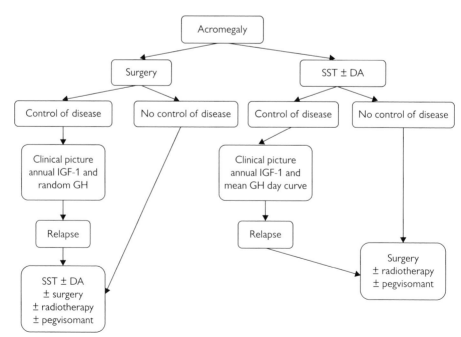

Fig 20.2 Management of acromegaly; DA, dopamine agonist; GH, growth hormone; SST, somatostatin analogue.

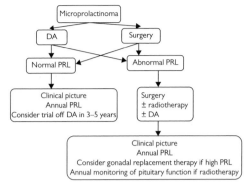

Fig 20.3 Management of microprolactinomas; DA, dopamine agonist; PRL, prolactin.

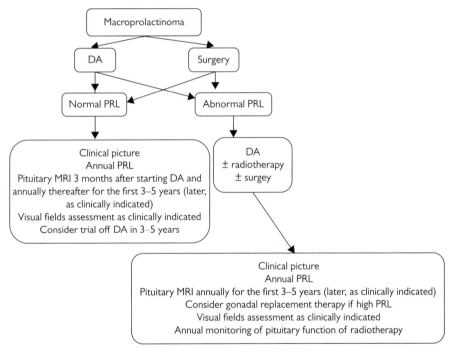

Fig 20.4 Management of macroprolactinomas; GTR, gross total resection; RT, radiation therapy.

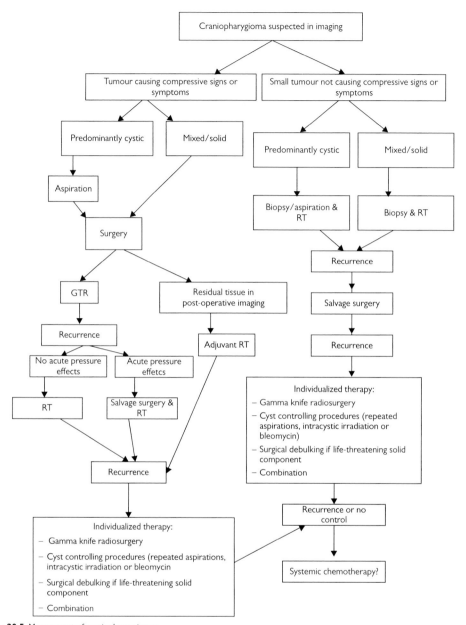

Fig 20.5 Management of craniopharyngiomas.
Reproduced from Karavitaki N, and Cudlip S, Craniopharyngiomas, Endocrine Reviews, Volume 27, Issue 4, pp. 371–397, https://doi.org/10.1210/er.2006-0002. Copyright (2006), by permission of Oxford University Press on behalf of the Endocrine Society.

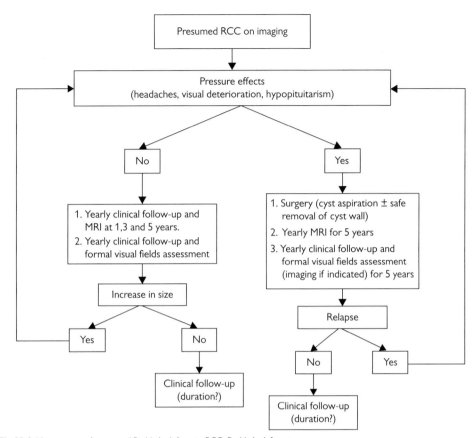

Fig 20.6 Management of presumed Rathke's cleft cysts; RCC, Rathke's cleft cyst.
Note: In case of multiple relapses, external irradiation may be considered.
Reproduced from Trifanescu R, Ansorge O, Wass JA, et al., Rathke's cleft cysts, *Clinical Endocrinology*, Volume 76, pp. 151–160, Copyright (2012), with permission from John Wiley and Sons.

20.5 Management of osteoporosis

Whom to treat

The NICE clinical guidelines propose that we target our assessment of risk for osteoporosis (http://cks.nice.org.uk/osteoporosis-prevention-of-fragility-fractures#!scenario). They propose that we consider assessment of fracture risk in all women aged 65 and over, and all men aged 75 and over. Women and men over 50 should be assessed for osteoporosis if they show any of NICE's proposed risk factors. The full list can be found on the NICE website, but can include previous fragility fracture; the current use or frequent recent use of oral or parenteral glucocorticoids; a history of falls or a family history of hip fracture (which could indicate low bone density); low BMI (<22; obesity protects against most fractures); smoking (currently); or alcohol intake (more than 14 units per week).

NICE do not recommend routinely assessing fracture risk in people under 50 unless major risk factors are present. This is because these individuals are at very low risk of fracture.

NICE proposed that we use fracture risk assessment tools such as FRAX (http://www.shef.ac.uk/FRAX/qrist) and QFracture (http://www.qfracture.org/) to predict fracture risk. The FRAX tool allows us to combine bone mineral density measurements with clinical risk factors and provides advice about treatment, based on guidelines from the National Osteoporosis Guideline Group (http://www.shef.ac.uk/NOGG/).

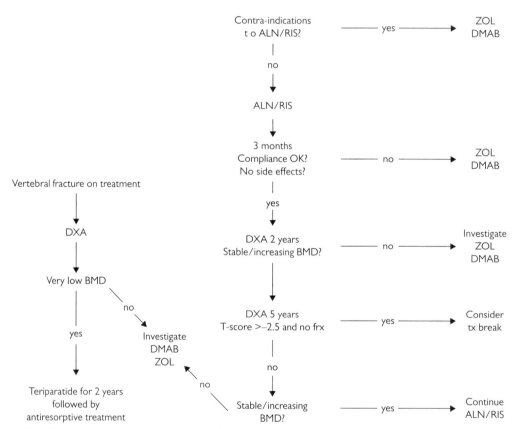

Fig 20.7 Algorithm for the treatment of postmenopausal osteoporosis; ALN, alendronic acid; BMD, bone mineral density; DMAB, denosumab; DXA, dual-energy x-ray absorptiometry; FRX, fracture; TX, treatment; ZOL, zoledronic acid.

How to treat

For men and women with an increased risk of fracture (T-score at spine or hip ≤−2.5), NICE recommend alendronic acid and risedronate as the first-choice treatments for postmenopausal osteoporosis in patients with or without prior fracture (http://cks.nice.org.uk/osteoporosis-prevention-of-fragility-fractures#!scenario:1). The reason for selecting these two oral bisphosphonates is that there is clinical trial evidence that they can reduce the frequency of spine, hip, and non-spine fractures. NICE recommend zoledronic acid as second-line treatment, although it can be used as first-line treatment if the fracture risk is high (10-year risk >10%). It is particularly useful if there is concern about gastric reflux and likely poor adherence with oral medication.

It is usual to start treatment with alendronic acid, 70 mg once a week, or risedronate, 35 mg once a week, and to ensure adequate intake of calcium (1000 mg daily if the diet provides inadequate levels) and vitamin D (800 IU daily in the elderly). These supplements are recommended, as they were included in almost all clinical trials. If the patient has an adequate intake of calcium, supplementation is not necessary. Alternatives to alendronate include raloxifene. If the bisphosphonate is not tolerated or not effective, parenteral treatments such zoledronic acid (5 mg intravenous once a year) or denosumab (60 mg subcutaneous once every 6 months) should be given. In the case of severe osteoporosis (e.g. vertebral fracture on treatment and a T-score <−3.5) then teriparatide (20 µg subcutaneous daily for 2 years) is given. See Figure 20.7 for details.

20.6 Autoimmune polyglandular syndromes

Definition

The term 'autoimmune polyglandular syndrome' is used to describe the co-occurrence of several autoimmune diseases affecting the endocrine system of a single patient. The most common subtypes are autoimmune polyglandular syndrome type 1 and autoimmune polyglandular syndrome type 2. Both of these are characterized by end-organ damage mediated by leucocytes in the presence of autoantibodies.

Autoimmune polyglandular syndrome type 3 is defined as the occurrence of autoimmune thyroid disease in combination with a second autoimmune condition other than Addison's disease or hypoparathyroidism.

IPEX (for *immune dysfunction, polyendocrinopathy, X-linked*) is a rare condition affecting infants. It is due to a mutation in *FOXP3* and is characterized by several endocrinopathies, including type 1a diabetes. Dermatitis and enteropathy are other features. Affected patients usually die by the age of 2.

Autoimmune polyglandular syndrome type 2

Autoimmune polyglandular syndrome type 2 is the most prevalent form of autoimmune polyglandular syndrome. It mostly affects female patients, and commonly presents after the age of 20. It is a genetic condition with a polygenic, HLA-associated, autosomal-dominant inheritance pattern with incomplete penetrance.

Clinical features

Autoimmune polyglandular syndrome type 2 consists of Addison's disease in combination with autoimmune thyroid disease or type 1a diabetes. It is associated with other autoimmune conditions such as vitiligo, alopecia, hypogonadism, pernicious anaemia, atrophic gastritis, and coeliac disease.

Autoimmune polyglandular syndrome type 1

Autoimmune polyglandular syndrome type 1 is a rare autosomal-recessive condition caused by a mutation in *AIRE*, which is involved in the elimination of autoreactive T-cells. This type usually presents in childhood.

Cardinal triad of autoimmune polyglandular syndrome type 1

The cardinal triad of autoimmune polyglandular syndrome type 1 consists of Addison's disease, chronic mucocutaneous candidiasis, and primary hypoparathyroidism. Two out of three of this triad suffice for a diagnosis. Other associations include alopecia, asplenia, vitiligo, hypothyroidism, hypogonadism, fat malabsorption, pernicious anaemia, atrophic gastritis, coeliac disease and hepatitis, and Sjögren's disease.

Diagnosis

See Boxes 20.2 and 20.3.

Screening

See Table 20.2. Since autoimmune polyglandular syndrome is genetically determined, family members of affected patients will need regular screening every 3–5 years (see Tables 20.3 and 20.4) with a clinical history and examination, a screen for adrenal, islet cell, and—if the index patient has thyroiditis—thyroid autoantibodies.

Box 20.2 Summary of common characteristics of autoimmune polyglandular syndrome type 1 and type 2

Autoimmune polyglandular syndrome type 1
Rare
Childhood or adolescence
AIRE (recessive; autoimmune regulator gene)
Diagnosis: *AIRE* mutations
Associated rheumatological diseases:
- Sjögren's syndrome
- systemic lupus erythematosus
- rheumatoid arthritis
- myasthenia gravis
- anti-phospholipid syndrome

Autoimmune polyglandular syndrome type 2
Common
Midlife
Polygenic (mainly HLA)
Diagnosis:
- antibodies
- clinical

Box 20.3 Diagnostic criteria and associated diagnoses for autoimmune polyglandular syndrome type 1 and type 2

Autoimmune polyglandular syndrome type 1
Addison's disease[†]
Hypoparathyroidism[†]
Mucocutaneous candidiasis[†]
Autoimmune thyroid disease
Type 1 diabetes mellitus
Vitiligo and alopecia
Hypogonadism
Pernicious anaemia
Pure red cell aplasia
Malabsorption syndrome
Asplenism
Chronic active hepatitis
Ectodermal dysplasia

Autoimmune polyglandular syndrome type 2
Two or more of any of the following:
- autoimmune thyroid disease
- type 1 diabetes mellitus
- vitiligo and alopecia
- hypogonadism
- pernicious anaemia
- idiopathic thrombocytopenia
- coeliac disease
- dermatitis herpetiformis
- idiopathic heart block
- serositis
- IgA deficiency

[†] Two or more.

Table 20.2 Target autoantigens in autoimmune polyendocrine syndrome type 1 and autoimmune polyendocrine syndrome type 2

Target organ	Autoantigen
Adrenal cortex	21-hydroxylase
Gonads/adrenal cortex	17α-hydroxylase
	Side-chain cleavage enzyme
Thyroid epithelium	Thyroid peroxidase
	TSH receptor
Langerhans' islets	Insulin
	Glutamic acid decarboxylase
	Tyrosine phosphatase-like protein IA-2
	Zinc transporter isoform 8
Gastrointestinal tract	H^+/K^+-ATPase
	Tryptophan hydroxylase
Liver	Cytochrome P450 1A2
	Cytochrome P450 2A6
Skin (melanocyte)	Tyrosinase

Reproduced from John A.H. Wass, Paul M. Stewart, Stephanie A. Amiel et al., *Oxford Textbook of Endocrinology and Diabetes, Second Edition*, Table 10.2.5.6, Copyright © 2011 with permission from Oxford University Press

Table 20.3 Screening in patients with autoimmune polyendocrine syndrome

What to screen	Frequency
Adrenal, thyroid, islet cell, and tTG autoantibodies	1–3 yearly
Ca	Yearly
TSH	
T4	
HBA1c	
Fasting glucose	
Vitamin B_{12}	
Cortisol	
ACTH	
PRA	
FSH	
LH	
Testosterone/estradiol	
FBC	
Blood film	
Intrinsic factor autoantibodies	5 yearly

Abbreviations: ACTH, adrenocorticotrophic hormone; Ca, calcium; FBC, full blood count; FSH, follicle-stimulating hormone; HBA1c, haemoglobin A1c; LH, luteinizing hormone; PRA, plasmin renin activity; T4, thyroxine; TSH, thyroid-stimulating hormone; tTG, tissue transglutaminase antibody.

Table 20.4 Screening in first-degree relatives of index patient with autoimmune polyendocrine syndrome

What to screen	Frequency
Adrenal, islet cell autoantibodies	3–5 yearly
If the index patient has thyroid disease: thyroid autoantibodies	3–5 yearly
Ca	3–5 yearly
TSH	
HBA1c	
Vitamin B_{12}	

Abbreviations: Ca, calcium; HBA1c, haemoglobin A1c; TSH, thyroid-stimulating hormone.

Biochemical screening should include levels of calcium, TSH, haemoglobin A1c, and vitamin B_{12}.

Further reading

Barker JM. Type 1 diabetes-associated autoimmunity: Natural history, genetic associations, and screening. *J Clin Endocrinol Metab* 2006; 91: 1210–17.

Betterle C, Dal Pra C, Mantero F, et al. Autoimmune adrenal insufficiency and autoimmune polyendocrine syndromes: Autoantibodies, autoantigens, and their applicability in diagnosis and disease prediction. *Endocr Rev* 2002; 23: 327–64.

Michels AW and Gottlieb PA. Autoimmune polyglandular syndromes. *Nat Rev Endocrinol* 2010; 6: 270–7.

20.7 Hyperglycaemia

Introduction

Insulin is a key hormone in glucose homeostasis. However, the actions of insulin are affected by several other hormones, including growth hormone, corticosteroids, adrenaline, and glucagon. Therefore, hyperglycaemia can occur with any pathological process which results in excess production of these 'counter-regulatory' hormones. Hyperglycaemia secondary to endocrine disease is typically mild, and often resolves entirely after effective treatment of the underlying endocrinopathy (Table 20.5). Current criteria are shown in Table 20.6.

Acromegaly

Pathogenesis of hyperglycaemia in acromegaly

Diabetes develops in ~20% and impaired glucose tolerance in up to 80% of patients with acromegaly. Growth hormone antagonizes several of the actions of insulin. One of the main metabolic functions of growth hormone is lipolysis, resulting in increased levels of circulating non-esterified fatty acids. These compete with glucose for uptake by muscle via the Randle cycle, which results in decreased glucose uptake and increased insulin resistance. In addition, growth hormone stimulates gluconeogenesis, and inhibits the activity of muscle glycogen synthase. Furthermore, drugs such as somatostatin analogues, which are used in the treatment of acromegaly, may worsen diabetes by inhibiting insulin secretion by the pancreatic beta cells.

Management of hyperglycaemia in acromegaly

The management of diabetes in acromegaly is comparable to the management of type 2 diabetes. Metformin (which improves insulin resistance) and sulfonylureas (which increase insulin secretion from pancreatic beta cells) are the first-line oral hypoglycaemic medications to control glycaemic levels in patients with acromegaly. Insulin should be started when oral medications are unable to maintain adequate control of dysglycaemia.

Glycaemic control is best achieved by treatment of underlying cause of growth hormone excess (e.g. neurosurgical removal of a pituitary adenoma which is secreting growth hormone). Insulin may be necessary during the perioperative period. Diabetes often resolves after 'cure' of acromegaly; therefore, it is important to monitor blood sugar levels in these patients and reduce or stop any anti-diabetic medications, to reduce the risk of hypoglycaemia. If diabetes persists after definitive treatment of acromegaly, hyperglycaemia should be managed according to standard guidelines for type 2 diabetes.

Cushing's syndrome

Pathogenesis of hyperglycaemia in Cushing's syndrome

Impaired glucose tolerance and diabetes are very common in Cushing's syndrome, and approximately 40% patients with Cushing's syndrome have diabetes at diagnosis. The pathogenesis of diabetes mellitus in patients with Cushing's syndrome involves increased insulin resistance (adipose tissue and skeletal muscle), and enhanced hepatic gluconeogenesis. Furthermore, glucocorticoids impair pancreatic beta-cell function. Impaired beta-cell function may be an important contributory factor in the development of diabetes in these patients, due to an inability to increase compensatory insulin secretion in response to insulin resistance.

Management of hyperglycaemia in Cushing's syndrome

The management of diabetes in Cushing's syndrome is similar to the management of type 2 diabetes. Oral hypoglycaemic agents which improve insulin sensitivity (e.g. metformin) and enhance insulin secretion (e.g. sulfonylureas and prandial secretagogues) can be used as first-line therapy. Insulin therapy may be necessary when oral medications cannot control glucose levels, and during the perioperative period. Glycaemic control is best achieved by controlling the underlying hypercortisolaemia. Diabetes usually resolves when cortisol levels are controlled; therefore, anti-diabetic medications may have to be reduced or stopped.

Neuroendocrine tumours

Pathogenesis of hyperglycaemia with neuroendocrine tumours

Diabetes develops in up to 80% of patients with an underlying glucagonoma (a slow-growing pancreatic alpha cell tumour). Elevated glucagon levels in these patients increase blood glucose levels, due to the effects of this hormone on gluconeogenesis and lipolysis. Patients with other gastroenteropancreatic neuroendocrine

Table 20.5 Frequency of diabetes mellitus or impaired glucose tolerance complicating endocrine conditions

Cause	Patients developing diabetes or impaired glucose tolerance (%)
Acromegaly	~20
Cushing's disease	~40
Neuroendocrine tumours	Up to 80
Phaeochromocytomas	35–50

Table 20.6 WHO glucose thresholds for diagnosis of diabetes mellitus and other stages of dysglycaemia

		Venous plasma glucose
Normal	Fasting *and* 2-hour glucose	<6.1 mmol/L (<110 mg/dL)
	During GTT	<7.8 mmol/L (<140 mg/dL)
Diabetes	Fasting *or* 2-hour glucose	>7.0 mmol/L (>126 mg/dL)
	During GTT	>11.1 mmol/L (>200 mg/dL)
IGT	Fasting *and* 2-hour glucose	<7.0 mmol/L (<126 mg/dL)
	During GTT	>7.8 mmol/L (>140 mg/dL) and <11.1 mmol/L (<200 mg/dL)
IFG	Fasting	>6.1 mmol/L (>110 mg/dL) and <7.0 mmol/L (<126 mg/dL)

Abbreviations: GTT, glucose tolerance test; IFG, impaired fasting glucose; IGT, impaired glucose tolerance.

Adapted from *Definition, Diagnosis and Classification of Diabetes Mellitus and Its Complications: Report of a WHO Consultation*, Department of Noncommunicable Disease Surveillance, pp. 1–66, Table 1. Copyright (1999) World Health Organization.

tumour subtypes may be at risk of surgically induced diabetes after partial or total pancreatectomy to remove the underlying pancreatic neuroendocrine tumour. Furthermore, somatostatin analogues are commonly used in the treatment of patients with neuroendocrine tumours, to improve morbidity and mortality. Somatostatin analogues can also impair glucose tolerance in these patients.

Management of hyperglycaemia in neuroendocrine tumours
The mainstay of treatment of diabetes in patients with a glucagonoma is surgical resection of the primary tumour. These patients often require insulin therapy to control hyperglycaemia until surgical intervention. Most patients show significant clinical improvement even with incomplete surgical resection.

Phaeochromocytomas

Studies suggest that approximately 35%–50% of phaeochromocytoma patients have hyperglycaemia. Adrenaline causes hyperglycaemia via its action on pancreatic beta cells and the liver. Adrenaline inhibits insulin secretion by the pancreas, and increases transient glycogenolysis and sustained gluconeogenesis in the liver. Adrenergic stimulation also induces insulin resistance of the muscles resulting in reduced peripheral glucose uptake.

Management of hyperglycaemia with phaeochromocytoma
The management of diabetes in patients with a phaeochromocytoma is similar to the management of type 2 diabetes. Metformin, sulfonylureas, and prandial secretagogues are the first-line oral hypoglycaemic agents. Alpha- and beta-adrenergic receptor blockers which effectively control cardiovascular symptoms do not appear to reverse the hyperglycaemic effects of catecholamines. Surgical removal of the underlying tumour is the definitive treatment of hyperglycaemia secondary to a phaeochromocytoma. Insulin may be needed during the perioperative period. Most of the metabolic abnormalities, including hyperglycaemia, do resolve following the surgical removal of the tumour. Close monitoring of blood glucose is mandatory, as patients may develop hypoglycaemia after removal of the phaeochromocytoma.

Autoimmune endocrinopathies

Pathogenesis of hyperglycaemia in autoimmune endocrinopathies
Diabetes associated with autoimmune endocrine disease (e.g. autoimmune polyendocrine syndromes) is most frequently type 1 diabetes. Hyperglycaemia in these patients arises secondary to autoimmune-mediated pancreatic beta-cell destruction and absolute insulin deficiency.

Management of hyperglycaemia associated with autoimmune endocrinopathies
It may be useful to assess pancreatic beta-cell autoantibodies (e.g. antibodies against glutamic acid decarboxylase, IA2 or islet cells) to confirm the diagnosis of autoimmune-mediated diabetes. Insulin should be started from diagnosis to prevent ketoacidosis. Typical insulin regimens include twice-daily biphasic/mixed insulin or the basal bolus regimen (i.e. rapid-acting insulin with each meal with background long-acting insulin). Education (e.g. injection technique; safe disposal of sharps; use of the glucometer; and recognition and treatment of hypoglycaemia) is paramount. Patients who start insulin should inform the DVLA.

Practical tips

- Management of hyperglycaemia associated with excess secretion of counter-regulatory hormones is similar to the management of type 2 diabetes.
- Hyperglycaemia usually resolves after definitive treatment of underlying endocrine disorder.
- Start with oral hypoglycaemic agents such as metformin (e.g. 500 mg twice daily, increasing usually to 1000 mg twice daily, with a maximum dose of 1000 mg three times daily) or consider sulfonylureas (e.g. gliclazide 80 mg once daily, increasing in 80 mg steps to a maximum of 160 mg twice daily). By using oral hypoglycaemic agents, it is usually possible to achieve good control of glucose levels, achieving target concentrations of haemoglobin A1c.
- Insulin should be introduced if oral agents do not control hyperglycaemia.
- Insulin therapy should be started from diagnosis in patients with autoimmune-mediated destruction of pancreatic beta cells and absolute insulin deficiency.

Further reading

American Diabetes Association. Diagnosis and classification of diabetes mellitus. *Diabet Care* 2012; 35: S64–71.

Resmini E, Minuto F, Colao A, et al. Secondary diabetes associated with principal endocrinopathies: The impact of new treatment modalities. *Acta Diabetol* 2009; 46: 85–95.

20.8 Hyperlipidaemia

Definition

Lipids transported in plasma are carried in macromolecules called lipoproteins. Lipoproteins conform to a general structure: a hydrophobic core containing triglycerides and cholesteryl esters, and an amphipathic surface containing free cholesterol, phospholipids, and apolipoproteins. The volume of the core determines the density of lipoprotein and this also provides insight into the nomenclature.

Very low density lipoprotein

Very low density lipoprotein (VLDL) is the main carrier of triglycerides. It is secreted as a macromolecule from the liver and contains apolipoprotein B (ApoB), triglycerides, some cholesterol, and a small amount of phospholipids. It thus provides a vehicle for triglyceride offloading and, in turn, the movement of fatty acids from the liver to adipose and muscle tissue. The triglyceride content of VLDL is removed from the lipoprotein particle by lipoprotein lipase, which lines the endothelium in adipose and muscle tissues. Lipoprotein lipase is the only triglyceride lipase to effectively remove triglycerides contained in VLDL particles. In healthy people, this removal is rapid and the major part of the triglyceride content is removed within 1–4 hours. This leads to the formation of a remnant lipoprotein particle (intermediate density lipoprotein and then LDL).

LDL

LDL is formed from VLDL, and is the main cholesterol carrier in plasma. It circulates for much longer than VLDL does—up to 2–3 days. In most people, LDL makes up about two-thirds of the total cholesterol content in plasma. Each VLDL and LDL particle contains one molecule of ApoB. The ApoB concentration is therefore largely reflective of the number of LDL particles in plasma. LDL particles are removed from plasma via the LDL receptor, which is highly expressed in the liver.

HDL

HDL is formed via a separate pathway. It contains apolipoprotein A1 (ApoA1) and apolipoprotein A2. ApoA1 is secreted from the intestine and the liver in small complexes with phospholipids and rapidly attracts free cholesterol, which is readily esterified by lecithin–cholesteryl acyltransferase into cholesteryl fatty acyl esters, which provide a core lipoprotein component and thereby allow for additional free cholesterol uptake. The ability of ApoA1 to attract free cholesterol supports the movement of cholesterol from peripheral tissues to the liver (reverse cholesterol transport). Some of the cholesteryl esters will be moved from the HDL particle to the VLDL particle by cholesteryl ester transfer protein.

Chylomicrons constitute a highly efficient transport vehicle of dietary triglycerides from the intestine (about 70–100 g /day on a typical Western diet). Chylomicrons are extremely large particles with a very rapid turnover via the lipoprotein lipase. Chylomicrons should not be present in plasma after an overnight fast and, in most people, there is very little dietary fat remaining in plasma 6–8 hours after food intake.

Assessment of lipids, lipoproteins, and apolipoproteins in plasma

Quantification of total cholesterol is independent of whether the sample has been taken after an overnight fast or is non-fasting. Some methods for determining lipoprotein subfractions (using the Friedewald formula (see below)) require a fasting sample. A random non-fasting triglyceride measurement can be useful: if it is low or normal, this implies that the fasting sample is also low or normal whereas, if an elevated concentration is observed, a fasting sample will be required to assess the degree of hypertriglyceridaemia.

There are readily available and commonly used methods to quantify HDL cholesterol, but the inter-laboratory variation is often rather unsatisfactory. Direct assessment of LDL cholesterol is becoming available but is still most often not used during routine clinical care. Instead, the LDL concentration is calculated using the Friedewald formula:

$$LDL - C = Total\ C - HDL - C - \frac{Triglycerides}{2.2},$$

(formula to be used for lipids measured in millimoles per litre), or

$$LDL - C = Total\ C - HDL - C - \frac{Triglycerides}{5},$$

(formula to be used for lipids measured in milligrams per decilitre), where *LDL-C* is the concentration of LDL cholesterol, *HDL-C* is the concentration of HDL cholesterol, *Total C* is the total cholesterol concentration, and *Triglycerides* is the triglyceride concentration.

Cholesterol and triglyceride concentrations are quantified in millimoles per litre or milligrams per decilitre. The equivalent concentration for cholesterol is 1 mmol/L = 38.7 mg/dL, whereas, for triglycerides, 1 mmol/L = 88.6 mg/dL. A convenient converter can be found at http://www.onlineconversion.com/cholesterol.

ApoB is often measured with good standardization between laboratories, and is normally given in grams per litre. Non-HDL cholesterol reflects the total burden of cholesterol positively associated with cardiovascular risk and does in most instances correlate closely with ApoB concentrations.

Classification of hyperlipidaemia

The classifications of hyperlipidaemia are based either on arbitrary cut-offs of measured lipid concentrations in lipoprotein subclasses (Frederickson's classification; see Table 20.7) or descriptive and disease-specific terms.

Table 20.7 Frederickson's classification of hyperlipidaemias (types 1–5)

Hypercholesterolaemia	Combined hyperlipidaemia	Hypertriglyceridaemia
Type 2a	Type 4	Type 4
	Type 2b	Type 1
	Type 5	
	Type 3	

Data from *Bulletin of the World Health Organization*, Volume 43, Classification of hyperlipidaemias and hyperlipoproteinaemias, 1970, pp. 891–915.

Hypercholesterolaemia

Hypercholesterolaemia is most often caused by an elevated level of LDL cholesterol. Occasionally, a normal level of LDL cholesterol can be seen in the context of a high level of HDL cholesterol, but this constellation is benign (see 'Hypertriglyceridaemia'). The elevated level of LDL cholesterol can be due to secondary factors of a polygenic nature (see 'Combined hyperlipidaemia') or, although only occasionally, the cause may be monogenic, as in familial hypercholesterolaemia (see 'Familial hypercholesterolaemia'); in the latter case, the elevation is often drastic.

Combined hyperlipidaemia

The combined elevation of cholesterol and triglyceride levels is common, and often seen as a consequence of obesity or type 2 diabetes. The level of HDL cholesterol is often low or very low. The cholesterol is contained in VLDL and/or LDL particles.

In type 4 hyperlipidaemia, the level of LDL cholesterol is low to normal in the context of hypertriglyceridaemia (increased levels of VLDL).

In type 2b hyperlipidaemia, the level of LDL cholesterol is high in the context of hypertriglyceridaemia. This phenotype is seen in what is called 'familial combined hyperlipidaemia'. Despite the name and suggestive pedigree structure of familial combined hyperlipidaemia, dominant genes explaining the actual cause of this disease have not been identified and it is likely the condition depends on an inherited aggregation of a large number of unfavourable genetic variants with small effect sizes.

Type 5 hyperlipidaemia is the very extreme progression of type 4 hyperlipidaemia, with very high triglyceride concentrations (typically >10 mmol/L (885 mg/dL)), and is often seen secondary to another cause (see below). A clear risk of pancreatitis is present when plasma triglycerides are >20 mmol/L (1770 mg/dL).

Type 3 hyperlipidaemia, also called dysbetalipoproteinaemia, is a specific hyperlipidaemia caused by homozygous carrier status of the ε2 variant of *APOE* (the typical population frequency of this is ~1%, but only 1%–10% of carriers actually get the hyperlipidaemia). The cholesterol elevation is due to an accumulation of extremely cholesterol-rich VLDL particles, but hardly any LDL particles. The precipitation of type 3 hyperlipidaemia requires a secondary factor, such as obesity, type 2 diabetes, alcohol, certain medications, or hypothyroidism. Cholesterol and triglyceride concentrations can be extreme (12–20 mmol/L (464–773 mg/dL) of cholesterol and 12–20 mmol/L (1062–1770 mg/dL) of triglycerides at the same time). This is one of the few hyperlipidaemic conditions that respond extremely well to monotherapy with fibrates (see 'Fibrates').

Hypertriglyceridaemia

Isolated hypertriglyceridaemia is a condition in which there is an increase in the level of VLDL with low or normal levels of LDL cholesterol. Type 4 hyperlipidaemia in its milder forms is classified as hypertriglyceridaemia; this condition is common and typically shows low-to-normal levels of LDL cholesterol, and triglyceride concentrations <5 mmol/L (443 mg/dL).

Pseudohypertriglyceridaemia is an unusual hypertriglyceridaemia variant. It is an X-linked recessive disorder (and therefore essentially only seen in men, with a population frequency in the range of 1/1000 to 1/10,000) caused by a loss-of-function mutation or deletion in *GK*, which encodes glycerol kinase. This leads to hyperglycerolaemia (not hypertriglyceridaemia), due to the lack of glycerol elimination by the liver. The background to the analytical error that leads to this condition being identified as hypertriglyceridaemia is that most triglyceride assays (which measure triglyceride levels by quantifying glycerol levels after a lipase reaction in plasma) do not blank for free glycerol. However, pseudohypertriglyceridaemia is a benign condition and should be left untreated.

Type 1 hyperlipidaemia is a rare form of extreme hypertriglyceridaemia caused by an absence of lipoprotein lipase activity. It is normally caused by homozygosity of recessive mutations in *LPL* (which encodes lipoprotein lipase), and therefore is more often seen as a consequence of consanguinity. Extreme hypertriglyceridaemia, also called chylomicronaemia, is seen in the fasting state and, in poorly managed conditions, plasma triglyceride concentrations can be seen in the range of 50–150 mmol/L (4425– 13,275 mg/dL). There is a very high risk of pancreatitis. In the acute setting with extreme hypertriglyceridaemia, pseudohyponatraemia can be seen, but this should not be corrected. The only effective treatment is an extremely low-fat diet.

Pathophysiology

Primary causes

Familial hypercholesterolaemia

Familial hypercholesterolaemia is caused by mutations in *LDLR*, *APOB*, or *PCSK9*, but other genes not yet discovered could be involved. LDLR is the receptor removing LDL from plasma, APOB is the lipoprotein carried ligand to the receptor and PCSK9 modulates the recirculation of the receptor back to the cell surface. About 90% of known cases are caused by heterozygous loss-of-function mutations in *LDLR*. The population frequency is often in the range of 1/300 to 1/500. The condition is dominant, and the loss of one functioning *LDLR* allele gives rise to a drastic rise in LDL cholesterol, due to impaired receptor-mediated removal by the liver. Typical untreated total-cholesterol concentrations are in the range of 7.5–14.0 mmol/L (290–541 mg/dL), with normal or near-normal plasma triglyceride concentrations. Additional cases are likely to be found among family members. Screening of family members has proven an effective way of identifying untreated patients. Genetic testing for familial hypercholesterolaemia can be helpful but is not required (see below for criteria). Untreated, the condition leads to a drastically high risk of early presentation of cardiovascular disease. Patients respond well to statin therapy and this should be started early—if not in childhood, then in young adulthood (but see 'Pregnancy'). Dietary and lifestyle treatment on its own is most often insufficient and is not recommended.

Homozygous familial hypercholesterolaemia is extremely rare (~1/1,000,000) and is normally picked up by paediatricians during the early presentation of heart disease.

The diagnostic criteria for familial hypercholesterolaemia (Simon Broome criteria) are as follows:

* definite familial hypercholesterolaemia: high cholesterol levels (in an adult, cholesterol >7.5 mmol/L (290 mg/dL) or LDL cholesterol >4.9 mmol/L (190 mg/dL)); in

a child under the age of 16, cholesterol >6.7 mmol/L (260 mg/dL) or LDL cholesterol >4 mmol/L (155 mg/dL)) plus at least one of the following:

- tendon xanthomas, in the patient or in a first-degree (i.e. parent, sibling, or child) or second-degree (i.e. grandparent, uncle, or aunt) relative
- DNA-based evidence of a mutation in *LDLR*, *APOB*, or *PCSK9*
- possible familial hypercholesterolaemia: high cholesterol levels (as above) plus at least one of the following:
  - a family history of myocardial infarction (occurring below the age of 50 in a second-degree relative or below the age of 60 in a first-degree relative)
  - a family history of raised total cholesterol (i.e. >7.5 mmol/L (290 mg/dL) in an adult first- or second-degree relative or >6.7 mmol/L (260 mg/dL) in a child or sibling under the age of 16)

Familial combined hyperlipidaemia and familial hypertriglyceridemia
Familial combined hyperlipidaemia and its subform, familial hypertriglyceridemia, are common (1/300), and index cases typically have raised levels of cholesterol, triglycerides, and ApoB, with a very high risk of early presentation of cardiovascular disease. Although there is a clear familial pattern for this disease, a defined molecular diagnosis does not exist; it is instead likely that the disease depend on the aggregation of a large number of genetic variants with adverse effects within the family. Cases and family members should be treated aggressively and early on. Familial hypertriglyceridaemia is much less common than familial combined hyperlipidaemia; it displays a level of cardiovascular risk that is similar to that seen in familial combined hyperlipidaemia but normally only with elevated triglyceride levels, which are rarely very drastically elevated (above >10 mmol/L (885 mg/dL)).

Type 1 hyperlipidaemia
Type 1 hyperlipidaemia is classically caused by homozygous null-allele variants in *LPL*. In addition, forms caused by mutations in *GPIHBP1*, *APOA5*, and *APOC2* have been described. Such mutations lead to extreme hypertriglyceridaemia and a significant risk of pancreatitis. Eruptive xanthomas, typically affecting the back, the arms, and chest, can be seen. As the condition is recessive, family members are often not affected. The mainstay of treatment is a very-low-fat diet but, on top of that, fibrates can be tested. In cases where the low-fat diet is difficult to implement, inhibition of fat absorption (via Xenical) can be tested.

Type 3 hyperlipidaemia
Type 3 hyperlipidaemia is caused by homozygous carrier status of *APOE-ε2*. This genetic background is carried by 1% of the population but only 1%–10% of those actually get the hyperlipidaemia; a precipitating factor is needed (see 'Secondary factors'). The hyperlipidaemia can be explosive, with a sudden onset of drastically elevated cholesterol and triglycerides (triglyceride levels >10 mmol/L (885 mg/dL) and cholesterol levels >10 mmol/L (387 mg/dL) can be seen). If long-standing, this may lead to a specific cutaneous manifestation (tuberoeruptive xanthomas), affecting elbows and knees first. The condition often responds rapidly and well to fibrates.

Elevation of lipoprotein(a)
Elevation of lipoprotein(a) (Lp(a)) is not normally considered to constitute a specific hyperlipidaemia, but is strongly determined by genetic background. The Lp(a) lipoprotein consists of an LDL-like particle carrying apolipoprotein(a) and ApoB but is not removed via the LDL receptor. A situation where elevated Lp(a) could be considered, and therefore tested for, is when moderate hypercholesterolaemia that appears treatment resistant to statins is found in a patient with premature cardiovascular disease.

Secondary causes
Diet
Hypertriglyceridaemia is closely linked to obesity. A diet rich in carbohydrates can increase the plasma triglyceride concentration. The strongest effect is seen with sucrose/fructose. A diet rich in saturated fat can raise the level of LDL cholesterol.

Alcohol
High alcohol consumption can, in some people, lead to significant hypertriglyceridaemia.

Obesity
Obesity is most often associated with raised triglyceride concentrations. Only abdominal obesity is associated with hyperlipidaemia. Paradoxically, the expanded fat mass has an inability to effectively store fat, and the spillover of excess fat to the liver fuels VLDL production and hypertriglyceridaemia. Obesity is very often seen with low levels of HDL cholesterol.

Type 2 diabetes
Hyperlipidaemia seen in type 2 diabetes is strongly dependent on glycaemic control.

Type 1 diabetes
Poorly controlled type 1 diabetes may lead to significant hypertriglyceridaemia.

Partial lipodystrophy
Partial lipodystrophy is most commonly seen in HIV/AIDS and antiretroviral treatment. Monogenic forms of partial lipodystrophy are almost invariably associated with hypertriglyceridaemia.

Hypothyroidism
Hypothyroidism is a common secondary cause of raised LDL cholesterol. TSH levels should be checked in suspected cases.

Cushing's syndrome and hypercortisolism
Cushing's syndrome and hypercortisolism are often associated with hypertriglyceridaemia.

Medication
A large number of pharmacological treatments may lead to hyperlipidaemia. These include retinoids, corticosteroids, antipsychotics, protease inhibitors, oral contraceptives, beta-adrenoceptor blockers, and thiazide diuretics.

Lipoproteins and the atherosclerosis disease process
ApoB-containing lipoproteins (LDL, VLDL, and Lp(a)) have all been associated with the development of cardiovascular disease. Elevated concentrations of these

lipoproteins in plasma will lead to greater deposition in the arterial subendothelial space, where the ApoB moiety itself will enhance retention. Retained lipoproteins may undergo modifications that lead to macrophage uptake. Macrophages full of cholesterol (foam cells) will trigger an inflammatory response to rebuild the injured artery. This may eventually lead to the build-up of an atherosclerotic plaque, which, upon rupture, can lead to the formation of an occlusive thrombus and infarction/ischaemia of the end organ.

HDL supposedly opposes this process, through either 'reverse cholesterol transport', or other qualities of HDL, but recent studies using Mendelian randomization raises doubt as to whether the plasma concentration of HDL (approximated by HDL cholesterol) is causally related to these processes.

Clinical features beyond cardiovascular disease

- Tendinous xanthomas are pathognomic for familial hypercholesterolaemia. In untreated patients, this sign may not become apparent until the age of 40. Lesions will regress upon effective treatment.
- Eruptive xanthomas are often seen in extreme hypertriglyceridaemia (triglycerides above 20 mmol/L (1770 mg/dL)).
- Tuberoeruptive xanthomas are pathognomonic for type 3 hyperlipidaemia.
- Extreme hypertriglyceridaemia can present with pancreatitis. This is a very serious condition and may imply the need for lifelong treatment with fibrates as protection.

Investigations

- The calculation of lipoprotein fractions via the Friedewald formula requires a fasting sample. Total levels of plasma cholesterol and ApoB do not change significantly after food intake, whereas triglyceride levels do. A low or normal non-fasting triglyceride measurement excludes hypertriglyceridaemia, whereas a high reading should be repeated under fasting conditions.
- Fasting glucose, TSH, and liver function tests are part of a lipid assessment. Anthropometric measurements are necessary.
- Genetic screening for mutations in familial hypercholesterolaemia can be helpful in diagnosis and family screening but are not absolutely necessary.
- *APOE* genotyping is needed to ascertain type 3 hyperlipidaemia.

Management: Treatment options and monitoring treatment (including frequency/subsequent action and troubleshooting)

The evidence base for using statins to lower cardiovascular disease risk in secondary prevention (including in type 2 diabetes) is strong. Statins, diet, and lifestyle management together with additional hypolipidaemic drugs, are used to lower elevated levels of LDL cholesterol, towards established targets. Current recommendations suggest a target total cholesterol of 4 mmol/L (155 mg/dL) and a target LDL cholesterol of 2 mmol/L (77 mg/dL). Elevated triglycerides can be treated with additional add-on therapy, if needed.

The evidence base for using statins to lower cardiovascular risk in primary prevention is also strong but, since the absolute cardiovascular risk is normally much lower than in secondary prevention, it is prudent to use a risk calculator (e.g. http://www.qrisk.org) to estimate the 10-year risk for cardiovascular disease and thus prioritize cases with increased risk.

There is currently little or no evidence for any benefit associated with raising levels of HDL cholesterol.

Patients with familial hypercholesterolaemia should be treated from a young age (see 'Familial hypercholesterolaemia'). It is inappropriate to use risk calculations in these cases.

If secondary causes for hyperlipidaemia can be identified (see 'Secondary causes'), these should be eliminated as far as possible

A diet rich in fibre lowers levels of LDL cholesterol. A diet switch away from saturated fat to mono- and polyunsaturated fats lowers levels of LDL cholesterol. Certain nutraceuticals, such as plant sterols/stanols have been proven to lower levels of LDL cholesterol (~15%, when used correctly).

Pharmacological lowering of hyperlipidaemia

Statins

Compared with other pharmacological agents, statins have unparalleled efficacy in lowering levels of LDL cholesterol, and unparalleled evidence for benefit in terms of reducing future cardiovascular events and overall mortality (see Table 20.8). The benefit appears to be proportional to the degree to which the level of LDL cholesterol is lowered. Statin therapy is the first-line pharmacological treatment in all cases except for type 3 hyperlipidaemia (see 'Type 3 hyperlipidaemia') or in cases with extreme hypertriglyceridaemia.

Although the risk for hepatotoxic effects in response to statins is small, it would be prudent to test ALT levels, both before and 3 months after commencing treatment.

Bile acid sequestrants

Bile acid sequestrants such as colesevelam, colestipol, and colestyramine disrupt enterohepatic recirculation of bile acid and give a modest reduction in levels of LDL cholesterol (~20%). They may be useful as an add-on therapy when the desired reduction in levels of LDL cholesterol has not been achieved with statins. They may increase the level of plasma triglycerides and interfere with vitamin K absorption.

Table 20.8 Approximate LDL reductions depend on the dose and type of statin

Type of statin	Response to the indicated daily dose (%)				
	5 mg	10 mg	20 mg	40 mg	80 mg
Atorvastatin	31	37	43	49	55
Rosuvastatin	38	43	48	53	58
Simvastatin	23	27	32	37	42
Fluvastatin	10	15	21	27	33
Lovastatin	—	21	29	37	45
Pravastatin	15	20	24	29	33

Ezetimibe

Ezetimibe reduces cholesterol absorption and gives modest lowering of levels of LDL cholesterol (15%–20%). It is useful as add-on therapy when the desired reduction in levels of LDL cholesterol has not been achieved with statins. The evidence base for using ezetimibe in this context is good. It should not be used in cases where there is impaired liver function.

Fibrates

Fibrates such as bezafibrate, ciprofibrate, fenofibrate, and gemfibrozil reduce levels of plasma triglycerides and are used as first-line therapies in cases of extreme hypertriglyceridaemia. They are useful as add-on therapies when the desired reduction in levels of LDL cholesterol has not been achieved with statins, or when residual hypertriglyceridaemia is seen in high-risk patients. However, there is an increased risk of side effects in muscles and liver when fibrates are combined with statins. If fibrates are to be used in combination with statins, it would be prudent to check ALT levels and to be particularly cautious with high doses of statins. Gemfibrozil interacts with a large number of pharmaceutical agents, including statins, so its use is limited. The evidence base for using fibrates in the secondary prevention of cardiovascular disease in the general population is questionable but is reasonably solid for patients with hypertriglycerideaemia (see Watts and Karpe, 2011).

PCSK9 inhibitors

Monoclonal antibody fortnightly injectable therapy that sequesters plasma PCSK9 and thereby lowers its plasma concentration. This promotes re-circulation of the LDL-R and increased removal of LDL cholesterol leading to a lowering of LDL cholesterol by 30–70%. Currently available therapies are evolocumab and alirocumab but additional compounds are under development including RNAi of PCSK9. These compounds do not appear to share the side effect pattern observed for statins. The first and only (2017) large-scale cardiovascular outcome RCT demonstrated reduced cardiovascular endpoints in expectation of the lipid lowering effect without any major adverse effects.

Niacin

Niacin, and acipimox, reduce levels of triglycerides (≥30%) and LDL cholesterol (~20%) and increases levels of HDL cholesterol (≥30%). However, the evidence base for using niacin for the prevention of cardiovascular disease is weak. In addition, it is associated with noticeable side effects such as skin flushing, an increased risk of diabetes, and gastrointestinal problems.

Fish oils

Highly concentrated forms of fish oils, such as Omacor, given at high doses (2–4 g per day), will reduce triglyceride levels (~30%). There is no proven benefit of using low doses of fish oils (e.g. 1 g/day).

Complications/risks of treatment

Myopathy

Myopathy in response to statin treatment is not uncommon and may range from generalized aches and stiffness to weakness and atrophy without pain. The level of creatinine kinase can be elevated. Severe reactions, such as rhabdomyolysis, are very rare and require hospitalization and immediate cessation of statin therapy. There is no clear difference between the statins in terms of their association with myopathy, except for simvastatin, at its highest dose (80 mg). Statins lower the muscular content of co-enzyme Q, but there is no evidence that the muscular side effects of statins can be ameliorated by supplementation with co-enzyme Q. Patients with milder forms of myopathy may tolerate an alternative statin, which is preferably used at a low dose. Myopathy can be precipitated or aggravated by combination therapy, for example statin plus fibrate.

Hepatotoxicity

Hepatotoxicity in response to statins is unusual, and with simvastatin is extremely rare; but, with the highest dose of atorvastatin (80 mg), it can be seen in up to 2% of treated patients (with a greater than threefold elevation of ALT levels). In such cases, changing to simvastatin is likely to be a safe option. Hepatotoxicity can be precipitated or aggravated by combination therapy, for example statin plus fibrate. A borderline elevated ALT level is not a contraindication for starting statin therapy.

Diabetes risk

Statins, particularly high doses of potent statins (rosuvastatin and atorvastatin), induce a small increase in the risk of type 2 diabetes. This increase is more evident in patients with additional risk factors for type 2 diabetes, such as a level of fasting glucose >5.6 mmol/L (101 mg/dL) or a raised BMI. At an individual level, the reduced risk for cardiovascular disease outweighs the risk of diabetes. Niacin increases the risk for type 2 diabetes.

Cancer and Alzheimer's disease

Long-term risk for any cancer or neurodegenerative disease has not been associated with any current hypolipidaemic therapy.

Skin reactions

Skin reactions in response to statins and fibrates are unusual. Skin flushing is very common after the intake of niacin and its derivatives. Forewarning patients about this side effect may help them to accept it and get used to it.

Pregnancy

Statins are potentially teratogenic. Effective contraceptive methods are required in fertile women taking statins. Women should stop statin therapy at least 1 month before a planned pregnancy. Fibrates can be foetotoxic and should not be used in pregnancy. Ezetimibe should not be used in pregnancy.

Drug interactions

Hypolipidaemic drugs interact with a large number of other drugs, so possible drug interactions must be checked before starting any therapy (see http://www.drugs.com/drug_interactions.html).

References and further reading

Bulbulia R and Armitage J. LDL cholesterol targets: How low to go? Curr Opin Lipidol 2012; 23: 265–70.

Durrington P. Dyslipidaemia. Lancet 2003; 362: 717–31.

Ewald N, Hardt PD, and Kloer HU. Severe hypertriglyceridemia and pancreatitis: Presentation and management. Curr Opin Lipidol 2009; 20: 497–504.

Gill PJ, Harnden A, and Karpe F. Familial hypercholesterolaemia. BMJ 2012; 344: e3228.

Johansen CT and Hegele RA. Genetic bases of hypertriglyceridemic phenotypes. Curr Opin Lipidol 2011; 22: 247–53.

Neuvonen PJ, Niemi M, and Backman JT. Drug interactions with lipid-lowering drugs: Mechanisms and clinical relevance. Clin Pharmacol Ther 2006; 80: 565–81.

Watts GF and Karpe F. Triglycerides and atherogenic dyslipidaemia: Extending treatment beyond statins in the high-risk cardiovascular patient. Heart 2011; 97: 350–6.

20.9 Hypertension

Introduction
Hypertension affects more than a quarter of adults, and over half of those over the age of 60 years. It is a major risk factor for ischaemic and haemorrhagic strokes, myocardial infarction, heart failure, chronic kidney disease, peripheral vascular disease, cognitive decline, and premature death. Above blood pressures of 115/70 mm Hg, every 20/10 mm Hg rise in blood pressure is associated with a doubling in the risk of cardiovascular events.

Definition of hypertension
Hypertension is present if the blood pressure during the consultation is 140/90 mm Hg or higher and subsequent ambulatory or home blood-pressure measurements demonstrate an average blood pressure of 135/85 mm Hg or higher.

Primary versus secondary hypertension
Primary hypertension (formerly known as 'essential hypertension') is sustained high blood pressure for which there is no obvious identifiable cause; this accounts for about 90% of cases of hypertension. The remaining 10% of cases are termed 'secondary hypertension', because the cause of the hypertension can be identified.

Suspect secondary hypertension in patients who have one or the following indications:
- are <40 years old
- experience a sudden worsening of hypertension
- present with accelerated hypertension (blood pressure >180/110 mm Hg, with papilloedema/retinal haemorrhage)
- respond poorly to treatment for hypertension (blood pressure >140/90 mm Hg despite treatment and concordance with three antihypertensive drugs)
- have a reduced eGFR (suggestive of renal or renovascular disease)
- have signs or symptoms of causes of secondary hypertension

Endocrinological causes of secondary hypertension include:
- phaeochromocytoma
- primary aldosteronism (hyperaldosteronism)
- Cushing's syndrome

More unusual endocrinological causes include:
- acromegaly
- hypothyroidism
- hyperthyroidism

The frequency of endocrinological causes for hypertension varies according to age: primary aldosteronism is the most common cause of hypertension in middle-aged adults; hypothyroidism is the most common cause of hypertension in those >65 years old; Cushing's syndrome and phaeochromocytomas are the most common causes of hypertension in those aged 40–64.

Management of hypertension
When identified, the underlying hormonal disorder can be treated, leading to an improvement in or even a cure of the hypertension.

In addition to the specific interventions for endocrine conditions listed below, many guidelines exist for the management of hypertension. Most recommend lifestyle modification before graduating to pharmacological intervention.

Lifestyle modifications
Lifestyle modifications include:
- weight loss (to BMI <25 kg/m^2)
- limiting alcohol intake (<140 g/week in men, <80 g/week in women)
- reducing sodium intake (to <5–6 g/day)
- regular aerobic exercise

Pharmacological interventions
Options for pharmacological interventions are as follows, depending on the co-morbidities present:
- heart failure: diuretics, beta blockers, ACE inhibitors, angiotensin-receptor blockers, aldosterone antagonists
- post myocardial infarction: beta blockers, ACE inhibitors
- high coronary disease risk: diuretics, beta blockers, ACE inhibitors, calcium-channel blockers
- diabetes: diuretics, beta blockers, ACE inhibitors, angiotensin-receptor blockers, calcium-channel blockers
- chronic kidney disease: ACE inhibitors, angiotensin-receptor blockers
- recurrent stroke: diuretics, ACE inhibitors

Combination therapy is usually required.

Hypertension in phaeochromocytoma
See also Chapter 6, Section 6.14. Phaeochromocytomas are rare and occur in 0.04%–0.1% of patients. However, 85%–90% of patients with a phaeochromocytoma will have hypertension. Adults with a phaeochromocytoma most commonly have sustained hypertension with severe high blood pressure during symptomatic episodes. Such paroxysms of severe hypertension occur in about 50% of adults with phaeochromocytomas.

Clinical pointers to phaeochromocytomas
The triad of tachycardia, headache, and sweating in a hypertensive patient has a sensitivity of 91% and specificity of 94% for a phaeochromocytoma. Other symptoms can include weight loss, facial flushing, nervousness, and oedema.

Patients with sustained hypertension due to a phaeochromocytoma usually experience a decrease in blood pressure after standing from a supine position. This fall in blood pressure can be so marked that it may cause symptomatic hypotension. Orthostatic hypotension is usually associated with a tachycardia.

Occasionally, phaeochromocytomas can be associated with a normal blood pressure despite elevated plasma concentrations of noradrenaline. This can be due to tachyphylaxis (which may be more common in the presence of certain polymorphisms of the gene for the beta-2 adrenoceptor), or due to co-secretion of dopamine (by dilating mesenteric and renal vessels).

Pathogenesis of hypertension in phaeochromocytoma
Adrenaline causes an increase in heart rate and contractility, whilst noradrenaline increases systemic vascular resistance.

Investigation of phaeochromocytoma in hypertensive patients

The screening tests for hypertensive patients with possible phaeochromocytomas are detailed in Chapter 6, Section 6.14.

Management of hypertension in phaeochromocytomas

The definitive treatment is surgical removal of the tumour, but severe hypertension can be induced by induction of anaesthesia without adequate medical treatment beforehand. The use of alpha and beta blockade as medical treatment is detailed in Chapter 6, Section 6.14.

Hypertension in primary aldosteronism

For discussions of hypertension in primary aldosteronism, see Chapter 6, Sections 6.4 and 6.5.

Hypertension in Cushing's syndrome

Cushing's syndrome occurs in 0.1%–0.6% of all patients. However, 80% of adults with Cushing's syndrome will have hypertension. In contrast, only 10%–20% of patients who receive exogenous steroids have hypertension.

Pathogenesis of hypertension in Cushing's syndrome

Cushing's disease is associated with normal plasma renin activity and deoxycorticosterone concentrations. Mechanisms of hypertension include increased production of angiotensin 2 due to increase glucocorticoid levels; increased hepatic synthesis of angiotensinogen; enhanced glucocorticoid-mediated vascular reactivity to vasoconstrictors; and inhibitions of vasodilatory systems such as kinins and prostaglandins (by inhibition of phospholipase A).

Ectopic production of adrenocorticotrophic hormone is usually accompanied by increased concentrations of adrenocorticotrophic-hormone-dependent steroids, such as corticosterone and deoxycorticosterone, along with increased mineralocorticoid activity and suppressed plasma renin activity. Hypokalaemia is common.

Investigation of Cushing's syndrome in hypertensive patients

The screening tests for hypertensive patients with possible Cushing's syndrome are detailed in Chapter 6, Section 6.8.

Management of hypertension in Cushing's syndrome

The definitive way to manage hypertension in Cushing's syndrome is to treat the Cushing's syndrome, if possible. The medical treatment of Cushing's syndrome is detailed in Chapter 6, Section 6.8. One year after a cure of Cushing's syndrome, ~30% of patients will still have persistent hypertension after 12 months; this appears to be related to the degree and duration of pretreatment hypercortisolaemia.

Hypertension in hypothyroidism

See also Chapter 2, Section 2.7. Hypothyroidism is associated with an increased diastolic blood pressure.

Pathogenesis of hypertension in hypothyroidism

The pathogenesis of hypertension in hypothyroidism is unclear. The reduced clearance of aldosterone is balanced by a reduction in its production, which results in a normal plasma concentration of aldosterone. Plasma renin activity and angiotensinogen production in the liver are reduced.

Although plasma sodium concentrations tend to be low (due to impaired water diuresis because of a decrease in the delivery of water to the distal nephron), total body sodium is increased, presumably bound to extracellular mucopolysaccharides. An increase in vasopressin concentrations also contributes to hyponatraemia, although there is an overall reduction in blood volume.

Hypothyroidism is also associated with endothelial dysfunction and increased systemic vascular resistance. Hypothyroid patients have a higher mean systolic blood pressure and increased variability in blood pressure, using ambulatory blood-pressure monitoring.

Although there is a statistically significant association between normal TSH concentrations and diastolic hypertension, it is unclear whether subclinical hypothyroidism is associated with hypertension.

Pregnancy-induced hypertension is two to three times more common in hypothyroid women.

Treatment of hypertension in hypothyroidism

After thyroid-replacement therapy, diastolic blood pressure returns to <90 mm Hg in over 30% of hypertensive hypothyroid patients.

Hypertension in hyperthyroidism

See also Chapter 2, Section 2.5. Hyperthyroidism can be associated with increased systolic blood pressure and a widened pulse pressure.

Pathogenesis of hypertension in hyperthyroidism

In hyperthyroidism, there is an increase in cardiac output and a decrease in peripheral vascular resistance, which results in an increased systolic blood pressure and increased pulse pressure. Tissue blood flow is increased in response to the accelerated metabolism and increased oxygen consumption. The cause for the reduced vascular resistance is unclear, but may be due to a direct action of thyroid hormone on the smooth muscle of blood vessels or to an increase in the concentrations of vasodilatory peptides (e.g. adrenomedullin). The increased cardiac output results from an increased stroke volume and heart rate. Whether subclinical hyperthyroidism is associated with hypertension is unclear.

Treatment of hypertension in hyperthyroidism

After treatment of hyperthyroidism, blood pressure returns to normal. See Chapter 2 for details.

Hypertension in acromegaly

Around 50% of patients with acromegaly have hypertension, usually with an increase in systolic blood pressure.

Pathogenesis of hypertension in acromegaly

Growth hormone directly increases sodium reabsorption and leads to an increase in intravascular volume, low plasma renin activity, and elevated aldosterone secretion. The resulting hypertension contributes to an increased risk of ischaemic heart disease, and this risk may be exacerbated by insulin resistance. Hypertensive acromegalic patients should have phaeochromocytoma excluded, especially prior to surgery.

Management of hypertension in acromegaly

The definitive treatment for hypertension in acromegaly is the management of the acromegaly. This is described in Chapter 3, Section 3.6.

Further reading

Funder JW, Carey RM, Fardella C, et al. Case detection, diagnosis and treatment of patients with primary aldosteronism: An Endocrine Society clinical practice guideline. *J Clin Endocrinol Metab* 2008; 93: 3266–81.

Laragh JH, Brener BM, and Kaplan NM, eds. *Endocrine Mechanisms in Hypertension*, 1989. Raven Press.

Mancia G, Fagard R, Narkiewicz K, et al. 2013 ESH/ESC guidelines for the management of arterial hypertension: The Task Force for the Management of Arterial Hypertension of the European Society of Hypertension (ESH) and of the European Society of Cardiology (ESC). *Eur Heart J* 2013; 34: 2159–219.

Melescu E and Koch CA. 'Syndrome of mineralocorticoid excess' in Koch CA, Chrousos GP, eds, *Endocrine Hypertension: Underlying Mechanisms and Therapy*, 2013. Springer, pp. 33–50.

National Clinical Guideline Centre. Hypertension: The clinical management of primary hypertension in adults. Available at https://www.ncbi.nlm.nih.gov/pubmedhealth/PMH0047679/ (accessed 19 Jan 2018).

Richards AM, Nicholls MG, Espiner EA, et al. Hypertension in hypothyroidism: Arterial pressure and hormone relationships. *Clin Exp Hypertens A* 1985; 7: 1499–514.

Chapter 21

Medico-legal aspects

Chapter contents

21.1 Medico-legal issues: Confidentiality, documentation, risk explanation, and consent

Introduction
Understanding the test for clinical negligence is key. It is important to remember that a mistake is not necessarily a negligent mistake and you cannot be held responsible for every adverse outcome.

The claimant must show that the standard of care that they received was below that which is expected to be reasonable in your area of medicine. They must also show that the substandard care was causative of damage.

An apology when things go wrong can often be enough. Patients often take legal action because they feel that their concerns have not been taken seriously or, worse, ignored.

Risk explanation, and consent
There is, of course, an inherent degree of risk in all medical treatment, and the law accepts this.

One of the key ways to avoid future disputes is to ensure that you communicate well with your patient and that your explanation of risk is as clear and precise as possible.

Drugs
- When prescribing drugs, ensure that you explain any potential side effects and what to do if side effects are experienced (e.g. serious side effects should be reported to the GP or hospital doctor as soon as possible).
- You should also explain the potential impact of mixing unprescribed medication with the drug(s) that you have prescribed.
- Ensure that you check whether the patient has any allergies; if so, take this into consideration when explaining the risks.
- You should keep a detailed note of risks explained.

Investigations
- When explaining the risks associated with a particular investigation, you have to ensure that the patient is able to come to an informed decision about the risks and benefits (i.e. informed consent). If the investigation itself carries a high degree of risk, this must be measured against the information which will hopefully be derived from it.
- You need to ensure that the patient is aware that an investigation may not result in a definitive diagnosis.
- You should keep a detailed note of risks explained.

Treatment
- Obtaining informed consent is essential when advising any form of treatment. Failure to obtain this is the source of many complaints about medical care.
- The law now emphasizes that the patient should be aware of any 'material risk' involved in the investigation and treatment, and any recommended alternatives. 'Material risk' is no longer the standard 'of a reasonable body of medical opinion' but is 'what is likely to be considered significant by a reasonable person in the patient's position, including the nature of the risk, the impact on the patient's life, the alternatives (including no investigation/treatment), and the associated risks'.
- Therefore, you should aim to ensure that the risks that you are warning of are focused on the individual in question rather than in general terms.
- Consider and remember the 1% issue (the clinician must tell the patient about any potential outcome, even if the chance of the outcome happening is very small, and also about any less serious risks or potential complications that occur frequently).
- Do not rely solely on the signed consent form to prove that the patient has provided informed consent. If you have not explained the potential complications in layman's terms, this may result in difficulties later on.
- The law also now states that, if time permits, the clinician should give the patient time to reflect upon the information provided and undertake their own research if they wish, before making a decision.

Confidentiality
Confidentiality is, of course, central to the doctor/patient relationship. However, in certain circumstances, there is a duty to disclose medical information to third parties. These circumstances are:
- when the patient provides consent (express or implied)
- where there is a statutory obligation, for example under the Public Health Act 1984, where the general public need to be protected
- to support the care of the individual patient (e.g. within the direct care team)
- for the protection of patients and others, or public interest
- for the purposes of medical research
- when the information is ordered to be disclosed by a court

With children and young people, the same rules of confidentiality apply. They may provide their own consent to disclosure of information to parents or authorities. However, if they withhold their consent, and the clinician believes that this will make them at risk of death or serious harm, then the clinician may make the disclosure. The reasons for the decision must be carefully recorded.

Documentation
- The basis of a good note is one which is comprehensive and clearly written in legible handwriting. The date, time, signature, printed name, and status should always be recorded.
- If you take advice from a senior colleague, make sure you make a careful note of what was discussed and what action was agreed. If necessary, read the note back to your senior colleague to ensure that your understanding is correct.
- Retrospective notes can sometimes appear to be suspicious. Make sure you always clearly state that it is a retrospective note, the time it is written, and why it is being made retrospectively, for example because it is about an emergency situation during which there had been no time to take notes.
- If carrying out an examination, clearly document this and, if helpful, draw a diagram.
- Do not rely on stating at a future date that '*it would be my normal practice to …*'. Instead, note what you did do.

Further reading
General Medical Council. Confidentiality: Good practice in handling patient information (2017). Available at http://www.gmc-uk.org/guidance/ethical_guidance/confidentiality.asp (accessed 19 Jan 2018).

21.2 DVLA regulations

The DVLA are legally responsible for ensuring that all drivers holding a driving licence are medically fit to drive, and employ specialist medical advisors to support the application of the medical standards.

Confidentiality

If you are unsure whether a patient is unfit to drive, you can seek the advice of a DVLA medical advisor. Although the driver has legal responsibility for informing the DVLA of any condition which may affect the ability to drive, if patients have a condition such as a visual disorder or diabetes, then you should explain that the condition may affect their ability to drive and that they have a legal duty to inform the DVLA of this condition. If they refuse to accept this, you can suggest that they seek a second opinion but advise them to not drive in the meantime. If they continue to drive against your advice, you should try to discuss with them further; and if they still refuse, you should then contact the DVLA and advise them that the patient is unfit to drive. This is in the public interest of safety and therefore justifies the potential breach in confidentiality.

Before contacting the DVLA, you should take all reasonable steps to advise your patient that you are obliged to disclose details of their medical condition to the DVLA, and confirm this in writing to them once you have done so. You should make a note in the patient's record.

Guidance in relation to hypoglycaemia and visual disorders

Hypoglycaemia

All insulin-dependent drivers must advise the DVLA about their condition. The DVLA will, however, consider several factors before considering whether to grant a licence. These are as follows:

- drivers must demonstrate satisfactory control and must recognize hypoglycaemia
- drivers must not have had more than one episode of hypoglycaemia requiring the assistance of another person in the preceding 12 months
- drivers must have appropriate blood glucose monitoring
- drivers must not be regarded as a likely source of danger to the public whilst driving
- visual standards for acuity and visual field must be met (standard requirement)

Drivers who are undergoing temporary insulin-treatment need not notify the DVLA, provided they are under medical supervision and have not been advised they are at risk of disabling hypoglycaemia. However, if they do experience disabling hypoglycaemia, the DVLA should be notified.

Where diabetes is managed by tablets which carry a risk of inducing hypoglycaemia, the driver must not have had more than one episode of hypoglycaemia requiring the assistance of another person within the preceding 12 months. You should consider monitoring blood glucose regularly and keep the patient under regular review. If this and the requirements set out in *Form INF188/2* are met, notification is not required.

For drivers managed by tablets other than those with a risk of inducing hypoglycaemia, or non-insulin injectable medication, if the requirements set out on Form INF188/2 are met and the drivers are under regular medical review, the DVLA need not be notified.

If diabetes is managed by diet alone, the DVLA need not be notified unless a relevant condition develops (e.g. diabetic eye problems).

If a patient's awareness of hypoglycaemia becomes impaired, they must stop driving and can only resume if a consultant or GP provides a report stating that this awareness has been regained.

If you think your patient needs to report their condition to the DVLA, direct them to http://www.direct.gov.uk/driverhealth.

Visual disorders

A driver must, by law, meet the following eyesight requirement: they must be able to read in good daylight (with the aid of glasses or contact lenses, if worn) a registration mark fixed to a motor vehicle at 20.0 or 20.5 metres, dependent upon the size of the characters.

Any driver that suffers from cataracts must be able to meet the above eyesight requirement.

Any driver that suffers from visual defects such as severe bilateral glaucoma or severe bilateral retinopathy must cease driving unless it is confirmed that he or she is able to meet the recommended national guidelines for visual field. These can be found on the DVLA website.

Please note this is just a guide to the DVLA regulations; for full details visit, their website (http://www.dft.gov.uk/dvla/medical/aag.aspx).

Further reading

General Medical Council. Confidentiality: Patients' fitness to drive and reporting concerns to the DVLA or DVA (2017). Available at http://www.gmc-uk.org/static/documents/content/Confidentiality_-_Patients_fitness_to_drive_and_reporting_concerns_to_DVLA_or_DVA.pdf (accessed 19 Jan 2018).

Index

Tables, figures, and boxes are indicated by an italic t, f, and b following the page number.

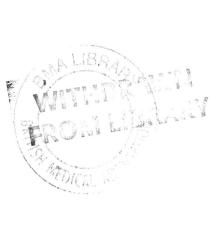